Pathology for Surgeons

Pathology for Surgeons

Patrick C. H. Watt, MD, FRCS

Senior Registrar,
Department of Histopathology,
Queen's University of Belfast

Roy A. J. Spence, MD, FRCS

Consultant Surgeon
Belfast City Hospital

with a Foreword by
Terence Kennedy

WRIGHT

BRISTOL
1986

Published under the Wright imprint by:
IOP Publishing Limited,
Techno House, Redcliffe Way, Bristol BS1 6NX

British Library Cataloguing in Publication Data
    Watt, Patrick C. H.
        Pathology for surgeons.
        1. Pathology, Surgical
        I. Title   II. Spence, Roy A. J.
        617'.07   RD57

ISBN 0 7236 0808 3

Typeset by
Bath Typesetting Ltd.
Printed in Great Britain by
Henry Ling Ltd, The Dorset Press, Dorchester.

TO EDWINA

    PCHW

TO DI, ROBERT AND ANDREW

        RAJS

Preface

This text is intended principally for surgeons in training who are preparing for the Pathology section of the final examination for admission as Fellows to one of the Royal Colleges of Surgeons. We hope it will also be of some use to the more senior surgeon who wants a summary of some subject outside his own field of interest.

Striking a balance as to what to include and what to leave out is difficult when writing a book about one speciality intended for readers of a different speciality; it is impossible to assess accurately how much pathology a junior surgeon should know. As relatively recent candidates for the FRCS, we have attempted to write the sort of book we would like to have had available at that time. To avoid overlap with books on clinical surgery, clinical details and the discussion of treatment have been kept to a minimum. To avoid overlap with books on general pathology, subjects such as shock, neoplasia, infections, etc., have been set aside.

P. C. H. Watt
R. A. J. Spence

Collaborators

This book has been written in collaboration with:

Barry T. Jackson MS, FRCS
Consultant Surgeon, St Thomas' Hospital, London
Member of the Court of Examiners,
Royal College of Surgeons of England

and

Ingrid V. Allen MD, DSc, FRCPath
Professor of Neuropathology,
Queen's University of Belfast

Herbert K. Graham MD, FRCS
Senior Registrar in Orthopaedic Surgery,
Royal Victoria Hospital, Belfast

J. M. Graham Harley MD, FRCOG
Professor of Obstetrics and Gynaecology,
Queen's University of Belfast

Claire M. Hill MD, FRCPI, MRCPath
Consultant Pathologist, Queen's University of Belfast and
Royal Victoria Hospital, Belfast

Elizabeth E. Mayne MD, MRCP, FRCPath
Consultant Haematologist,
Royal Victoria Hospital, Belfast

Francis V. O'Brien MB, BDS, FDSRCS
Professor of Dental Surgery,
Queen's University of Belfast

Acknowledgements

The first group of people we would like to thank are those who gave extensive assistance with various chapters. Mr Barry Jackson gave extensive advice and help from the outset of the project and collaborated closely with us on the chapters on Breast, Oesophagus, Intestines and Anal Region. Professor Graham Harley, Dr Claire Hill, Dr Elizabeth Mayne and Mr Kerr Graham each contributed an entire chapter on their respective speciality subjects. Professor Ingrid Allen and Professor Frank O'Brien collaborated with us on the chapters on the Nervous System and on the Oral Cavity, Salivary Glands and Neck respectively.

We would like to thank the following for reading and giving advice on various parts of the manuscript: Dr A. B. Atkinson, Professor P. C. Bornman, Dr M. E. Callender, Dr N. Campbell, Dr C. M. Hill, Mr R. Johnston, Mr T. L. Kennedy, Mr A. Leonard, Dr J. M. Sloan, Mr M. Stevenson and Professor J. Terblanche.

Dr J. M. Sloan gave us access to his large collection of histological slides, from which we took material for some of the photomicrographs. Dr E. McIlrath and Dr M. Mills lent us radiographs for some of the illustrations. Others who provided illustrations, are acknowledged individually in the text.

Mr Roy Creighton, Miss Karen McPherson and Mr Gary White of the Photographic Unit, Institute of Pathology, Queen's University of Belfast, made all the photomicrographs and most of the prints of macroscopic specimens. Mr Brendan Ellis, Miss Cathy Gilmartin and Mr Mark Hamilton drew the line diagrams and the staff of the Medical Illustrations Department, Royal Victoria Hospital, Belfast, and of the Photographic Unit, Institute of Pathology, Queen's University of Belfast, photographed them.

We would like to thank Mr Peter Hamilton who gave considerable assistance with the manuscript, especially in the finding and checking of references.

Mrs Sheena Watson typed many drafts of the manuscript accurately and tolerated our many changes. Miss May Weller typed Professor Harley's chapter.

Finally, we would like to thank the staff of John Wright & Sons, especially Mr Roy Baker who gave invaluable assistance from the outset of the project.

Contents

Foreword   XV

Chapter   **1**   The Oral Cavity, Salivary Glands and Neck
             In collaboration with Professor F. O'Brien   1

  2   The Oesophagus
        In collaboration with Mr Barry Jackson   29

  3   The Stomach and Duodenum   52

  4   The Intestines
        In collaboration with Mr Barry Jackson   81

  5   The Anal Region
        In collaboration with Mr Barry Jackson   132

  6   The Liver   143

  7   The Biliary System   173

  8   The Pancreas   192

  9   The Kidney, Ureter and Bladder   218

  10   The Male Genitalia   260

  11   The Breast
        In collaboration with Mr Barry Jackson   291

  12   The Heart   319

  13   The Blood Vessels   351

  14   The Lung, Pleura and Mediastinum   377

  15   The Lymphoreticular System   420

  16   The Endocrine Glands   450

  17   The Skin   493

  18   The Soft Tissues   524

  19   The Bones and Joints
        By Mr Kerr Graham   542

Chapter 20   The Nervous System
In collaboration with Professor Ingrid Allen   597

21   Renal Transplantation
By Dr Claire Hill   643

22   Gynaecological Emergencies
By Professor Graham Harley   658

Appendix   Surgery and Haemostasis
By Dr Elizabeth Mayne   675

Index   685

Foreword

Terence Kennedy
MD (Hon) (Belf.), MS (Lond.), FRCS, FRCSI
The Royal Victoria Hospital and Queen's University Belfast

Notwithstanding the astonishing technical advances that have been made during the past few decades, a sound knowledge of pathology remains the fundamental basis of all surgical practice. The link between the surgeon and the pathologist is indissoluble.

In surgical training in the British tradition pathology has been, and continues to be, an extremely important subject, forming a major part of the Fellowship examinations of all our Royal Colleges. This book has been written primarily for fellowship candidates but it will also, without doubt, be widely welcomed by more senior surgeons as a reference book. The authors are two outstanding young men, both trained in the generality of surgery as well as pathology. Both are young enough to remember the problems of the examination candidate and to present the subject with this in mind.

The format of the book is traditional and the material is laid out in a way that is easy to read and assimilate, aided as it is by many illustrations of gross as well as microscopic appearance. 'General Pathology', as such, is not included as it is well covered in at least one other popular British text. Where relevant, however, aspects of general pathology, as well as relevant physiology, anatomy and embryology, are included in chapters that deal with individual organs or systems.

Throughout the book the authors have paid much attention to recent advances and areas of controversy. Examples include – early gastric cancer, lobular carcinoma-in-situ of the breast, dysplasia and its relationship to cancer, and the adverse late effects of splenectomy. The authors have received specialist help with the chapters on bone pathology, the central nervous system, and gynaecological emergencies. The chapter on renal transplantation is, in a way, a tribute to the outstanding success in this area of the Belfast team.

The contents of this book far exceed the minimum requirements of the fellowship candidate. In every chapter both common and lesser known or rare conditions are described sufficiently comprehensively to make this a useful reference book for all surgeons, however experienced they may be.

The late Sir John Henry Biggart, father of pathology in the Belfast School, once wrote: 'The study of things caused must precede the study of the causes of things and, in the case of the surgeon, their treatment.' What he meant was that a proper understanding of pathology is essential to the practising surgeon.

It is with pride for the Belfast Medical School, which celebrates its 150th anniversary this year, that I commend this book as I know that John Henry Biggart himself would have been absolutely delighted with this result of his influence. I just wish that there had been a book like this around when I was working for my fellowship!

Chapter 1

The Oral Cavity, Salivary Glands and Neck

THE ORAL CAVITY

Normal Structure

The oral cavity is lined by squamous epithelium which tends to be keratinized in areas, such as the palate, which are subject to greatest friction. The squamous epithelium lies on the lamina propria which is composed of connective tissue. The lamina propria is attached loosely to the underlying tissue in areas, such as the floor of the mouth, where the mucosa is mobile. It is tightly bound to the underlying tissue in areas, such as the hard palate, where it is immobile.

The surface of the tongue is covered by papillae. The filiform papillae are small, and keratinized surface projections give them a white appearance. The fungiform papillae are larger, non-keratinized and red in colour. The circumvallate papillae form a V-shaped row which divides the anterior two-thirds from the posterior one-third of the tongue. There are no glands on the dorsum of the anterior two-thirds of the tongue. The nodular appearance of the mucous membrane of the posterior one-third of the tongue is due to masses of mucous and serous glands and aggregates of lymphoid tissue which are part of Waldeyer's ring. The anterior two-thirds of the tongue derives from the first and second branchial arches and the posterior one-third originates from the third arch. Distributed throughout the oral cavity are numerous accessory salivary glands.

Traumatic Lesions

Traumatic ulcers

These are simple ulcers often due to trauma from ill-fitting dentures or sharp teeth. They are frequently linear and after removal of the cause they usually heal within two weeks. If healing does not occur, biopsy is recommended to exclude malignancy.

Fibrous hyperplasia

This term embraces a group of lesions which exhibits a fibro-epithelial proliferative response to trauma, although sometimes no obvious cause can be found. They normally do not recur after local excision.

DENTURE INDUCED HYPERPLASIA: This lesion occurs in soft tissues usually at the buccal site of insertion of the lower or upper limit of a denture flange.

FIBROUS EPULIS: A lump in the gum which forms as a response to a combination of low grade trauma (from filling or tooth) and non-specific infection. Histologically it consists of a mass of connective tissue with a covering of squamous epithelium.

FIBRO-EPITHELIAL POLYP: A polypoid lesion usually found in the buccal mucosa as a result of cheek biting. The histology is the same as a fibrous epulis.

Pyogenic granuloma

These are common in the mouth and are benign. They occur in any part of the oral cavity but are most common on the gingiva (*see Fig.* 1.1). They appear as small red lesions which bleed easily. Histologically they are composed of vascular granulation tissue and as such may be confused with capillary haemangioma. Occasionally pyogenic granulomas occur on the gingiva of pregnant women (so called 'pregnancy tumours'); they usually regress after delivery.

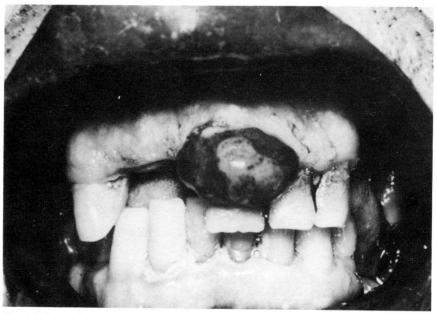

Fig. 1.1. Pyogenic granuloma.

Oral Infections

Viral

Acute herpetic stomatitis is due to primary infection with the type I herpes simplex virus. The condition is most common in children and young adults, who develop an acute gingivitis. Vesicles are seen on the oral mucosa and these rupture to produce ulcers. Recurrent herpes simplex infection is characterized by groups of small clear vesicles on a red base. The virus is present in nerve ganglia and can form lesions, usually on the lips (cold sores), in response to trauma, emotional stress, sunshine, etc. The Coxsackie A virus may cause an acute oropharyngitis with vesicles and this is known as herpangina. It is a self-limiting condition lasting about a week.

Bacterial

The oral cavity is well protected from infection by antibacterial agents in saliva and by local immunoglobulin production. However, occasionally the oral flora may cause an infective disease if the patient is compromised by nutritional deficiency, immunodeficiency, etc.

Acute necrotizing ulcerative gingivitis (also termed Vincent's disease or fusospirochetosis) seems to be due to invasion of oral tissues by several symbiotic organisms (including *Borrelia vincentii* and *Fusiformis fusiformis*) which are normally present in the mouth. The disease affects the interdental papillae and free gingival margin but may spread to involve other oral tissues. In severely compromised children suffering from kwashiorkor or parasitic disease, the infection may rapidly spread to the cheeks, lips and jaws, which become necrotic (noma or cancrum oris).

The mouth may occasionally be involved in syphilis or tuberculosis. Cervicofacial actinomycosis arises from invasion of the oral mucous membrane or a tooth socket by the organism *Actinomyces israelii* (or rarely by other species of Actinomyces). The infection may lead to involvement of the jaw with sinus tracks to the skin. Typical sulphur granules are seen in the pus. Microscopically, these sulphur granules are clumps of organisms.

Ludwig's angina is a spreading infection of the submandibular spaces due to apical pathology of the lower molar teeth. The cellulitis produces swelling of the floor of the mouth and elevation of the tongue. Oedema of the glottis may require tracheostomy although nowadays the condition usually responds to extraction of the offending tooth and antibiotic therapy.

Fungal

Candida albicans is a normal inhabitant of the mouth which may invade the tissues to produce candidiasis (thrush) if there is a predisposing cause (e.g. debility, oral antibiotics, AIDS). Clinically, white patches are seen on the oral mucosa and these are easily rubbed off to produce a raw oozing surface. Other fungal infections of the mouth (e.g. histoplasmosis and coccidioidomycosis) are rare.

White Lesions

White sponge naevus

This is an inherited condition in which part of the oral mucosa (usually the cheeks) forms thick white folds. Microscopically there may be hyperkeratosis and intracellular oedema. The lesion is harmless and its main importance is that it may be confused with leukoplakia.

Lichen planus

Lichen planus affects both the skin and mucous membranes. Typically it appears as white lacy striae on the buccal mucosa or tongue, although it may appear as a white plaque. Histologically the characteristic features are degeneration of the basal layer of the epidermis and a band-like lymphocytic infiltrate in the upper dermis. Very rarely, malignant transformation has been reported.

Leukoplakia

Leukoplakia now has a WHO accepted definition which is 'a white patch or plaque on the oral mucous membrane which cannot be removed by scraping and cannot be classified clinically or microscopically as another disease entity' (e.g. lichen planus, candidiasis, etc.). Leukoplakia is therefore a clinical term with no histological inference. Pathologists do not use the term leukoplakia as a definitive diagnosis but rather report the actual findings seen histologically, which range from a simple hyperkeratosis to squamous carcinoma (*see Fig.* 1.2).

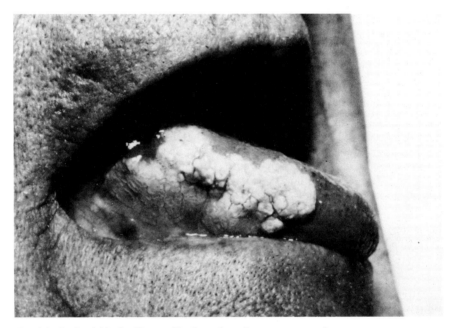

Fig. 1.2. Leukoplakia. In this case, histology showed a squamous carcinoma.

Leukoplakia appears grossly as a homogeneous white plaque (homogeneous type) or as white nodular areas, side by side with red areas (nodular or speckled type). The white areas may be smooth or they may be furrowed and fissured. It is a common condition and the majority of cases occur in men of middle age. Waldron and Shafer (1975) reviewed 3256 cases of oral leukoplakia. In a quarter of these cases the lesion was on the mandibular mucosa or sulcus; one-fifth were on the buccal mucosa; the lips, maxillary mucosa and palate each accounted for 10%; the tongue and floor of the mouth each accounted for less than 10%. About 20% of their cases of leukoplakia showed significant epithelial abnormality. This was mild to moderate dysplasia in 12% and severe dysplasia, carcinoma-in-situ or squamous carcinoma in 8%. The remaining 80% showed varying combinations of hyperkeratosis, acanthosis (increased thickness of the prickle cell layer of the squamous epithelium) and parakeratosis (retention of cell nuclei in the keratinized layer of the epithelium). Dysplastic epithelium was more commonly seen in the nodular type of leukoplakia than in the homogeneous type.

Follow-up study suggests that about 5% of patients with leukoplakia eventually develop carcinoma. Since different histological features may be seen in different parts of a leukoplakia patch, an excisional biopsy, or failing that, multiple incisional biopsies, should be performed. Several factors are associated with a higher risk of malignancy including female sex, iron deficiency and excessive alcohol or tobacco consumption.

Erythroplakia

As has been stated, leukoplakia may be homogeneous or speckled, the latter being a combination of red and white. When the red plaque is the predominant component, the term used is erythroplakia. A similar range of histological findings may be seen, although dysplastic changes are much more frequent than in leukoplakia.

Tumours of the Mouth

Tumours of the mouth may be classified under the following headings:
—covering epithelium
—odontogenic epithelium
—glandular epithelium (discussed later under salivary glands)
—connective tissue

Tumours of the Covering Epithelium

Squamous papilloma

These benign tumours are not uncommon within the oral cavity and may appear as broad based sessile or pedunculated growths. Microscopically they consist of fronds of neoplastic squamous epithelium with connective tissue cores. The lesion is presumed to be viral in origin and sometimes occurs in association with warts on the hand.

Epithelial dysplasia and carcinoma-in-situ

Just as not all cases of leukoplakia show dysplasia, not all cases of dysplasia appear macroscopically as leukoplakia. Microscopically, the epithelial cells show atypical changes such as pleomorphism, nuclear hyperchromasia and increased numbers of mitoses. If these changes are severe, the lesion is termed carcinoma-in-situ. In practice, the differentiation between severe dysplasia and carcinoma-in-situ is difficult.

The significance of oral epithelial dysplasia is not yet clear, although it appears that like cervical dysplasia it may regress, remain static, or progress to invasive carcinoma. Progression to malignancy appears to be more common in lesions of the tongue and floor of the mouth than in other areas.

Squamous carcinoma of the oral mucosa

Ninety per cent of all malignant tumours of the oral cavity are squamous carcinomas.

Epidemiology and aetiology

Oral cancer accounts for 2–5% of all cancers in Western countries, although in some areas of India up to 50% of cancers are oral squamous carcinomas. The condition is more common in men than women and is rarely seen in patients under 45 years old. Pipe and cigar smokers have a four times greater risk of developing oral cancer than the rest of the population; cigarette smokers also have a slightly increased risk. In the past half century, lung cancer has increased by about fivefold, whereas oral cancer has halved in frequency. This has been attributed to the replacement of pipe smoking by cigarette smoking. Up to one-third of patients who continue to smoke after treatment of an oral cancer will develop a second primary whereas those who stop smoking immediately after excision only have a slightly increased risk. In tobacco chewers, cancers arise in the buccal mucosa where the quid is kept lodged (Friedell and Rosenthal 1941). In India the habits of reverse smoking (with the lighted end inside the mouth) and chewing a mixture of tobacco, betel nut and slaked lime, both strongly predispose to oral cancer.

Alcoholics have six times the risk of developing oral cancer compared with the general population and there is evidence that alcohol and tobacco act synergistically. There is an association between liver cirrhosis and oral cancer, presumably on the basis of alcohol.

There is a weak association between syphilis and oral cancer. An association between poor oral hygiene and oral cancer is not proven. Leukoplakia and lichen planus have already been discussed. Patients with the Plummer–Vinson syndrome (*see* p. 40) may develop oral cancer as well as post-cricoid cancers. Submucous fibrosis is a specific entity which occurs in Indians as a dense fibrosis of the palate and buccal mucosa and it gives rise to squamous carcinoma in up to 50% of cases. Finally, strong sunlight predisposes to cancer of the lower lip.

Morphology

The early macroscopic changes of oral cancer may simply be a change of colour in the mucous membrane and some cases of leukoplakia are already carcinoma at the time of presentation. In Mashberg and Meyers' (1976) study of early squamous carcinoma of the mouth, erythroplakia was found to be the predominant mucosal change. Later cases present as ulcers or as exophytic lesions.

The distribution of squamous cancers given by Lucas (1984) is lip 25% (almost all on the lower lip), floor of the mouth 15%, gingiva 10%, tongue 30%, cheek 10% and palate 10%. The distribution of early asymptomatic cancer is strikingly different. A study by Mashberg and Meyers (1976) of 222 early lesions (excluding the lips) showed that 97·1% were found in three high risk areas: the floor of the mouth, the ventral and lateral surfaces of the tongue and the soft palate complex. These authors suggest that a mucosal alteration in any of the 'high risk areas' of more than 14 days duration should be biopsied.

Biopsy of any suspicious oral lesion is necessary prior to treatment. If possible, local anaesthetic should be avoided, as an increase in local tissue pressure may spread the tumour. If general anaesthetic is used, an assessment of the extent of spread can be made by palpation as well as taking a biopsy. The edge of the lesion, rather tnan the necrotic centre, should be biopsied.

Histologically, the tumour is usually a well differentiated squamous carcinoma. Strands of squamous epithelium break through the basement membrane into the underlying connective tissue where they form epithelial nests and keratin pearls (*see Fig.* 1.3). The cells show various degrees of nuclear hyperchromatism and pleomorphism, depending on the degree of differentiation. Well differentiated tumours have to be distinguished from benign lesions, such as simple epithelial hyperplasia (which does not show any cellular atypia). Poorly differentiated tumours are difficult to distinguish from lymphomas and metastatic deposits.

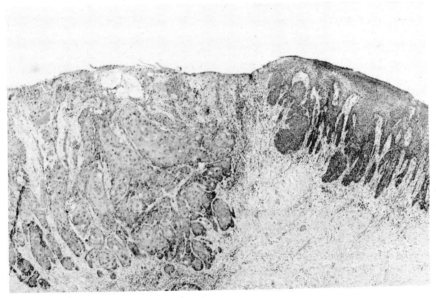

Fig. 1.3. Squamous carcinoma of tongue. (H and E × 30)

Pathological changes may also be seen as a result of therapy. The side effects of radiotherapy include dental caries and osteoradionecrosis. It may also be difficult to diagnose local recurrence after radiotherapy as it may be impossible to know if deep induration represents viable tumour cells or a post-radiation fibrosis. If radiotherapy fails it does so in the deepest part of the tumour where oxygen tension is lowest.

The TNM system of staging is given in *Table* 1.1.

Table 1.1. TNM classification of oral cavity cancer

T1	≤ 2 cm
T2	2–4 cm
T3	> 4 cm
T4	Extension to bone or muscle
N1	Ipsilateral movable nodes
N2	Contralateral or bilateral movable nodes
N3	Fixed nodes
M0	No distant metastases
M1	Presence of distant metastases

LIP: Squamous carcinomas here are usually well differentiated and have a good prognosis, especially if on the lower lip. In cases without nodal involvement, five year survival is 80–85% (Cross *et al.* 1948). Spread is first to the submental and submandibular nodes and then to the deep cervical nodes. Involvement of nodes reduces the five year survival rate to 40%.

FLOOR OF MOUTH: These are most common in the anterior part of the floor of the mouth. The tumours are usually well differentiated and tend to develop metastases late. Five year survival rate is about 50%. Direct spread is limited by the mylohyoid diaphragm and lymphatic spread involves the submandibular and cervical nodes.

TONGUE: These tumours often appear as a malignant ulcer with raised edges, although, characteristically, palpation reveals a much wider area of infiltration than is appreciated visually. The commonest site is the middle third of the lateral border. The lymphatic drainage of the anterior two-thirds of the tongue is via the submental and submandibular nodes to the lower deep cervical nodes, while the posterior third drains to the upper deep cervical nodes. Tumours of the anterior two-thirds tend to metastasize to one side of the neck as there is little lymphatic anastomosis across the midline in this part of the tongue. Tumours of the posterior one-third metastasize bilaterally as there is a good anastomosis across the midline in this region. Prognosis for tumours of the anterior tongue is therefore better than for tumours of the posterior third. The average five year survival rate for all sites is approximately 25%.

BUCCAL MUCOSA: These tumours most frequently occur opposite the lower molar teeth and often develop from leukoplakia. Spread is to the submandibular and deep cervical nodes. It is an aggressive tumour affecting older patients, and three macroscopic types have been described: exophytic, ulcerative and verrucous, the verrucous type being the least common and least aggressive (*see* below). Death is usually due to a local recurrence rather than distant metastases. Affected patients have a five year survival rate of about 20–30%.

GINGIVA: These tumours are usually well differentiated growths of the molar or premolar areas of the lower jaw. Spread is to the submandibular and deep cervical nodes. They also tend to spread locally within the mucosa and half the cases involve the underlying bone. Average five year survival rate is 40%.

PALATE: Carcinomas are more common on the soft palate than on the hard palate. They are well differentiated but may directly invade the maxillary sinus or nasal cavities. Lymphatic spread is to the submandibular and upper cervical nodes. Prognosis is poor with five year survival of only 5–10%.

Variants of squamous carcinoma of the oral mucosa

Verrucous carcinoma (Jacobson and Shear 1972)

This variant of squamous carcinoma is discussed separately because its behaviour is markedly different from that of ordinary squamous carcinoma. The lesion typically occurs in elderly men as a slowly growing cauliflower-like growth with folds and deep clefts. Microscopically, it is composed of bulbous pegs of squamous epithelium which appear to be pushing into the surrounding connective tissue. The epithelium is exceedingly well differentiated and therefore the distinction from a benign lesion may be exceedingly difficult. It is essentially a clinicopathological diagnosis and failure to provide adequate clinical details may result in an incorrect report. It infiltrates locally although it only rarely gives rise to distant metastases. Prognosis is very good although it can recur after local excision. Radiotherapy is contraindicated as it may cause anaplastic change.

Just as verrucous carcinoma may appear to mimic a benign lesion histologically, so it should be observed that some local reactive lesions of the mouth may histologically mimic a carcinoma. This is due to the occurrence of pseudoepitheliomatous hyperplasia—an excessive degree of epithelial hyperplasia in response to irritation—which may occur in denture-induced hyperplasia. It is also seen in association with a granular cell myoblastoma (see p. 13).

Spindle cell carcinoma (Leifer et al. 1974)

This variant occurs as a polypoid fleshy tumour of the mouth. Histologically it is composed of hyperchromatic pleomorphic spindle cells. Demonstration of an origin from the squamous epithelium confirms the diagnosis of carcinoma rather than sarcoma. Spindle cell change may occur in a squamous carcinoma after irradiation and in these cases it is difficult to distinguish a benign proliferation of reactive fibrous tissue from a recurrence of the carcinoma.

Malignant melanoma·

Malignant melanoma accounts for 1–2% of all malignant oral tumours. They may arise in a pre-existing benign naevus of the oral mucous membrane, or they can arise de novo. They are often preceded by non-neoplastic intra-oral pigmentation of several months or years duration.

The commonest site is the hard palate, although they can also occur on the lower jaw, buccal mucosa, tongue and lips. The tumour appears as a painless, pigmented swelling which later ulcerates and bleeds. Occasionally they are non-pigmented. They rapidly invade local structures and metastasize to lymph nodes. Histologically they are similar to melanomas of the skin (see p. 509). The prognosis is poor with a five year survival rate of approximately 30%, although this drops to only 5% if lymph nodes are involved at the time of presentation.

Cysts and Tumours of Odontogenic Epithelium

The epithelium which contributes to tooth formation disintegrates to leave remnants of epithelial cells which may undergo stimulation in later life to produce a dentigerous cyst (which envelops the crown of an unerupted tooth), a dental cyst (which occurs at the apex of a root of a dead tooth), or an odontogenic keratocyst. The latter is lined with squamous epithelium showing various degrees of keratinization and its main relevance to the surgeon is its high recurrence rate and tendency to be multiple. Multiple odontogenic keratocysts may be seen with multiple basal cell carcinomas of the skin, a variety of skeletal anomalies and intracranial calcifications (Gorlin's syndrome).

The ameloblastoma is the most common of the rare tumours of odontogenic epithelium. It may be classified with basal cell carcinoma as a tumour of intermediate malignancy and it shares with basal cell carcinoma some histological features, notably the palisading arrangement of the epithelial cells at the periphery of each island of tumour. It is a relatively slow growing tumour, usually first discovered at X-ray in this country. It eventually produces swelling and facial deformity due to its capacity for local invasion.

Connective Tissue Tumours

These tumours are similar to connective tissue tumours elsewhere in the body and are much rarer than epithelial oral tumours. It is not proposed to discuss them individually here. Mention will be made, however, of two lesions which are generally regarded as hamartomas rather than neoplasms.

Haemangioma

Small haemangiomas may occur on the insides of the lips or on the buccal mucosa. They are of surgical importance when they occur in the substance of the tongue since, if they become enlarged, they may produce obstruction of the airway.

When such small lesions are multiple, one of the angiomatous syndromes such as the Rendu–Weber–Osler disease should be considered. Finally, angiomatous-like lesions may occur in the mouth, particularly the palate, as part of the Kaposi's sarcoma component of the acquired immunodeficiency syndrome (AIDS—see p. 539).

Lymphangioma

Similar in many respects to the haemangioma this has, however, a greater predilection for the tongue. Due to its deeply ramifying nature, similar to the cystic hygroma (its counterpart in the neck), it may present difficulties in surgical management.

Extra-oral Malignancies Presenting in the Mouth

Carcinoma of the maxillary sinus

The initial presentation of carcinoma of the maxillary sinus may be in the hard palate where it produces pain, swelling and ulceration. Consequently, the differential diagnosis of a malignant ulcer in the upper jaw should include squamous carcinoma of oral mucosa, carcinoma of maxillary sinus and adenocarcinoma of minor salivary gland origin.

Trotter's syndrome

This is a clinical condition characterized by pain in the lower jaw, asymmetry and displacement of soft palate and deafness due to nasopharyngeal tumour (usually carcinoma). The symptoms are due to involvement by the tumour of the mandibular nerve in the area of the foramen ovale. With the progression of the tumour, trismus may eventually develop.

Miscellaneous Conditions

Aphthous ulcers

These are very common lesions of oral mucosa (usually the non-keratinized areas) and differ from traumatic and neoplastic ulcers in that they are multiple and recurrent. Hence the synonym 'recurrent oral ulceration'. They occur in both minor and major forms.

The minor form is the more common variety and consists of small shallow ulcers with a white central slough surrounded by a red halo. They are found in the 10–40 year age group, are extremely painful, last 4–10 days and heal without scarring.

The major form is of similar appearance except the ulcers are very much larger, more painful, last 10–40 days and heal with scarring.

The cause of recurrent oral ulceration is unknown. Trauma, stress and hormonal factors have been suggested. Attempts have been made to implicate various micro-organisms without complete success. Immune responses appear to be involved in some undefined way and 75% of affected patients have a high serum level of antibody to fetal oral mucosa. Interestingly, the ulcers are extremely rare in smokers.

A minority of these patients on investigation suffer from a haematological abnormality such as deficiency of vitamin B_{12}, folic acid or iron. Rarely, such lesions may presage or occur as part of Behçet's syndrome, ulcerative colitis or Crohn's disease.

Crohn's disease

Oral manifestations occur in about 10% of all cases of Crohn's disease. The initial lesion appears to be oedema of the mucosa, usually the cheek lining. This produces characteristic bulging which forms a cobblestone appearance. With passage of time, the inflammatory infiltrate produces a firm consistency and at the base of the cobblestones small non-specific ulcers develop. Histological examination reveals oedema, capillary dilatation, a lymphocytic infiltrate and granuloma formation. The lesions usually post-date bowel involvement but may precede it. Oral ulceration may also be associated with ulcerative colitis.

Median rhomboid glossitis

This lesion appears clinically as a red rhomboid or oval shaped area anterior to the circumvallate papillae. It is devoid of filiform papillae. Traditionally it has been regarded as due to failure of withdrawal of the tuberculum impar before fusion of the lateral halves of the tongue. However, recent work has shown that it may be due to Candida infection. It should not be misdiagnosed as a carcinoma which would be unusual at this site.

Geographic tongue

In this not uncommon condition, the dorsal surface of the tongue shows smooth red areas due to atrophy of the filiform papillae. The fungiform papillae consequently stand out as red elevations. As one area returns to normal, another area in a different part of the tongue may become affected. It is a harmless condition of unknown aetiology.

Necrotizing sialometaplasia (Fechner 1977)

This very rare condition is easily mistaken for malignancy, both macroscopically and microscopically. It forms a deep ulcer, usually on the hard palate. Microscopically, as the name suggests, there is squamous metaplasia of the ducts of a minor salivary gland and necrosis of the salivary acini. The nests of squamous metaplasia lying beneath the epithelium may suggest a squamous carcinoma histologically. The aetiology is unknown although trauma is suspected. It is benign and will heal in 6–10 weeks without treatment, although many undergo excision biopsy to exclude carcinoma.

Dermoid cyst

About 2% of dermoids occur in the region of the floor of the mouth and they most commonly present in teenagers and young adults. When situated above the geniohyoid they are predominantly intra-oral, whereas those below the geniohyoid appear as submental swellings. Microscopically they are lined by squamous epithelium and skin appendages are usually present. Rarely, other tissues such as respiratory or gastrointestinal epithelium may be seen. They are benign.

Giant cell epulis

An epulis is defined as 'any benign tumour-like condition of the gum'. They are classified as fibrous (discussed under fibrous hyperplasia), pregnancy (discussed under pyogenic granuloma), congenital (discussed below) and giant cell.

The giant cell epulis is also known as a peripheral giant cell tumour or peripheral giant cell granuloma. It forms a small mass in the subepithelial connective tissue of the gum. It may become pedunculated to form a soft red lesion on the gingival or alveolar mucosa.

Histologically it consists of a mixture of spindle and giant cells. Osteoid and bone formation may be seen. It is benign and does not recur if completely excised.

Congenital epulis

This occurs in the newborn, commonly in the anterior part of the maxilla. It is about ten times more common in females than males and presents as a soft, sessile or pedunculated mass. Histologically it is very similar to a granular cell myoblastoma (*see* below), but it does not have the associated pseudo-epitheliomatous hyperplasia. The cell of origin is unknown. It does not recur if completely excised.

Granular cell myoblastoma

These tumours are frequently seen on the tongue but also occur in other parts of the oral cavity, the breast, skin and skeletal muscle. Typically they form a painless circumscribed mass which is very slow-growing and can arise in any age group. The structure is similar to congenital epulis but they may be of different histogenesis.

Histologically the tumour is composed of large cells which have an eosinophilic granular cytoplasm. They are arranged in sheets and nests and have a delicate connective tissue stroma. The overlying epithelium often shows pseudo-epitheliomatous hyperplasia (*see* p. 9). The cell of origin is controversial, although Schwann cells are the most likely candidates. The lesion is benign.

SALIVARY GLANDS

Normal Structure

The parotid, submandibular and sublingual glands constitute the three major pairs of salivary glands. Accessory glands are scattered throughout the oral mucosa and are termed the minor salivary glands.

The parotid is the largest of the major salivary glands. It is wedged between the ramus of the mandible anteriorly, the mastoid process behind and the styloid process medially. The base of the wedge is superficial and extends forward over the masseter. The gland lies within the parotid sheath which is derived from the deep cervical fascia and swellings of the parotid cause tension and consequent discomfort. From the anterior border emerges the parotid duct and the five divisions of the facial nerve. The parotid duct (Stensen's duct) passes forward across the masseter and pierces the buccinator to open onto the mucous membrane of the cheek opposite the second upper molar tooth. A detached part of the gland, the accessory lobe, is often found lying on the masseter between the parotid duct and the zygomatic arch.

The parotid is supplied by branches of the external carotid artery and venous drainage is to the retromandibular vein. Lymphatic drainage is to nodes within the parotid sheath and then to the anterior superior group of deep cervical nodes. Secretomotor fibres arise in the otic ganglion and reach the gland via the auriculo-temporal nerve. Injury to the auriculo-temporal nerve (e.g. during parotid surgery) may produce Frey's syndrome, in which the skin anterior to the ear sweats during eating (gustatory sweating).

The submandibular gland lies in the submandibular fossa, partially under the mandible. It has superficial and deep parts which communicate round the posterior border of the mylohyoid muscle. The submandibular duct (Wharton's duct) emerges from the anterior part of the deep lobe and runs forward between the mylohyoid and hyoglossus muscles, to open onto the sublingual papilla in the floor of the mouth near the frenulum. The submandibular duct is longer and narrower than the parotid duct and is more prone to stone formation. Blood supply is from the facial artery, venous drainage is to the common facial vein and lymphatic drainage is to the submandibular glands. Secretomotor fibres are from the facial nerve and travel to the gland via the chorda tympani and the submandibular ganglion.

The sublingual gland lies below the mucous membrane of the floor of the mouth. It has about fifteen ducts, half opening into the sublingual papilla and the remainder opening into the submandibular duct. It is supplied by the lingual artery and submandibular ganglion.

The major glands are divided into lobules by connective tissue septa and each lobule contains many secretory units. The septa act as barriers to the spread of infection between lobules. The parotids produce mainly serous secretion, the sublinguals mainly mucous secretion and the submandibulars produce a mixture of both.

The secretory unit consists of a tubulo-acinar structure, composed of serous or mucous cells or a mixture of the two. The acini are surrounded by myoepithelial cells which contract to force the secretion into the duct system. The acini drain into the intercalated ducts which are also lined by secretory cells. The intercalated ducts drain into the striated ducts, so-called because of the striated appearance of the cells on light microscopy which is due to infoldings of the plasma membranes. The ionic composition of the saliva is altered in the striated ducts and it then drains into the intra- and interlobular ducts (*see Fig.* 1.4).

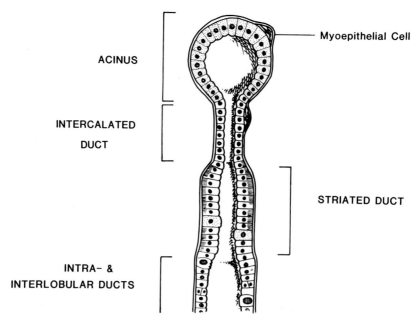

Fig. 1.4. Schematic diagram of the structure of normal salivary gland. (Adapted from Conley 1975.)

Salivary Gland Biopsy

Most authors agree that a discrete salivary gland mass should not be subjected to incisional biopsy. Most single parotid masses are due to a pleomorphic adenoma and incisional biopsy may later produce local recurrence. Therefore superficial parotidectomy is more acceptable. If, however, there is skin involvement and obvious malignancy, incisional biopsy is acceptable.

A parapharyngeal mass should not be biopsied through the pharynx. If the mass is a chemodectoma, then severe bleeding will ensue, while if it is a salivary gland tumour, there will be a high risk of recurrence.

A diffuse enlargement of a salivary gland is probably not due to a tumour and an incisional biopsy is permissible if the diagnosis cannot be attained by other means. If a benign lymphoepithelial lesion is suspected then a labial biopsy to examine the minor salivary glands is useful.

More recently, fine needle aspiration biopsy has been applied to salivary gland swellings. In one series of 271 fine needle aspiration biopsies, recognition of a neoplasm was 98% accurate, recognition of benign tumour was 91% accurate and recognition of a malignant tumour was 89% accurate (Webb 1982). However, as with fine needle aspiration cytology elsewhere, an experienced cytologist is required. Frozen section material from salivary gland tumours is particularly difficult to interpret.

Mucocoele

These cysts frequently form in the submucosa of the mouth, the most common sites being the lower lip and the floor of mouth. In the latter site they are termed ranulas. They may be retention cysts due to obstruction of a salivary gland duct (in which case they are lined by epithelium) or more commonly extravasation cysts due to rupture of a salivary gland duct with consequent leakage of mucus into the surrounding tissue (in which case they do not have a lining of epithelium). In most cases the lining consists of compressed granulation tissue or connective tissue. The cysts can be readily removed under local anaesthesia but if the associated gland is not removed, the lesion may recur. In the case of a ranula the extravasated material may penetrate deeply into the tissue planes of the floor of the mouth forming submandibular or parapharyngeal extensions (the so-called plunging ranula).

Inflammatory and Calculus Disease of the Salivary Glands

Acute sialadenitis

In adults this occurs most commonly as acute parotitis, occurring in post-surgical or debilitated patients. There is a sudden onset of swelling of the gland with pain and a purulent discharge from Stensen's duct, associated with a systemic reaction with pyrexia and leucocytosis. It probably arises as a result of retrograde infection, due to the increase in oral bacteria which is known to take place in the post-operative phase. Pathologically there is an infiltration of acute inflammatory cells into the parenchyma of the gland and small abscesses form which are separated from each other by the fibrous septa of the gland.

Chronic recurrent sialadenitis

This occurs more frequently in the parotid than in the submandibular glands. It presents clinically as recurrent attacks of swelling with associated discomfort. When it occurs in children, there is usually no obvious obstruction of the salivary ducts and there is a tendency for the disease to terminate spontaneously at puberty. In adults, however, there is usually duct obstruction. Studies have shown that, in adults with recurrent parotitis, the glands produce a reduced quantity of secretion. This is thought to lead to retrograde infection with consequent metaplasia of ductal epithelium, which is associated with obstruction due to mucous plugs, strictures and calculi. The cause of the reduction in secretion may be a pre-existing viral infection or repeated low-grade ascending infections. Grossly, dilatation of the ductal system (sialectasis) may be demonstrated on a sialogram. Histologically, as well as the ductal dilatation and metaplastic changes of the ductal epithelium, there is a lymphocytic infiltrate of the parenchyma which tends to replace the acini.

Calculi

The aetiology is unknown; there is no correlation with plasma calcium levels, dietary habits or oral sepsis. The majority of salivary gland calculi (80–90%) occur in the submandibular gland and less than 20% occur in the parotid gland, although calculi are present in approximately two-thirds of patients who have chronic parotitis. The calculus is usually solitary, occurs in middle-aged patients and is slightly more common in men than women; they are rare in children. The classical clinical presentation of submandibular calculi is recurrent episodes of pain and swelling in the submandibular region occurring after eating and lasting 2–3 hours. Parotid gland calculi usually cause symptoms which are not related to food but may be prolonged for several days due to the higher incidence of secondary infection in these cases.

The calculus is composed mainly of calcium phosphate and may be present either in the ducts or the gland parenchyma. In the latter position it is less likely to cause symptoms.

The surgical management of a parotid stone may be expectant or alternatively a buccal approach with ductoplasty may be used. Superficial parotidectomy is rarely required (Hobsley 1981).

If a submandibular gland stone is palpable anteriorly in the duct, it is easily removed via an incision in the floor of the mouth. If the stone is posterior, a direct oral approach may injure the lingual nerve and therefore excision of the whole gland via a cervical approach is preferable.

Benign Lymphoepithelial Lesion, Sicca Syndrome, Sjögren's Syndrome and Mikulicz's Disease

The terminology of these conditions is confusing. The following account is based on the terminology used by Lucas (1984).

The histological findings in a salivary gland of a diffuse lymphocytic infiltrate, acinar destruction and ducts which have undergone metaplasia to form epithelial islands are together known as the 'lymphoepithelial lesion' (see Fig. 1.5). If the condition is confined to the salivary glands, with no other manifestation, the term

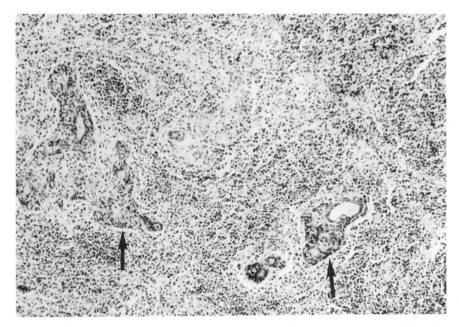

Fig. 1.5. Lymphoepithelial lesion. A diffuse lymphocytic infiltrate with epimyoepithelial islands (arrows). (H and E × 30)

'benign lymphoepithelial lesion' is used without further qualification (although this term has been criticized since the onset of lymphoma has been described; *see below*). If there are ocular and salivary symptoms due to the involvement of both the salivary and lacrimal glands, the term 'sicca syndrome' is used. If there are ocular and salivary manifestations, together with a systemic autoimmune disease such as rheumatoid arthritis, the term 'Sjögren's syndrome' is used. In all cases the salivary gland histology is identical. It is unclear whether or not the benign lymphoepithelial lesion can progress to Sjögren's syndrome, or whether it is a completely different disease process which merely has identical histological findings to Sjögren's syndrome.

Mikulicz, in 1892, published a case of a man with bilateral lacrimal, parotid and submandibular swellings of uncertain aetiology. The terms 'Mikulicz's disease' and 'Mikulicz's syndrome' have since then been applied to various salivary disorders, to the extent that they are now considered by some authorities to be meaningless. Mikulicz's syndrome can, however, be used as a clinical term to describe bilateral lacrimal and salivary enlargement from whatever cause, for example leukaemia, lymphoma and Sjögren's syndrome.

Symptoms of the benign lymphoepithelial lesion are usually mild and may not require treatment. Xerostomia is the most common salivary symptom in Sjögren's syndrome. Painless gland enlargement may occur in the sicca syndrome and may be unilateral or bilateral and can be confused with tumour. The parotids are the most commonly affected glands. The ocular symptoms include dryness of the eye, pain and photophobia. The systemic symptoms of Sjögren's syndrome depend on the associated autoimmune disease which is most commonly rheumatoid arthritis, but can also be systemic lupus erythematosus, polymyositis, etc.

The aetiology of the various conditions is unknown, although genetic, viral and immunological factors have been implicated.

Macroscopically the affected glands are not necessarily enlarged. The involvement may be diffuse or nodular and the affected areas are white and rubbery.

Microscopically the early findings are infiltration of lymphocytes around the salivary ducts with atrophy of the acini but preservation of the ducts. More commonly, the fully developed lesion is seen. This characteristically shows a diffuse lymphocytic infiltrate which has destroyed the salivary acini. Within this infiltrate, irregular islands of epithelial tissue termed 'epimyoepithelial islands' are found. These islands often contain hyaline material and arise from ducts, the epithelium of which has undergone metaplasia and proliferation.

Patients with the sicca syndrome and Sjögren's syndrome require careful follow-up since the lymphocytic proliferation may develop into a lymphoma. The relative risk of lymphoma is forty times that of the general population, and both extra- and intrasalivary lymphomas may occur. The onset of lymphoma is more common in those patients who have a salivary swelling (Moutsopoulos *et al.* 1980). Malignant lymphoma has also been described in association with the benign lympho-epithelial lesion (Azzopardi and Evans 1971).

Histological diagnosis and monitoring of patients with Sjögren's syndrome can be carried out by biopsy of the minor salivary glands, for example in the lip, since these reflect the activity in the other glands.

Tumours of the Salivary Gland

The annual incidence of salivary gland tumours is in the region of one per 100 000 of the population. Approximately 80–85% are in the parotids, 10–15% are in the submandibular glands and 5% are in the sublingual and minor glands. The commonest tumour is the pleomorphic adenoma which accounts for approximately 75% of parotid tumours and 60% of submandibular tumours. Submandibular tumours are more commonly malignant (30%) than parotid gland tumours (10%).

Most parotid tumours occur in the superficial lobe. Paralysis of the facial nerve and fixation of the tumour are indicative of malignancy.

A submandibular mass is more likely to be due to a benign inflammatory disorder than to a tumour. Nerve involvement is less common than in the parotid but the tumour may involve the cervical branch of the facial, the lingual or the hypoglossal nerves.

Several studies have reported an association between breast cancer and salivary gland tumours. Salivary gland cancers are slightly more common in patients who have had previous head and neck radiotherapy. No other definite aetiological agents have been identified.

Classification

The WHO classification of epithelial tumours is given in *Table* 1.2. Non-epithelial tumours of various types, such as fibrosarcoma, lymphoma, etc., are occasionally seen.

Table 1.2. WHO classification of epithelial tumours of the salivary glands

	Parotid*	Submandibular*
Adenoma		
Pleomorphic adenoma	76·2	60·0
Monomorphic adenoma		
Adenolymphoma	4·7	2·4
Oxyphilic adenoma	1·0	0·6
Other types	—	—
Mucoepidermoid tumour	4·1	3·6
Acinic cell tumour	3·0	0·6
Carcinoma		
Adenoid cystic	2·3	15·0
Adenocarcinoma	2·4	—
Epidermoid	0·3	7·0
Undifferentiated	3·9	9·0
Carcinoma in pleomorphic adenoma	1·5	1·8

*Percentage of each tumour type in Eneroth's (1971) study of 2158 parotid and 170 submandibular tumours.

Adenomas

Pleomorphic adenoma (mixed salivary tumour)

Clinically these are typically slowly growing painless tumours (*see Fig.* 1.6). Males and females are affected equally and the peak incidence is in the fifth decade. There may be sudden periods of rapid growth, followed by quiescent periods and, therefore, a rapid increase in size is not necessarily indicative of malignant change. The commonest site is the parotid gland near the angle of the jaw. They are usually unilateral, although bilateral tumours have been reported. Pleomorphic adenomas of the minor salivary glands are most frequently found on the palate. Tumours of the deep lobe of the parotid may present as a pharyngeal mass.

Grossly, pleomorphic adenomas have a smooth and lobulated surface. The capsule has a tendency to be incomplete and satellite nodules of the tumour can become walled off outside the main mass, although some of these nodules are pseudopods of the tumour which appear to be detached on tangential section. These isolated nodules can be responsible for recurrences, particularly multiple recurrences. The appearance of the cut surface depends on the constituents of the tumour and so it may be mucoid, cartilaginous or fleshy.

Histologically, pleomorphic adenomas characteristically show both epithelial and mesenchymal-like components and one of these may predominate. The epithelial component typically consists of ducts lined by large epithelial cells, surrounding which are smaller dark-staining (probably myoepithelial) cells which form mantels and sheets. The tumour is therefore pleomorphic, both with respect to having epithelial and mesenchymal-like components and also in having different

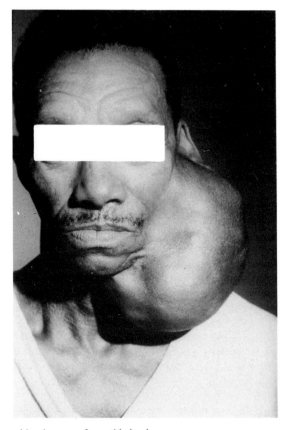

Fig. 1.6. Pleomorphic adenoma of parotid gland.

epithelial cell types (*see Fig.* 1.7). Strands of the myoepithelial-like cells tend to merge into the background mesenchymal-like tissue which may be myxoid, chondroid or hyaline. Great variation is seen, however, and some tumours may consist of tubules and sheets of cells in which a careful search is necessary to find a mesenchymal-like element. Ten per cent are highly cellular and these are more liable to local recurrence than the usual type.

The cell of origin of pleomorphic adenomas is controversial although most authorities now consider that the tumour is purely epithelial rather than a mixture of epithelial and true mesenchymal elements. Ultrastructural studies have demonstrated both ductal and myoepithelial cells and are known to have the ability to differentiate into fibroblasts, chondroblasts, etc.

Since pleomorphic adenomas have pseudopods and satellite tumours which are separate from the main mass, simple enucleation will leave these behind, causing a characteristic multicentric recurrence which may be of a more aggressive histological type. Also, the plane of cleavage in enucleation procedures often forms actually within the tumour, leaving a rim of tumour behind. Therefore, many surgeons treat pleomorphic adenomas of the parotid by formal parotidectomy (Stevens and

Hobsley 1982), although other surgeons advocate simple enucleation and radio-therapy which reduces the risk of facial nerve damage (Armitstead *et al.* 1979). In submandibular tumours, the entire gland should be removed.

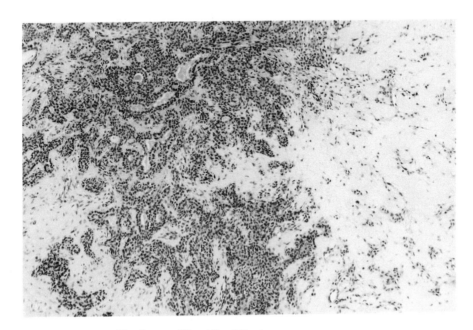

Fig. 1.7. Pleomorphic adenoma. (H and E × 30)

Monomorphic adenomas

In monomorphic adenomas the epithelial component is arranged in a regular fashion throughout the tumour. They differ from pleomorphic adenomas in two main respects: (1) they do not have mesenchymal-like tissue and (2) they do not show the two different (ductal and myoepithelial) epithelial cell types.

ADENOLYMPHOMA: These occur in patients aged 50–70 years old and up to 90% are found in males. They occur commonly in the lower third of the parotid gland and present as a soft or fluctuant mass. Rarely they are located within a lymph node in the upper part of the neck, outside the parotid gland. They are exceedingly rare in the other salivary glands. Five to ten per cent are bilateral. An individual tumour can vary greatly in size at different times. (Also known as Warthin's tumour.)

Macroscopically they are rounded masses which, on cut section, character-istically show cystic spaces containing a dark-brown tenacious material. They are rarely more than 5 cm in diameter.

Microscopically they have a very characteristic pattern, consisting of cyst-like spaces lined by a double layer of epithelium (*see Fig.* 1.8). The intervening tissue has a very heavy lymphocytic infiltrate with many germinal centres. Although the tumour has epithelial and lymphoid components, it is classified as a monomorphic adenoma since only the epithelial part is considered to be neoplastic. If the cyst's contents come into contact with the stroma, granulomas may form.

Adenolymphomas are thought to arise from duct epithelium. Those outside the salivary glands probably arise from nests of ectopic salivary tissue which are frequently seen in the lymph nodes surrounding the major glands.

If excision is complete, it is curative and malignant transformation is exceedingly rare.

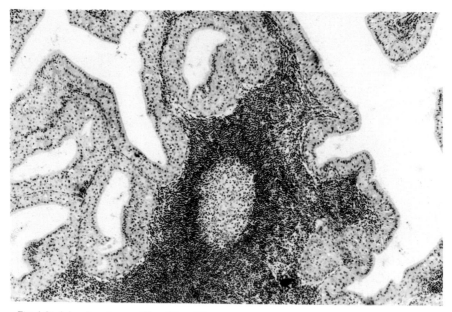

Fig. 1.8. Adenolymphoma. (H and E × 75)

OXYPHILIC ADENOMA (Gray *et al.* 1976): Like the adenolymphoma, this tumour occurs in older patients. It is well encapsulated and measures up to 5 cm in diameter. Microscopically it consists of large polygonal cells with strikingly eosinophilic granular cytoplasm. These are arranged in columns, acini or small tubules. The tumours arise from ductal epithelium which has altered to form large eosinophilic cells (oncocytes). Foci of these cells are commonly seen distributed throughout the salivary glands of elderly people (oncocytosis).

Although malignant oxyphilic cell tumours have occasionally been reported, the tumour is considered benign and does not recur after excision.

OTHER TYPES OF ADENOMA: Other rare monomorphic adenomas are well recognized. Some are classified according to the cell type (clear cell or basaloid) and others according to the architecture (tubular, trabecular or canalicular). Malignant forms of some of these have been described but are rare. They usually do not recur if completely excised.

Mucoepidermoid tumours

These are tumours composed of squamous (epidermoid) and mucus secreting cells. Ninety per cent involve the parotid gland and they occasionally occur in the minor salivary glands of the palate.

They occur in all age groups but are commonest in patients aged 20–60 years. It is the commonest salivary gland tumour of children. The sex distribution is even. Although in some cases they present as an obvious malignant growth with skin ulceration and fixation and facial nerve paralysis, more often they are clinically indistinguishable from pleomorphic adenomas.

Macroscopically they are firm and ill-defined masses, sometimes showing infiltration of the surrounding gland, and cut section typically shows mucoid containing cysts. Histologically mucoid cells, epidermoid cells and cells intermediate between the two are seen. Both the mucoid and epidermoid cells can line the cystic spaces or form solid clumps. Some tumours are almost completely solid.

All mucoepidermoid tumours are considered to have malignant potential, although this is low grade and the majority neither metastasize nor recur if adequately treated, that is, surgically removed with a wide margin (Thackray and Lucas 1974). The histological appearance of the tumour is only a rough guide to the malignant potential. The five year cure rate in recent reports is up to 90% (Fu et al. 1977), although it can be as low as 40% for intermediate and high grade tumours.

Acinic cell tumours

These tumours are commoner in women than men. The peak age is in the fifth decade, although they can occur in childhood. Although growth is slow and clinically the tumour is like a pleomorphic adenoma, recurrences and metastases have been described. About 3% are bilateral.

It appears as a single, often encapsulated, solid tumour. Satellites may be present outside the main mass and these can result in multiple recurrences if enucleation is carried out.

Microscopically the typical feature is the presence of cells which have a granular basophilic cytoplasm. These cells resemble the normal serous cells of the salivary glands and are arranged in acini or solid sheets. Clear spaces appear between the cells and are due to the accumulation of serous secretion which cannot escape as the tumour does not contain ducts.

The prognosis after complete removal is good with a five year survival rate of over 80%. Metastases are exceedingly rare.

Carcinomas

Adenoid cystic carcinoma

This is the commonest true malignant tumour of the salivary gland. It is more common in the minor than in the major glands and it has a predilection for hard palate. The tumour is composed of duct and myoepithelial cells arranged in a cribriform pattern. Sex incidence is equal and the maximum age incidence is the sixth decade.

The tumour is slow growing and has a propensity to ulcerate and to involve nerves, causing pain and facial paralysis. Bony involvement is also early although it may not be recognizable on X-ray since the spread tends to be along marrow cavities.

Grossly, it appears as a well defined mass, often with some infiltration visible macroscopically at the edge. The cut surface is fleshy without the mucoid change seen in pleomorphic adenomas.

Microscopically, clumps of tumour cells are seen. These clumps contain multiple, small, cyst-like spaces which are lined either by duct-type epithelium or more commonly by small dark cells, presumably myoepithelial in type. Perineural invasion is frequently seen, as is invasion of the rest of the gland substance and surrounding tissue (*see Fig.* 1.9).

Prognosis is related to the feasibility of complete resection as cure is very unlikely if resection is incomplete. If resection is incomplete, metastases eventually occur to long bones and lung via vascular dissemination. Nevertheless, the course of the disease is slow with 10 and 20 year survival rates of 70% and 20% respectively being reported (Lucas 1984).

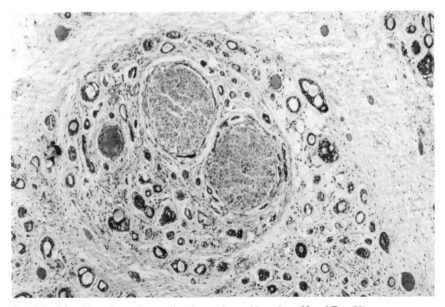

Fig. 1.9. Adenoid cystic carcinoma showing perineural invasion. (H and E × 30)

Adenocarcinoma, squamous carcinoma and undifferentiated carcinoma

These present with the characteristic features of malignancy, that is, a fixed mass with nerve paralysis and occasionally skin ulceration. Adenocarcinomas are usually well differentiated and have a relatively good prognosis compared with adenocarcinomas elsewhere in the body. Sex incidence is equal and about one-quarter have facial nerve palsy. Squamous carcinomas probably arise after squamous metaplasia in salivary gland ducts and have a marked male predominance. They are rare and aggressive with rapid growth, facial pain and facial nerve palsy. Half of the patients have positive lymph nodes at the time of presentation. The undifferentiated carcinomas are either spheroidal or spindle cell and have a poor prognosis. They may be difficult to differentiate from sarcomas.

Carcinoma arising in a pleomorphic adenoma

Carcinoma may occur in association with a pleomorphic adenoma in two ways: (1) as a malignant change in a long-standing pleomorphic adenoma; (2) as a malignant tumour from the outset. Less than 10% of all pleomorphic adenomas undergo malignant change.

When malignancy arises in a pre-existing adenoma it changes its character in that it enlarges, it may involve the facial nerve and it becomes fixed. The malignancy may occur in an unresected tumour or in the recurrences following unsuccessful surgery. Malignant change is most common in the parotid gland.

Grossly, on the cut surface, an area of typical pleomorphic adenoma adjoins a hard fleshy infiltrating area of carcinoma. Histologically the type of carcinoma which develops is one of the types previously described. Adenocarcinoma and undifferentiated types are the most common, although mucoepidermoid and adenoid cystic carcinomas can also occur. Malignancy in a pleomorphic adenoma is recognized microscopically by infiltrating areas of hyperchromatic pleomorphic cells showing necrosis and mitotic activity. The presence of pleomorphic adenoma tissue in an extensive carcinoma may be difficult to detect and in these cases it may not be realized that the tumour arose in a pleomorphic adenoma.

The prognosis for tumours arising in a pre-existing adenoma is poor with a high incidence of metastases and a high recurrence rate. Five year survival is less than 40%.

Tumours which are malignant from the outset show a basic structure similar to the pleomorphic adenoma and are considered to be its malignant counterpart. They are very rare.

Non-epithelial tumours of the salivary glands

Benign non-epithelial tumours are rare. Haemangiomas and lymphangiomas have been described. Lipomas are unilateral and tend to lie lateral to the parotid.

Sarcomas such as fibrosarcomas are very rare. Lymphomas may invade the salivary glands from surrounding lymph nodes or may arise within the salivary gland in association with Sjögren's syndrome or the sicca syndrome.

The parotid may be involved by metastatic spread of head and neck tumours, especially by malignant melanoma.

THE NECK

Most causes of lumps in the neck have been dealt with elsewhere. In this section, only branchial cysts, branchial fistulas and sinuses and carotid body tumours will be considered.

Branchial Cysts

The aetiology of branchial cysts is unknown. Some authorities consider it likely that those rare branchial cysts which have an internal opening are derived from remnants of the first or second branchial pouch, whereas the more common ones with no internal opening are due to epithelial inclusions in lymph nodes which undergo cyst formation.

Branchial cysts are more common in men than in women and the peak age of presentation is between 20 and 30 years old, this being in favour of the second acquired theory of aetiology. Clinically they are fluctuant swellings most commonly situated just anterior to the sternomastoid in the upper third of the neck. Rarely they are bilateral.

On sectioning, the cysts characteristically contain straw-coloured fluid and within this, cholesterol crystals can be seen. The wall of the cyst is lined by squamous or columnar epithelium and it typically contains a heavy infiltrate of lymphoid tissue (*see Fig.* 1.10). Branchial cysts may become infected. Branchiogenic carcinoma is exceedingly rare.

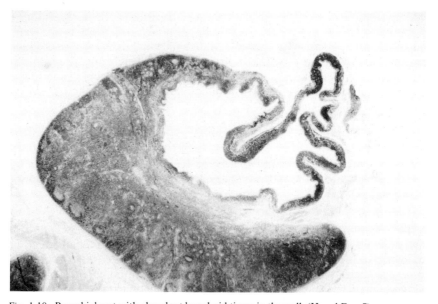

Fig. 1.10. Branchial cyst with abundant lymphoid tissue in the wall. (H and E × 7)

Branchial Fistulas and Sinuses

These may represent a persistent second branchial cleft. The tract of a complete branchial fistula runs from the internal opening which is situated on the anterior aspect of the posterior pillar of the fauces to the external opening which is situated just anterior to the lower part of the sternomastoid. Complete branchial fistulas are, however, rare and most end blindly deep in the neck near the pharyngeal wall. Histologically a branchial fistula is lined by ciliated columnar epithelium which is often lost if chronic inflammation is present.

Incision of an inflamed branchial cyst will give rise to a sinus in this region.

Carotid Body Tumours

The carotid bodies are small reddish-brown structures about 7 mm × 3 mm, situated either just behind the bifurcation of the common carotid artery or else wedged in the fork of the bifurcation. They are chemoreceptors which respond to changes in blood oxygen and carbon dioxide tension. Histologically, identical tissue which probably has a chemoreceptor role has also been identified in the jugular bulb (the jugulo-tympanic body) in close association with the inferior (nodose) ganglion of the vagus nerve (the vagal body) and in the adventitia of the aortic arch and pulmonary arteries. Tumours of this tissue are termed chemodectomas or para-gangliomas.

Chronic hypoxia leads to carotid body hyperplasia and the incidence of carotid body tumours is higher than average in high altitude regions such as Peru.

Clinically, carotid body tumours usually present as a painless lump in the neck and a transmitted impulse may be palpable (*see Fig.* 1.11). Occasionally, they present as a pharyngeal mass. The sex distribution is equal and most cases occur in patients aged between 30 and 60 years. In almost 10% there is a family history and in these cases they are more likely to be bilateral.

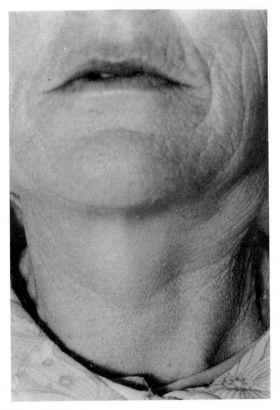

Fig. 1.11. Left sided carotid body tumour.

Grossly, they are partially encapsulated tumours which are tan coloured on cut section. The tumour is adherent to the bifurcation of the common carotid artery and typically causes widening of the bifurcation which can be seen on angiography.

Histologically, the main feature is the presence of cells which are polygonal or ovoid in shape and have a moderate amount of eosinophilic cytoplasm. These cells are arranged in clusters (or zellballen) which are surrounded by a highly vascular stroma. All chemodectomas have a similar structure.

In one series, carotid body tumours were malignant in 9% of cases and vagal body tumours were malignant in 15% of cases (Lack *et al.* 1979). Histologically the malignant examples showed areas of necrosis, a high mitotic rate and evidence of the tumour invading vascular spaces.

Carotid body tumours are slow growing and some authorities may only recommend removal if there is an indication such as aggressive growth, symptoms (for example, interference with speech or swallowing), or presentation as a small tumour in a young healthy individual. Others recommend surgery whenever possible.

References

Armitstead P. R., Smiddy F. G., Frank H. G. (1979) Simple enucleation and radiotherapy in the treatment of the pleomorphic salivary adenoma of the parotid gland. *Br. J. Surg.* **66**, 716–17.

Azzopardi J. G., Evans D. J. (1971) Malignant lymphoma of parotid associated with Mikulicz disease (benign lymphoepithelial lesion). *J. Clin. Pathol.* **24**, 744–52.

Conley J. (1975) *Salivary Glands and the Facial Nerve.* Stuttgart, Georg Thieme.

Cross J. E., Guralnick E., Daland E. M. (1948) Carcinoma of the lip. A review of 563 case records of carcinoma of the lip at Pondville Hospital. *Surg. Gynaecol. Obstet.* **87**, 153–62.

Eneroth C. M. (1971) Salivary gland tumours in the parotid gland, submandibular gland and the palate region. *Cancer* **27**, 1415–18.

Fechner R. E. (1977) Necrotizing sialometaplasia: a source of confusion with carcinoma of the palate. *Am. J. Clin. Pathol.* **67**, 315–17.

Friedell H. L., Rosenthal L. M. (1941) The etiological role of chewing tobacco in cancer of the mouth: report of 8 cases treated with radiation. *J. A. M. A.* **116**, 2130–5.

Fu K. K., Liebel S. A., Levine M. L., Friedlander L. M., Boles R., Phillips T. L. (1977) Carcinoma of the major and minor salivary glands: analysis of treatment results and sites and causes of failures. *Cancer* **40**, 2882–90.

Gray S. R., Cornog J. L. Jr., Seo I. S. (1976) Oncocytic neoplasms of salivary glands: a report of fifteen cases including two malignant oncocytomas. *Cancer* **38**, 1306–17.

Hobsley M. (1981) Surgery of the salivary glands. In: Hadfield J., Hobsley M., (eds.) *Current Surgical Practice,* Vol. 3, pp. 8–31. London, Edward Arnold.

Jacobson S., Shear M. (1972) Verrucous carcinoma of the mouth. *J. Oral Pathol.* **1**, 66–75.

Lack E. E., Cubilla A. L., Woodruff J. M. (1979) Paragangliomas of the head and neck region. A pathologic study of tumours from 71 patients. *Human Pathol.* **10**, 191–218.

Leifer C., Miller A. S., Putong P. B., Min B. H. (1974) Spindle-cell carcinoma of the oral mucosa. A light and electron microscopic study of apparent sarcomatous metastasis to cervical lymph nodes. *Cancer* **34**, 597–605.

Lucas R. B. (1984) *Pathology of tumours of the oral tissues.* Edinburgh, Churchill Livingstone.

Mashberg A., Meyers H. (1976) Anatomical site and size of 222 early asymptomatic oral squamous cell carcinomas: a continuing prospective study of oral cancer. II. *Cancer* **37**, 2149–57.

Moutsopoulos H. M., Chused T. M., Mann D. L. *et al.* (1980) Sjögren's syndrome (Sicca syndrome): current issues. *Ann. Intern. Med.* **92**, 212–26.

Stevens K. L., Hobsley M. (1982) The treatment of pleomorphic adenomas by formal parotidectomy. *Br. J. Surg.* **69**, 1–3.

Thackray A. C., Lucas R. B. (1974) Tumours of the major salivary glands. *Atlas of Tumor Pathology.* Second Series, Fascicle 10. Washington DC, Armed Forces Institute of Pathology.

Waldron C. A., Shafer W. G. (1975) Leukoplakia revisited. A clinicopathologic study of 3256 oral leukoplakias. *Cancer* **36**, 1386–92.

Webb A. J. (1982) Surgical aspects of aspiration biopsy cytology. In: Russell R. C. G. (ed.) *Recent Advances in Surgery II*, pp. 39–69. Edinburgh, Churchill Livingstone.

Chapter 2

The Oesophagus

Normal Structure and Function

The oesophagus measures 25 cm in length and extends from the cricoid cartilage (level C6) to the cardia (level T11). It pierces the right crus of the diaphragm (level T10) and the last two centimetres are intra-abdominal. In the adult, the endoscopist sees the cricopharyngeus muscle sphincter, which is normally closed, at 15 cm from the incisor teeth and the squamo-columnar junction at 40 cm. The squamo-columnar junction is recognised by an irregular line (the Z line) above which is the pale oesophageal mucosa and below which is the red gastric mucosa.

The oesophageal wall consists of a mucosa, a submucosa and a muscular layer (muscularis propria). Only the intra-abdominal part has a serosa and anastomotic healing is tenuous in the intra-thoracic part because the serosa is absent. The mucosa consists of an epithelium, a lamina propria and a muscularis mucosa. The latter separates the mucosa from the submucosa. The epithelium is of a non-keratinizing, stratified squamous type. It has a basal zone of regularly arranged dark-staining cells which divide and replace the surface cells which are continually lost. The cells progress towards the surface and become flattened with pale cytoplasm due to the accumulation of glycogen. Loss of this maturation sequence is seen in dysplasia. Connective tissue papillae containing capillaries extend upward into the epithelium from the lamina propria. These papillae form longitudinal ridges which are visible endoscopically in the lower oesophagus.

The submucosa contains oesophageal mucous glands, the ducts of which pass to the lumen. It also contains an extensive network of lymphatic channels which aid submucosal spread of tumour.

The muscle layer has an inner circular and outer longitudinal coat. In the upper third the muscle is skeletal and this merges with smooth muscle in the middle third, while only smooth muscle is found in the lower third.

The oesophageal muscle is supplied by branches of the vagi which enter the upper oesophagus. The supply reaches the lower oesophagus via intramural plexuses and, thus, a thoracic vagotomy does not normally interfere with oesophageal motor function. Part of the oesophageal blood supply is from vessels arising directly from the aorta which may cause troublesome bleeding during mobilization.

Peristalsis may be initiated by swallowing (primary peristalsis) or by distension from a bolus of food (secondary peristalsis). Peristalsis occurs because the latent period between stimulation and muscle contraction increases from the upper to the lower oesophagus, causing a wave of contraction to progress in an orderly downward direction. It is not clear whether this increasing latent period is a function of the nerve supply or of the muscle itself. Primary peristalsis is mediated by a swallowing centre in the medulla and the motor response is carried in the vagus. Secondary peristalsis is probably independent of vagal function.

A lower oesophageal sphincter is present in the distal end of the oesophagus and separates the positive intragastric pressure from the negative oesophageal pressure.

Congenital Oesophageal Disorders

The oesophagus develops from the foregut which lies between the fourth pharyngeal arch and the yolk sac. During the third week of intra-uterine life, the laryngotracheal groove develops in the floor of the ventral part of the foregut, giving rise to the lung buds at its distal end. Folding in and fusion of the lateral walls of the foregut forms a septum which separates the primitive respiratory and oesophageal tubes. The oesophagus elongates rapidly and, at eight weeks, its caudal end is marked by the developing stomach. The oesophagus is initially lined by columnar epithelium which proliferates until the lumen is almost obliterated; it then breaks down so that recanalization is complete by 10 weeks. Squamous epithelium appears during the fifth fetal month, although islands of columnar epithelium may persist after birth.

Oesophageal atresia and tracheo-oesophageal fistula

Oesophageal atresia (OA) occurs with or without tracheo-oesophageal fistula (TOF) in about 1 in 3000 births. The cause is unknown, although persistence of the obliterative phase of the oesophageal lumen has been suggested as a cause of OA, whereas defects in the septum between oesophagus and trachea have been suggested as a cause of TOF. In approximately 50% of cases there is an associated abnormality, such as congenital heart disease or other gastrointestinal anomalies. One well recognized pattern of defects is known as the VATER syndrome (*Ver*tebral defects, *A*nal atresia, *T*racheo-o*E*sophageal fistula and *R*enal dysplasia). OA with distal TOF is the most common variety (87%) (Ashcraft and Holder 1976). The atretic segment may be long or short and the TOF may occur at or above the tracheal bifurcation. Both OA and TOF may occur in isolation. The main types are shown in *Fig.* 2.1.

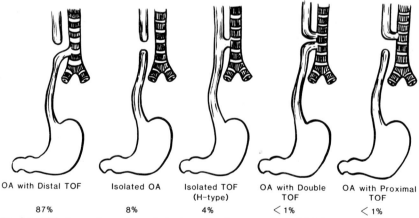

OA with Distal TOF	Isolated OA	Isolated TOF (H–type)	OA with Double TOF	OA with Proximal TOF
87%	8%	4%	<1%	<1%

Fig. 2.1. Main types of oesophageal atresia and tracheo-oesophageal fistulas.

Major pulmonary complications can be minimal if surgery is carried out between 12–18 hours after birth and, if this is the case, survival can be as high as 90%.

Oesophageal stricture occurs after surgery in up to 80% of cases and appears to be most common after a two-layer anastomosis. Chronic respiratory problems may persist into adult life as a result of aspiration secondary to stricture and oesophageal motility disorders. These motility disorders appear to be an intrinsic part of the abnormality and they persist after surgery.

Duplications and cysts

Although true duplication of a segment of oesophagus can occur, a more common disorder is the oesophageal duplication cyst which presents as a mediastinal mass. The cyst is attached to the oesophagus, has a full muscle coat and is lined with columnar or, less commonly, squamous epithelium. They cause pressure on the oesophagus and trachea with resultant dysphagia and dyspnoea. They are often associated with vertebral abnormalities. One theory suggests that the foregut becomes adherent to the notochord and, as the oesophagus lengthens, the connection becomes a diverticulum which eventually separates forming an enteric cyst. The cyst may then expand due to an accumulation of secretions from the lining epithelium.

Congenital oesophageal web and stenosis

Oesophageal webs occur most commonly in the upper oesophagus and at the junction between the middle and lower thirds. They may occur in combination with single or multiple oesophageal stenoses. Both conditions are thought to be due to an abnormal recanalization of the oesophageal lumen. They can be distinguished from the more common peptic stricture by the normal range of oesophageal pH monitoring and by the fact that they rarely recur after dilatation.

Motor Disorders

Achalasia

Achalasia is characterized by three abnormalities: (1) absent oesophageal peristalsis, (2) incomplete relaxation of the lower oesophageal sphincter, and (3) increased resting pressure of the lower oesophageal sphincter to about twice normal. In addition, some patients, especially in the early stages of the disease, have vigorous non-peristaltic contractions associated with chest pain.

The disease affects males and females equally and presents most commonly between the ages of 35 and 45 years.

Pathogenesis

The skeletal and smooth muscle of the oesophagus is supplied by neuronal fibres which originate in the vagal dorsal motor nuclei and pass down the vagal trunks to the ganglia of Auerbach's plexus between the circular and longitudinal layers of the oesophageal muscular coat. Post-ganglionic cells then supply the muscle fibres.

Microscopic abnormalities have been identified at all levels from the vagal nuclei to the oesophageal muscle. The most likely site of primary damage is in the ganglion cells of Auerbach's plexus in which case the changes in the vagal trunks and nuclei may be explained by subsequent retrograde degeneration. Auerbach's plexus contains two types of ganglion cells: non-argyrophil (non-silver staining) cells which directly supply muscle and argyrophil cells which exert a controlling influence on the non-argyrophil cells. Smith (1970) has shown that in achalasia the argyrophil cells are specifically lost and has suggested that damage to these cells could explain both the motor disorder and the degenerative findings in the vagal trunks and nuclei.

Morphology (see Fig. *2.2*)

At endoscopy, the oesophagus appears as a dilated cavity containing food debris; the mucosa may be ulcerated and the endoscope passes easily into the stomach. At autopsy, the body of the oesophagus is grossly dilated with tapering of the lower end. The muscle of the oesophageal body is hypertrophied, but in advanced cases the oesophageal wall may appear thin due to massive dilatation.

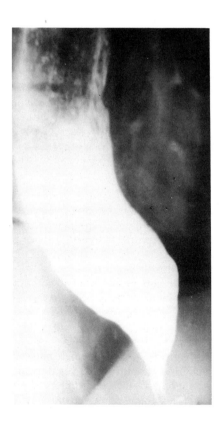

Fig. 2.2. Barium contrast X-ray showing achalasia.

Histologically, there is diminution in number or absence of ganglion cells in Auerbach's plexus, noticeable particularly in the dilated segment rather than in the tapered lower end. A mild inflammatory infiltrate may be seen in Auerbach's plexus with fibrosis in advanced cases. The muscle shows a non-specific sclerosis due to denervation. The number of cell nuclei in the dorsal nucleus of the vagus is reduced and electron microscopy has demonstrated degenerative changes in the axons of the vagal trunk.

Complications

Overspill into the lungs produces pulmonary complications, especially aspiration pneumonia and lung abscess.

A study of 1318 cases seen in the Mayo Clinic demonstrated the presence of oesophageal carcinoma 6·5 times more often than would be expected in a normal population (Wychulis *et al.* 1971). On average, the achalasia had been present 28 years before the diagnosis of malignancy. An associated carcinoma tends to be diagnosed late as the symptoms are often wrongly ascribed to the achalasia.

The standard surgical operation for achalasia is Heller's cardiomyotomy. The resulting incompetence of the lower oesophageal sphincter may give rise to reflux oesophagitis with peptic stricture and return of dysphagia. Some surgeons, therefore, advocate an anti-reflux procedure at the time of cardiomyotomy in order to prevent gastro-oesophageal reflux.

Secondary achalasia

A form of achalasia with manometric findings identical to those seen in primary achalasia may occur in patients who have various types of malignancy. It most commonly occurs in association with tumours of the gastro-oesophageal junction, typically in patients over 50 years of age who have a short history of dysphagia. The cause is probably direct invasion of the myenteric plexus. Secondary achalasia has also been described in association with pancreatic and bronchogenic carcinomas, in which case it may be caused either by direct invasion or by a neuropathy. Malignancy should, therefore, be excluded in elderly patients who appear to develop primary achalasia.

Diffuse oesophageal spasm

This condition is defined as the triad of chest pain, dysphagia and high amplitude, non-peristaltic contractions which occur during at least 30% of swallows. The clinical symptoms are necessary for the diagnosis as the manometric abnormalities can occur in the absence of symptoms. In 70% of patients the lower oesophageal sphincter is normal. In 30% of patients, however, abnormal relaxation and high resting pressures of the lower oesophageal sphincter make the condition difficult to distinguish from achalasia. Cohen (1979) considers that the two conditions form the opposite ends of a spectrum and, in fact, 3–5% of patients with diffuse oesophageal spasm progress to achalasia. Diffuse oesophageal spasm has the clinical features of chest pain and dysphagia with preservation of some peristaltic activity, regardless of lower oesophageal sphincter function, whereas achalasia involves total aperistalsis and abnormal lower oesophageal sphincter relaxation, regardless of clinical features. Cohen (1979) maintains that most cases of motor dysfunction can be fitted into this spectrum.

Histologically, the ganglion cells are present but infiltrated by an inflammatory reaction and the vagal fibres show degeneration. Diffuse oesophageal spasm may, therefore, be a patchy form of the neuronal dysfunction which occurs in achalasia.

Chagas' disease

This is caused by the protozoan *Trypanosoma cruzi* which destroys the myenteric ganglia of the oesophagus and other parts of the gut. This causes an aperistalsis similar to that seen in achalasia, although the lower oesophageal sphincter pressure may be normal. Histologically, there is a reduction in the number of ganglion cells, although no organic stricture develops. The condition may be associated with cardiomyopathy, megacolon and megaureter.

Connective tissue diseases

About 75% of patients with systemic sclerosis (scleroderma) have oesophageal involvement and the condition may be entirely confined to the gastrointestinal tract. The smooth muscle of the lower two-thirds of the oesophagus is involved, giving rise to reduced peristalsis and reduced resting pressure of the lower oesophageal sphincter. This produces incompetence, with subsequent gastro-oesophageal reflux.

Reflux Oesophagitis

Symptoms of reflux oesophagitis are extremely common. One study found, on detailed questioning, that 7% of 'normal' individuals have daily heartburn and over one-third of 'normal' individuals experience heartburn at least once per month (Nebel *et al.* 1976). Prolonged oesophageal pH monitoring has shown that most normal asymptomatic individuals have acid reflux during the day, and in some subjects it also occurs at night (Spence *et al.* 1985).

Pathogenesis

In any one individual, reflux of gastric contents into the oesophagus occurs when the anti-reflux mechanisms fail, either because they are inefficient or because they are overwhelmed by reflux promoting factors or by a combination of both. Once gastric juice is in the oesophagus, the resultant symptomatology depends on other factors, such as the length of time it is in contact with the oesophageal mucosa, the tissue resistance and the composition of the juice. The subject has been comprehensively reviewed by Dodds *et al.* (1981).

ANTI-REFLUX MECHANISMS: Classically, the factors which prevent gastro-oesophageal reflux are extrinsic compression of the oesophagus by the diaphragmatic crura; oesophageal compression by the oblique smooth muscle fibres of the stomach which act as a sling; valvular action by gastric mucosal folds at the cardia; and the acute angle of oesophageal entry into the stomach (the cardiac angle of

His). More recently, however, it has become apparent that two additional factors are paramount in preventing reflux of gastric contents into the oesophagus.

1. An intrinsic physiological lower oesophageal sphincter (LOS) which is 3–5 cm long and maintains a resting pressure of between 10–30 mmHg. Only recently has thickened muscle been demonstrated in the LOS providing anatomical confirmation of a sphincter (Liebermann-Meffert *et al.* 1981). This muscle is tonically contracted at rest but relaxes on swallowing, an opposite response to swallowing to that given by the rest of the oesophageal muscle. The muscle of the LOS is more sensitive to neuronal and hormonal influences than the rest of the oesophagus. Dopaminergic receptors may be of importance in controlling basal tone and dopaminergic inhibitory drugs, such as metoclopramide, produce a rise in sphincter pressure. The role of gastrin may not be as important as was suggested by some early studies which used pharmacological rather than physiological doses. Cigarette smoking, particularly when associated with alcohol consumption, lowers the LOS pressure.
2. The intra-abdominal oesophagus which acts as a flutter valve. The intra-abdominal pressure is higher than the intra-oesophageal pressure and this causes closure of the intra-abdominal oesophagus. This closing mechanism is reinforced during abrupt rises in intra-abdominal pressure, such as occur during coughing or straining.

Clark (1982) has suggested that the LOS may be important in preventing supine reflux while the intra-abdominal oesophagus prevents reflux while upright. Patients with a mean LOS pressure of less than 5 mmHg or a mean abdominal segment length of less than 1 cm are especially likely to reflux.

FAILURE OF ANTI-REFLUX MECHANISMS: The intra-abdominal portion of the oesophagus is dragged into the chest by the sliding type of hiatus hernia and is then no longer subject to intra-abdominal pressure. This has been suggested as the cause of reflux in patients with hiatus hernia. In addition, a sphincter disturbance caused by tension on the phreno-oesophageal ligament, as a result of the herniation, has been implicated as the cause of reflux in some of these patients. It is currently believed, however, that the presence of a hiatus hernia is relatively unimportant in the clinical evaluation of a patient with reflux. The majority of patients with a hiatus hernia have no reflux symptoms and many patients with mild reflux oesophagitis have no demonstrable hernia, although a hiatus hernia usually accompanies severe reflux.

Reflux in some patients may be due to an intrinsic defect in the LOS and, in support of this suggestion, the LOS pressure tends to be lower in patients with reflux than in controls, although there is much overlap. Recently, continuous monitoring of the LOS pressure has demonstrated the existence of transient relaxations of 5–30 seconds duration. These relaxations account for the episodes of reflux which are known to occur in normal individuals and they are thought to account for the symptomatic reflux in patients who have an otherwise normal lower oesophageal sphincter pressure. This phenomenon explains the overlap in basal sphincter pressure which occurs between controls and patients with reflux. It also underlines the necessity for prolonged pH monitoring of the lower oesophagus in clinical evaluation.

The LOS pressure normally rises in response to gastric contractions and failure of this compensatory rise may cause reflux in some patients. Other factors which may result in failure of the anti-reflux mechanisms include an increased intra-abdominal pressure (e.g. due to pregnancy), which can overcome a feeble LOS, and defects in gastric emptying.

FACTORS IN THE OESOPHAGUS: Once gastric contents are in the oesophagus, several other factors are important in determining whether or not symptoms occur.

1. *The potency of the reflux material.* Pepsin, hydrochloric acid, bile and pancreatic juice can all cause oesophagitis in experimental animals. Recently, bile has been implicated in those patients who have reflux symptoms in the absence of a lowered oesophageal pH (so called alkaline reflux oesophagitis). Bile also occurs in gastric juice of low pH and may therefore also play a role in acid reflux oesophagitis, since a mixture of bile and acid is particularly harmful.

2. *Oesophageal clearance.* Patients with oesophageal reflux tend to have prolonged oesophageal clearance although there is substantial overlap with controls. Gravity, peristalsis and saliva all contribute to the speed of oesophageal clearance. Abnormal oesophageal motility may, therefore, be a contributory factor in the development of oesophagitis, although any observed motility disorder might be a secondary phenomenon.

3. *Tissue resistance.* Reduced secretory output of oesophageal glands, reduced epithelial cell turnover accompanying ageing and a decrease in mucosal blood flow may all affect tissue resistance, making some patients prone to oesophagitis.

In summary, the pathogenesis of reflux oesophagitis is a complex matter and patients with reflux may have any one or more of a heterogeneous group of abnormalities.

Clinical features

The chief symptom of reflux oesophagitis is heartburn which is worse after meals and is associated with bending and with cigarette smoking. Many of the patients are obese, middle-aged women. Dysphagia is a later feature and is often transitory. Initially, it may be related to spasm rather than to a fibrous stricture. Chest pain, indistinguishable clinically from angina, occurs in 10% of patients. Rarely, haematemesis or melaena may occur as a result of bleeding from the inflamed oesophageal mucosa. Scoring systems have been devised in an attempt to quantify the symptomatology of reflux oesophagitis, but there is often poor correlation between symptomatology, endoscopic findings and histology.

Morphology

Severe ulcerative oesophagitis is easily recognized at endoscopy as a reddened lower oesophagus with greyish-white areas of necrotic slough. The ulcerated areas may be longitudinal, giving rise to a striped appearance. These endoscopic features correspond well with severe reflux symptoms and with ulceration and inflammation seen histologically. Lesser degrees of oesophagitis, which may merely appear as areas of subjective redness, do not correlate well with symptomatology or with histology.

The initial response of the oesophagus to damage caused by reflux is an increase in cell turnover which causes hyperplasia of the basal cell layer. Subsequent desquamation of the superficial layer of the epithelium causes the papillae of the lamina propria (which normally extend to less than one-third of the epithelial thickness) to come near the surface. These features have been used to establish two histological criteria for the diagnosis of oesophagitis, namely a basal zone thickness of greater than 15% of the total epithelial thickness and papillae extending for more than two-thirds of the thickness of the epithelium (*see Fig.* 2.3). These criteria correspond well, but not perfectly, with both symptoms and acid reflux (Ismail-Beigi *et al.* 1970). In more severe cases, a dense inflammatory infiltrate with ulceration is seen. Eventually, the whole epithelium is destroyed and the oesophagus becomes lined by granulation tissue.

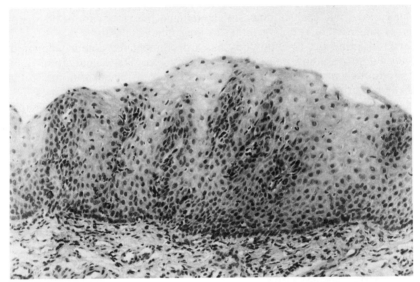

Fig. 2.3. Oesophageal biopsy showing positive criteria for oesophagitis (Ismail-Beigi *et al.* 1970—*see* text). (H and E × 75)

Complications of reflux oesophagitis

Fibrous stricture

Although in some patients the inflammatory process heals by resolution, in others it heals by fibrosis with subsequent stricture formation. The fibrosis initially occurs in the submucosa and eventually goes on to involve the muscle coat and peri-oesophageal tissues, making dissection difficult at the time of surgery. The condition is usually associated with a long history of reflux oesophagitis, although occasionally it may be caused by prolonged nasogastric intubation.

Peptic ulceration

This may occur in squamous epithelium or in an area of columnar cell metaplasia in which case it is termed a 'Barrett's ulcer'. Oesophageal peptic ulcers may be associated with haemorrhage or stricture, but perforation is uncommon.

Barrett's oesophagus

In this condition, columnar cell epithelium is found in the lower oesophagus. It was initially considered to be a congenital condition in which a short oesophagus had the effect of dragging the stomach into the thorax. This theory has been discounted in favour of an acquired aetiology as a result of gastro-oesophageal reflux. There is good correlation between the condition and the symptoms of reflux and 2–11% of patients with reflux develop a Barrett's oesophagus. Presumably, ulceration of the oesophagus is followed by regeneration of pluripotential basal cells which can form a columnar epithelium. There are two broad areas of evidence for the acquired nature of the condition. Firstly, the lesion can be produced in experimental animals and has been shown to be progressive. Secondly, columnar epithelium occurs in what is both the physiological oesophagus (above the lower oesophageal sphincter) and the anatomical oesophagus (as demonstrated by the presence of oesophageal submucosal glands) and therefore cannot be of stomach origin as suggested by the congenital short oesophagus theory.

Barrett's epithelium at endoscopy has a prominent red colour compared with the normal surrounding pale oesophageal mucosa. The demarcation is usually sharp, although recognition may be more difficult if the surrounding squamous epithelium is erythematous due to gastro-oesophageal reflux. Herlihy *et al.* (1984) have demonstrated that Barrett's oesophagus can either line the whole circumference of the lower oesophagus for a variable distance in continuity with the gastric mucosa, or it can occur in islands. These authors excluded from their studies the common condition in which tongues of red gastric mucosa extend up from the squamo-columnar junction but remain in continuity with it.

Histologically, the pathologist looks at three aspects of a biopsy from a case of possible Barrett's oesophagus: (1) the surface pattern which may range from flat,

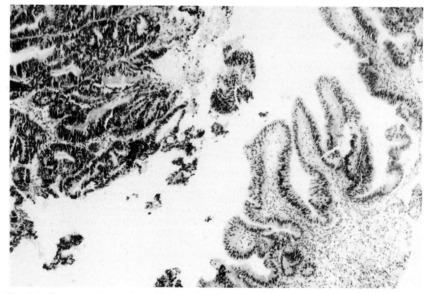

Fig. 2.4. Fragmented oesophageal biopsy showing adenocarcinoma on the left and dysplastic Barrett's type oesophageal mucosa on the right. The adenocarcinoma presumably arose in Barrett's epithelium. (H and E × 30)

like the stomach, to villous, like the intestine; (2) the surface columnar epithelium which may be composed of simple mucus secreting cells, similar to the stomach, or goblet and absorptive cells, as in the intestine; (3) the specialized glands immediately under the epithelial surface which, again, may be either gastric or intestinal in type. These features can occur in any combination in any one biopsy and a mosaic of different patterns occurs in any one oesophagus. If an oesophageal biopsy shows a pattern not normally seen in the stomach, then the diagnosis can be made on histological grounds alone. If gastric-like epithelium is seen, then the diagnosis can only be made if the endoscopist is confident that the biopsy was indeed taken in the oesophagus and not from the stomach as might occur in a case of hiatus hernia.

Dysplastic changes are frequently seen in Barrett's oesophagus and it is widely accepted that the condition is pre-malignant. The associated tumour is an adeno-carcinoma and develops in up to 8·5% of cases (*see Fig.* 2.4). However, since a carcinoma can obliterate any remaining Barrett's epithelium, it may be difficult to determine whether a given adenocarcinoma arose in gastric epithelium at the cardia or in a true Barrett's oesophagus. The risk of carcinoma is sufficient for many authorities to recommend regular endoscopic screening of a patient diagnosed as having a Barrett's oesophagus. Treatment of reflux rarely causes regression of columnar to squamous epithelium and long-term follow-up is recommended, even after fundoplication (Skinner and Little 1982).

Hiatus Hernia

In a sliding hiatus hernia, the lower oesophageal sphincter is displaced into the chest because of weakening of its diaphragmatic attachment. Contributory factors include increases in intra-abdominal pressure, obesity and pregnancy. One theory suggests that the inflammation and fibrosis caused by gastro-oesophageal reflux has the effect of causing contraction of the longitudinal muscle in the oesophageal wall so that the sphincter is dragged into the chest. It is a common condition, par-ticularly in patients over 40 years of age. The association between a sliding hiatus hernia and reflux oesophagitis is discussed on p. 35.

In a paraoesophageal hiatus hernia (rolling hernia) the cardia is usually below the diaphragm and the fundus of the stomach rotates anticlockwise into the mediastinum, so that the greater curvature lies uppermost. This type of hernia is not usually associated with reflux, but causes pressure effects on surrounding structures, including the oesophagus itself. The complications tend to be mechani-cal; stricture and bleeding seldom occur.

A combined sliding and paraoesophageal hernia may also occur.

Sliding Hiatus Hernia Presenting in Infancy

This condition is also termed 'partial thoracic stomach'. It occurs in about one in 400 births and usually presents in the first week of life with persistent vomiting. The vomitus is characteristically blood-stained. The absence of an abdominal segment of oesophagus results in gastro-oesophageal incompetence and reflux oesophagitis. Occasionally, a stricture occurs and, rarely, a Barrett's oesophagus develops. Most patients respond to conservative management, although some develop aspiration pneumonia as a complication.

Paterson–Kelly Syndrome

The association of post-cricoid dysphagia, glossitis, koilonychia and iron deficiency anaemia is known as the Paterson–Kelly or Plummer–Vinson syndrome. It is described most commonly in women aged 40–50 years. The dysphagia is often, but not always, associated with a post-cricoid web which consists of a fold of squamous epithelium with a connective tissue core. In long-standing cases, the dysphagia may be associated with an upper oesophageal stricture in addition to the web. Although the association of these factors is well accepted, there is no conclusive evidence that the iron deficiency anaemia causes the dysphagia or the stricture. The syndrome is associated with a high incidence of post-cricoid carcinoma. In one follow-up study of 49 patients with post-cricoid web, 5% developed malignancy (Chisholm *et al.* 1971). Histological studies have shown that the epithelium on the web is relatively normal but that abnormalities occur in the epithelium of adjacent structures (Entwistle and Jacobs 1965). Biopsies should, therefore, be taken not only from the web, but also from the surrounding mucosa. Correction of the anaemia may relieve the dysphagia in patients with small webs, but those with large webs may require dilatation. It is unclear whether correction of the iron deficiency anaemia prevents the development of cancer.

Oesophageal Varices

Bleeding oesophageal varices account for about 5% of the admissions for haematemesis and melaena to non-specialized UK centres. The majority of cases are associated with liver cirrhosis which in over 60% of cases is alcohol induced. Less than 50% of patients with proven varices will develop variceal haemorrhage.

The venous blood of the oesophagus drains through either branches of the left gastric vein into the portal vein (portal system) or through branches of the azygos, hemiazygos and inferior thyroid veins into the superior vena cava (systemic system). These two venous networks form an anastomosis in the oesophageal wall. If one system becomes obstructed, all venous blood is channelled into the other system, overloading it, and causing venous dilatation (oesophageal varices). If the superior vena cava becomes obstructed (e.g. due to mediastinal fibrosis), blood flows downwards to the portal system, causing 'downhill varices', which are often in the upper oesophagus. If the portal system becomes obstructed, blood drains upwards to the systemic system, causing 'uphill varices' which are always in the lower oesophagus, although they may eventually extend to include the full length of the oesophagus. For practical purposes, only oesophageal varices due to portal hypertension (*see* Chapter 6) are of importance.

Morphology (see Fig. 2.5)

At endoscopy, oesophageal varices are seen as large blood vessels, protruding longitudinally into the oesophageal lumen. If superficially placed, they appear blue or red, but if deeply placed, they may appear white in colour. Careful inspection of the surface in some patients will reveal the presence of small red blebs known as 'cherry-red spots' or 'varices upon varices'. The significance of these is discussed below.

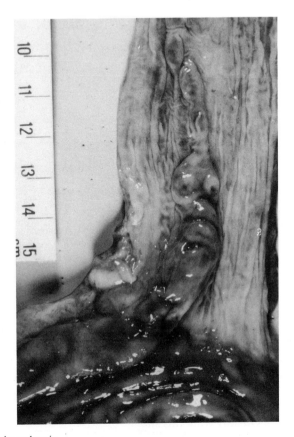

Fig. 2.5. Oesophageal varix.

Microscopy shows large venous channels in the oesophageal lamina propria and submucosa. Recently, histological examination of rings of oesophagus, taken at the time of oesophageal transection in patients with varices, has demonstrated the presence of small vascular channels actually within the squamous epithelium (Spence *et al.* 1983)—*see Fig.* 2.6. These vessels only rarely occur in the normal oesophagus and it is likely that they represent the 'cherry-red spots' described above.

Pathogenesis of variceal bleeding

When varices bleed, the haemorrhage almost invariably occurs from the lower third of the oesophagus, even if the varices extend into the middle or upper third.

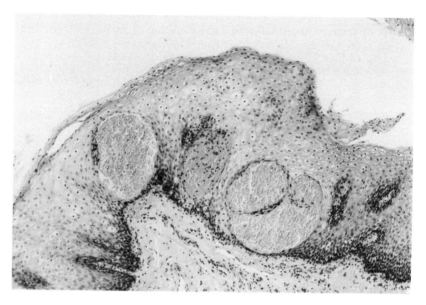

Fig. 2.6. Oesophageal varices. Intraepithelial channels in a ring of oesophageal mucosa taken at the time of oesophageal transection (H and E × 30)

Also, many patients with documented varices never bleed. Two questions, therefore, arise.

1. *Why does variceal bleeding occur at the lower end of the oesophagus?* Anatomical studies of the venous anatomy of the lower oesophagus have shown that veins in the stomach and proximal oesophagus lie mainly in the submucosa. In the distal 2–5 cm of oesophagus, however, they rise nearer the surface and extend into the lamina propria (Spence 1984). This may explain why variceal bleeding occurs mainly from this site.
2. *What initiates variceal bleeding?* The two traditional suggestions have been 'erosion from without' by gastric contents which have been refluxed into the oesophagus and 'explosion from within' by the increased portal venous pressure. Recent study of oesophageal rings taken at oesophageal transection, however, has shown little evidence to support the theory of oesophagitis initiating haemorrhage. There is also no direct relationship between bleeding and the level of portal venous pressure.
   Attention has recently been focused on the cherry-red spots described above which are thought to be the intra-epithelial vascular channels seen microscopically. These only occur in a proportion of patients with varices. Rupture of these vascular channels may initiate bleeding, as they are separated from the oesophageal lumen by only a few cells, and join with the much larger mucosal and submucosal vascular channels via the papillae of the lamina propria. It may be the case that those patients with varices who bleed are the ones who have developed intra-epithelial extensions of their varices.

Endoscopic recognition of these cherry-red spots might help to identify those patients likely to bleed and who might therefore benefit from prophylactic surgery (Inokuchi 1984).

Prognosis

In some series, approximately 50% of patients admitted to hospital with bleeding varices will die during their first admission and, of the survivors, most will rebleed within one year. Overall, only 25% survive two years (Editorial 1984). In general, patients with extrahepatic portal hypertension have good liver function and a good prognosis, while patients with liver cirrhosis have poor liver function and a poor prognosis. Child's classification, based on nutritional status, serum bilirubin, encephalopathy, the presence or absence of ascites and serum albumin, separated patients into prognostic groups A, B and C (Child and Turcotte 1964). Pugh *et al.* (1973) have developed a scoring system using encephalopathy, ascites, serum bilirubin, serum albumin and prothrombin time and their score correlates with prognosis. More recently, Garden *et al.* (1985), using multivariant analysis, have shown that only prothrombin ratio, serum creatinine and the presence of encephalopathy on admission have independent significance.

Oesophageal Perforation

Instrumental perforation is probably the commonest and occurs during rigid oesophagoscopy, dilatation of strictures, attempted intubation and variceal tamponade. Spontaneous perforation (Boerhaave's syndrome) occurs mainly in men after alcoholic excess or in association with severe vomiting. It produces severe pain with mild haematemesis (in contrast with the Mallory–Weiss syndrome, in which there is mild pain, greater haematemesis and only rarely a full thickness perforation—*see* p. 79). The ingestion of fish bones and various foreign bodies, accounts for a number of perforations. These usually lodge at one of three levels: (1) at the cricopharyngeus in the neck; (2) adjacent to the aortic arch in the chest; (3) in the distal oesophagus, just above the cardia. Occasionally, operative trauma or injection sclerotherapy produce perforations. Benign ulcers of the oesophagus, especially the penetrating Barrett's type, may also perforate.

Since the intrathoracic oesophagus has no serosa, it is more liable to rupture at pressures lower than the rest of the gastrointestinal tract, especially if the strong mucosal layer is perforated. The pressure in the thoracic cavity is less than atmospheric and thus the pressure gradient across the oesophageal wall tends to favour rupture, especially if the intra-oesophageal pressure is high, as when vomiting. As there is little soft tissue surrounding the mid- and lower oesophagus, spread of contamination and rupture into the pleural cavities can easily occur. Mediastinitis, empyema and surgical emphysema are therefore common complications.

Perforation of the cervical oesophagus carries the best prognosis and treatment is usually with antibiotics, drainage and cessation of feeding. If patients with perforation of the intra-thoracic oesophagus are treated within 24 hours, the mortality rate is around 10%. If the treatment is delayed over 24 hours, however, the mortality rises to 50% due to the associated mediastinitis and toxaemia.

Oesophageal Infections

Candida oesophagitis

This infection is usually caused by *Candida albicans*, although other Candida species may be involved. The disease may occur with or without associated infection of the mouth, usually in patients with a predisposing factor such as achalasia, oesophageal tumours, neutropenia or the administration of immunosuppressive drugs. The classical presentation is that of a neutropenic patient with dysphagia and retrosternal pain. In the early stages, white mucosal plaques are seen at endoscopy, but in the later stages, the mucosa becomes necrotic and ulcerated. Membranes composed of mycelia and necrotic debris are then seen lying on a red friable mucosa. Histologically, the organism is seen together with associated tissue necrosis, but often there is little surrounding inflammation. About 30% of cases present with upper gastrointestinal bleeding. Aspiration pneumonia due to poor motility of the oesophagus is a further complication.

Herpes simplex oesophagitis

The herpes simplex virus may cause oesophageal infection, either by direct spread from the mouth or by reactivation of the virus in the sensory ganglia of the vagus nerves. Initially, an intra-epithelial vesicle is formed which ruptures at an early stage to form an ulcer. Multiple ulcers may coalesce. Histologically, the characteristic feature is the presence of an intra-nuclear inclusion body in cells taken from the edge of the ulcer. Confirmation of the diagnosis is obtained by culture of the virus. In otherwise normal individuals, the disease is often self-limiting, but patients on immunosuppressive therapy may require a reduction in their drug dosage.

Diverticula of the Oesophagus

An oesophageal diverticulum is defined as a pouch lined by epithelium. This may be the result of pressure from within (pulsion diverticulum) or traction from without (traction diverticulum).

Pharyngeal diverticulum (pouch)

This is a pulsion diverticulum which protrudes between the oblique fibres of the inferior constrictor muscle and the transverse fibres of the cricopharyngeus. This area of weakness is known as Killian's dehiscence. Contributory factors include a high pressure developing in the proximal oesophagus as a result of diffuse oesophageal spasm and constant impingement of food on the weak area of the hypopharynx. The diverticulum enlarges, first lying posterior and then to the left of the oesophagus. The sac consists of mucosa and submucosa only. Complications may arise from aspiration of pouch contents which cause chest infection and lung abscess. Occasionally, a carcinoma occurs in the pouch.

Lateral pharyngeal diverticulum

This is an uncommon condition and may represent a congenital lesion derived from the second, third or fourth branchial clefts. It arises from the tonsillar fossa or the pyriform recess. Acquired lateral diverticula also arise from the pyriform recess and pierce the thyrohyoid membrane. The are usually symptomless.

Mid-oesophageal traction diverticulum

This arises at the level of the bifurcation of the trachea and is usually the result of traction from inflamed adherent lymph nodes, classically tuberculous. Occasionally, it may be caused by a motor disorder in which case it is of pulsion type. Symptoms are rare but dysphagia may occur if a large diverticulum presses on the oesophageal wall.

Epiphrenic diverticulum

This develops from a mechanical or functional obstruction in the lower oesophagus which causes the formation of a pulsion sac consisting of mucosa and submucosa. It occurs in association with achalasia, diffuse oesophageal spasm and hiatus hernia.

Schatzki's Ring

This is an incomplete web of mucosa situated in the lower oesophagus. It consists of an upper layer of squamous epithelium, a fibrous core and a lower layer of columnar epithelium. Schatzki (1963) therefore believed that it marked the oesophago-gastric junction. It causes dysphagia which is characteristically episodic, and occurs in middle-aged individuals. It is possibly developmental in origin but usually manifests late in life when oesophageal motor power reduces. It may require dilatation but rarely surgical removal is needed.

Benign Tumours of the Oesophagus

Squamous papilloma

This is rare and appears as a sessile papillary mass. It is composed of papillary projections of squamous epithelium with connective tissue cores. It does not undergo malignant change.

Fibrous polyp

Fibrous polyps are relatively common and may occur anywhere within the oesophagus. They occur as a fleshy pedunculated polyp and vary markedly in size. Rarely, they become dislodged into the laryngopharynx where they can cause acute dyspnoea. They may ulcerate and cause haemorrhage. Histologically, they consist of a connective tissue core covered by a simple squamous epithelium. They are totally benign.

Leiomyoma

A leiomyoma is the most common benign tumour of the oesophagus. It usually occurs in the lower oesophagus and is more common in men than in women. It arises either in the muscularis mucosa, in which case it forms a pedunculated intraluminal mass, or in the muscularis propria, in which case it grows in the oesophageal wall and may present as a mediastinal mass. The cut surface is characteristically white and whorled in appearance. Histologically, leiomyomas consist of bundles of regular, spindle-shaped, smooth muscle cells. As with gastric smooth muscle tumours, their behaviour can be difficult to predict from the histological appearance. The presence of mitoses seems to be the most reliable indicator of malignancy (see p. 76).

Oesophageal Carcinoma

Epidemiology and aetiology

Squamous carcinoma of the oesophagus is characterized by a varying geographical incidence ranging from less than 10 per 100 000 in the UK to over 100 per 100 000 in high risk zones—the littoral zone of Russia and Iran around the Caspian Sea, the Henan province of Northern China and the Transkei region of South Africa are examples. Even within these regions, the incidence can vary up to fifty-fold within 300 miles. In the UK, squamous tumours of the middle and lower third occur between 1·5 and 4 times more commonly in men than in women. This male predominance pertains to most countries, although in a few high risk areas the sex ratio is reversed.

The varying incidence suggests that environmental factors may play a role in aetiology. Poor nutrition is common in the high risk areas of Iran and China where deficiencies of vitamins A and C have been implicated. Resultant poor cellular nutrition may hinder the normal replacement and maturation of squamous epithelium (Correa 1982). Fresh vegetables are scarce in these high risk areas, leading to riboflavin deficiency which has been shown to cause oesophageal atrophy in experimental animals, a condition which may be pre-malignant. Another factor which may be relevant in Iran is that food is eaten dry due to the lack of rainfall, with the result that silica particles, present in flour because of grinding by stones, constantly abraid the oesophageal mucosa, causing mechanical damage. N-nitroso compounds specifically cause oesophageal cancer in some experimental animals and high levels of these compounds have been noted in some foods (especially pickled vegetables) in high risk zones of China and in alcoholic drinks of other high risk areas. Opium smoking has been implicated in Iran without definite proof.

Chemical damage may be caused by lye ingestion which produces a stricture and a high incidence of oesophageal cancer after a lag period of about 20 years. Tannins, which may be carcinogenic, occur in some alcoholic drinks and there is a strong association between excessive alcohol intake and oesophageal cancer. Heavy alcohol intake may also be implicated through associated dietary deficiencies. Smokers of cigarettes, cigars and pipes all have a higher incidence of oesophageal cancer than non-smokers which may be associated with the tannins that occur in tobacco smoke.

Genetic influences appear to be of minor importance although patients with inherited tylosis (a keratosis of the palms and soles) have a high incidence of oesophageal cancer.

Pathogenesis

Oesophageal cancer may be preceded by various pre-malignant conditions.

DYSPLASIA: Dysplasia implies the presence, within the squamous epithelium, of atypical cells with large pleomorphic hyperchromatic nuclei. Initially, the basal part of the squamous epithelium is affected (mild dysplasia). The atypical cells then progress to involve almost the entire thickness of the epithelium (severe dysplasia) and eventually the whole thickness (carcinoma-in-situ). The condition becomes an invasive carcinoma when the basement membrane is breached (Thompson 1982).

Mass screening studies have shown that dysplasia is very common in asymptomatic patients in high risk areas and that it occurs in patients about 7–8 years younger than those who have oesophageal cancer.

Studies in China have shown that dysplasia may either regress to a normal epithelium, or progress to invasive carcinoma. Invasive carcinoma occurs 140 times more commonly in those patients with severe dysplasia than in the normal population of the same geographical region.

OESOPHAGITIS: The association between reflux oesophagitis, Barrett's oesophagus and carcinoma has already been discussed on p. 39. Another type of oesophagitis has been described in the high risk area of Iran (Crespi *et al.* 1979). It occurs in 80% of asymptomatic individuals screened by endoscopy and differs from the reflux oesophagitis more commonly seen in Western countries in two respects: it is not associated with heartburn and it spares the lowest part of the oesophagus. It is, therefore, an oesophagitis which may predispose to malignancy but which apparently is not caused by gastro-oesophageal reflux. It may be due to the dietary factors discussed earlier.

OTHER PRE-MALIGNANT CONDITIONS: Achalasia and the Paterson–Kelly syndrome have already been discussed.

Clinical features

The typical presentation is of an elderly patient who gives a short history of dysphagia in the absence of pre-existing symptoms of reflux oesophagitis. In Western countries, oesophageal cancer presents late since the oesophagus is distensible and dysphagia does not occur until almost the entire circumference is involved.

Morphology (see Fig. 2.7)

Carcinoma of the oesophagus may either be a squamous carcinoma or an adenocarcinoma. The oesophagus is traditionally divided into upper, middle and lower thirds and about half of squamous carcinomas arise in the middle third. One-third arise in the lower third of the oesophagus and one-fifth in the upper third (although upper third tumours are much less common if post-cricoid lesions are excluded). If adenocarcinomas arising at the cardia are included, however, the lower third becomes the most common site of oesophageal cancer.

Screening studies in China have shown that in the early stages of oesophageal cancer it may present as a small polyp, a mucosal plaque or a superficial depression. Three types of more advanced tumours are recognized: fungating, which occurs as an intra-luminal growth (60%), ulcerative (25%) and infiltrating, which spreads extensively beneath the surrounding intact mucosa (15%) (Ming 1973). Satellite nodules are often seen close to the main tumour and are caused by

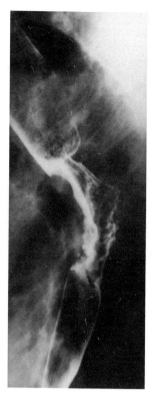

Fig. 2.7. Barium contrast X-ray of oesophageal carcinoma.

submucosal lymphatic spread. It is not possible to distinguish between a squamous carcinoma and an adenocarcinoma on macroscopic appearance alone.

Histologically, well differentiated squamous carcinomas of the oesophagus are easily recognized as nests of squamous cells with central keratin pearls which have breached the basement membrane of the epithelium. In poorly differentiated tumours, however, the pathologist may have to rely on more subtle features such as intercellular bridges in order to classify the tumour as squamous. The degree of differentiation is a poor indicator of prognosis. Within the submucosa, columns of malignant cells may be seen within lymphatics some distance away from the main tumour. This often underlies normal epithelium and therefore may be missed in a superficial biopsy (*see Fig.* 2.8).

Adenocarcinomas are composed of glandular structures formed by irregular columnar cells with mucus secretion. Most adenocarcinomas are thought to arise from the columnar epithelium on the gastric side of the oesophago-gastric junction with upward invasion into the oesophagus, and, strictly speaking, these are not oesophageal carcinomas. However, true adenocarcinomas of the oesophagus have been described arising high in the oesophagus, and these probably arise from submucosal glands or Barrett's oesophagus.

Some tumours show both adeno- and squamous patterns. This may occur as a simple squamous metaplasia in an adenocarcinoma (adeno-acanthoma) or as an adenosquamous carcinoma in which both elements are malignant. The latter may

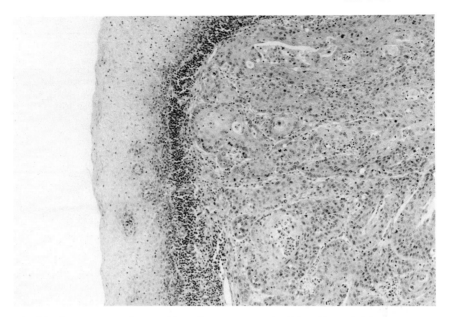

Fig. 2.8. Squamous carcinoma. Normal mucosa on the left with underlying squamous carcinoma which has spread from an adjacent tumour. A superficial biopsy here may miss the carcinoma. (H and E × 30)

occur due to simultaneous carcinogenic stimulation of both squamous and columnar epithelium, although origin from submucosal glands has also been suggested. The adenosquamous form is highly malignant.

Spread

Lymphatic spread occurs early due to the rich submucosal lymphatic network. It occurs first within the oesophageal wall, often producing satellite lesions, and progresses to lymph nodes in the neck, mediastinum and abdomen. The tumour is often more widespread than suspected clinically. Local mediastinal structures, especially the bronchi and trachea, are often invaded, giving rise to fistulas. Occasionally, invasion of the aorta results in fatal haemorrhage. One necroscopy study showed that abdominal lymph nodes were involved in 40% of upper third tumours and that cervical nodes were involved in 60% of lower third tumours (Mandard *et al.* 1981). The lung and liver are the most common sites of distant blood-borne spread. In view of the extensive submucosal spread, at least 10 cm clearance at surgery is advised. Some surgeons advocate near-total oesophagectomy in order to avoid local recurrence.

Staging and prognosis

The TNM system of clinical staging is given in Table 2.1.

In Western series the prognosis is poor, with a five year survival rate in the region of 5% regardless of the method of treatment. Prognosis is related to size, especially the length, and degree of spread at the time of treatment rather than to any histological feature, although adenocarcinomas tend to have a worse prognosis than squamous carcinomas.

Table 2.1. TNM—pre-treatment clinical classification

Tis — Pre-invasive carcinoma (carcinoma-in-situ)
T0 — No evidence of primary tumour
T1 — Tumour involving 5 cm or less of the oesophageal length, producing no obstruction, does not involve the entire circumference of the oesophagus and which shows no evidence of extra-oesophageal spread
T2 — Tumour involving more than 5 cm of the oesophageal length and with no evidence of extra-oesophageal spread, or tumour of any size producing obstruction and/or involvement of the entire circumference of the oesophagus but with no extra-oesophageal spread
T3 — Tumour with evidence of extra-oesophageal spread, such as recurrent laryngeal, phrenic or sympathetic nerve involvement, fistula formation, involvement of trachea or bronchial tree, vena cava or azygos vein obstruction or malignant effusion

Cervical oesophagus
N0 — No evidence of regional lymph node involvement
N1 — Evidence of involvement of moveable unilateral regional nodes
N2 — Evidence of involvement of moveable bilateral regional nodes
N3 — Evidence of fixed regional nodes

Thoracic oesophagus
N0 — No evidence of regional node involvement on exploration or mediastinoscopy
N1 — Involved regional nodes

Distant metastases
M0— No evidence
M1— Presence of distal metastases

Other Malignant Oesophageal Tumours

Carcinosarcoma

This is a tumour in which both epithelial and connective tissue stromal elements are malignant. The epithelial component is usually squamous in type and is interspersed with a malignant stroma containing pleomorphic and bizarre spindle shaped cells. Although rare, it has three features of importance to the clinician. First, it grows as an intra-luminal polypoid mass, unlike most other malignant tumours of the oesophagus. Secondly, it has a much better prognosis than other malignant tumours because it metastasizes late, and thirdly, when it does metastasize, it is usually the sarcomatous portion which does so.

Leiomyosarcoma

This tumour is rare and differs from leiomyomas in having bizarre cell forms with many mitoses, although borderline lesions may occur in which the behaviour cannot be predicted. The prognosis is much better than for carcinoma as it grows mainly by infiltration and rarely metastasizes. It is also radiosensitive.

Malignant melanoma

Melanomas rarely occur as a primary tumour of the oesophagus but may do so since melanoblasts occur in the normal oesophageal tissue in some people. Primary oesophageal melanomas occur as pigmented pedunculated masses, usually in the lower oesophagus of elderly patients. They have a poor prognosis.

References

Ashcraft K. W., Holder T. M. (1976) Esophageal atresia and tracheoesophageal fistula malformations. In: Hendren W. H. (ed.) *Surgical Clinics of North America: Pediatric Surgery.* Vol. 56, No. 2, 299–315. Philadelphia, W. B. Saunders.

Child C. G., Turcotte J. G. (1964) Surgery and portal hypertension. In: Child C. G. (ed.) *The Liver and Portal Hypertension.* Philadelphia, W. B. Saunders.

Chisholm M., Ardran G. M., Callander S. T., Wright R. (1971) A follow-up study of patients with post-cricoid webs. *Quart. J. Med.* **40**, 409–20.

Clark J. (1982) The lower oesophageal closure mechanism. In: Russell R. C. G. (ed.) *Recent Advances in Surgery No. 11*, pp. 153–68. Edinburgh, Churchill Livingstone.

Cohen S. (1979) Motor disorders of the oesophagus. *N. Engl. J. Med.* **301**, 184–92.

Correa P. (1982) Precursors of gastric and oesophageal cancer. *Cancer* **50**, 2554–65.

Crespi M., Grassi A., Amiri G. *et al.* (1979) Oesophageal lesions in Northern Iran: A premalignant condition? *Lancet* **2**, 217–21.

Dodds W. J., Hogan W. J., Helm J. F., Dent J. (1981) Pathogenesis of reflux oesophagitis. *Gastroenterology* **81**, 376–94.

Editorial (1984) Bleeding oesophageal varices. *Lancet* **1**, 139–41.

Entwistle C. C., Jacobs A. (1965) Histological findings in the Paterson-Kelly syndrome. *J. Clin. Pathol.* **18**, 408–13.

Garden O. J., Motyl H., Gilmour W. H., Utley R. J., Carter D. C. (1985) Prediction of outcome following acute variceal haemorrhage. *Br. J. Surg.* **72**, 91–5.

Herlihy K. J., Orlando R. C., Bryson J. C., Bozymski E. M., Carney C. N., Powell D. W. (1984) Barrett's oesophagus: Clinical, endoscopic, histologic, manometric and electrical potential difference characteristics. *Gastroenterology* **86**, 436–43.

Inokuchi K. (1984) Prophylactic portal nondecompression surgery in patients with oesophageal varices. An interim report. *Ann. Surg.* **200**, 61–5.

Ismail-Beigi F., Horton P. F., Pope C. E. (1970) Histologic consequences of gastroesophageal reflux in man. *Gastroenterology* **58**, 163–74.

Liebermann-Meffert D., Heberer M., Martinoli S., Allgoewer M. (1981) Are there muscular structures which may contribute to closure of the gastroesophageal junction? *Scand. J. Gastroent.* **16** (Suppl. 67), 123.

Mandard A. M., Chasle J., Marnay J., *et al.* (1981) Autopsy findings in 111 cases of oesophageal cancer. *Cancer* **48**, 329–35.

Ming S. C. (1973) Tumours of the oesophagus and stomach. In: *Atlas of Tumour Pathology*, 2nd ed. Armed Forces Institute of Pathology.

Nebel O. T., Fornes M. F., Castell D. O. (1976) Symptomatic gastroesophageal reflux: incidence and precipitating factors. *Am. J. Dig. Dis.* **21**, 953–6.

Pugh R. N., Murray-Lyon I. M., Dawson J. L., Pietroni M. C., Williams R. (1973) Transection of the oesophagus for bleeding oesophageal varices. *Br. J. Surg.* **60**, 646–9.

Schatzki R. (1963) The lower oesophageal ring. Long-term follow-up of symptomatic and asymptomatic rings. *Am. J. Roentgen.* **90**, 805–10.

Skinner D. B., Little A. G. (1982) New concepts in esophageal surgery. In: Cohen S., Soloway R. D. (eds.) *Diseases of the Esophagus*, pp. 287–97. New York, Churchill Livingstone.

Smith B. (1970) The neurological lesion in achalasia of the cardia. *Gut* **11**, 388–91.

Spence R. A. (1984) The venous anatomy of the lower oesophagus in normal subjects and in patients with varices: an image analysis study. *Br. J. Surg.* **71**, 739–44.

Spence R. A., Johnston G. W., Parks T. G. (1985) Prolonged ambulatory pH monitoring in patients following oesophageal transection and control subjects. *Br. J. Surg.* **72**, 99–101.

Spence R. A. J., Sloan J. M., Johnston G. W., Greenfield A. (1983) Oesophageal mucosal changes in patients with varices. *Gut* **24**, 1024–9.

Thompson J. J. (1982) Esophageal cancer and the premalignant changes of esophageal diseases. In: Cohen S., Soloway R. D. (eds.) *Diseases of the Esophagus*, pp. 239–76. New York, Churchill Livingstone.

Wychulis A. R., Woolam G. L., Andersen H. A., Ellis F. H. (1971) Achalasia and carcinoma of the oesophagus. *J.A.M.A.* **215**, 1638–41.

Chapter 3

The Stomach and Duodenum

Normal Structure

The stomach is divided anatomically into four parts. The cardia is the area surrounding the oesophagogastric junction; the fundus lies above a horizontal line drawn through the cardia; the body is between the fundus and the incisura; and the antrum is between the body and pylorus. The area just proximal to the pylorus is termed the pyloric channel.

The fundus and body are recognized endoscopically as having thick vertical mucosal folds or rugae. Beyond the incisura, which is usually obvious as a transverse ridge, the antral mucosa becomes flat.

The wall of the stomach consists of mucosa, submucosa, muscularis propria and serosa. These are shown in Fig. 3.1. The mucosa has three parts: (1) mucus secreting epithelial cells which cover the surface and line the gastric pits, (2) the lamina propria which contains the gastric glands of specialized cells and lies between the basement membrane of the surface epithelium and the muscularis mucosa, and (3) the muscularis mucosa which divides the mucosa from the submucosa.

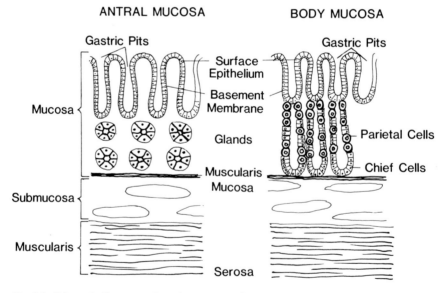

Fig. 3.1. Schematic diagram to show the structure of antral and body gastric mucosa.

Three types of mucosa are seen in the stomach depending on the type of specialized cells making up the gastric glands.

1. Cardiac mucosa—this is a simple mucosa consisting of mucus secreting gastric glands.
2. Body and fundal mucosa—the gastric glands here are single, elongated and test-tube like. They contain parietal cells and chief cells. Parietal cells which produce acid and intrinsic factor are eosinophilic and triangular in shape. Chief cells which produce pepsin are basophilic and lie mainly in the bases of the glands.
3. Antral or pyloric mucosa—the gastric glands here are branched and are composed mainly of mucus secreting cells. Gastrin producing (G-cells) and other endocrine cells are also found in this area.

The histological division between body and antral mucosa does not correspond to the anatomical division but is more irregular. Normally, a tongue of antral mucosa extends up the lesser curve and the length of this tongue increases with age. This is of importance in determining the high site of gastric ulcers in elderly patients (see p. 59).

The blood supply of the stomach is from the coeliac axis. The main arteries are the left and right gastric arteries and the left and right gastroepiploic arteries. The short gastric arteries supply the fundus. Venous drainage is eventually to the portal vein.

The lymphatic drainage runs with the arterial supply to the left and right gastric nodes, the sub-pyloric nodes, the pancreaticosplenic nodes and the right gastro-epiploic nodes. Hence it drains to the coeliac nodes.

Gastric Secretion

Acid is produced by parietal cells and pepsin is produced by chief cells. At the cellular level, acetylcholine and gastrin increase acid secretion but both appear to act, at least in part, through histamine which stimulates H_2 receptors on the parietal cell wall to produce cyclic AMP. The cyclic AMP in turn causes acid secretion by a mechanism not fully understood.

Prostaglandins antagonize the release of acid by histamine and in addition protect cells against acid/pepsin digestion, possibly by stimulating them to produce mucopolysaccharides. The actual quantity of acid produced may, therefore, depend on the balance between histamine and prostaglandins in the region around the parietal cells.

Control of acid secretion is by cephalic, gastric and intestinal factors. The cephalic phase starts with the sight or thought of food and is mediated by the vagus which stimulates parietal cells through acetylcholine. It also stimulates antral G-cells to produce gastrin. During the gastric phase, distension of the antrum or contact with peptides from food causes further gastrin release. The low pH produced by these factors has a direct inhibitory effect on parietal cells and also inhibits antral G-cells, thus providing a negative feedback mechanism. In the intestinal phase, food entering the duodenum causes further gastrin release from duodenal G-cells. However, acid entering the duodenum inhibits gastric acid secretion by hormonal mechanisms and by local neuronal reflexes.

Secretion of pepsin is increased by the vagus and by gastrin, and in this respect it mirrors acid secretion. However, cholecystokinin and secretin which reduce acid secretion seem to stimulate pepsin secretion. Pepsin is secreted in the form of pepsinogens of which there are two types. The pepsinogens are converted to active pepsin in the presence of acid and are inactive in an achlorhydric environment.

Gastric Biopsy

It is important that an adequate number of biopsies from the correct site be taken at the time of endoscopy. At least six (some endoscopists maintain up to twelve) should be taken from any significant lesion in order to minimize sampling error. In the case of an ulcer, biopsy from the edge gives more yield than from the base which may be covered with necrotic slough. Well taken biopsies which are orientated on a card will often give the full thickness of mucosa and make diagnosis easier. Lesions deep to the mucosa may not be diagnosed with ordinary techniques. Repeated biopsies from the same site (well biopsy technique) may assist in the diagnosis of such conditions as linitis plastica or submucosal lesions such as lymphoma, although there is a danger of perforation. This technique is also useful in large fungating carcinomas which have a thick covering layer of necrotic slough. Brush biopsy is said to increase diagnostic accuracy in the case of carcinoma although the technique depends on the availability of an experienced cytologist. Lavage cytology can be used but extraneous cells may make interpretation difficult. In the case of pedunculated polyps, it is essential that they are removed *in toto*, usually by a snare technique, in order to facilitate histological examination.

Congenital Conditions

Stenosis and atresia

Atresia implies complete loss of continuity and stenosis is narrowing without loss of continuity. Both are extremely rare in the stomach.

Duodenal atresias account for 40% of small bowel atresias and are associated with Down's syndrome. Since it is an upper gastrointestinal atresia, the mother may have hydramnios. The atresia may be in the form of a septum (type I), a string of fibrous tissue between the two ends (type II), or a complete loss of contact between the ends (type III). Stenosis may be in the form of a perforated diaphragm or a length of narrow duodenum.

Duplications

Gastric duplications are exceedingly rare and many of the examples described in the literature are now thought to be the result of previous inflammatory conditions. Duodenal duplications are also exceedingly rare.

Ulcers and Erosions

An erosion is a mucosal defect which does not penetrate the muscularis mucosa. An acute ulcer has penetrated the muscularis mucosa for a variable distance but there is no attempt at repair and therefore no fibrous tissue is seen. A chronic ulcer is one in which fibrous tissue has formed and therefore the normal architecture cannot be restored. These are illustrated in *Fig.* 3.2.

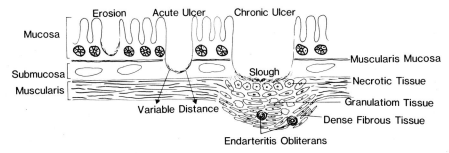

Fig. 3.2. Schematic diagram to show the differences between an erosion, an acute ulcer and a chronic ulcer.

Acute erosions and ulcers (Crawford *et al.* 1971)

Some causes of acute erosions and ulcers are given in *Table* 3.1. Aspirin and indomethacin can damage the gastric mucosa both directly and by acting systemically; they tend to cause erosions rather than acute ulcers. Aspirin at the low pH of gastric juice is fat soluble and can, therefore, be absorbed by cell membranes and damage them directly. Both aspirin and indomethacin, acting systemically, inhibit prostaglandin synthesis. As discussed earlier, prostaglandins appear to have a protective effect on gastric mucosa. Aspirin has also been implicated in the aetiology of chronic gastric ulcers.

Cushing's ulcers occur as a result of neurosurgical trauma or surgery. They differ from other acute lesions in that they are associated with an increased gastric acid/pepsin secretion, possibly caused by direct pressure on the vagal nuclei. They have a greater tendency to perforate than other acute ulcers.

The aetiology of non-Cushing's stress ulcers is obscure. They are not due to increased acid/pepsin secretion. Mucosal ischaemia appears to be the most important factor and many patients have had a prolonged period of hypotension. One theory suggests that sympathetic stimulation and circulating catecholamines open

Table 3.1. Causes of acute erosions and ulcers

1.	Drugs—aspirin, indomethacin
2.	Cushing's ulcers
3.	Stress ulcers:
	—trauma
	—surgery
	—sepsis
	—burns (Curling's ulcer)
	—myocardial infarction
	—respiratory failure

up arterio-venous fistulas in the submucosa, thus diverting blood from the mucosa. In some patients, diffuse intravascular coagulation results in microthrombi which lodge in the mucosal blood vessels and add to the ischaemia. The gastric mucosa is easily damaged by ischaemia since it lacks glycogen supplies, has a high metabolic rate and cannot use anaerobic glycolysis.

The ischaemic mucosa is prone to attack from hydrogen ions and bile. There is evidence that both bile and acid are necessary for the formation of stress ulcers and that duodeno-gastric reflux is increased in patients with stress ulcers.

Acute erosions and ulcers usually occur in the stomach although Cushing's and Curling's ulcers also occur in the duodenum. Unlike chronic peptic ulcers, they have no predilection for antral as opposed to body or fundal mucosa. At endoscopy, erosions appear as small lesions up to half a centimetre across, with slightly raised edges due to oedema. They may be white due to slough or dark brown due to altered blood if they have been bleeding. The rim appears red and the surrounding mucosa is also often red due to petechial haemorrhages. Endoscopic studies have shown that within 24 hours of severe trauma, foci of pallor appear in the gastric mucosa. At 48 hours, erosions form and by three to four days, some have formed into acute ulcers.

Acute ulcers are larger than erosions. The penetration of the muscularis mucosa and contact with submucosal vessels means that bleeding is more severe than if only erosions are present. Bleeding is about nine times more common than perforation. An acute ulcer can be difficult to distinguish from a chronic ulcer on a purely morphological basis at the time of operation.

Microscopy of these lesions reveals necrosis of the mucosa which extends into the submucosa if the lesion is an acute ulcer. There is a surrounding acute inflammatory reaction but no substantial granulation or fibrous tissue is present.

There is no evidence that acute ulcers lead to chronic peptic ulcers. The prognosis for drug induced erosions is much better than for stress erosions.

Chronic peptic ulcer

Epidemiology

The epidemiology of chronic peptic ulcer is difficult to study since many patients with the condition do not attend hospital and most patients do not die of it. One method of assessing changes in the prevalence of peptic ulcers is to study the number of hospital admissions due to perforation. Mackay (1966; 1978) studied hospital admissons in the West of Scotland for perforated ulcer and found that the incidence increased from the early part of the century until 1950 (with a peak at the beginning of World War II) and that it is now declining. The ratio of males to females in the study fell from 19 : 1 between 1924 and 1943, to 4 : 1 between 1964 and 1973. This was due to both a declining incidence in men and a slightly increased incidence in women. One study carried out in Leeds calculated that approximately 13% of men and 5% of women over the age of 35 years have been treated for duodenal ulceration (Watkinson 1960). Bonnevie carried out a study in Copenhagen county which has both an urban and a rural population. Between 1963 and 1973 he found that the mean annual incidence rate for duodenal ulcer per 1000 people over the age of 15 years was 1·83 for men and 0·84 for women. The same figures for gastric ulcer were 0·51 and 0·38 (Bonnevie 1975 a and b).

Although there is no conclusive evidence for emotional causes of peptic ulcer, there is evidence that there is an increased incidence during war time, although this was not confirmed by a study carried out in Belfast during the time of maximum stress caused by civil violence.

Duodenal ulcer is more common in patients who have blood group O with non-secretory status and in the relatives of duodenal ulcer patients than in the rest of the population. Gastric ulcer is more common in relatives of gastric ulcer patients. There is no crossover in heredity between the two ulcer types. It appears that some duodenal ulcer patients inherit a large parietal cell mass.

Gastric ulcer patients have excess mortality from chronic bronchitis and emphysema. Duodenal ulcer patients have excess mortality from liver cirrhosis and cancer of the pancreas. All peptic ulcer patients have excess mortality from lung cancer. There is an association between peptic ulcer and hyperparathyroidism.

Aetiology and pathogenesis

Peptic ulceration occurs when there is a disturbance in the balance between the secretion of acid/pepsin and the mucosal resistance.

DUODENAL ULCER (Grossman 1978): Increased secretion of acid and pepsin seems to be more important in the pathogenesis of duodenal ulcer than abnormalities of mucosal resistance. It has been shown that duodenal ulcer patients have, *on average*, an increased basal secretion of acid/pepsin and an increased response to stimuli such as pentagastrin. However, there is considerable overlap with normal and many duodenal ulcer patients have secretion within the normal range.

The elevated secretion may be due to increased numbers of parietal cells and Cox (1952) found twice as many acid secreting cells in duodenal ulcer patients compared with controls. Whether this is the result of work hypertrophy (i.e. a secondary phenomenon) or hereditary factors is unknown. Several other mechanisms of increased gastric secretion have been suggested.

1. *Excessive secretory drive.* This may be vagal or gastrin mediated. 'Vagal tone' cannot be measured, although the fact that excessive acid secretion can occur in the presence of a normal serum gastrin at least suggests that a factor such as increased vagal tone may be responsible. The fasting serum gastrin in duodenal ulcer patients is normal but there is an exaggerated and prolonged gastrin response to eating. Other studies have shown an increased number of antral G-cells in duodenal ulcer patients.
2. *Defective inhibition.* Acidification of the gastric antrum in duodenal ulcer patients results in less inhibition of gastrin secretion than normal, suggesting a defect in the hormonal feedback mechanism.
3. *Increased sensitivity of parietal cells.* The amount of pentagastrin required for half maximum stimulation of parietal cells is less in duodenal ulcer patients, suggesting that they may be more sensitive than normal.

There is little evidence of a mucosal barrier to acid in the duodenum similar to that in the stomach. There is, however, evidence that entry of acid into the duodenum in duodenal ulcer patients does not cause the same reduction of gastric secretion and brake on gastric emptying found in normal subjects. Duodenal pH is, therefore, at a lower level for longer periods than normal. Defective feedback inhibition by hormones such as gastric inhibitory peptide (GIP) has been implicated.

Bicarbonate produced by duodenal mucosa and by the pancreas is the main neutralizer of gastric acid but recent evidence suggests that production is normal in duodenal ulcer patients.

It is likely that duodenal ulcer patients do not form a homogeneous group and that different pathogenic factors are active in different patients.

GASTRIC ULCER (Avery Jones 1979): Since the secretion of acid and pepsin is normal or even low in gastric ulcer patients, it is usually considered that defective mucosal resistance is the more important factor in the pathogenesis of gastric ulcer. Some secretion of acid/pepsin is required and benign ulcers generally do not develop in achlorhydric patients. Mucosal resistance is determined by a number of factors.

1. *Vascular.* There is some evidence that the arteries crossing the muscularis mucosa into the mucosa in the lesser curve and first part of the duodenum are end arteries. Contraction of the stomach wall could lead to local ischaemia in those areas of the stomach and duodenum most prone to ulceration.
2. *Mucus.* A recent concept is that a thin layer of mucus termed the 'unstirred layer' coats the surface of the stomach. Bicarbonate which is secreted into this layer is trapped within the mucus glycoprotein polymer. This reacts with hydrogen ions to give carbon dioxide and water, thus neutralizing the acid, and it may form part of a barrier to back diffusion of hydrogen ions. Although back diffusion of hydrogen ions is considered important in the genesis of ulceration, no defective secretion of mucus has been demonstrated in gastric ulcer patients.
3. *Cell regeneration.* There is evidence that the lipoprotein cell membrane of the epithelial cells is the most important part of the mucosal barrier and disruption of this allows digestion of the mucosa by bile or acid/pepsin. A peptide isolated from urine (urogastrone) has a trophic effect on human cell cultures and a similar peptide has been found in gastric juice. Deficiency of such a factor may be important in the pathogenesis of ulceration.
4. *Prostaglandins.* These can increase mucosal blood flow, bicarbonate secretion and mucus secretion. Abnormalities of prostaglandin production have been proposed in the pathogenesis of gastric ulcer.

When the gastric mucosal resistance is compromised it is more prone to attack from:

1. *Drugs.* One study (Piper *et al.* 1981) has shown an association between the consumption of analgesics containing aspirin and chronic gastric ulcer. Aspirin and other ulcerogenic drugs, such as indomethacin may act by inhibiting prostaglandins which have an active mucosal protective effect. There is no convincing evidence that alcohol is a cause of chronic gastric ulcer.
2. *Bile and pancreatic lysolecithin.* These may reflux into the stomach and cause low grade damage leading to gastritis and finally ulceration. A defect in antro-duodenal motility has been incriminated as a cause of duodenogastric reflux and increased concentrations of bile acids have been found in the gastric juice of gastric ulcer patients. The gastritis and the duodenogastric reflux persist after healing of the ulcer suggesting that they are primary rather than secondary phenomena.

3. *Cigarettes*. Smoking is more common in peptic ulcer patients than controls and although it may not cause ulceration, it does reduce peptic ulcer healing.

Morphology

Gastric ulcers usually occur on the antral side of the border zone between the acid secreting body mucosa and the non-acid secreting antral mucosa along the lesser curve. Since the antral mucosa extends upwards with age, gastric ulcers tend to be high in elderly patients and it may be necessary to excise a 'tongue' of lesser curve to include the ulcer at the time of gastrectomy. One study found 88% on the lesser curve, 5% on the greater curve, 6% on the posterior wall and 1% on the anterior wall (Sun and Stempien 1971). Fifty per cent are less than 2 cm and 75% less than 3 cm across. Size is not a good guide as to whether or not an ulcer is malignant. Chronic gastric ulcers are round or ovoid in shape with sharply defined edges which often overhang slightly to give a flask shape in profile (*see Fig. 3.3*). Contraction of scar tissue causes radiating mucosal folds which are characteristic and helpful in distinguishing benign from malignant ulcers at endoscopy. The floor is white due to necrotic slough and the edges appear red. A blood clot may be present and active bleeding from a basal vessel may occasionally be seen. Endoscopy may be difficult to interpret if there is a severe fibrous reaction in a mid lesser curve ulcer causing an hour glass deformity of the stomach.

Ninety per cent of duodenal ulcers occur in the first part of the duodenum, just distal to the junction of pyloric and duodenal mucosa; they are most common on the anterior wall. Duodenal ulcers are multiple in 10–15% of cases and if present

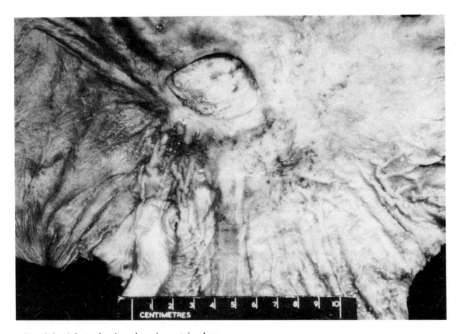

Fig. 3.3. A large benign chronic gastric ulcer.

on both anterior and posterior walls, are termed 'kissing ulcers'. At endoscopy they appear as white excavated areas with oedematous red edges. Deformity of the pylorus suggests the presence of an active or healed duodenal ulcer. There may be associated scarring in the form of ridges and pseudodiverticula of the duodenum. Distortion and radiating folds of mucosa or white mucosal scars suggest previous ulceration.

At laparotomy there may be no external evidence of peptic ulcer, although there is usually thickening and redness of the serosa and invagination of the finger allows palpation of the ulcer crater. Often surrounding lymph nodes are swollen and this does not necessarily indicate malignancy. Fibrous tissue is plentiful in gastric ulcers and may make identification of the left gastric artery difficult. Fibrous adhesions to adjacent organs such as the pancreas can cause difficulties with dissection.

Microscopically, four zones are seen in chronic peptic ulcers: (1) exudate on the surface of the ulcer, (2) necrotic tissue, (3) granulation tissue with young fibroblasts and immature blood vessels, and (4) mature and dense fibrous tissue at the base (see Fig. 3.2).

Vessels in the base of the ulcer often have organizing thrombus and endarteritis obliterans is usually seen (gross thickening of the vessel wall). In gastric ulcers there is a tendency for the muscularis propria to curl up and blend with the muscularis mucosa and this feature helps to distinguish benign from malignant ulcers. The mucosa surrounding a chronic peptic ulcer invariably shows gastritis or duodenitis and in the stomach there may be intestinal metaplasia.

Complications

HAEMORRHAGE: Up to 20% of patients who have been seen at hospital with a peptic ulcer eventually have a haematemesis; it is the commonest complication. Posterior postbulbar duodenal ulcers are especially likely to bleed due to the close proximity of the gastroduodenal artery. Angiography in these cases usually demonstrates bleeding from its supraduodenal branch. Stomal ulcers also have a marked tendency to bleed. The relative frequency of the various causes of haematemesis are given in *Table* 3.2. The miscellaneous category includes a number of relatively uncommon conditions. Leiomyomas and various polyps of the stomach may bleed. Mallory–Weiss tears are discussed on p. 79. Aorto-enteric fistulas which may follow aortic grafting procedures usually occur in the third part of the duodenum but may involve the stomach. Angiodysplasia and haemangiomas may be diagnosed by angiography. Connective tissue diseases may occasionally cause haematemesis and can be diagnosed by the presence of other characteristic lesions (coarse yellow skin around the neck and axilla in the Ehlers–Danlos syndrome;

Table 3.2. Causes of haematemesis (in the UK)

Duodenal ulcer	35%
Gastric ulcer	20%
Acute gastric erosions	21%
Gastric carcinoma	3%
Oesophageal varices	5%
Miscellaneous	16%

lax skin and joints in pseudoxanthoma elasticum). Bleeding into the biliary tree (haematobilia) due to liver trauma, biopsy or tumour may rarely present as haematemesis and is characteristically associated with biliary colic and jaundice.

Several factors have been identified which affect mortality after haematemesis due to peptic ulceration. Recurrent haemorrhage following hospital admission is associated with a marked increase in mortality. Mortality is also increased with patients over 60 years old, with chronic rather than acute ulcers, with gastric rather than duodenal ulcers, when there are associated medical conditions such as chronic respiratory or cardiac disease and when the first bleed was severe as indicated by hypotension, low haemoglobin and large transfusion requirement.

Rebleeding is more common with gastric than duodenal ulcers and in patients who present with haematemesis rather than melaena. If a patient rebleeds within two days of hospital admission, he is likely to have a further haemorrhage. At endoscopy, evidence of likely rebleeding include adherent clot in an ulcer, a vessel seen in the base of an ulcer and the presence of fresh blood.

There is currently considerable interest in treating haematemesis from bleeding peptic ulcer by endoscopic techniques. Actual tissue contact is required for electrocoagulation since an 'active' high frequency current electrode is applied to the bleeding lesion. The high energy density at the electrode/tissue contact point causes heat which results in coagulation. Tissue contact is not required in laser photocoagulation in which an intense coherent monochromatic light is directed at the bleeding area. Energy is absorbed and the heat results in coagulation of protein and tissue shrinkage. Potential dangers include damage to the gut wall or to the operator's eye.

PERFORATION: Mackay's (1966) study found duodenal perforations to be nine times more common than gastric perforations. The site of duodenal perforation was the anterior wall in 92%, the posterior wall in 2% and the pyloro-duodenal junction in 6%.

The overall mortality for perforated peptic ulcer is about 13% (Williams and Cox 1969). However, many of the deaths are due to failure to recognize the correct diagnosis. The mortality of those coming to operation is less than 3% (Booth and Williams 1971). The mortality after perforated gastric ulcer is higher than for duodenal ulcer. At the time of surgery, it can be exceedingly difficult to tell whether an ulcer is acute or chronic and, therefore, the decision regarding definitive surgery will often depend on a clinical history of chronicity.

Perforated gastric ulcers must be biopsied as 5–10% are malignant. Ideally they should be examined immediately so that radical gastrectomy can be carried out if necessary. There is some evidence that if a resected 'benign' ulcer turns out to be malignant on histological examination, re-operation with a more radical clearance will improve prognosis. Occasionally ulcers may chronically penetrate adjacent organs such as the liver and pancreas, and penetration of the latter causes severe continuous backache. Acute perforation of a posterior gastric ulcer into the lesser sac may cause atypical symptoms.

MALIGNANT TRANSFORMATION: The incidence of malignant change in gastric ulcers was previously exaggerated because gastric glands trapped in the edge of a healing ulcer may look like malignant infiltration on histological examination. Also, scirrhous carcinomas have a marked fibrous reaction which may be mistaken for the base of a previous ulcer. The incidence of cancer arising in gastric ulcers is now thought to be less than 1%. Malignant transformation in duodenal ulcer virtually never occurs.

PYLORIC STENOSIS: This is discussed on p. 65.

Pre-pyloric ulcers

These are often considered biologically similar to duodenal ulcers. However, although increased secretion of acid may be present, there is evidence that this in itself may lead to increased duodenogastric reflux. There is, therefore, a two-pronged attack on the antral mucosa. Since pre-pyloric ulcers are by definition gastric, the same caution regarding biopsy as is observed for other gastric ulcers must be practised.

Duodenitis

A group of patients who have typical duodenal ulcer symptoms but no actual ulcer has been identified as having duodenitis or 'pseudo-ulcer'. At endoscopy, the duodenum may be red, oedematous and friable and biopsy shows an inflammatory infiltrate in the superficial duodenal mucosa. In more severe forms there are superficial erosions and loss of duodenal villi. Gastric metaplasia of the surface epithelium may also occur. A follow-up study of 14 patients with duodenitis (as diagnosed by endoscopy) over a period of one to three and a half years showed that six developed duodenal ulceration (Thompson *et al.* 1977). Therefore, many clinicians regard duodenitis as part of the duodenal ulcer diathesis.

Pathology in the Postoperative Stomach

After surgery for benign ulcer disease, a series of abnormalities may occur in the stomach, jejunum or duodenum.

Lesser curve necrosis

After proximal gastric vagotomy, devascularization of the lesser curve may rarely lead to lesser curve necrosis. The presence of a fundoplication makes the condition more likely, possibly because it allows the stomach to distend with gas. Lesser curve necrosis presents with perforation between three days and one week after operation.

Afferent loop obstruction

This occurs after Pólya gastrectomy or gastrojejunostomy and may be acute or chronic. The acute variety usually occurs soon after surgery but may not appear for several years. It may be caused by internal herniation of the afferent loop or by oedema around the stoma due to jejunal ulcer or by intussusception of jejunal mucosa into the stomach. This retrograde intussusception of jejunum presents as an intragastric mass. If the acute obstruction is unrelieved, the afferent loop may perforate.

The chronic variety manifests as severe bile vomiting after a meal. Secretion of bile and pancreatic fluid is stimulated by a meal and accumulates under pressure in the afferent loop which is partially obstructed by adhesions, herniation or kinking. When the obstruction is overcome there is a sudden rush of bile into the stomach and consequent vomiting.

Postoperative bile gastritis

The term 'bile gastritis' is confusing. To the endoscopist it means red, inflamed-looking bile stained mucosa but to the pathologist it means an inflammatory infiltrate in the mucosa. Clinically it implies reflux of bile causing symptoms of burning epigastric pain and bile vomiting. Unfortunately, the endoscopic, histological and clinical pictures do not correlate well. However, the following points can be made.

1. Postoperative patients with bile vomiting have larger amounts of bile acids refluxing into the stomach in the fasting state than do asymptomatic post-operative patients (Alexander-Williams 1981).
2. There is a very poor correlation between gastric mucosal histology and symptomatology.
3. Diversion of bile from the stomach by Roux-en-Y loop or closure of a gastrojejunostomy causes a good improvement of symptoms but does not necessarily improve the inflammatory changes seen on gastric histology.

Recurrent ulcer

Recurrence after duodenal ulcer surgery occurs at the stoma or in the duodenum. Rarely, recurrence occurs in the stomach due to stasis consequent upon inadequate drainage. After proximal gastric vagotomy or vagotomy and pyloroplasty, recurrence is invariably in the duodenum, whereas after vagotomy and gastroenterostomy or Pólya gastrectomy, it is more common at the stoma. After gastric ulcer surgery, recurrence is rare if gastrectomy was performed and usually occurs in the stomach. Causes of recurrence are given in *Table* 3.3. Although inadequate vagotomy is undoubtedly a cause of recurrent ulcer, the fact that gastric acid secretion initially falls and then may rise again substantially some months or years after vagotomy leads to the theory that regrowth of the vagus is responsible in some cases. Ulcer recurrence in the presence of a high serum gastrin level may be due to a retained antrum, the Zollinger–Ellison (Z–E) syndrome or antral G-cell hyperplasia. If, during Pólya gastrectomy, the distal stomach is transected instead of the duodenum, then a portion of the antrum which contains gastrin

Table 3.3. Causes of recurrent ulceration

1.	Inadequate surgery
2.	Possible regrowth of vagus
3.	Antral G-cell hyperplasia
4.	Zollinger-Ellison syndrome
5.	Retained antrum

secreting cells is retained. This portion of the antrum comes in contact only with alkaline secretion and, therefore, it is constantly stimulated to secrete gastrin. This in turn stimulates a high acid output from the remaining stomach. The Z–E syndrome is discussed on p. 214. Hyperplasia of antral G-cells is a controversial disorder since there is difficulty in counting gastrin secreting cells accurately.

Post-gastric surgery carcinoma

Stump cancer is often used in this context but the term is unsatisfactory since the condition has also been described following vagotomy and drainage in which case there is no gastric stump.

There are still conflicting reports in the literature as to whether or not surgery for benign ulcer disease leads to an increased incidence of cancer of the stomach. Schrumpf *et al.* (1977) endoscoped 108 patients 20–25 years after gastrectomy and found four gastric cancers, more than expected in the normal population. A long-term follow-up study of gastrectomy patients in Edinburgh failed to show any increase in mortality from gastric cancer (McLean Ross *et al.* 1982), whereas a similar study of vagotomy and drainage patients in Belfast did show an increased mortality from gastric cancer (Watt *et al.* 1984). Several authorities are convinced that the association between gastric surgery and gastric cancer is strong enough to recommend regular endoscopy and biopsy even in asymptomatic post-gastric surgery patients.

Cancer of the postoperative stomach most frequently arises around the stoma. It seems to be rather more aggressive than the normal type of cancer and has a poor prognosis (*see Fig.* 3.4). Therefore, postoperative patients who are found to have dysplastic mucosal changes should be particularly closely followed up.

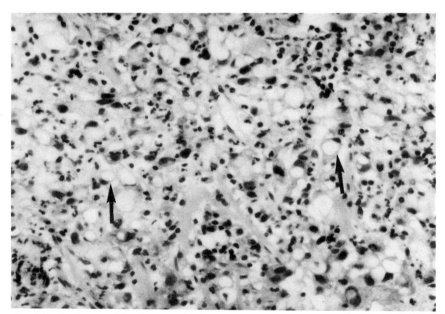

Fig. 3.4. Carcinoma arising in stomach after previous partial gastrectomy. Diffuse type with signet ring cells (arrows). (H and E × 150)

Two theories exist to explain the aetiology of post-gastric surgery cancer.

1. The hypochlorhydric condition of the post-operative stomach may lead to the formation of N-nitroso compounds in gastric juice (*see* p. 70).
2. The bacteria which proliferate in high pH conditions metabolize bile into unconjugated and secondary bile acids, some of which have been shown to have a promoting effect on cancer formation in experimental animals.

Neither theory has, as yet, been fully accepted or rejected.

Gastric Outlet Obstruction

Pyloric stenosis

Peptic ulcer
Of all peptic ulcer patients seen in general practice, approximately one per cent develop stenosis (about 6% will eventually perforate and 14% will bleed). Frequently the obstruction is due to oedema and spasm thus justifying initial conservative treatment. However, continued vomiting usually indicates that fibrotic stenosis has occurred. Since the fibrosis is more common in the first part of the duodenum rather than in the pylorus itself, some surgeons advocate duodenoplasty rather than pyloroplasty. The stomach normally compensates for outlet obstruction by hypertrophy of its muscle wall.

Infantile hypertrophic pyloric stenosis (Spicer 1982)
This condition occurs in 2·5 per 1000 live births in the UK and the incidence appears to be rising. It is four times more common in boys than in girls and the average age of onset of symptoms is 3·5 weeks. Heredity is an important factor since 20% of the sons and 7% of the daughters of an affected mother develop the condition. Since some studies have identified a peak incidence in spring and autumn, a viral aetiology has been proposed but not proven. Other suggested aetiologies include immaturity or degeneration of ganglion cells.

The pylorus is increased in length and diameter and the 'tumour' ends abruptly at the duodenum. The stomach is dilated. Microscopically, the circular muscle is up to four times thicker than normal due to both hypertrophy and hyperplasia of muscle cells. The longitudinal muscle is attenuated. There is also an increase in the number of autonomic nerve fibres and Schwann cells, although ganglion cells are reduced in number.

Pyloromyotomy (Ramstedt's procedure) through the relatively avascular anterior-superior surface is usually successful.

Carcinoma and other gastric tumours
A short history of pyloric stenosis raises the suspicion of a malignant cause. Endoscopic biopsy is essential.

Adult hypertrophic pyloric stenosis
In this condition, the pylorus is grossly thickened and microscopy shows hyperplasia of the circular muscle layers similar to that seen in the infantile type,

although the relationship between the two conditions is unclear. Some patients give a history dating back to childhood and the condition appears to be hereditary in some cases.

Pre-pyloric web

This may be due to incomplete canalization of the pyloric channel. On X-ray the appearance is of two duodenal bulbs.

Annular pancreas

This condition is a very rare cause of pyloric outlet obstruction (see p. 195)

Wilkie's syndrome (Lundell and Thulin 1980)

Compression of the third part of the duodenum may occur between the superior mesenteric artery and the aorta. Other abnormalities may contribute such as a short ligament of Treitz or an acute angle of origin between the aorta and superior mesenteric artery. A fat pad between the superior mesenteric artery and the aorta helps to keep the angle open and, therefore, emaciation is an acquired cause of the condition. Immobilization in the supine position is a further cause. In cases where no mechanical obstruction can be found, defects in the myenteric plexus and smooth muscle have been noted and the term 'megaduodenum' is used. The syndrome therefore appears to have diverse pathophysiology. It is commonest in females in the second and third decades of life.

Other conditions of the duodenum such as tumours and Crohn's disease may present as obstruction and are dealt with elsewhere.

Gastritis, Atrophy, Intestinal Metaplasia and Dysplasia

These terms often appear in pathological reports of endoscopic biopsies and the relationship between them may lead to confusion. Gastritis implies an inflammatory reaction in the gastric mucosa characterized by either neutrophils (acute gastritis) or mononuclear cells (chronic gastritis). When gastritis is associated with pernicious anaemia it is termed 'type A' and other forms are termed 'type B'. Atrophy implies loss of the specialized cells of the gastric glands, either the acid and pepsin producing cells of the body and fundus, or the mucous and endocrine cells of the antrum. Intestinal metaplasia implies change of gastric epithelial cells into intestinal cells and dysplasia implies cellular atypia of the gastric epithelial cells, without invasion through the basement membrane.

Acute gastritis

This condition occurs when there is a widespread acute inflammatory infiltrate in the gastric wall. This may lead to multiple gastric erosions and it then represents a widespread form of acute erosions (acute erosive or acute haemorrhagic gastritis). Causes are, therefore, similar to those discussed under 'acute erosions and ulcers' (see p. 55). Endoscopically, the mucosa is red and oedematous with or without multiple erosions. Since erosions by definition do not reach the submucosal blood vessels, the bleeding tends to be self-limiting and therefore conservative treatment is in order.

When the full thickness of the mucosa is affected by the inflammatory reaction, the term 'acute phlegmonous gastritis' is used. This results mainly from streptococcal infection of the stomach wall and may lead to necrosis, perforation and peritonitis. It is rare.

Chronic gastritis and atrophy (*see Fig.* 3.5)

These conditions are considered together as they are closely linked. When the chronic inflammatory cells are confined to the superficial part of the lamina propria, especially that part between the gastric pits, without any atrophy of specialized cells, the term 'chronic superficial gastritis' (CSG) is used. If the chronic inflammatory cells extend through the entire lamina propria, there is invariably atrophy of some of the specialized glands and replacement by connective tissue. This is called 'chronic atrophic gastritis' (CAG). It may affect body or antral mucosa. Eventually virtually all specialized glands disappear and the inflammatory reaction resolves. This is termed 'gastric atrophy'. The epithelium covering the gastric pits in gastric atrophy, and to a lesser extent in CAG, has frequently undergone intestinal metaplasia. There is evidence that there is a gradual progression from CSG through CAG to gastric atrophy which represents an end stage.

The endoscopic findings of CSG may be normal and there is poor correlation between histology and gross appearance. In CAG and in gastric atrophy, the mucosa becomes paler, blood vessels become more easily visible, the rugal folds become flatter and are absent on inflation of the stomach.

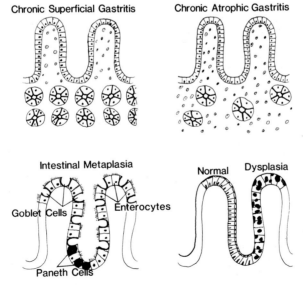

Fig. 3.5. Schematic diagram to demonstrate the main features of chronic superficial gastritis, chronic atrophic gastritis, intestinal metaplasia and dysplasia.

CSG, CAG and gastric atrophy are divided into types A and B (Strickland and Mackay 1973).

TYPE A: This is associated with pernicious anaemia and affects mainly the body and fundus. These patients have antibodies to parietal cells and possibly also to intrinsic factor. It is the loss of intrinsic factor, secreted by parietal cells, which leads to vitamin B_{12} deficiency. The serum gastrin is very high since the antrum, where the gastrin secreting cells are situated, is spared and the inhibitory effect of acid is absent. Carcinoma is three to four times more common in patients with pernicious anaemia than in normals and it occurs in the body and fundus, as is expected from the distribution of the gastritis.

TYPE B: This is most common in the antrum. It may be idiopathic or occur as a result of gastric surgery (see Postoperative Bile Gastritis), chronic aspirin ingestion and possibly chronic alcoholism. It is very common in the mucosa surrounding gastric ulcers and gastric carcinoma.

There is generally a very poor correlation between gastrointestinal symptoms and histological gastritis.

The evidence for pre-malignant potential is more definite. One study found an increased incidence of gastric cancer in patients with chronic atrophic gastritis followed up over a long period (Siurala et al. 1966). The intestinal metaplasia associated with gastric atrophy may also be pre-malignant.

Intestinal metaplasia (IM) (see Fig. 3.5)

In intestinal metaplasia the gastric epithelium changes to an intestinal-type epithelium which has three hallmarks: (1) intestinal absorptive-type cells which have a brush border (enterocytes), (2) goblet cells, and (3) Paneth cells which have bright red granules on H & E staining.

IM is common in the general population and there is a marked increase in incidence with age. Endoscopically, since it is commonly associated with atrophy, it may appear as a thin white mucosa. There is evidence that intestinal-type cancers arise in areas of intestinal metaplasia because: (1) intestinal metaplasia is a common finding in the mucosa surrounding intestinal-type gastric cancer, (2) populations at high risk for gastric cancer have an increased incidence of intestinal metaplasia, and (3) first degree relatives of patients with gastric cancer have an increased incidence of intestinal metaplasia.

Since IM is so common, its occurrence in any one patient is of little significance since obviously only a small proportion of patients with IM progress to gastric cancer. However, sub-typing of IM has distinguished varieties which are more strongly associated with gastric cancer than intestinal metaplasia in general. Two main types are recognized by mucin staining; (1) complete or small intestinal and (2) incomplete or colonic which stains positively for colonic sulphated glycoproteins. The complete or colonic variety has a much stronger association with gastric cancer than in the small intestinal type.

Dysplasia (Morson et al. 1980) (see Fig. 3.5)

This condition cannot be recognized endoscopically. It commonly occurs in epithelium which has undergone intestinal metaplasia but it may also occur in ordinary gastric-type epithelium. Epithelial cells which have undergone dysplasia become irregular in shape and their nuclei become larger, hyperchromatic and pleomorphic. Branching and budding of the gastric pits are seen. The relationship between these changes and early gastric cancer is discussed later. There is no definite evidence that gastric dysplasia progresses to invasive carcinoma and some cases of dysplasia may regress. However, evidence from other organs, such as cervix and colon, suggest that patients with dysplasia should be closely followed up. Some clinicians advocate gastrectomy when severe dysplasia is found by endoscopic biopsy in a relatively young patient, although this question remains extremely controversial.

Gastric Polyps

Epithelial polyps

Two main types are recognized

HYPERPLASTIC OR REGENERATIVE POLYPS: These are sessile and occur throughout the stomach. They may arise as part of an inflammatory reaction and there is often associated gastritis. Microscopically, they are covered with mucosa which has elongated gastric pits, and little or no epithelial dysplasia. Cyst formation occurs in the deep layers. They do not have significant pre-malignant potential.

NEOPLASTIC OR ADENOMATOUS POLYPS: These are mainly sessile polyps which usually adopt a villous pattern (see p. 113). The surface is often covered with epithelium which has undergone intestinal metaplasia and shows varying degrees of dysplasia. These lesions have considerable pre-malignant potential which is directly proportional to their size, malignancy being unusual in polyps less than 2 cm diameter.

In the case of pedunculated polyps, it is essential that they be removed completely with as much stalk as possible. This enables the pathologist to describe accurately whether or not malignant invasion into the stalk has occurred. Sessile polyps may require a segmental resection of stomach and if multiple adenomas are present, distal gastrectomy may suffice since the majority occur in the antrum.

It has recently become apparent that up to 80% of patients with polyposis coli have gastric adenomatous polyps as well as colonic polyps. Regular lifelong gastroscopy is therefore required in these cases.

Other polyps

Early carcinomas and most of the other tumours of the stomach described later may present as polyps. In addition several other conditions of the stomach may present as gastric polyps.

HETEROTOPIAS (presence of tissues not normally found in the area): The most important of these is aberrant pancreatic tissue which may form elevated sessile areas in the antrum. They are quite common, are usually submucosal and consist of normal pancreatic tissue. They may be the site of origin of some endocrine secreting tumours of the stomach.

HAMARTOMAS (abnormal development of tissues which are normally found in the area): Peutz–Jeghers' and juvenile polyps may occur in the stomach (*see* p. 108 and 112).

INFLAMMATORY FIBROID POLYPS: These occur as small sessile or pedunculated polyps in the antrum and consist of vascular tissue with fibroblasts and inflammatory cells. If eosinophils are present they are called eosinophilic granulomatous polyps.

Gastric Cancer

Epidemiology and aetiology

The incidence of gastric cancer is declining in Western countries but the reason is unknown. The maximum incidence is in the 55–65 age group and the male to female ratio is 3 : 2.

ENVIRONMENT: The incidence of gastric cancer varies between and within countries and is similar in that respect to cancers of other organs, such as the colon, which are directly exposed to environmental carcinogens. This is in contrast to organs such as the pancreas and breast which are not directly exposed and where geographical variation is less. Diet has been incriminated in various high risk areas. Smoking of mutton in Iceland produces 3–4 benzpyrine which is carcinogenic. A decline in this technique of cooking mirrors a decline in gastric carcinoma in that country. In Japan, high risk has been associated with the consumption of raw fish and talc rice. The latter contains a compound chemically similar to asbestos. However, recently contradictory evidence has been produced by the demonstration that talc rice is eaten widely in low risk areas such as the Philippines.

N-nitroso compounds (N-nitrosamines and N-nitrosamides) are potent carcinogens in experimental animals and have been suggested as a cause of gastric carcinoma. Exogenous N-nitroso compounds are known to occur in certain foods. Recently, attention has been focused on endogenous formation of N-nitroso compounds. In human gastric juice, N-nitroso compounds may be formed at low pH by purely chemical means and at high pH by bacteria. In theory, bacteria enzymatically reduce dietary nitrate to nitrite and then further reduce nitrite to N-nitroso compounds by combining it with dietary amines or amides. It has been suggested that bacterial formation of N-nitroso compounds accounts for the excess incidence of gastric cancer found in conditions of high intragastric pH, such as chronic atrophic gastritis, pernicious anaemia, and after gastric surgery. In addition, epidemiological data (e.g. Hill *et al.* 1973) have linked gastric cancer with high environmental levels of nitrate. In practice, there is general agreement that hypochlorhydria leads to high levels of gastric juice nitrite. Unfortunately, N-nitroso compounds are difficult to assay and it is unclear whether or not they are also present in large amounts. The formation of N-nitroso compounds at high pH does not, therefore, convincingly explain the increased incidence of gastric carcinoma in hypochlorhydric states.

Further evidence for environmental factors in the aetiology of gastric cancer comes from the study of people who have migrated from Japan (high risk area) to the USA (low risk area). These people have a gradual fall in incidence of gastric cancer which is more marked in the second generation suggesting that environmental factors act early in life.

GENETICS: There is a greater than normal incidence of gastric cancer in people with blood group A. First degree relatives of patients with gastric cancer have a higher than normal incidence. They also have a higher than normal incidence of atrophic gastritis, dysplasia and achlorhydria.

'EPIDEMIC' VERSUS 'ENDEMIC' GASTRIC CARCINOMA: This important concept has arisen out of histological studies in different geographical areas. Lauren (1965) divided gastric cancer into intestinal and diffuse types based on microscopic findings. In high risk countries the high incidence seems to be due almost entirely to the intestinal type, whereas the diffuse type has the same incidence in low and high risk countries. This has led to the concept that there are two distinct types of gastric cancer: (1) an intestinal or epidemic type due to environmental factors, and (2) a diffuse or endemic type related to genetic factors.

PRE-MALIGNANT CONDITIONS: Gastric polyps, atrophic gastritis, intestinal metaplasia, dysplasia, pernicious anaemia and gastric surgery are dealt with elsewhere.

Morphology

Gastric cancers have a predilection for central-type mucosa and are, therefore, more common in the pyloric channel, the antrum and the tongue of antral mucosa which extends up the lesser curve. There is a further concentration at the cardia. Morson and Dawson (1979) examined 206 cases and found 47% in the pylorus and antrum, 23% in the body, 21% in the cardia and 2% in the fundus. Seven per cent occurred as linitis plastica.

The tumour can grow into the lumen, through the wall or within the wall. This gives a series of different appearances, given different names by different authors. In Morson and Dawson's (1979) 206 patients, 44% were nodular, 7% were fungating, 40% were ulcerating, 7% were linitis plastica and 2% were superficial spreading. Other authors give widely different percentages probably due to differences in definition. Any of these gross types has the ability to produce mucin and this gives a rather gelatinous form termed 'colloid' carcinoma. Nodular and fungating growths are usually obvious endoscopically and the surface may be necrotic or ulcerated. The ulcerating type differs from benign ulceration in that the ulcer has heaped up irregular edges with infiltration of the surrounding mucosa. The mucosal folds, however, do not radiate away from the edge in contrast to those around a benign ulcer. In linitis plastica there is widespread submucosal involvement of the stomach wall. This is important to recognize endoscopically since biopsy of the overlying mucosa may not give the diagnosis. The endoscopic features are rigidity and contraction of the gastric wall, failure of the stomach to inflate and loss of peristalsis. The superficial spreading type spreads in the mucosa and submucosa early and invades the deep tissues later. The term is not synonymous with early gastric cancer (see later). It appears as a thickened puckered area of the mucosa. The macroscopic types described above have little influence on prognosis. Borrmann (1926), however, in an attempt to relate macroscopic findings to prognosis, has suggested four types with increasing infiltration or malignancy and, therefore, reducing prognosis: type 1—polypoid or fungating; type 2—ulcer with no infiltration of surrounding mucosa; type 3—ulcer with infiltration of surrounding mucosa; type 4—diffuse infiltration (which eventually leads to linitis plastica).

The histological classification by Lauren (1965) into intestinal and diffuse types is widely accepted.

INTESTINAL: These tumours show attempts at intestinal type gland formation. The glands are lined by irregularly shaped columnar cells with hyperchromatic, pleomorphic and stratified nuclei (*see Fig.* 3.6). The growth tends to be expansive rather than infiltrative and at the margin there is an inflammatory reaction. The surrounding mucosa commonly has undergone intestinal metaplasia.

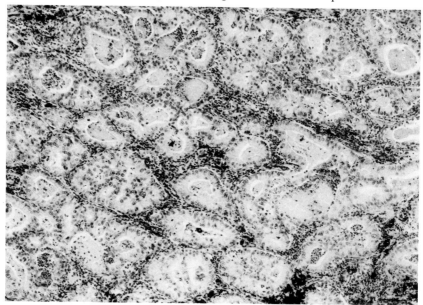

Fig. 3.6. Adenocarcinoma of stomach. Intestinal type showing good gland formation. (H and E × 75)

DIFFUSE: The cells are small and uniform and gland formation is poor. Individual cells or small groups of cells occur scattered throughout the large amount of stroma. There is usually mucin secretion and the mucin is dispersed throughout the stroma and within cells (signet ring cells—*see Fig.* 3.4 earlier). At the edges there is no well defined margin and no inflammatory reaction. The surrounding mucosa does not have an increased incidence of intestinal metaplasia.

Purely squamous carcinomas rarely occur in the stomach, although some tumours have both adeno- and squamous components (adeno-squamous carcinoma).

Spread

Direct spread through and within the gastric wall occurs early. The transverse mesocolon is often involved, making resection difficult and the transverse colon itself is occasionally invaded, giving rise to a malignant gastrocolic fistula. Spread by lymphatics also occurs early. The lymphatic vessels in the gastric wall form submucosal and subserosal plexuses. From the submucosal plexus, vessels enter the lamina propria by penetrating the muscularis mucosa and this may account for the early spread through the wall. The submucosal plexus does not extend across the pylorus but invasion of the duodenum can occur via the subserosal vessels. Further lymphatic drainage to the nodes follows the arterial supply of the gastric and gastroepiploic arteries. From here, spread is directly or via the sub- and suprapyloric nodes, to the coeliac axis and porta hepatis.

The Japanese have suggested that lymph nodes surrounding a gastric tumour be divided into three concentric rings termed N_1, N_2 and N_3, the last being furthermost from the tumour. Gastric resections are termed R_1, R_2 and R_3 to correspond. Frozen section examination of different nodes determines which resection to use. If N_1 nodes are positive, an R_2 resection is done. An R_3 resection is carried out if N_2 nodes are positive. However, if N_3 nodes are positive, the procedure is usually palliative and only an R_1 resection is carried out. Frozen section examination can also give information as to whether limits of excision are clear since palpation is not a good indicator.

For blood spread the most important sites are the liver and the lung. Bone metastases are rare.

Transperitoneal spread is important in gastric carcinoma since tumour cells may spread to the ovaries causing Krukenberg tumours, which may be the presenting feature of gastric carcinoma. Peritoneal seedlings found at laparotomy indicate incurability.

Prognosis

The prognosis of early gastric cancer is good. The overall five year survival rate for advanced gastric cancer is only 5–10% although this may rise to 25% in those patients who have had a 'curative' resection. Absence of lymph node involvement and metastases also greatly improves prognosis. The actual histological appearance of the tumour appears to have little influence on prognosis. However, the presence of a host reaction around the tumour, in the form of a lymphocytic infiltrate and fibroblastic reaction, does seem to be a favourable prognostic sign.

Early gastric cancer (EGC) (Green et al. 1981)

This term is widely used in Japan and the importance of the concept is now recognized in the West. It is defined as gastric cancer confined to the mucosa and submucosa irrespective of lymph node metastases. It is divided into two types— intramucosal and submucosal (see Fig. 3.7).

Intramucosal carcinoma (see Fig. 3.8) does not cross the muscularis mucosa but there is definite invasion of malignant cells across the basement membrane of the epithelium into the lamina propria. Where there is gross abnormality of the epithelial cells but no demonstrable invasion of the lamina propria, the lesion is termed 'severe dysplasia' rather than EGC. It is often difficult to assess whether or not invasion across the basement membrane has occurred, and in this case the term 'borderline lesion' (see Fig. 3.7) is used.

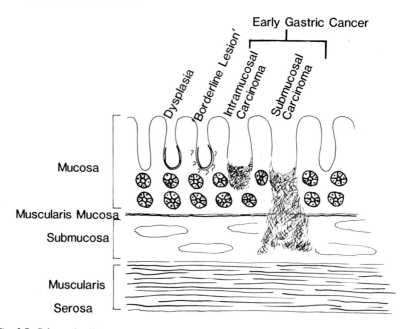

Fig. 3.7. Schematic diagram to demonstrate the differences between dysplasia, 'borderline lesion', intramucosal carcinoma and submucosal carcinoma.

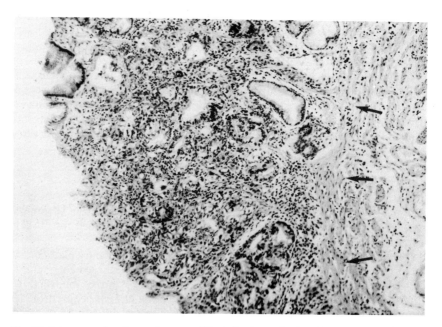

Fig. 3.8. Intramucosal early gastric cancer. The lesion is confined to the mucosa and does not extend below the muscularis mucosa which is arrowed. (H and E × 30)

EGC has been classified into three types (*see Table* 3.4) and type 2 has three subtypes. The more elevated lesions tend to have a more differentiated cell type. The more depressed or ulcerated lesions tend to have a less differentiated cell type and a worse prognosis. Very small polyps or plaques seen at endoscopy may be EGCs and should be biopsied. Type 2B, being flat, is especially difficult to see and may appear as a slight reddening of the mucosa. The Japanese, through mass screening procedures, now find that up to 30% of gastric cancers are resected at the EGC stage, whereas the figure in the West is less than 10%. The Japanese claim a 95% cure rate for EGC, thus emphasizing the importance of detecting this lesion.

Table 3.4. Classification of early gastric cancer

1	Protruded	— polypoid, similar to a benign polyp
2	Superficial	— discoloured plaques on the gastric mucosa
		A elevated
		B flat
		C depressed
3	Excavated	— small ulcers

Other Gastric Tumours

Carcinoid tumours

Gastric carcinoids account for about 6% of all gastrointestinal carcinoids. They appear as well defined tumours and are confined to the mucosa and submucosa until late in the disease process. They are yellow or grey in colour. Microscopically, the cells grow in ribbons and trabeculae. They may give rise to the carcinoid syndrome, and even when there are metastases the lesions are of low grade malignancy.

Other endocrine tumours

These may arise from the endocrine cells in the gastric epithelium or possibly from pancreatic nests in the gastric wall. They are microscopically and macroscopically similar to other endocrine tumours of the gut. They may be functional or non-functional and are a rare cause of the Zollinger–Ellison syndrome.

Smooth muscle tumours

Leiomyomas and leiomyosarcomas are considered together to emphasize the fact that there can be difficulty distinguishing between them. The majority are small, obviously benign, masses, 2–3 cm in diameter and cause no symptoms. They are usually found incidentally at endoscopy. They arise from the muscularis propria and rarely the muscularis mucosa. They may grow into the gastric lumen (intragastric) or outwards through the gastric wall (extragastric) or they may grow on both sides of the gastric wall (dumb-bell tumours). When large, they form soft rubbery masses, grey or pink in colour, which on cutting have a fleshy and whorled appearance. The surface often has a characteristic ulcer giving the whole lesion a volcano-like appearance. Bleeding gives rise to haematemesis or to chronic anaemia. Microscopically, there are spindle shaped smooth muscle cells arranged in whorls (*see Fig.* 3.9). Bizarre cells do not necessarily indicate malignancy and so distinction between leiomyoma and leiomyosarcoma has to rely on size, the number of mitotic figures, infiltration by the tumour and presence or absence of metastases.

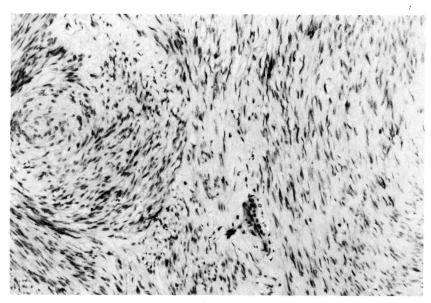

Fig. 3.9. Leiomyoma of stomach. (H and E × 30)

The 'epithelioid smooth muscle tumour' is of smooth muscle origin and is also termed 'leiomyoblastoma' or 'bizarre smooth muscle tumour'. Macroscopically, they are identical to other smooth muscle tumours. Microscopically, the cells are polygonal rather than spindle shaped. Although the tumour cells are epithelial-like, electron microscopy has confirmed that they are derived from smooth muscle cells. The diagnosis will not be made until microscopy is done. Most are benign and have an excellent prognosis.

Tumours of lymphoid tissue
It is important to distinguish true lymphoma from pseudolymphoma.

Pseudolymphoma (Anderson *et al.* 1980)
This is a mass of lymphoid tissue lying in the lamina propria and only rarely extending through the muscularis mucosa. It occurs as an area of nodular polypoid thickening of the stomach wall and may ulcerate. The presence of well developed lymphoid follicles and a mixture of inflammatory cells suggests pseudolymphoma rather than true lymphoma.

Lymphoma (Gray *et al.* 1982)

These are most common in the body of the stomach and may be polypoid, ulcerated or diffusely infiltrating. In the latter case there is characteristic rugal hypertrophy producing giant folds in the region of the tumour. Some are multicentric. On gross examination they can be difficult to distinguish from carcinoma but they tend to be softer on palpation. Histologically, most gastric lymphomas are of follicle centre cell origin (*see* p. 432). A diffuse infiltrate of uniform basophilic cells is seen. The lymphoma cells tend to invade the gastric glands and pits and this feature is helpful in the diagnosis.

Tumours of neural origin

Neurilemmomas or schwannomas arise from the sheath of nerve plexuses in the gastric wall. They occur in the submucosa and project into the stomach. Ulceration may produce haemorrhage. Neurofibromas may occur singly or as part of neurofibromatosis. They also project into the lumen and may become pedunculated. Up to 10% undergo sarcomatous change.

Glomus tumours

These usually present as a mass around the pylorus. Microscopically, they have many vascular spaces interspersed with masses of pericytes and are similar to glomus tumours of the skin (p. 517). They may present with haematemesis.

Miscellaneous Conditions

Acute dilatation of the stomach

The pathogenesis of this condition is unclear although reflex inhibition of intrinsic electrical pacemaker activity has been proposed. It can follow any surgery, especially splenectomy. Occasionally it occurs in chronic illness with no prior surgery and it has been reported during prolonged immobilization. Additional predisposing factors include aerophagia, gastric distension due to ventilation or endoscopy and administration of opiate narcotics which delay gastric emptying. Early symptoms include hiccup and vomiting. Later, pain or collapse from hypovolaemia occurs, associated with copious effortless vomiting. If recognition is early, treatment by nasogastric intubation and intravenous fluids is usually successful.

Ménétrier's disease

This condition is of unknown aetiology. The term 'giant hypertrophic gastritis' is inappropriate since there is no evidence that it is inflammatory. Patients may present with symptoms of protein loss, dyspepsia or, occasionally, haematemesis. At endoscopy, there are giant rugal folds either along the greater curve or throughout the body and fundus. The antrum is not affected. The folds remain after inflation of the stomach. Ménétrier's disease may be confused with other causes of large rugae, such as the Zollinger–Ellison syndrome, duodenal ulcer and certain types of lymphoma. Microscopic examination shows that the gastric pits are greatly elongated. The gastric glands may also be elongated and loss of parietal cells accounts for the hypochlorhydria often found. At endoscopy, it is important to take a biopsy as deeply as possible since a superficial one may be normal.

Volvulus

The factors that predispose to gastric volvulus are: (1) abnormal bands or adhesions around which the volvulus can occur, and (2) an abnormal space for herniation, most commonly paraoesophageal. The twisting can occur around one of two axes; (1) organoaxial, that is, around a line joining the cardia to the pylorus —the stomach becomes upside down and may enter a paraoesophageal space to form a paraoesophageal hernia; (2) mesenterico-axial, that is, twisting around the line of the mesenteric axis which is at right angles to the organoaxial line. This type is less common.

The volvulus may be acute or chronic. An acute volvulus presents as an acute abdomen and usually occurs around the organoaxial axis (mortality 50%). Chronic volvulus may occur around either axis and presents with pain, vomiting and bloating.

Complications may arise, especially within paraoesophageal hernias. Ulceration, haemorrhage, complete obstruction and strangulation leading to gangrene and perforation have all been described.

Diverticula

Gastric diverticula are rare and are most commonly found near the cardia. In this position they are usually lined by normal gastric mucosa and are probably due to a congenital weakness of the muscle wall of the stomach. Other gastric diverticula may occur in the region of the pylorus and these are more likely to be acquired due to previous peptic ulceration.

Duodenal diverticula may be intraluminal or, more commonly, extraluminal. The intraluminal variety is due to ballooning out of the wall of a congenital duodenal diaphragm in a distal direction and this usually results in duodenal obstruction and vomiting. Extraluminal diverticula are more likely to be acquired and occur at points of weakness in the duodenal wall. They often present as an incidental finding on barium studies. Their clinical importance lies in the complication of perforation, which due to their position, occurs retroperitoneally and may not be obvious at laparotomy. Ulceration of the diverticulum may cause haemorrhage. Obstruction of the common bile duct or pancreatic duct may rarely occur and bacterial proliferation within the diverticulum may cause malabsorption.

Bezoars

These are intragastric masses of hair (trichobezoars) or plant material (phytobezoars). They may present as a puzzling epigastric mass and complications such as gastric ulceration or perforation may ensue. Phytobezoars occur in conditions associated with decreased motility and trichobezoars occur in young females who have no other gastrointestinal disease.

Brunner's gland hyperplasia (Kaplan *et al.* 1968)

Brunner's glands which lie beneath the muscularis mucosa of the duodenum may rarely, and for unknown reasons, undergo hyperplasia. This results in sessile or polypoid projections in the first part of the duodenum which can easily bleed and occasionally cause obstruction. Surgical excision is rarely required. It is unclear whether they are the result of 'overstimulation' or are merely hamartomas. Microscopically, large numbers of well differentiated Brunner's glands are seen.

Mallory–Weiss syndrome (Baker *et al.* 1982)

This causes upper gastrointestinal bleeding from a linear mucosal tear in the region of the cardia (*see Fig.* 3.10). In over 75% of cases the lacerations are confined to the gastric mucosa. In 5% the tear is confined to oesophageal mucosa and the remaining 20% extend across the gastro-oesophageal junction. The linear tear extends 3–13 mm in the long axis of the stomach and results from a large rise (120–160 mmHg) in intragastric pressure usually caused by vomiting, coughing or abdominal trauma. A number of the patients have an associated hiatus hernia and the condition is common in alcoholics. Other causes include status asthmaticus, convulsions, gastroscopy, childbirth and cardiac massage. The majority (85%) present with haematemesis and in the UK the condition accounts for 1–3% of all haematemeses. Endoscopy is essential for diagnosis. Most cases respond to conservative measures and in those cases coming to surgery, suture of the tear gives good results. Infusion of pitressin into the left gastric artery, Sengstaken intubation and endoscopic coagulation have all been reported with success.

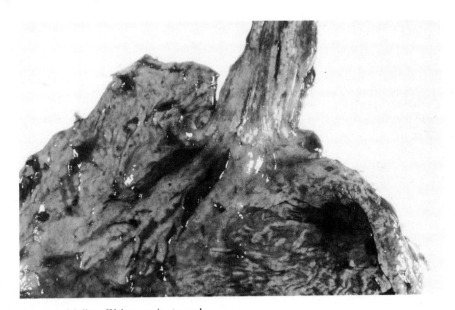

Fig. 3.10. Mallory-Weiss tears in stomach.

References

Alexander-Williams J. (1981) Duodenogastric reflux after gastric operations. *Br. J. Surg.* **68**, 685–7.
Anderson J. R., Lee D., Naysmith A., Busuttil A. (1980) Gastric pseudolymphoma. *Br. J. Surg.* **67**, 672–4.

Avery Jones F. (1979) Pathogenesis of gastric ulcer. In: Truelove S. C., Willoughby C. P. (eds.) *Topics in Gastroenterology 7*, pp. 35–45. Oxford, Blackwell Scientific Publications.

Baker R. W., Spiro A. H., Trnka Y. M. (1982) Mallory-Weiss tear complicating upper endoscopy: Case reports and review of the literature. *Gastroenterology* **82**, 140–2.

Bonnevie O. (1975a) The incidence of gastric ulcer in Copenhagen County. *Scand. J. Gastroent.* **10**, 231–9.

Bonnevie O. (1975b) The incidence of duodenal ulcer in Copenhagen County. *Scand. J. Gastroent.* **10**, 385–93.

Booth R. A., Williams J. A. (1971) Mortality of perforated duodenal ulcer treated by simple suture. *Br. J. Surg.* **58**, 42–4.

Borrmann R. (1926) Geshwulste des Magens und Duodenums. In: Henke F., Luabarsh O. (eds.) *Handbuch der Spezieller Pathologischen Anatomie und Histologie*. Vol. 4, pt. 1, p. 865. Berlin, Springer.

Cox A. J. (1952) Stomach size and its relation to chronic peptic ulcer. *Arch. Pathol.* **54**, 407–22.

Crawford F. A., Hammon J. W. Jr., Shingleton W. W. (1971) The stress ulcer syndrome. A Clinical and pathological review. *Am. J. Surg.* **121**, 644–9.

Gray G. M., Rosenberg S. A., Cooper A. D., Gregory P. B., Stein D. J., Herzenberg H. (1982) Lymphomas involving the gastrointestinal tract. *Gastroenterology* **82**, 143–52.

Green P. H. R., O'Toole K., Weinberg L. M., Goldfarb, J. P. (1981) Early gastric cancer. *Gastroenterology* **81**, 247–56.

Grossman M. I. (1978) Abnormalities of acid secretion in patients with duodenal ulcer (editorial). *Gastroenterology* **75**, 524–26.

Hill M. J., Hawksworth G., Tattersall G. (1973) Bacteria, nitrosamines and cancer of the stomach. *Br. J. Cancer.* **28**, 562–7.

Kaplan E. L., Dyson W. L., Fitts W. T. (1968) Hyperplasia of Brunner's glands of the duodenum. *Surg. Gynaecol. Obstet.* **126**, 371–5.

Lauren P. (1965) The two histological main types of gastric carcinoma: diffuse and so-called intestinal-type carcinoma. An attempt at a histoclinical classification. *Acta. Path. Microbiol. Scand.* **64**, 31–49.

Lundell L., Thulin A. (1980) Wilkie's syndrome—a rarity? *Br. J. Surg.* **67**, 604–6.

Mackay C. (1966) Perforated peptic ulcer in the West of Scotland: a survey of 5343 cases during 1954–63. *Br. Med. J.* **1**, 701–5.

Mackay C. (1978) Unpublished data cited in: Watkinson G. (1979) Epidemiological aspects. In: Truelove S. C., Willoughby C. P. (eds.) *Topics in Gastroenterology 7*. Oxford, Blackwell Scientific Publications.

McLean Ross A. H., Smith M. A., Anderson J. R., Small W. P. (1982) Late mortality after surgery for peptic ulcer. *N. Engl. J. Med.* **307**, 519–22.

Morson B. C., Dawson I. M. P. (1979) *Gastrointestinal Pathology*, 2nd ed. Oxford, Blackwell Scientific Publications.

Morson B. C., Sobin L. H., Grundmann E., Johansen A., Nagayo T., Serck-Hanssen A. (1980) Precancerous conditions and epithelial dysplasia in the stomach. *J. Clin. Pathol.* **33**, 711–21.

Piper D. W., McIntosh J. H., Ariotti D. E., Fenton B. H., MacLennan R. (1981) Analgesic ingestion and chronic peptic ulcer. *Gastroenterology* **80**, 427–32.

Schrumpf E., Serck-Hanssen A., Stadaas J., Aune S., Myren J., Osnes M. (1977) Mucosal changes in the gastric stump 20–25 years after partial gastrectomy. *Lancet* **2**, 467–9.

Siurala M., Varis K., Wiljasalo M. (1966) Studies of patients with atrophic gastritis: a 10–15 year follow up. *Scand. J. Gastroent.* **1**, 40–8.

Spicer R. D. (1982) Infantile hypertrophic pyloric stenosis: a review. *Br. J. Surg.* **69**, 128–35.

Strickland R. G., Mackay I. R. (1973) A reappraisal of the nature and significance of chronic atrophic gastritis. *Am. J. Dig. Dis.* **18**, 426–40.

Sun D. C. H., Stempien S. J. (1971) Site and size of the ulcer as determinants of outcome. *Gastroenterology* **61**, 576–84.

Thompson W. O., Joffe S. N., Robertson A. G., Lee F. D., Imrie C. W., Blumgart L. H. (1977) Is duodenitis a dyspeptic myth? *Lancet* **1**, 1197–8.

Watkinson G. (1960) The incidence of chronic peptic ulcer found at necropsy: a study of 20 000 examinations performed in Leeds in 1930–49 and in England and Scotland in 1956. *Gut* **1**, 14–30.

Watt P. C. H., Patterson C. C., Kennedy T. L. (1984) Late mortality after vagotomy and drainage for duodenal ulcer. *Br. Med. J.* **288**, 1335–8.

Williams J. A., Cox A. G. (1969) *After Vagotomy*, p. 334. London, Butterworth.

Chapter 4

The Intestines

Normal Structure

The small intestine consists of the duodenum, jejunum and ileum. The jejunum and ileum together extend from the duodenum to the ileocaecal valve. The jejunum accounts for the proximal 40% and the ileum for the distal 60%, although the point of division between them is arbitrary.

The wall of the small bowel consists of mucosa, submucosa, muscularis propria and serosa. The mucosa is composed of an epithelial layer, a lamina propria and a muscularis mucosa. The mucosa has a basal layer; villi project upwards from this layer and crypts of Lieberkühn descend downwards from it. The villi can be narrow and finger-like or broad and leaf-like. Each consists of a core of lamina propria and a covering of epithelial cells which are either absorptive-type cells (enterocytes) or goblet cells which secrete mucus. The crypt linings contain Paneth cells and endocrine cells in addition to the enterocytes and goblet cells. The mucosal surface is thrown up into folds (valvulae conniventes) which are visible macroscopically and on plain abdominal X-ray when the small bowel is distended with gas as in intestinal obstruction. The submucosa consists of loose connective tissue; the muscularis propria or muscle coat consists of an inner circular and an outer longitudinal layer.

The whole of the jejunum and ileum is supplied by the superior mesenteric artery and venous drainage is to the portal vein. The lymphatics drain to the superior mesenteric nodes.

The large bowel consists of caecum, ascending colon, hepatic flexure, transverse colon, splenic flexure, descending colon, sigmoid colon and rectum. The caecum is that part below the ileocaecal valve. The sigmoid colon extends from the brim of the pelvis to the rectum. The rectum starts opposite the sacral promontory and has a complete longitudinal muscle layer in contradistinction to the remainder of the large bowel. This is of importance in the distribution of diverticula.

The large bowel wall, like the small bowel wall, consists of a mucosa, a submucosa, a muscularis propria and a serosa. The epithelium of the mucosa forms tubules which are non-branching, are parallel to each other and extend down to the muscularis mucosa. There are no villi. The surface cells are mainly absorptive in type while the crypts are lined mainly by goblet cells and occasional endocrine cells.

Very few lymphatics pass through the submucosa into the lamina propria and this is of importance in the pathology of malignant disease (*see* p. 117). The muscularis propria has an inner circular and outer longitudinal layer. The longitudinal coat of muscle is condensed into three bands termed 'taeniae coli' although a thin layer of longitudinal muscle is continuous between the taeniae. The large bowel is characterized by sacculations or haustra which appear on X-ray as incomplete septa projecting into the gas shadow when the colon is distended.

The colon from the caecum to the splenic flexure is supplied by the superior mesenteric artery. The rest of the colon is supplied by the inferior mesenteric artery. The rectum is supplied by the superior rectal artery (a branch of the inferior mesenteric), the middle rectal artery (a branch of the internal iliac), and the inferior rectal arteries (from the internal pudendal). Lymphatic drainage is first to the paracolic or pararectal nodes and then follows the course of the arteries.

Developmental Abnormalities

Rotational abnormalities

During the sixth week of fetal life the gut herniates into the umbilical cord. When it returns it undergoes complex rotation, failure of which may lead to anatomical abnormalities. For example, the small bowel may be entirely to the right of the midline with the caecum in the left iliac fossa. In these cases the midgut tends to be on a long narrow mesentery which is prone to undergo torsion with resultant volvulus.

Atresia and stenosis

Atresia indicates complete discontinuity of the lumen for a variable distance whereas stenosis indicates narrowing. These abnormalities are most common in the ileum (60%) but also occur in the jejunum and duodenum (40%) (see p. 54). They may be associated with Down's syndrome.

Duplications and cysts

The aetiology of these conditions is discussed on p. 31. Duplications may be complete or partial and communication with the main gastrointestinal tract is variable. Some have their own mesentery while others are incorporated into the mesentery of the main gut. Enterogenous cysts may occur in the wall of the bowel, in the mesentery or else completely separate from the bowel. The lining of these cysts is alimentary in type.

Duplications or cysts may occasionally cause obstruction, haemorrhage or intussusception.

Meckel's diverticulum

The vitello-intestinal duct connects the midgut to the yolk sac in embryological life. If the proximal portion remains it forms a Meckel's diverticulum. This is present in about 2% of the population and it lies on the anti-mesenteric border of the ileum, approximately 90 cm from the ileocaecal valve. It measures up to 8 cm in length. The tip may be connected to the umbilicus by a fibrous cord although it is usually free. A terminal branch of the superior mesenteric artery crosses the ileum to supply the diverticulum and this distinguishes the condition from an ileal duplication.

The muscle coat of the diverticulum is continuous with that of the ileum. The lining mucosa is usually small bowel in type, although gastric and duodenal linings are occasionally seen. Gastric epithelium may give rise to peptic ulceration, either in the diverticulum or in the adjacent ileum. This is prone to bleeding and perforation.

Moses (1947) reviewed 1605 cases of complicated Meckel's diverticulum and reported haemorrhage in 30·9%, intestinal obstruction in 23·8%, perforation in 13·8%, herniation (Littre's hernia) in 11·7% and diverticulitis in 10·3%. Intestinal obstruction may be caused by associated fibrous cords or by the diverticulum inverting and causing an intussusception. Acute inflammation is usually associated with obstruction of the mouth of the diverticulum by oedema, food residue or foreign body, but is relatively uncommon because the mouth is wide.

Soltero and Bill (1976) calculated that a patient with a Meckel's diverticulum has a 4% chance of developing a complication in a lifetime. This low figure led them to challenge the tradition of excising a Meckel's diverticulum if found incidentally at laparotomy.

If the vitello-intestinal duct remains completely patent, it causes an umbilical fistula. This can be diagnosed by the finding of intestinal mucosa on umbilical biopsy.

Hirschsprung's disease

Hirschsprung's disease is a condition in which the ganglion cells in a segment of large bowel are absent. The abnormality starts at the anus and extends proximally for a variable distance. It occurs in about one in 20 000 births and is about five times more common in males than females.

Hirschsprung's disease may present in the neonatal period, in infancy or in later life—the so-called adult Hirschsprung's disease. The age of presentation depends on the length of bowel affected.

During normal embryological development, preganglionic parasympathetic nerve fibres from both the vagal and sacral outflow grow into the bowel. Ganglion cells later migrate from the neural crest and pass along these fibres, to take up their place in the submucosal and intermuscular plexuses. In Hirschsprung's disease, there is a partial failure of ganglion cell migration. Their absence stimulates an abnormal proliferation of those nerve fibres which are present.

The condition is often classified into ultra-short, short, usual, long and total colonic disease (according to the length of the aganglionic segment). The lumen of the aganglionic segment is narrow and the proximal bowel is grossly dilated. The region between the narrow and dilated segments is classically funnel shaped on contrast radiology.

Microscopically, the diagnosis may be made on either a full thickness rectal biopsy or a partial thickness suction biopsy. The two cardinal histological features are a complete absence of ganglion cells and an increase in non-myelinated nerve fibres in the submucosa and between the longitudinal and circular muscle layers. Since these nerve fibres are cholinergic, an increase in acetylcholinesterase activity in specially stained sections is a helpful diagnostic aid and many authorities are now prepared to make the diagnosis by demonstrating increased acetylcholinesterase activity in superficial biopsies which contain mucosa alone. Anorectal manometry is also helpful in the diagnosis.

The site of the biopsy must be more than 2 cm from the anal verge, above the dentate line, since there is a normal hypoganglionic region below this point (Lake 1983). Biopsies taken at the time of operation can be examined using frozen tissue section techniques so that normal bowel can be identified and the amount of resection determined.

A serious complication is the development of enterocolitis. The cause is unknown although both *Clostridium difficile* toxin and sensitivity to *Escherichia coli* endotoxin have been suggested. Ischaemic necrosis and perforation of the bowel above the aganglionic segment may develop and cause a presentation similar to neonatal necrotizing enterocolitis.

Conditions Occurring in Childhood

Neonatal necrotizing enterocolitis

This condition usually affects premature infants in the first week of life who have often undergone some form of stress, such as perinatal hypoxia.

The aetiology is unknown. The most likely explanation is that the bowel becomes ischaemic and is then secondarily invaded by the bacterial flora of the bowel lumen. The reason for the ischaemia is uncertain although it is possible that blood is redistributed away from the splanchnic circulation during periods of perinatal stress, resulting in mesenteric hypoperfusion.

The terminal ileum and right colon are the most commonly affected sites and show gross vascular congestion with mucosal haemorrhages, ulceration and necrosis. Small submucosal gas bubbles may be seen on careful macroscopic examination.

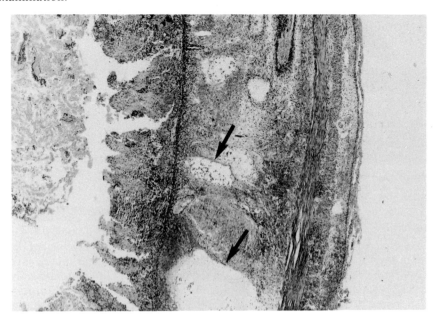

Fig. 4.1. Neonatal necrotizing enterocolitis. Note the widespread necrosis of the mucosa and the large spaces in the submucosa (arrows). (H and E × 75)

Microscopically, there is marked vascular congestion and oedema, with necrosis of the mucosa. A pseudomembrane of necrotic epithelium and debris is commonly present. Gas bubbles appear as cyst-like spaces in the submucosa and are important in diagnosis, both radiologically and microscopically (*see Fig.* 4.1). Surgical resection may be required and in those patients who survive without resection a stricture may form in the affected part of the bowel.

Intussusception

Intussusception is the invagination of one part of the small or large bowel into the next part. It almost invariably occurs in a forward direction, although retrograde intussusception has been described.

Intussusception is the commonest cause of intestinal obstruction in children between 2 months and 5 years old. Seventy per cent occur in children aged between 4 and 11 months and 60–70% occur in boys. It is more common in spring and autumn and in fat rather than thin infants. Only 10% of cases in children have an obvious anatomical cause, such as an intestinal polyp, an inverted Meckel's diverticulum or a food bolus. In adults, at least 85% of patients have a predisposing anatomical cause sited at the apex of the intussusception (*see Fig.* 4.2). The aetiology of intussusception in children is not entirely clear. The most likely explanation is that hypertrophy of the lymphoid tissue of Peyer's patches acts as a starting point for the intussusception. The cause of the hypertrophy may be a viral infection since many patients have a pre-existing upper respiratory tract infection and Gardner *et al.* (1962) showed that adenovirus antibodies were present in 80% of children with intussusception compared with 18% of controls.

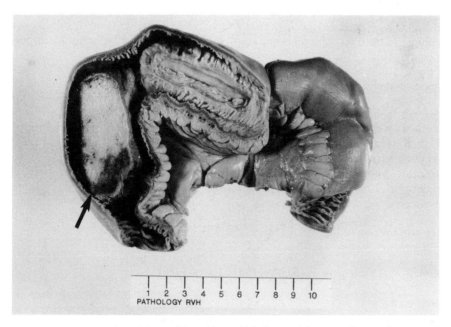

Fig. 4.2. Intussusception of the small bowel in an adult due to a leiomyoma (arrowed).

The site may be enteric (ileoileal, jejunoileal or jejunojejunal), colic (colocolic) or ileocolic. The latter accounts for over 70% of cases. The invaginated segment is termed the intussusceptum and the receiving segment is termed the intussuscepiens. When the process starts the intussusceptum acts as a bolus stimulating further peristalsis and invagination becomes progressive to the extent that occasionally the apex protrudes through the anus. Pressure on the invaginated mesentery causes occlusion of veins with resultant haemorrhagic infarction of the bowel and this may not be appreciated in cases where non-operative reduction has taken place.

Recurrence of idiopathic intussusception in children occurs in about 5% of cases after reduction.

Inflammatory Bowel Disease (IBD)

Epidemiology

Both ulcerative colitis (UC) and Crohn's disease (CD) now have an annual incidence in Western populations in the region of five per 100 000. This rate has remained constant for UC although over the past 20 years there has been a rise in the incidence of CD which may now have plateaued. Both conditions are more common in the United States and Northern Europe than in Africa and India.

Both UC and CD have a peak incidence early in adult life with some studies reporting a second peak in patients over 55 years old. This second peak may include some cases of ischaemic bowel disease and is therefore not as convincing as the earlier one.

Close relatives of patients both with UC and with CD have an increased incidence of the disease. In CD the risk for siblings is increased by up to thirty-fold. There is also a cross-over risk in that relatives of CD patients are more likely to develop UC than the general population, and vice versa. The inheritance appears to be polygenic.

Several studies have been carried out to look for clustering of cases of CD which, if present, might suggest an infective aetiology, but no convincing clustering has been found. A detailed study of the diet of 30 UC patients showed no significant difference from controls (Thornton et al. 1980).

Patients with Crohn's disease have a higher sugar consumption than controls, although the significance of this is unclear. Dietary fibre is believed to be unimportant in the aetiology of CD.

Recent studies have shown an association between non-smoking and UC (Logan et al. 1984) and between smoking and CD (Somerville et al. 1984). The significance of these reports is uncertain. One suggestion is that there is a genetic predisposition to inflammatory bowel disease and the patient's smoking habit determines which of the two diseases develops.

Aetiology and pathogenesis (Rhodes 1981; Jewell 1980)

Infectious agents

Several animal studies have shown that homogenates of Crohn's tissue injected into mice cause granulomatous inflammation and it has been suggested that this is

strong evidence for the presence of a transmissible agent in CD. However, no definite organism has been identified and other studies have given conflicting results. A
similar transmissible agent has been suggested in UC but has not been proved.

Some studies have shown a cytopathic effect of both CD and UC tissue on tissue
culture monocell layers suggesting a viral infection (Strickland and McLaren
1981). Philpotts *et al.* (1979), however, were unable to confirm these findings.

The granulomatous reaction of CD led to a search for a mycobacterial cause and
Burnham *et al.* (1978) isolated *Mycobacterium kansasii* from one patient. Further
studies were unable to repeat this finding.

In summary, the evidence for a transmissible agent in IBD remains controversial
and unproven.

Immunological factors

Mucosal permeability is increased in IBD and luminal antigens therefore gain contact with various immune mechanisms in the bowel wall, thus setting up a series of
immunological mechanisms which lead to inflammatory reaction and damage. It is
unclear whether the immune reactions are simply secondary phenomena or
whether there is an underlying immunological abnormality.

IMMUNOLOGICAL MECHANISMS OF DAMAGE: Hypersensitivity of types I–IV have all
been implicated in causing damage in IBD.

1. *Type I*: In this process, antibody is bound to the membranes of mast cells.
   Contact with an antigen causes degranulation of the mast cells with release
   of histamine, bradykinin and other agents which mediate the immediate or
   type I hypersensitivity reaction. Evidence for type I hypersensitivity in IBD
   includes the electron microscopic demonstration of mast cell degranulation
   in CD and an increased incidence of positive skin tests to food allergens.
   The weight of evidence, however, suggests that type I reactions are secondary
   phenomena in IBD.
2. *Type II*: In the type II hypersensitivity reaction, antibody combines with
   antigen on the target cell. Death of the cell follows either by complement
   fixation or by 'antibody dependent cell-mediated cytotoxicity'. In the latter
   case, lymphocytes, monocytes and macrophages are attracted to the antibody
   coated target cells and destroy them (i.e. they act as killer or K-cells).

   The most likely target cell in IBD is the colonic epithelial cell and high
   circulating levels of anti-colonic epithelium antibodies have been found in
   both UC and CD. These anti-colonic antibodies cross-react with a
   lipopolysaccharide present in *E. coli* and it has been suggested that an initial
   immunological reaction against *E. coli* might lead to cross-reaction with
   colonic epithelium and cause IBD, possibly by the mechanism of antibody
   dependent cell-mediated cytotoxicity.

   Anticolon antibodies, however, also occur in such diseases as amoebic colitis, thus suggesting that they may be secondary to the inflammatory process.
3. *Type III*: This type of reaction is caused by the combination of antibody with
   soluble antigen to form antigen-antibody complexes, which in turn cause
   inflammation mainly by activating complement. This is manifest by the
   Arthus' reaction or by serum sickness. In the Arthus' reaction injection of

antigen into a previously sensitized animal leads to an inflammatory response, the histology of which is very similar to UC. If antibody is present in excess, granulomas may form. In serum sickness, generalized abnormalities may occur which are similar to the extra-intestinal manifestations of IBD.

The evidence for type III reactions in the pathogenesis of IBD include an increased amount of immunoglobulin in the colonic mucosa of patients with both UC and CD and the demonstration of circulating immune complexes in patients with IBD.

Again, it is not clear whether type III reactions are primary or secondary phenomena.

4. *Type IV*: This is cell-mediated immunity which is mediated by T cells sensitized to antigen. The similarity of Crohn's granulomas to those found in tuberculosis and sarcoidosis stimulated an interest in type IV hypersensitivity in CD, although granulomas can occur in antibody-mediated reactions. Type IV hypersensitivity has also been implicated in UC. It can be demonstrated that there are increased numbers of T cells in the bowel mucosa of patients with IBD and, furthermore, animals which are sensitized to dinitrochlorobenzene, a known inducer of T cells, develop a colitis on subsequent challenge, indicating that type IV reactions can cause bowel damage.

DEFECTS OF THE IMMUNE MECHANISM IN IBD: There is some evidence that patients with IBD have an intrinsic abnormality of the immune system.

Antibody responses to bacteria and viruses are normal in patients with IBD and there are no differences in complement levels, although a diminished lymphocyte responsiveness is seen in many patients with CD and in a few patients with UC. Patients with IBD may, therefore, have an impaired cellular immunity, but the significance of this is unclear.

Defects in the immune regulatory system have also been suggested in IBD and, in particular, abnormalities of suppressor T cells have been found. In simplistic terms, it might be suggested that a defect of suppressor T cells in the gut wall might lead to an uncontrolled cellular hypersensitivity and associated inflammatory response.

There is also evidence for a defect of the local immune system in the gut.

Despite the obvious confusion in the literature on the aetiology and pathogenesis of IBD, Kirsner and Shorter (1982) have suggested the following hypothesis.

1. UC and CD are prototypes of a single disease process, the differing manifestations of which depend on the site involved, the nature of the antigens and the genetic influences.
2. An external agent (bacterial, viral or dietary) cross-reacts with a host antigen.
3. Sensitization to the particular antigen takes place during infancy before the full development of the immune system.
4. After the initial priming, any insult (e.g. antibiotic therapy or viral illness) that increases the intestinal mucosal permeability to bacteria or other gut antigens can precipitate an immunological response in the bowel wall.

Ulcerative colitis

The commonest form of UC is the chronic intermittent type in which the symptoms are episodic. Each episode may be mild with four or less motions per day and no constitutional symptoms, moderate, or severe with more than eight motions per day and marked constitutional symptoms. Severe attacks may be complicated by acute dilatation of the colon (toxic megacolon). A less common presentation is the chronic continuous type of UC. In less than 5% of cases, only one attack occurs.

Morphology

During endoscopy, the appearance and the geography of the abnormal mucosa are documented. The early changes observed are erythema of the mucosa and haziness of the submucosal vascular pattern. In more severe disease, diffuse small ulcers on a red granular mucosa are seen, the mucosa is friable and bleeds on contact and the vascular pattern is lost. Inflammatory polyps are seen in some cases. In quiescent disease, the mucosa may be normal or it may be smooth and atrophic with loss of mucosal folds.

The abnormal mucosa affects the rectum and extends proximally in a continuous fashion involving the entire circumference of the lumen. The condition tends to be worse distally and it may have a slightly patchy distribution, giving the false impression of skip lesions. Biopsies from the apparently normal areas are, however, abnormal; it is therefore important to take multiple biopsies.

Operation is carried out for failed medical treatment in severe attacks or for the complications of toxic dilatation, perforation or haemorrhage. Occasionally, resection is performed as prophylaxis against cancer. At laparotomy the colon is shortened but the serosal surface has its usual glistening appearance. The serosa may have increased vascularity, but no exudate is seen. Examination of the opened

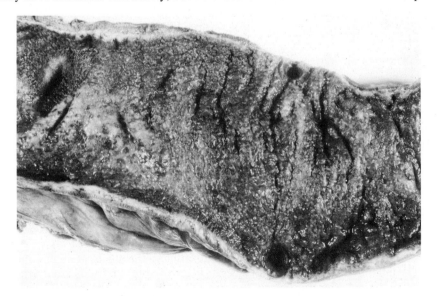

Fig. 4.3. Colon in ulcerative colitis. Numerous small ulcers are seen.

specimen, if removed during an acute exacerbation, reveals a red, granular, friable, ulcerated mucosa which is spongy and oozing blood (*see Fig.* 4.3). Characteristically, the mucosa between the ulcers is diseased. Inflammatory polyps (pseudopolyps) may be prominent. In 10% of cases the ileum is involved and shows the same macroscopic appearance as the colon (backwash ileitis). In these cases there is usually an incompetent ileocaecal valve.

Histologically, in active UC there is an inflammatory reaction in the mucosa and superficial submucosa. This is associated with capillary congestion and a chronic inflammatory cell infiltrate throughout the lamina propria. Polymorphs are seen invading the bases of the glandular crypts forming crypt abscesses (*see Fig.* 4.4). Crypt abscesses are, however, not specific to UC. These crypt abscesses may rupture, either into the lumen causing pus in the stool, or into the submucosa causing desloughing of the overlying mucosa with ulceration. The mucosa at the margins of these ulcerated areas is undermined and raised above the surrounding mucosa to form inflammatory polyps. Depletion of goblet cells and distortion of the crypts are other characteristic features of the acute phase.

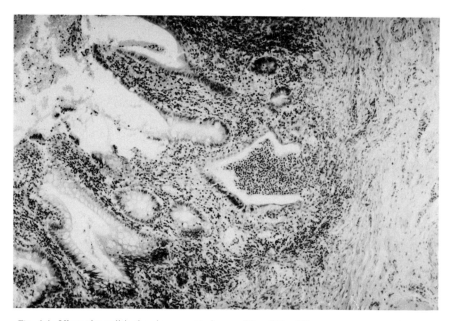

Fig. 4.4. Ulcerative colitis showing a crypt abscess. (H and E × 75)

In resolving colitis, the ulcerated areas become re-epithelialized. The epithelium becomes regenerative and the resulting heaping up and loss of polarity may be mistaken for dysplastic change. This is further discussed on p. 94.

In the quiescent phase of UC, between acute attacks, the mucosa remains abnormal. The inflammatory exudate and ulceration resolve but the crypts are shortened and do not reach the muscularis mucosa. They also lose the normal parallel arrangement and become branched.

Crohn's disease

Crohn's disease may affect any part of the gastrointestinal tract, although it has a propensity to occur in the small bowel, especially the terminal ileum, and colon. The commonest clinical presentation is a gradual onset of diarrhoea with or without a right iliac fossa mass. Abdominal pain is not uncommon. The macroscopic and microscopic features are similar in both the large and small intestine.

Morphology

The small bowel only is affected in 66% of cases, small and large bowel together in 17% of cases and the large bowel only in 17% (Morson and Dawson 1979).

Endoscopically, the earliest feature is the aphthoid ulcer, a small punched-out lesion which lies on an otherwise normal mucosa. Later, deep linear ulcers are seen but, in contrast to UC, the intervening mucosa is often normal. In some cases interlacing ulcers form a cobblestone appearance (*see Fig.* 4.5), and pseudopolyps are frequently seen. The mucosa eventually becomes thickened and oedematous but is not as friable as in UC. The mucosal abnormalities are typically discontinuous and asymmetrical.

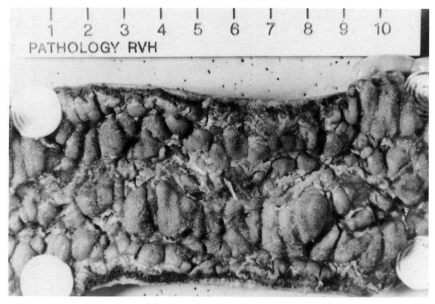

Fig. 4.5. Crohn's disease of colon. Linear ulcers and a cobblestone pattern are seen.

The affected bowel is thickened due to fibrosis and oedema forming, in some cases, a classical hose-pipe segment. The strictures (skip lesions) are usually multiple. The serosal surface often has a fibrinous exudate and there is a tendency for several loops of gut to be matted together, possibly with concomitant abscess and fistula formation. These features are not seen in UC. The associated mesentery is often oedematous with enlarged lymph nodes caused by reactive hyperplasia.

An important feature of small and large bowel CD is the discontinuity of the disease which is not seen in UC.

Perianal lesions, such as fistulas, fissures and abscesses, are much more common in CD (75%) than in UC (25%). The anal lesions are seen in both small bowel and large bowel CD, but are more common in the latter. One study of 112 patients with CD and anal fistulas reported that the disease was confined to the small bowel in only 13 cases (Marks *et al.* 1981).

Histological abnormalities affect all layers of the bowel wall which is grossly thickened due to fibrosis and oedema, mainly in the submucosa. Granulomas are present in 50–70% of cases and consist of collections of epithelioid cells (ovoid cells with abundant pink cytoplasm) and Langhans' giant cells (with peripheral nuclei) (*see Fig.* 4.6). Granulomas help to distinguish the disease from UC, although foreign body granulomas may be seen in the latter. Morson and Dawson (1979) regard fissuring as 'almost pathognomonic of Crohn's disease'; the fissures are seen as deep clefts lined with granulation tissue penetrating into the submucosa. Aggregates of lymphocytes and dilatation of lymph channels are also characteristic of CD. Close inspection of the inflammatory infiltrate in the mucosa may show it to be more focal than in ulcerative colitis. Crypt abscesses, although present, tend also to involve the crypts focally, unlike the diffuse involvement in UC. Within the crypts, goblet cell depletion is not seen to the same extent as in UC.

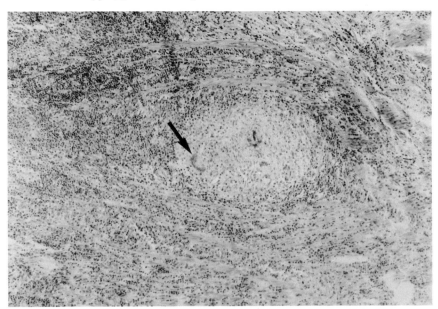

Fig. 4.6. Crohn's disease. Granuloma with giant cells (one of the giant cells is arrowed). (H and E × 30)

Prognosis of IBD

The prognosis of UC has improved with better medical therapy and earlier colectomy. The overall mortality from the first attack is between about 3% and 10%, depending on severity. Patients with extensive disease have an increased mortality during the first year of disease and then the mortality approaches that of the general population. About 5–10% of patients have either a long-term (15 year) or a complete remission after the first attack. A further 10% experience continuous symptoms and the remainder have remissions and exacerbations over the ensuing years. At the time of presentation, approximately one-quarter of patients have proctitis only and one-quarter have extensive colitis. If patients with proctitis are followed up over 10 years, the disease will spread to involve the sigmoid in 30% and the entire colon in 5–10%. Overall, about one-fifth of all patients require proctocolectomy at some stage of their disease.

In CD, actuarial methods show that recurrence rates after a first attack are high: over 30% at 5 years and over 50% at 10 years. Although wide resection was popular in the past, it has now been shown that minimal resections are appropriate because the high recurrence rate often necessitates further excision at a later date. It has also been shown that the presence of microscopic disease at the margin of the excision does not appear to alter the incidence of symptomatic recurrence (Heuman *et al.* 1983). The overall mortality attributed to CD or its complications ranges from 5–18%.

Complications of IBD

External fistulas in CD

External fistulas occur in about one quarter of patients with CD. Irving (1983) recognizes two types. Type I arises from a diseased segment of bowel, often ileum, and is associated with an abscess. These nearly always require operation. Type II fistulas occur after breakdown of an anastomosis. Most of them heal spontaneously without the need for surgical operation.

Toxic megacolon

Acute dilatation of the colon occurs in 2–4% of all UC patients and is a surgical emergency. It occurs equally commonly in the first attack and in severe subsequent relapses. It may also occur in CD and in other forms of colitis. The underlying cause is unknown, although predisposing factors such as anti-diarrhoeal agents, anti-cholinergic drugs and barium enema examination have been implicated.

In toxic megacolon the inflammation is always transmural. At operation, a dilated bowel, usually the transverse colon and less commonly the sigmoid colon, is seen. The serosa is dull and congested and has a fibrinoid or purulent exudate. The wall is classically likened to wet blotting paper. The mucosa is grossly ulcerated leaving only small islands which stand out on plain radiographs as nodular filling defects in the dilated colonic lumen.

Histologically, gross ulceration with deep penetrating clefts is seen (*see Fig.* 4.7). The muscular layers show extensive lysis (myocytolysis). Vascular engorgement is marked. It is often impossible, even after resection, to distinguish whether the underlying condition is UC or CD.

Cancer in UC

Patients with extensive UC of more than ten years standing have an increased risk of developing colorectal cancer. The risk is greater in patients who develop the disease at an early age. Lennard-Jones *et al.* (1977) found that the increased risk of

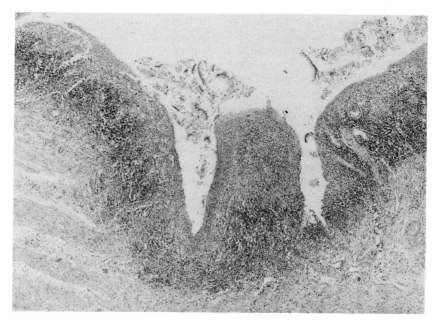

Fig. 4.7. Toxic megacolon due to ulcerative colitis. The mucosa is extensively ulcerated and deep penetrating ulcers extend into the muscularis propria. (H and E × 30)

developing cancer is twenty-three-fold in the second decade and thirty-two-fold in the third decade of the disease. One in four patients with extensive UC will develop colorectal cancer during the third decade of their disease.

Cancers complicating UC are more evenly distributed than colorectal cancer arising *de novo*. Only about 45% arise in the rectum and sigmoid colon. They tend to be flat and infiltrating and may form fusiform strictures. Microscopically they are adenocarcinomas and are often poorly differentiated.

Prophylactic proctocolectomy may be avoided in some cases by meticulous follow-up which includes: (1) frequent sigmoidoscopy with rectal biopsy to determine if dysplasia is present, and (2) regular colonoscopy with biopsy.

Severe epithelial dysplasia is seen in the rectum of 73–87% of patients who have UC complicated by colorectal cancer and, conversely, 60% of patients with severe dysplasia have a concomitant cancer. Negative rectal biopsy, especially if multiple and performed on several occasions, is therefore a reasonably good indicator that the patient does not have cancer. However, it is not a perfect indicator and this is why regular colonoscopy is also recommended.

Rectal (or colonoscopic) biopsies in UC may be random or 'target orientated'. Although severe dysplasia may only be detected microscopically in some cases, in others it may be seen as a plaque or small polyp.

Microscopically, dysplasia is recognized by cytological abnormalities such as nuclear pleomorphism and hyperchromasia and also by architectural abnormalities, such as complex branching of glands.

Lennard-Jones *et al.* (1977) recommend the screening of patients with UC by annual rectal biopsy starting five years after the onset of symptoms. In addition, colonoscopy at 1–3 year intervals may be performed. Proctocolectomy is carried out if severe dysplasia is seen at several sites over a period of several months.

Cancer in CD

SMALL BOWEL: Small bowel cancer complicating CD tends to involve sites of macroscopic disease; it also occurs in a younger age group than normal, suggesting a true association. Greenstein and Sachar (1983) reported that small bowel cancer occurs 85 times more frequently in CD than in the normal population, although this figure is based on small numbers.

The tumours are often not suspected clinically since the symptoms and signs of obstruction, abdominal mass and weight loss are put down to the CD. At operation, the tumour is not always obvious and may only be detected histologically. Occasionally, the cancer arises at a site distant from the macroscopic CD, such as in the stomach or oesophagus.

LARGE BOWEL: Greenstein and Sachar (1983) quote a seven-fold increase in risk for large bowel cancer in patients with CD. The cancer occurs at a younger age group than does ordinary colorectal cancer. Screening of patients with CD for rectal dysplasia is not yet of proven efficacy.

Extra-intestinal manifestations of IBD

Liver and biliary
Mild abnormalities of liver function tests are common in patients with both CD and UC and may improve after surgical resection of the affected bowel. However, several specific liver complications are described, particularly in UC. Fatty change may be seen especially in patients with toxic megacolon. More than 75% of patients with sclerosing cholangitis have underlying UC (*see* p. 183), although the association with CD is rare. Colectomy has little effect on the progression of sclerosing cholangitis. Pericholangitis in which there is inflammation and fibrosis around intra-hepatic ducts is believed to be part of the spectrum of sclerosing cholangitis. Cirrhosis occurs in 1–5% of UC patients but is only rarely seen in CD. The development of bile duct carcinoma has been described in patients with long-standing UC. Gallstones occur with increased frequency in CD affecting the terminal ileum due to reduction in bile acid absorption, causing a relative rise in the cholesterol concentration of bile.

Skin
Erythema nodosum appears as raised, red, tender nodules, classically on the anterior tibial aspect of the leg in 2–4% of patients with UC and less commonly in CD. Pyoderma gangrenosum, which also occurs more commonly in UC than in CD, appears as a large, deep ulcer with central necrosis. It usually, but not always, improves with colectomy.

Eyes
Episcleritis is more common in CD than UC. Uveitis is a more serious condition which presents with pain and blurring of vision. It may or may not be related to exacerbations of the bowel disease.

Joints

Patients with IBD may develop arthritis. This usually occurs during exacerbations of the colitis and runs a self-limiting course. The knees are most frequently affected and in general the joints are asymmetrically affected. Between 2% and 6% of cases of both UC and CD are associated with ankylosing spondylitis.

Urinary tract

Amyloid of the kidney occurs rarely in both CD and UC. Urinary calculi occur in up to 10% of patients with IBD, especially in those with an ileostomy. Diarrhoea and ileostomy discharge cause a low volume of concentrated urine which predisposes to stone formation. Oxalate stones may occur if the terminal ileum is resected or affected by CD. Normally, dietary oxalate binds to calcium in the small bowel and is excreted in the faeces as an insoluble salt. In malabsorption due to terminal ileum malfunction, the calcium binds to the excess fat leaving free oxalate which is absorbed in the colon.

Colitis indeterminate

In some cases of acute IBD, a rectal biopsy may show features of both CD and UC to the extent that it is impossible to determine which is the true disease. The term 'colitis indeterminate' is applied to these cases. Sequential biopsies taken during quiescent phases may elucidate the diagnosis. In 5–10% the diagnosis of colitis indeterminate remains.

Idiopathic proctitis

This is a disease in which macroscopic and histological findings identical to UC are found restricted to the rectum. Many authorities consider that it differs from UC only in the extent of bowel involvement. It tends to run a relapsing course. Follow-up of patients shows that less than 10% will develop extensive colitis after 10 years and the prognosis for an individual patient is, therefore, good.

Other Inflammatory Conditions of the Intestines

Yersinia enteritis

Yersinia is a coccobacillus and two forms, *Y. pseudotuberculosis* and *Y. enterocolitica*, may cause acute enteritis with fever and diarrhoea. There is an acute ileitis, the differential diagnosis being CD. Yersinia infection may also present with features indistinguishable from acute appendicitis. At laparotomy, the appendix is usually normal but the mesenteric glands are swollen and inflamed. The terminal ileum and caecum may also be inflamed and oedematous with an abnormal mucosa containing superficial ulceration. Histologically the bowel wall has an inflammatory infiltrate and granulomas, often with central microabscesses, are characteristic. The ileitis resolves in a few weeks and transition to CD has not been reported. Diagnosis can be made by isolation of the organism from blood or lymph nodes or by the demonstration of specific antibodies in rising titres.

Infective colitis

Infective colitis may present as an acute illness with bloody diarrhoea which can be difficult to distinguish from UC and CD. The organisms responsible include Shigella, Salmonella, certain strains of *E. coli* and Campylobacter. Campylobacter organisms have recently been accepted as an important cause of diarrhoeal illness. They are Gram-negative bacilli, probably spread by dogs and cats. Barium enema and endoscopic findings may be identical to other forms of colitis.

Rectal biopsy can often distinguish infective colitis from other forms of colitis. The prominent histological findings in infective colitis are oedema of the lamina propria with a predominantly polymorphonuclear infiltrate (unlike UC and CD which have both acute and chronic inflammatory cells).

The toxic megacolon which has been described as a complication of Salmonella infection may mimic ulcerative colitis.

Amoebic dysentery

Amoebic dysentery is caused by the protozoan parasite *Entamoeba histolytica*. The disease occurs in the large bowel and may be confused with both UC and CD.

Small, yellow lesions are seen on the mucosa. These break down to form ulcers which are typically flask-shaped with overhanging edges, the long axis being at right angles to that of the colon. Diagnosis is by identification of the organism in the warm stool or in a rectal biopsy. The early microscopic changes in the rectal biopsy are similar to other forms of infective colitis but biopsy of an ulcer will show the amoebae as large cells with small, dark nuclei. Rarely, the colon perforates or an amoeboma forms which presents as a fibrous stricture. This can be confused with a carcinoma on digital examination. Very occasionally, amoebic dysentery is complicated by toxic megacolon.

Pseudomembranous colitis

This condition may develop after major abdominal surgery but is more commonly seen as a complication of antibiotic administration. It is especially associated with lincomycin and clindamycin although it has been reported as a complication of a wide range of antibiotics. The organism *Clostridium difficile* and its toxin can be isolated from the stool in over 90% of patients and is, therefore, believed to be the cause. The organism requires special culture techniques and demonstration of its toxin is the basis of a laboratory screening test for the disease.

C. difficile is not a normal commensal in the gut and it is unclear why it should proliferate in the gut of patients with pseudomembranous colitis. The selection of a resistant organism appears not to be the reason since isolates of *C. difficile* from affected patients are usually sensitive to conventional antibiotics. It is likely that pseudomembranous colitis arises when two coincidental events occur: (1) an increased susceptibility of the bowel to bacterial colonization brought about by antibiotics or by major surgery, and (2) the presence of virulent strains of *C. difficile* in the environment. This theory is supported by the fact that small epidemics of the disease sometimes occur.

Macroscopically, the mucosal surface has yellow plaques of different sizes which may become confluent. They are easily seen on sigmoidoscopy, although sometimes the rectum is spared.

Microscopically, the yellow plaque consists of a group of partially disrupted epithelial crypts on the surface of which is a cap of epithelial debris, mucin, fibrin and polymorphs (*see Fig.* 4.8). Later in the disease there is complete mucosal necrosis with an overlying necrotic membrane. At this stage the histological features are no longer diagnostic.

C. difficile is sensitive to vancomycin which is the treatment of choice. Occasionally, pseudomembranous colitis is complicated by a toxic megacolon.

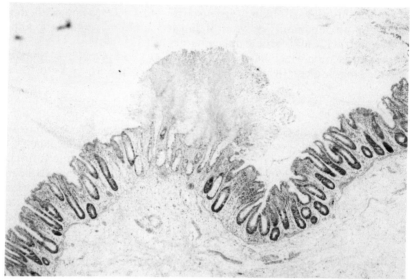

Fig. 4.8. Pseudomembranous colitis. A group of partially disrupted crypts with a surface cap of debris, mucin, fibrin and polymorphs. (H and E × 30)

Tuberculosis

Gastrointestinal tuberculosis most frequently involves the terminal ileum and caecum. It may be primary, due to infection with the bovine bacillus, or secondary due to swallowed sputum in patients with open pulmonary tuberculosis.

Macroscopically, in the early stages of the disease, a tuberculous ulcer is seen. These ulcers lie transversely to the long axis of the bowel and often have raised edges. At a more advanced stage, fibrosis occurs and this leads to the development of single or multiple strictures. The differential diagnosis then includes lymphoma, Crohn's disease and ischaemic colitis.

Microscopically, caseating granulomas are seen in the early stages. In chronic disease, the fibrosis causes destruction of normal tissues and the features may be those of a fibrous stricture with few, if any, granulomas. Distinction from Crohn's disease and ischaemic stricture by histology may be difficult.

Diverticular Disease of the Colon

Diverticulosis is the presence of multiple colonic diverticula. It is often asymptomatic. Alternatively, it may cause irregularity of bowel habit and abdominal pain without constitutional upset. Occasionally, it is complicated by haemorrhage. Diverticulitis indicates inflammation of one or more of the diverticula and this gives rise to both local and systemic symptoms. Diverticulitis may be complicated by perforation, abscess, fistula formation, peritonitis, intestinal obstruction and haemorrhage. Diverticular disease occurs much less frequently in the small bowel where complications include malabsorption.

Epidemiology

The major epidemiological features of diverticular disease are an increasing incidence with age, an increasing incidence since the early part of the twentieth century and a marked geographical variation.

Autopsy studies have shown that the incidence rises with age, to the extent that in the UK at least one in three persons over 60 years of age has colonic diverticula. The condition is slightly more common in females than males.

The incidence of diverticular disease has been increasing steadily throughout this century. In 1910, autopsy studies showed an incidence of only 5%. The fact that this figure has risen so dramatically is attributed to the introduction of roller milling of wheat flour in 1880 which resulted in a decreased consumption of crude grain. Diverticular disease is very much more common in Western countries than in Africa, India, South America and Japan. It has been postulated that this is due to high dietary fibre intake in the latter areas. Some of this geographical variation may be due to genetic influences, although the rapid emergence of the disease in Japanese immigrants to Hawaii and in urban South African blacks is in favour of environmental factors.

Further evidence for the importance of dietary factors comes from the study of Oxford vegetarians who had a 12% incidence of diverticulosis compared with 33% in controls (Gear *et al.* 1979).

Right-sided diverticular disease is occasionally seen, especially in the Japanese and Chinese races. The patients tend to be younger than those who have the Western pattern of left-sided disease.

Aetiology and pathogenesis

It is generally accepted that acquired colonic diverticula are pulsion in type, the aetiology of which depends on both the intraluminal pressure and the strength of the colonic wall.

Several studies using open tipped catheters showed that patients with diverticular disease had an exaggerated pressure response in the sigmoid colon to food ingestion. These high pressure waves coincided with contractions which occluded short segments of the colon. It was therefore postulated that the ingestion of a low residue diet which requires greater force to propel the faecal stream leads to work hypertrophy of the muscle layer of the colon. The thickened, circular muscle forms semilunar folds which protrude into the lumen and overlapping of these folds of muscle during bowel contraction causes segments of the colon to be sealed off from each other. The pressure therefore rises in these closed off segments and diverticula are pushed out through the colonic wall.

More recent studies, however, have only been able to detect motility disorders in symptomatic patients with diverticulosis, suggesting that a hypermotility disorder is not essential for the development of diverticula. The earlier work which showed hypermotility disorders in all diverticulosis patients may have used selected symptomatic patients, thus explaining the discrepancy. Other factors of uncertain importance are an increase in low amplitude fast waves and shortening of the longitudinal muscle with consequent exaggeration of the haustral pattern found in the colon of patients with diverticular disease. In addition, aging is associated with an increase in type I collagen and a decrease in type II collagen with a consequent decrease in the tensile strength of the colonic wall.

In summary, the development of colonic diverticula depends on the balance between the intraluminal pressure and the strength of the colonic wall.

Morphology

The condition is most common in the sigmoid colon but the proximal colon may be involved for a variable distance. The rectum is not involved, due to its full investing layers of both muscle coats. The diverticula appear in rows between the one mesenteric and the two antimesenteric taeniae at points of weakness where blood vessels enter (*see Fig.* 4.9). The diverticula consist of pouches of mucosa which have herniated through the circular muscle. They often contain a faecolith.

Antimesenteric Border

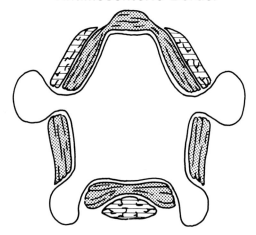

Mesenteric Border

Fig. 4.9. Schematic cross section of colon to show the position of diverticula (*see* text).

The circular muscle is greatly thickened and firm. It forms folds which protrude into the lumen, giving the saw-toothed appearance on barium contrast radiographs. The mouths of the diverticula are found between these folds (*see Fig.* 4.10). It has been shown, using X-ray studies, that the muscle abnormality may precede the formation of diverticula (the pre-diverticular state).

The affected bowel is often greatly shortened, probably due to contraction of the taeniae coli. This results in redundant folds of mucosa which, in combination with the muscle thickening and fibrosis, may cause stenosis. The shortening may cause difficulty in mobilization of the colon during operation.

Histologically, in uncomplicated diverticular disease, the presence of extraluminal diverticula lined by mucosa of normal appearance is confirmed. Marked thickening of the circular muscle is also seen.

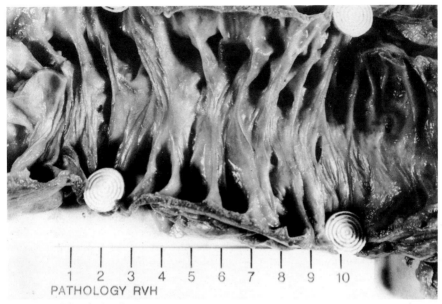

PATHOLOGY RVH

Fig. 4.10. Diverticular disease.

Complications of diverticular disease

Inflammation (acute diverticulitis)

There are two possible explanations for the onset of acute diverticulitis. In the first a faecolith abrades the mucosal lining or obstructs the neck of a diverticulum and an inflammatory response occurs. This results in localized pain and a systemic response to the inflammatory process. Alternatively, an individual diverticulum undergoes mechanical rupture as the primary event with subsequent inflammation which is controlled by surrounding adhesions. The inflammatory process then spreads along the external surface of the bowel to affect other diverticula. This would explain why histological examination often shows the inflammation to be worse in the outer wall of a diverticulum than in the epithelium.

Perforation

Diverticula expand greatly during contraction and segmentation of the colon and some cases of perforation may be due to simple mechanical rupture during contraction. Other cases are caused by a faecolith obstructing the neck of a diverticulum. The consequent inflammation causes necrosis and perforation of the wall. The perforation may be contained, forming an abscess, or it may cause generalized peritonitis.

Obstruction

The inflammatory process of acute diverticulitis heals by fibrosis and the fibrous tissue contracts leading to stenosis of the bowel. Contraction of the taeniae coli and thickening of the circular muscle add to the stenosis. This may cause chronic or acute intestinal obstruction.

Haemorrhage

Haemorrhage usually occurs in diverticulosis rather than in diverticulitis and therefore it may not be preceded by colonic symptoms. Since the diverticula protrude through the colonic wall where blood vessels enter, it is perhaps not surprising that erosion or ulceration of the wall of the diverticulum will lead to massive haemorrhage.

Selective mesenteric angiography performed during bleeding has shown that diverticular disease is not as common a cause of colonic bleeding as was once thought and that lesions such as polyps, vascular ectasia, caecal ulcers and ischaemia account for a large number of cases (Goligher 1984).

Fistula

A pericolic abscess may perforate into the bladder, uterus, vagina, ureter, small intestine or to the skin with the formation of a fistula. Colovesical fistulas are the commonest type. In the UK, approximately 4% of cases of diverticular disease are complicated by colovesical fistula, which typically present with pneumaturia and cystitis. Patients rarely pass urine per rectum as the colonic pressure is higher than the bladder pressure.

Ischaemic Disorders of the Intestine

Ischaemic disorders of the intestine are due to a reduction or absence of intestinal blood flow. This may be caused by arterial disease, venous disease, systemic hypotension or a combination of all three.

Causes of reduced intestinal blood flow

Arterial obstruction

Arterial disease causing intestinal ischaemia is most commonly found in the superior mesenteric artery which must be narrowed considerably before ischaemia will occur. The most common cause of obstruction is atheroma which typically affects the ostium and the first few centimetres while sparing the more peripheral branches. Predisposing factors include hypertension and diabetes mellitus. Sudden occlusion of the superior mesenteric artery may be due to bleeding into an atheromatous plaque, the development of a superimposed thrombus on an atheromatous plaque or an arterial embolism.

Arterial obstruction may also be associated with arteritis (as seen in collagen diseases or after radiation), dissecting aneurysm and tumours which compress or invade the arteries. Angiography may occasionally be complicated by superior mesenteric artery occlusion.

Venous occlusion

Venous occlusion may result from a local cause such as compression within a hernial sac or from an abdominal or pelvic infection. Alternatively, a generalized disease which precipitates intravascular thrombosis, such as polycythaemia, may be associated with venous occlusion. Some cases have been reported in association with the contraceptive pill (Civetta and Kolodny 1970). Venous occlusion may present acutely, in which case it is indistinguishable from other sudden causes of intestinal ischaemia, or with a slow onset of gradually increasing abdominal pain.

Hypotension

Hypotension may occur as a result of severe blood loss or left ventricular failure. Both cause massive splanchnic vaso-constriction. This may cause intestinal ischaemia, especially if there is associated vascular obstruction.

Classification and morphology

Marston (1977) has classified intestinal ischaemia into four main categories.

Acute intestinal failure

Sudden complete occlusion of the superior mesenteric artery rapidly leads to necrosis and gangrene of the small intestine and ascending colon unless the obstruction is relieved by operation. The condition is due to sudden arterial or venous occlusion or to severe hypotension. There may be a history of abdominal angina. Patients present as an abdominal emergency with severe pain and later circulatory collapse.

At the time of operation, the serosal surface of the affected bowel is deep red in colour in the early stages and in the later stages it becomes green or black. The serosal surface loses its sheen, peristalsis ceases and, in arterial occlusion, mesenteric pulsation is absent.

Histological examination shows vascular congestion and necrosis of the intestinal wall.

Ischaemic colitis

Acute ischaemia of the colon most often affects the splenic flexure. Here the blood supply is normally somewhat tenuous, being between the areas supplied by the superior and inferior mesenteric arteries. If the ischaemia is severe, full thickness necrosis ensues and the presentation is as an abdominal emergency characterized by severe left sided abdominal pain. In less severe cases, or transient cases, there is partial thickness necrosis and presentation is with colicky abdominal pain and bloody diarrhoea.

In severe cases with full thickness necrosis, the pathology is similar to that described under acute intestinal failure.

In less severe cases, the serosal surface of the colon may show red patches or it may be normal. Gross inspection of the mucosal surface shows it to be haemorrhagic and ulcerated. Between the ulcerated areas, oedema causes submucosal swelling which causes the thumb-printing sign that may be observed on abdominal radiographs. Altered blood is often present in the lumen and necrosis of the mucosa causes a grey slough which forms a pseudomembrane.

If the bowel remains viable, it enters a reparative phase. Colonoscopy at this stage shows granulation tissue and the appearance may resemble Crohn's disease.

Eventually, an ischaemic stricture with thickening of the colonic wall and mucosal ulceration results. This may also resemble Crohn's disease.

Histologically, in the acute stage the mucosa and submucosa show oedema, vascular congestion and haemorrhage. Necrosis of the epithelium is at first focal and then widespread with ulceration (*see Fig.* 4.11). Later, an inflammatory reaction is seen and fibrin thrombi are characteristically present in the mucosal and submucosal capillaries. The thickness of the colonic wall affected depends on the severity of the ischaemia.

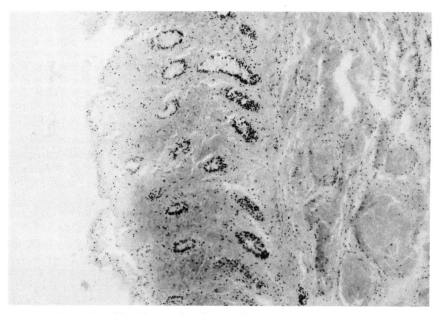

Fig. 4.11. Ischaemic colitis with necrosis and congestion of the mucosa. (H and E × 75)

In the reparative phase, the mucosa is replaced by granulation tissue which is gradually covered by regenerating epithelium. Haemosiderin laden macrophages are numerous and help to distinguish ischaemia from Crohn's disease.

At the stage of ischaemic stricture, the granulation tissue is organized by fibrosis, although mucosal ulceration may still be present. Again, the histological appearance may resemble Crohn's disease.

Chronic intestinal ischaemia

This causes the symptoms of abdominal angina which is characterized by colicky abdominal pain occurring about thirty minutes after eating. It is usually ascribed to atheroma of the superior mesenteric artery. A large post-mortem study of the mesenteric arteries, however, demonstrated that although mild degrees of stenosis were common, the incidence of critical stenosis was rare and no correlation between the degree of stenosis and previous gastrointestinal symptoms could be found. The authors concluded that the radiological demonstration of a stenosed visceral artery was of dubious clinical significance (Croft *et al.* 1981).

Focal ischaemia of the small bowel

A relatively small area of the small bowel may be subject to ischaemia as in a strangulated hernia or after pelvic irradiation. Depending on the severity and the speed of onset, the ischaemia may resolve or cause acute necrosis or produce a stricture.

Vascular Abnormalities

Haemangiomas

Haemangiomas of the intestine may be single or multiple and may occur in both the small and large bowel. Some cases are associated with haemangiomas outside the gastrointestinal tract as in hereditary telangiectasia (Rendu–Weber–Osler disease). They may present with gastrointestinal haemorrhage, anaemia, obstruction or intussusception and are considered to be developmental in origin.

Cavernous haemangiomas may be large and extend circumferentially around the bowel wall, or may be small, polypoid masses projecting into the bowel lumen. Capillary haemangiomas consist of masses of capillaries in the submucosa and are normally found in the small bowel; they may also project into the lumen.

Haemangiomas may be the cause of obscure gastrointestinal bleeding in patients with negative barium radiographs. Angiography or labelled red cell scintiscanning may be required to reveal the site of the lesion. In some cases phleboliths are seen on plain abdominal radiographs.

Angiodysplasia

Angiodysplasia is a condition in which small vascular lesions, consisting of dilated mucosal and submucosal vessels, occur in the bowel. Most commonly they are found in the caecum and ascending colon of elderly patients, although they have also been reported in the small bowel, stomach and left colon. Sometimes they occur in young patients. They are the cause of many cases of obscure gastrointestinal haemorrhage. The most likely cause of angiodysplasia is intermittent chronic partial obstruction of veins as they pass outwards through the muscular coat of the colon. The obstruction causes a rise in pressure, secondary dilatation and eventually degenerative structural abnormalities in the mucosal and submucosal vessels. The tension in the colonic wall is greatest in the caecum (law of Laplace—*see* p. 123) and thus venous obstruction occurs principally in this region, explaining the predilection of angiodysplasia for the caecum.

Examination of colons at autopsy has shown that various degrees of angiodysplasia are common findings in the elderly and therefore the clinical demonstration of angiodysplasia in an individual elderly patient with rectal bleeding is not necessarily proof that it is the site of the bleeding (Boley *et al.* 1977).

Diagnosis is by angiography, in which tortuous early filling arteries, vascular lakes and early filling veins are seen. At colonoscopy, the lesions appear as small cherry-red areas, 2–5 mm in diameter. Each lesion has a large central vessel and radiating peripheral vessels.

In order to confirm the diagnosis after resection, Rees and Wright (1984) suggest that the specimens should be sent fresh to the laboratory with the vascular pedicle marked. The vessels should then be flushed with heparin and saline and injected with a barium–gelatin mixture and fixed in formalin for 24 hours. The bowel is opened and the mucosa examined with a dissecting microscope. The lesions are seen most commonly on the antimesenteric border opposite the ileocaecal valve.

Microscopically, dilated vessels are seen in the submucosa and mucosa. In advanced lesions, there is atrophy of the mucosal glands and in some cases only a single layer of endothelial cells separates the vessels from the caecal lumen.

Small lesions causing chronic bleeding may be treated by electrocoagulation during colonoscopy. More severe bleeding requires right hemicolectomy. Rebleeding after operation for angiodysplasia is well recognized. It may be due to missed pathology at the original operation, inadequate resection of the angiodysplasia or to the formation of new angiodysplasia.

Solitary Rectal Ulcer Syndrome

Although the term solitary rectal ulcer has been used extensively it can be misleading in that the lesion is not necessarily ulcerated or single. It is a localized abnormality of the rectum, with specific histological features, seen in younger patients (usually under 40 years of age). Of the 40 patients reported by Ford *et al.* (1983), rectal bleeding and passage of mucus was present in 39. Difficulty in the initiation of defaecation was also very common.

The aetiology of the condition is not fully understood, although trauma secondary to a partial rectal prolapse is implicated in most cases. Martin *et al.* (1981) recorded varying degrees of prolapse, from complete rectal prolapse to bulging of the anterior rectal wall, in 91% of their 51 cases. In their series, the lesions were always found on the redundant migratory part of the rectal wall. Identical histological abnormalities have been found in cases of rectal prolapse, further suggesting that prolapse and subsequent trauma are important in the pathogenesis. In the solitary rectal ulcer syndrome, electromyographic studies have shown that the normal relaxation of the puborectalis muscle which occurs during defaecation, is replaced by overactivity of the muscle. This may explain the difficulty with defaecation. Although some patients practise insertion of the finger into the rectum to aid defaecation, there is no definite evidence that this is the primary cause and this theory is now discredited.

Macroscopically, the lesion is seen on sigmoidoscopy, usually at about 7–10 cm from the anal verge on the anterior wall of the rectum. In the study of Ford *et al.* (1983), ulceration was seen in 27 out of 40 patients, the remaining 13 having erythematous areas in the mucosa or a nodular mucosa.

Microscopically, the typical feature is the presence of smooth muscle fibres extending upwards from a thickened muscularis mucosa into the lamina propria with associated fibrosis (*see Fig.* 4.12). This may be present with or without ulceration of the mucosa. At the edge of any ulcerated area, the colonic epithelium tends to become misplaced into the submucosa and this appearance may be confused with invasive carcinoma.

Follow-up of patients has shown that symptoms can persist even after the ulcer has healed. Excision of the lesion is usually followed by recurrence. Regulation of bowel habit helps a few patients and Martin *et al.* (1982) reported some success with an Ivalon sponge rectopexy to remedy the prolapse.

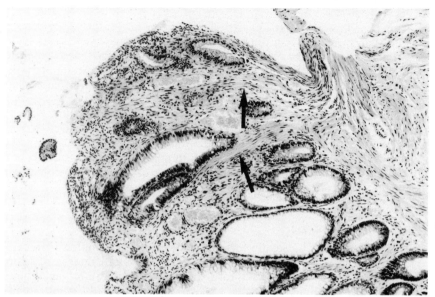

Fig. 4.12. Solitary rectal ulcer. Note the bands of smooth muscle rising upwards from the muscularis mucosa (arrows). (H and E × 75)

Small Bowel Tumours

Primary tumours of the small bowel are rare and are seen in only 0·5% of autopsies.

The common benign tumours are adenoma, leiomyoma and lipoma. They are often incidental findings.

The relative frequency of malignant tumours depends upon factors such as whether tumours of the duodenum are included and whether carcinoids are considered malignant. Perzin *et al.* (1983) quote the following figures: adenocarcinoma (including those of the ampulla of Vater) 59%, lymphoma 20%, carcinoid 15%, leiomyosarcoma 6%.

Benign small bowel tumours

Adenomas

Small bowel adenomas have the same gross and histological features as large bowel adenomas. They occur with decreasing frequency from the duodenum to the ileum. Patients with familial polyposis coli or Gardner's syndrome (*see* p. 117) may develop multiple small bowel adenomas and carcinomas. As with colonic adenomas, small bowel adenomas are premalignant and malignant change is associated with the villous, rather than the tubular pattern.

Leiomyomas

There may be considerable difficulty in distinguishing benign from malignant smooth muscle tumours and therefore both are discussed together under the heading 'smooth muscle tumours' (*see* p. 111).

Peutz–Jeghers polyps

Peutz–Jeghers polyps are hamartomas rather than true neoplasms. They occur as part of the Peutz–Jeghers syndrome which consists of pigmented spots in the mucous membrane of the oral cavity and skin together with multiple hamartomatous polyps of the gastrointestinal tract. The commonest sites for polyp formation are the jejunum and ileum although they can also occur in the stomach and large bowel. Inheritance is autosomal dominant.

Macroscopically, they appear as lobulated polyps, either sessile or occasionally pedunculated. They do not have the smooth surface of juvenile polyps (*see* p. 112).

Microscopically, there is proliferation and branching of the muscularis mucosa. The covering epithelium is normal and non-dysplastic. Morson and Dawson (1979) believe the polyps represent a malformation of the muscularis mucosa. Malignant change has been described but the risk is very small.

Carcinoma of the small bowel

Carcinomas of the small bowel are forty to sixty times less common than carcinomas of the large bowel. Perzin and Bridge (1981) found evidence of a pre-existing adenoma in 25% of their 130 cases and suggested that most small bowel carcinomas arise in adenomas. Patients with coeliac disease and Crohn's disease have an increased risk of developing adenocarcinoma. Many patients present with partial or complete small bowel obstruction but chronic non-specific abdominal pain and anaemia are also very common.

Macroscopically the common type is annular and the rest are polypoid.

Microscopically the appearances are similar to other carcinomas of the gastrointestinal tract. The presence of lymph node metastases is the most important prognostic feature.

Endocrine tumours of the small intestine

The endocrine cells of the intestine are triangular in shape and have a clear or granular cytoplasm. They are wedged between the surface epithelial cells and the basement membrane and are distributed throughout the gastrointestinal tract. They share features in common with certain other cells of the body, in particular the C cells of the thyroid, the pancreatic islet cells, the chromaffin cells of the adrenal medulla and some cells in the pituitary, skin, bronchi and sympathetic ganglia, etc. These cells have been termed APUD cells (*A*mine *P*recursor *U*ptake and *D*ecarboxylation), although this term is not always appropriate since some of them do not have the capacity for amine precursor uptake and decarboxylation. Originally all these cells were considered to be of neural crest origin, but there is now strong evidence that the gut endocrine cells are endodermal in origin.

An endocrine cell of the gut secretes predominantly either an amine such as 5-hydroxytryptamine (5HT) or a polypeptide hormone such as gastrin or somatostatin. The individual cells can be identified by the shape of the secretory granules on electron microscopy and by immunohistochemistry, in which antisera to the individual hormones are used in the staining of histological sections.

The gut endocrine cells can be divided according to their silver staining characteristics. The argentaffin reaction is a silver staining process which detects only those granules containing 5HT. Tumours of these cells are therefore known as argentaffinomas or carcinoid tumours. The argyrophil reaction is a different silver staining technique which stains nearly all gut endocrine cells, including the 5HT containing cells.

Carcinoid tumours (argentaffinomas)

The common site for small bowel carcinoids is the distal ileum. Appendiceal carcinoids are dealt with separately on p. 128. All small bowel carcinoids are of low grade malignancy as they have the potential to metastasize. They present as an incidental finding at laparotomy, as a result of local complications or as a consequence of the effect of their secretory products.

Local complications include intussusception, haemorrhage and small bowel obstruction, which is likely to be due to kinking of the bowel associated with local thickening of the mesentery and muscularis propria. Annular constricting carcinoids are uncommon.

Most of these tumours are functional and secrete several amines, especially 5HT, but also 5-hydroxytryptophan, histamine and bradykinin. 5HT is degraded in the urine to 5-hydroxyindoleacetic acid (5HIAA) which can be detected in the urine and can be used for diagnostic purposes. These amines may have local effects on the small bowel muscle causing diarrhoea. The carcinoid syndrome occurs when the amount of amine secretion overwhelms the body's ability to degrade it. This usually occurs only when liver metastases are present because of the large tumour bulk and because the amines are then secreted into the systemic system, thus bypassing the liver where most degradation takes place.

The carcinoid syndrome is characterized by paroxysms of flushing, wheezing and diarrhoea. Pulmonary stenosis and tricuspid insufficiency may develop because of the effects in the right heart (see p. 345). 5HT appears to be responsible for the diarrhoea. The cause of the flushing is unknown, although bradykinin has been incriminated.

Grossly carcinoid tumours appear as nodular growths in the mucosa and submucosa. They may be ulcerated. On cut section they have two characteristic features: they are yellow and the thickened muscularis propria is clearly seen traversing the tumour (see Fig. 4.13). Ischaemia or even infarction of the surrounding small bowel may be seen due to the changes in mesenteric blood vessels (see below).

Four histological types of endocrine tumours have been described (see p. 212). Small bowel carcinoids are characteristically type A (insular pattern), consisting of solid islands of closely packed uniform cells with darkly staining nuclei. Cords of cells are seen between the islands (see Fig. 4.14). The cytoplasm usually contains argentaffin positive granules because of the contained 5HT. The muscle hypertrophy, seen macroscopically, is confirmed. Thickening of mesenteric blood vessels, probably the result of amine secretion, may also be seen. This may lead to ischaemic changes in the surrounding bowel.

Carcinoid tumours spread into the mesentery causing thickening and fibrosis and angulation of the bowel. They also spread via the blood stream to the liver and lungs. Metastases usually do not show the yellow appearance.

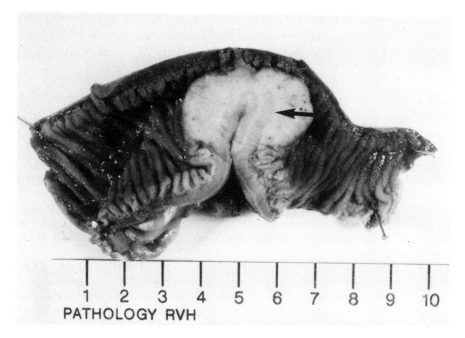

PATHOLOGY RVH

Fig. 4.13. Carcinoid tumour of ileum. Note the kinking of the bowel wall and the characteristic thickening of the muscular layer seen actually within the tumour (arrow).

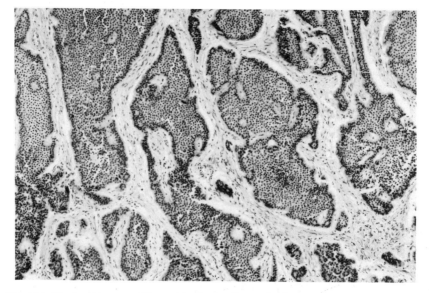

Fig. 4.14. Carcinoid tumour of ileum. Islands of uniform cells. (H and E × 30)

Other endocrine cell tumours

Tumours which contain and/or secrete polypeptide hormones, such as gastrin, enteroglucagon, ACTH and somatostatin, have been described in the midgut, although they are exceedingly rare compared with carcinoids.

Small bowel lymphomas

The distinction between primary and secondary small bowel lymphomas is difficult. Wright and Isaacson (1983) define primary small bowel lymphomas as 'those presenting in the gastrointestinal tract necessitating the direction of diagnostic investigation and treatment to that site'.

Morson and Dawson (1979) divide primary small bowel lymphomas into those with and those without preceding abnormalities.

Lymphomas arising without pre-existing abnormalities arise in the mucosal lymphoid nodules of the gut which are most frequent in the terminal ileum. The tumour may present with intussusception, obstruction, perforation or haemorrhage. Macroscopically, they appear either as rubbery, polypoid masses with secondary ulceration, or as plaque-like thickenings due to infiltration of the muscle coat of the bowel. This latter type occasionally may be confused with Crohn's disease or tuberculosis of the terminal ileum. If lymphoma is found at laparotomy, the surgeon should carry out a lymph node and liver biopsy to aid staging.

Microscopically, the majority are follicle central cell lymphomas (*see* p. 432) Fissuring and ulceration are common. The lymphoma cells rarely form follicular patterns but appear more commonly as sheets of monotonous cells. A diagnostic feature of all gut lymphomas is the invasion of epithelial glands by the tumour cells.

Small bowel lymphomas may also arise in a preceding abnormality. Alpha chain disease and multiple lymphomatous polyposis both predispose to lymphoma. Coeliac disease predisposes to a particular type of lymphoma known as malignant histiocytosis of the intestine. Patients are usually over 50 years of age and the onset of the lymphoma may be the primary indication of the coeliac disease. Presenting features include abdominal pain, weight loss and recurrent steatorrhoea while still on a gluten-free diet.

Malignant histiocytosis arises in the macrophages of the intestine. Macroscopically, the tumours appear as single or multiple circumscribed nodules or ulcers. Histologically, they consist of masses of malignant histiocytes which, in well differentiated cases, have characteristically indented nuclei and abundant cytoplasm.

Smooth muscle tumours

These arise from the muscularis propria or, less commonly, from the muscularis mucosa. They are often incidental findings but they may produce obstruction, bleeding and intussusception. The behaviour of smooth muscle tumours is difficult to predict and therefore Morson and Dawson (1979) use 'leiomyomatous tumours' as a general term rather than separating them into benign leiomyomas and malignant leiomyosarcomas.

Macroscopically they appear as circumscribed tumours which may project into the lumen and eventually become pedunculated. Growth onto the serosal surface can produce a dumb-bell appearance. The cut surface is typically white or grey with a whorled appearance. Microscopically bundles of smooth muscle cells are seen. Histologically, benign tumours may show considerable pleomorphism and malignant tumours may appear innocuous. Indications of malignancy are a large size (greater than 5 cm in diameter), an infiltrating edge and a high mitotic rate. Some authorities believe that the presence of metastases is the only absolute indication of malignancy.

Colonic Polyps

A polyp is a circumscribed lesion which projects above the surrounding mucous membrane. It may or may not have a stalk. In the colon polyps can be hamartomatous, metaplastic, inflammatory or neoplastic. Benign non-epithelial tumours such as lipomas and neuromas may also present as polyps.

Hamartomatous polyps

Hamartomas are disorders of growth and consist of an abnormal mixture of those tissues normally found in the organ concerned. They are not true neoplasms. The two hamartomas encountered in the colon are Peutz–Jeghers polyps (discussed on p. 108) and juvenile polyps.

Juvenile polyps

These occur in children and less often in adolescents with a peak age incidence of 5 years. They are usually solitary (85%) and are commonly sited in the rectosigmoid region (85%). They usually present with bleeding. Auto-amputation with passage of the polyp per rectum occasionally occurs. Grossly, they have a red, smooth surface and on cut section, cystic dilated glands may be seen.

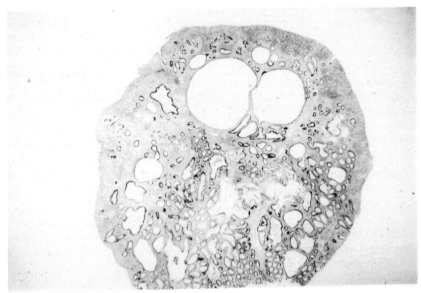

Fig. 4.15. Low power view of a juvenile polyp. (H and E × 7)

Microscopically, the surface is ulcerated and the lesion consists of cystic dilated glands lying in an excess of inflamed lamina propria (*see Fig.* 4.15). The cells lining the glands are not dysplastic. The polyp has no malignant potential.

Juvenile polyposis is becoming increasingly recognized as a syndrome. Cases which present in infancy have large collections of juvenile polyps in the colon, stomach and small intestine. Haemorrhage or intussusception may be fatal. There is no family history. Cases presenting in older children may or may not have a family history and some have colonic polyps only. Juvenile polyposis may be associated with an increased incidence of gastrointestinal malignancy which generally does not arise in the polyps themselves. Prophylactic removal, therefore, is not an effective measure against the onset of malignancy.

Metaplastic polyps

These polyps are very frequently observed during lower gastrointestinal endoscopy. They are said to be present in 75% of people aged over 40 years. They appear as sessile polyps, 2–5 mm in diameter, often on the tips of mucosal folds. They have a similar, or slightly redder colour, than the surrounding mucosa. Histologically, they consist of a focal enlargement of crypts with crowding of cells, although the normal parallel orientation of the crypts is maintained. Towards the mouths of the crypts the epithelium is characteristically serrated.

Metaplastic polyps are unrelated to adenomatous or neoplastic polyps and are benign.

Inflammatory polyps

Included in this section are the inflammatory polyps seen in inflammatory bowel disease which were discussed on p. 90 and inflammatory polyps of the rectum (benign lymphoid polyps) which are considered on p. 123.

Neoplastic polyps

The term adenoma is used to describe a neoplastic polyp. Morson and Dawson (1979) define an adenoma as 'a sharply demarcated circumscribed elevation of dysplastic epithelium which is usually small but can cover a large surface area and may or may not have a stalk or pedicle'. It is important to realize that the proliferating epithelium is abnormal, i.e. dysplastic. Adenomas are classified as tubular, villous and tubulo-villous according to their histological appearance.

The incidence of colonic adenomas varies depending on the exact definition of a polyp. One American autopsy study of 1000 colonic specimens found polyps in 35% overall, ranging from 14·3% in the 20–29 year age group to 44·4% in those aged 80 years or more. They were slightly more common in males than in females (Arminski and McLean 1964).

Colonic adenomas tend to be commonest in those countries with a high incidence of colonic cancer, although this correlation is strong only when large polyps are considered.

Gillespie *et al.* (1979) reported the St Mark's Hospital experience of 1049 colonic adenomas removed during colonoscopy from 620 patients. The sigmoid and descending colon were the commonest sites, accounting for 47·5% and 21·5%

respectively; 20% were in the transverse colon and the remainder were more or less equally distributed throughout the caecum, ascending colon, hepatic and splenic flexures and rectum. Half were under 1 cm in diameter, one-third were between 1 and 2 cm in diameter and the remainder (17·3%) were over 2 cm.

Tubular adenomas tend to be lobulated, spherical, pedunculated and small, whereas villous tumours tend to be large and sessile with fronds covering part of the colonic mucosa. Mixed patterns are seen in tubulovillous adenomas (*see Fig.* 4.16).

In the series of Gillespie *et al.* (1979), about three-quarters were tubular, one-fifth were tubulo-villous and less than 5% were purely villous. Tubular adenomas consist of closely packed epithelial tubules, separated from each other by lamina propria. Tubules are often cut in cross-section and they may be branched and have cystic dilatations. The villous pattern consists of fingers of lamina propria covered with dysplastic epithelium. A mixture of these patterns is seen in the tubulo-villous adenoma (*see Fig.* 4.17).

The overlying dysplastic epithelium which is seen in all types of colonic adenomas shows hyperchromatic, pleomorphic crowded nuclei with an increased mitotic rate. The dysplasia may be mild, moderate or severe and different grades can be seen in one adenoma. Severe dysplasia is associated with irregular branching and budding of the glands. Dysplasia tends to be more severe in villous adenomas than in tubular adenomas.

The muscularis mucosa separates the proliferating epithelium from the stalk of the polyp and absence of malignant epithelial elements from the stalk ensures that the lesion is non-invasive, although in some cases pseudocarcinomatous invasion of the stalk is seen, possibly as a result of twisting or haemorrhage.

Malignancy arising in adenomas

Most authorities now accept the concept that the vast majority of colonic carcinomas arise in pre-existing colonic adenomas. The evidence for this so-called 'adenoma–carcinoma sequence' is as follows (Morson and Dawson 1979):

1. One-third of all colonic specimens resected for cancer contain polyps. The presence of adenomas in the resected specimen indicates a greater likelihood of developing a second carcinoma (metachronous carcinoma).
2. Seventy-five per cent of patients with two colonic tumours (synchronous carcinomas) have associated polyps.
3. Malignant change is commonly seen in an otherwise benign adenoma.
4. Contiguous, benign, adenomatous tissue is much more likely to be seen in early rather than late carcinomas, suggesting that as the carcinoma grows progressively, more of the adenoma is destroyed.
5. Distribution of adenomas throughout the colon is roughly similar to that of carcinomas.

In order to make a diagnosis of malignancy in a colonic polyp, it is necessary to demonstrate that malignant epithelial cells (as distinct from pseudoinvasion) have traversed the muscularis mucosa into the stalk. Severe dysplasia while confined to the mucosa has very little potential for metastasis because lymphatics very rarely cross the muscularis mucosa into the mucosa.

The most important indicator of the malignant potential of an adenoma is its

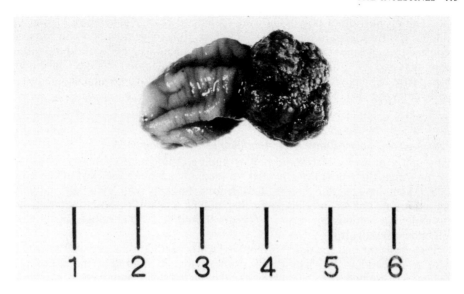

Fig. 4.16. Polyp removed by colonoscopic snare. Histology showed a tubulo-villous adenoma.

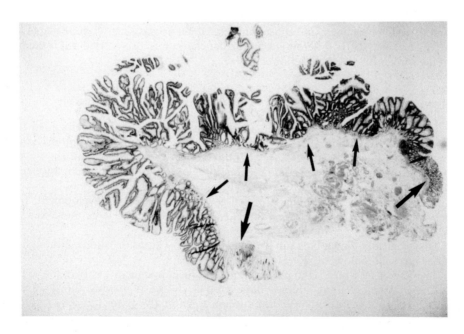

Fig. 4.17. Tubulo-villous adenoma. Note the strip of normal colonic mucosa at either end (large arrows). None of the dysplastic glands have breached the muscularis mucosa which can be seen in places as a faint line (small arrows). (H and E × 7)

size. The proportion of polyps showing malignant change in relation to size is as follows: less than 1 cm in diameter 1%; 1–2 cm 10%; over 2 cm 50%. In the series reported by Gillespie *et al.* (1979) 18% of villous adenomas, 5·8% of tubulo-villous adenomas and 2·2% of tubular adenomas showed malignant change. This finding may partly be explained by the larger size of villous adenomas. The chances of malignancy are also increased with increasing grades of dysplasia.

Pathological considerations in the treatment of colonic polyps

Although a minority of colonic polyps undergo malignant change, it is usually accepted that the risk is large enough to recommend snare removal of the polyp unless there are exceptional contraindications. Patients who have had one polyp excised are at risk of developing further polyps and follow-up is required. It is probable that colonoscopy every 2–3 years should be done although this policy is still under investigation.

It is important that the polyp is removed whole so that it may be well orientated prior to embedding for histological examination in order that the anatomy is maintained and the extent of any invasion of the stalk can be accurately assessed.

If malignant change is diagnosed in a colonic polyp, the further management is debatable. St Mark's Hospital carry out no further treatment if excision of the polyp is complete and the contained carcinoma is moderately or well differentiated. If the carcinoma is poorly differentiated, however, further resection is carried out regardless of whether the excision was complete or incomplete. This policy is based on the fact that colonic carcinomas which are confined to the submucosa (i.e. the core of the polyp) have only a one in ten chance of having lymph node metastases, and those tumours which do have lymph node metastases are invariably poorly differentiated. Further excision is also carried out if the base of the stalk is involved by tumour.

Familial polyposis coli

This is an inherited autosomal dominant disease in which multiple polyps (by definition, over 100) arise in the colon in early adult life. Presenting symptoms consist of the passage of diarrhoea, mucus and blood. Recent work has shown that occasionally there are associated adenomatous polyps in the stomach, duodenum or small bowel which also have a propensity to become malignant.

Macroscopically, the polyps are seen at different stages of development, from very small to large. The average number is 1000 and they tend to be more common in the distal colon.

Histologically, the polyps can be tubular, tubulo-villous or villous, although the latter are uncommon.

The aim of treatment is to prevent colonic cancer arising not only in the patient but also in relatives as siblings have a 50% chance of having the disease. If untreated, 10% of patients will develop cancer within five years and 20% within 20 years of onset. Eventual development of cancer is said to be invariable in all untreated patients. Surveillance of the siblings of patients should start at about 14 years of age.

Gardner's syndrome

In this syndrome familial polyposis coli is associated with extraintestinal manifestations. It is not yet clear whether this syndrome is distinct from the typical polyposis coli described above. The extraintestinal manifestations include osteomas, especially of the skull, desmoid tumours of the abdominal wall and mesentery, lipomas, fibromas and epidermoid cysts. Periampullary carcinomas also occur with an increased incidence. These patients have the same risk of developing colonic cancers as those with simple polyposis coli. Panoramic radiographs of the jaws are a useful screening test to detect the presence of osteomas in relatives of patients (Jarvinen *et al.* 1982).

Turcot's syndrome

In this rare syndrome, which has an autosomal recessive inheritance, colonic polyposis is associated with central nervous system malignancy.

Colorectal Cancer

The essential criterion for the diagnosis of colorectal cancer is the presence of malignant glands or cells which have infiltrated across the muscularis mucosa into the submucosa. When limited to the mucosal side of the muscularis mucosa, the lesion is referred to as severe dysplasia and it has virtually no potential to metastasize as lymphatics do not (or at least very rarely) cross the muscularis mucosa into the mucosa. This feature is in marked contrast to the stomach where lymphatics do cross the muscularis mucosa and the entity of intramucosal carcinoma does exist. Biopsy of colorectal tumours must, therefore, be sufficiently adequate to include the muscularis mucosa and some submucosa.

Epidemiology

Colorectal cancer is second only to carcinoma of the bronchus as the commonest cause of death from malignant disease in the UK. Each year there are 20 000 new cases in England and Wales and 16 000 deaths (colon 10 000; rectum 6000). Colonic and rectal cancers have different sex distributions with a slight female predominance for the colon and a marked male predominance for the rectum. Colorectal cancer is three times more common in first degree relatives of affected patients than in the general population. This may be partly due to environmental influences as spouses of patients with colorectal cancer also have an increased incidence.

The geographical distribution points strongly to the importance of environmental factors. Colorectal cancer is common in wealthy countries (except Japan) and much less common in Africa and Asia. Within Third World countries, those patients who do develop colorectal cancer tend to be in high socio-economic groups, while in Japan colorectal cancer patients are those who have adopted a Western type of diet. Migrant populations to high risk areas, such as the Japanese to Hawaii, acquire a high incidence, often within their lifetimes. The reason for this wide geographical variation is thought to be dietary.

Aetiology and pathogenesis

The aetiology of colorectal cancer has been reviewed by Stubbs (1983). He identifies three theories which have been postulated to date.

1. *Fibre hypothesis.* This is championed by Burkitt who suggests that a large intake of dietary fibre reduces intestinal transit time so that carcinogens spend less time in contact with the bowel wall and bacteria have less time in which to produce carcinogens. Three problems have arisen with this theory. Firstly, several studies have shown no decrease in transit time with increased fibre in the diet. Secondly, although Modan *et al.* (1975) did report an association between low dietary fibre and colorectal cancer, other studies have found no association. Thirdly, bran has no protective effect against experimentally induced colorectal cancer in rats.

2. *Animal fat hypothesis.* The geographical distribution of colorectal cancer has led to the implication of animal fats in the aetiology as these tend to be eaten in higher income areas. A correlation between the incidence of colorectal cancer and the per capita intake of animal fats has been observed and it is suggested that increased dietary fat leads to an increased concentration of bile acids in the faeces. The bile acid deoxycholic acid has a similar structure to the carcinogen methylcholanthrene and dehydrogenation of the steroid nucleus of deoxycholic acid could, theoretically, produce methylcholanthrene. The anaerobic bacterium *Clostridium paraputrificum* is capable of this dehydrogenation and has been termed a nuclear dehydrogenating clostridium (NDC). Anaerobic organisms and degraded bile acids are more common in faeces in high risk areas, thus suggesting that bacteria do indeed produce carcinogens from bile acids in the colon.

3. *Vegetable hypothesis.* There is evidence that colorectal cancer is less common in those who eat cabbage, brussel sprouts and other similar vegetables. These vegetables contain indoles which induce activity of the enzyme aryl-hydrocarbon hydroxylase which is known to degrade noxious environmental chemicals.

As discussed on p. 114, most, if not all, colorectal cancers are believed to arise from pre-existing polyps. Hill *et al.* (1978) have combined the epidemiological data and the adenoma–carcinoma sequence to suggest that three different, as yet unidentified, environmental substances are responsible for (1) adenoma development, (2) adenoma growth, and (3) carcinomatous change in a large adenoma.

The association between colorectal cancer and familial polyposis coli, ulcerative colitis and Crohn's disease is discussed elsewhere. There is also some evidence that patients who have had a previous cholecystectomy have an increased risk of developing right-sided colonic cancer (Turnbull *et al.* 1981) although this is not yet generally accepted. The explanation could be the carcinogenic effect of secondary bile acids which are present in increased concentration after cholecystectomy.

Patients with a previous ureterosigmoidostomy have an increased incidence of colorectal cancer in the region of the anastomosis, possibly as a result of the formation of N-nitroso compounds. It has been recommended that annual sigmoidoscopy or limited barium studies should be performed five years after this operation (Thompson *et al.* 1979).

Morphology

Half of all colorectal cancers occur in the rectum and rectosigmoid areas; 25% occur in the sigmoid; the remaining 25% are equally distributed between the caecum, ascending, transverse and descending colon (Morson and Dawson 1979). Up to three-quarters of these tumours are, therefore, within reach of the rigid sigmoidoscope if introduced to the full length. In recent years, this left-sided dominance has reduced with relatively more occurring in the right colon. Between 2–5% of patients have more than one colorectal cancer (synchronous tumours). Patients who have had one colorectal cancer resected have a 3–5% chance of developing another subsequent colorectal tumour (metachronous tumours). These figures justify investigation of the entire large bowel in any patient presenting with a rectal cancer.

Colorectal cancers tend to be ulcerating and infiltrating; less commonly they are polypoid in type (*see Fig.* 4.18). Although all are thought to arise in pre-existing adenomas, the adenoma may be completely destroyed and not evident. The polypoid form tends not to be as invasive as the ulcerating/infiltrating type and has a better prognosis. The ulcerating/infiltrating type shows the typical raised everted irregular edges and necrotic centre of a malignant ulcer. When it grows around the circumference of the colon it forms an annular, constricting cancer, liable to cause intestinal obstruction. This is more common in left-sided cancers. Occasionally much mucin production gives a gelatinous or colloid appearance. A linitis plastica pattern is occasionally seen in the rectum, but when it does occur it is more likely to be due to a secondary carcinoma from the stomach.

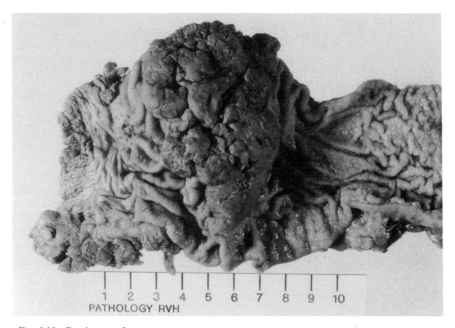

Fig. 4.18. Carcinoma of rectum.

Histologically, the vast majority of colorectal cancers are adenocarcinomas (*see Fig.* 4.19). They may be well differentiated (good glandular formation 20%), moderately well differentiated (some gland formation 60%), or poorly differentiated (no gland formation 20%). The epithelial cells lining the glands show nuclear stratification, pleomorphism, hyperchromasia and a high mitotic rate. Extensive intramural spread beyond the macroscopic limit is unusual.

Squamous carcinoma and adenosquamous carcinomas are rare in the colon although squamous metaplasia in an adenocarcinoma is seen more commonly.

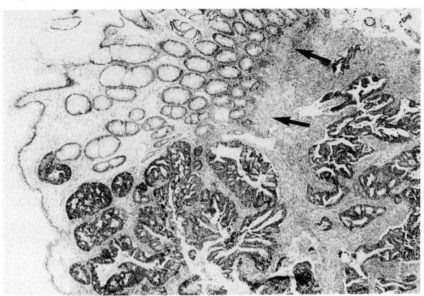

Fig. 4.19. Rectal biopsy. Carcinoma below and normal mucosa above. A definite diagnosis of carcinoma can be made since invasion is seen across the muscularis mucosa (the muscularis mucosa is arrowed). (H and E × 75)

Spread

Direct spread takes place laterally through the colonic wall, especially at points where blood vessels enter. Longitudinal spread is not a marked feature and distal intramural spread of more than 1 cm beyond the gross margins of the tumour is unusual (Williams 1984). Reduction of the traditional 5 cm distal margin has thus facilitated low anterior resections with sphincter preservation for rectal cancer. The peritoneum provides a tough defence but once penetrated, peritoneal dissemination may occur. The ovaries are likely to be involved in these cases (Krukenberg tumours). Lymphatic spread takes place in a contiguous fashion, that is, if one node is involved all the intervening nodes between it and the tumour are also involved. If lymphatic obstruction occurs, retrograde metastases may occur. Vascular spread is associated with hepatic metastases.

A characteristic feature of colorectal cancer is the occasional development of implantation metastases. Malignant cells shed from a tumour can implant at a distant ulcerated site, e.g. in an anal fistula, a haemorrhoidectomy wound or in an abdominal incision after operation. Implantation may be responsible for some suture line recurrences, although most of these are due to inadequate excision.

Staging and Prognosis

Up to half of patients with colorectal cancer are cured by appropriate surgical resection alone.

Prognosis depends to a large extent on staging. The staging of colorectal cancer is based on the Dukes classification which, unfortunately, is confusing due to many subsequent modifications. Originally, Dukes described three stages (*see Fig.* 4.20). A—tumour spread as far as, but not through, the muscularis propria; B—tumour spread through the bowel wall into perirectal tissues; C—those with lymph node involvement. Dukes himself later divided his group C into C_1 (only local lymph nodes involved) and C_2 (mesenteric nodes involved at the level of ligation of the vascular pedicle). A significant modification of the Dukes classification was made by Astler and Coller (1954) (*see also Fig.* 4.20). A—intramucosal only; B_1—tumour into, but not beyond, the muscularis propria; B_2—spread through the wall into peritoneal tissue; C_1—lymph nodes involved but tumour confined to bowel wall; C_2—lymph nodes involved and tumour through bowel wall. It is important to note that Astler and Coller grade A is not an invasive carcinoma, and that their C_1 and C_2 stages are different from Dukes' own modification of stage C into C_1 and C_2.

DUKES (Original Classification)

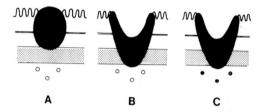

A   B   C

ASTLER/COLLER MODIFICATION

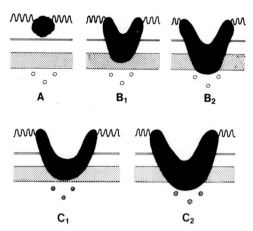

A B_1 B_2

C_1 C_2

Fig. 4.20. Staging of carcinoma of the rectum by the Dukes Original Classification and by the Astler/Coller Modification. Unshaded circles represent uninvolved lymph nodes and shaded circles represent involved lymph nodes.

Wood *et al.* (1981) have clearly shown that local extramural spread is of major prognostic importance.

Recently, Phillips *et al.* (1984) in a study of 2518 patients who had undergone curative surgery for colorectal cancer showed that histological grade, lymph node status and vascular invasion all contributed independently to prognosis within each Dukes' stage, although they were to some extent inter-related.

HISTOLOGICAL GRADE: Those tumours which are poorly differentiated tend to have a more advanced Dukes' stage than those which are well differentiated. However, even after stratifying for Dukes' stage, poorly differentiated tumours still have a worse prognosis than do moderately or well differentiated tumours, each of which appear to have equal prognosis.

LYMPH NODE STATUS: The presence of involved lymph nodes significantly worsens prognosis. This is particularly so if more than four nodes are involved or if the apical node at the site of vascular ligation is involved.

VASCULAR INVASION: Talbot *et al.* (1980) found venous invasion in 53% of their cases. Invasion of extramural veins, particularly those with a thick wall, considerably worsened the prognosis. Venous invasion is also associated with a higher incidence of hepatic metastases, although these are not invariable. Invasion of submucosal intramural veins does not appear to affect prognosis.

Venous invasion parallels local spread and lymph node involvement, although it appears to exert an influence on prognosis independent of these two factors. Demonstration of the importance of venous spread has prompted some authors to support the 'no-touch' technique of surgical resection and it provides a basis for the early ligation of veins in colorectal resection.

DURATION OF SYMPTOMS: One major study has shown that, contrary to popular belief, the duration of symptoms has little bearing on the stage of colonic cancer and does not appear to have a major influence on prognosis (McDermott *et al.* 1981).

CARCINO-EMBRYONIC ANTIGEN: Pre-operative levels of carcino-embryonic antigen (CEA) tend to reflect the extent of the underlying disease. Estimations of pre-operative CEA levels are only of limited value in predicting prognosis after curative resection for colorectal cancer (Lewi *et al.* 1984). Postoperative estimations may be of help in diagnosing recurrences before overt symptoms and signs are manifest.

Complications of colorectal cancer

INTESTINAL OBSTRUCTION: Annular growths in the left side of the colon where the faeces are solid predispose to intestinal obstruction. This is the presenting feature of colorectal cancer in 20% of cases. The proximal colon becomes dilated and thick walled due to work hypertrophy.

PERFORATION: Goligher (1984) states that the commonest type of perforation in the absence of obstruction is of the tumour itself. Stercoral ulcers may occur proximal to an obstructing tumour. These are probably ischaemic in origin due to dilatation of the bowel wall and they occasionally perforate.

If the ileocaecal valve remains closed during intestinal obstruction (closed loop obstruction), the caecum dilates massively as it is the most distensible part of the colon. Since the tension of the wall increases with the radius (law of Laplace), caecal perforation may eventually occur.

Perforation of the tumour may give rise either to peritonitis or to a localized pericolic abscess. If this should burst into another organ, such as the bladder, a malignant fistula arises.

Other Tumours of the Large Bowel

Endocrine tumours

Endocrine cells containing 5HT and polypeptide hormones occur throughout the large bowel and they may give rise to endocrine tumours, especially in the caecum and rectum. They have similar features to endocrine tumours of the small bowel. Caecal carcinoids tend to metastasize but rarely cause the carcinoid syndrome. The rectum is the commonest site of hindgut endocrine tumours. They may be an incidental finding on rectal examination, or may present as a large ulcerating or polypoid growth. The larger tumours commonly metastasize. Clinical syndromes of hormone production are rare.

Lymphoid tumours

Benign

Small benign lymphoid polyps are a common finding in the lower rectum. They may be sessile or pedunculated. They are probably inflammatory and consist of normal lymphoid tissue with lymphoid follicles.

Occasionally overgrowth of the lymphoid follicles of the rectum and colon gives rise to multiple nodules, a condition known as benign lymphoid polyposis (not to be confused with multiple lymphomatous polyposis—see p. 111). Clinically it may be confused with familial polyposis coli.

Malignant

Lymphomas of the rectum and colon may be primary or secondary. Primary lymphomas are more common in the caecum and rectum than in the rest of the colon. They have similar pathological features to small bowel lymphomas.

Smooth muscle tumours

These are rare. Colonic lesions account for 3% and rectal lesions for 7% of all smooth muscle tumours of the intestine (Golden and Stout 1941). The pathology is similar to small bowel smooth muscle tumours.

Lipomas

These are more common in the right colon than in the left and are usually submucosal. Although normally symptomless, larger lesions may provoke intussusception or may ulcerate and cause haemorrhage. Microscopically they consist of mature adipose tissue.

Miscellaneous Conditions

Volvulus

The sigmoid colon is the commonest part of the colon to undergo volvulus. Twisting of the small intestine may, rarely, occur around a band or adhesion and volvulus of the caecum together with terminal ileum and ascending colon is also described. Volvulus of the transverse colon is exceedingly rare; it usually has no predisposing cause, although some cases have been reported in association with distal obstruction (Anderson *et al.* 1981).

Sigmoid volvulus

This is a relatively rare cause of acute intestinal obstruction in Western Europe but is more common in Africa. This geographical variation has been related to differences in dietary fibre intake. In one British study, half of the patients were over 65 years old and two-thirds had associated medical or psychiatric conditions (Anderson and Lee 1981). Anatomical predisposing factors include a large redundant sigmoid loop and binding together of the two ends of the sigmoid loop by peritoneal adhesions.

The clinical presentation is that of acute large bowel obstruction with gross abdominal distension. The twist is usually in an anticlockwise direction. This initially causes venous obstruction and then arterial insufficiency with resulting ischaemia, necrosis of the colonic wall, perforation and peritonitis.

Without elective operation, about 50% of patients have a recurrence within three years.

Caecal volvulus

Although the term caecal volvulus is used, the terminal ileum and ascending colon are also normally involved. In most cases there is a failure of the normal fixation of the right colon to the posterior abdominal wall. Wolfer *et al.* (1942) found that 11·2% of cadavers had a caecum sufficiently mobile to undergo torsion.

The patients present with acute intestinal obstruction. Torsion of the mesentery causes ischaemia of the caecal wall with subsequent necrosis and perforation.

Pneumatosis cystoides intestinalis

Gaseous cysts may occur anywhere in the bowel either in the submucosa or subserosa. They contain oxygen and nitrogen under pressure and are more common in the small than in the large bowel. The aetiology is unknown but possibilities include entry of gas-forming bacteria into the bowel wall and dissection of air from ruptured pulmonary alveoli through the mediastinum and retroperitoneum and along the mesenteric vessels to the bowel wall.

Pneumatosis usually occurs in middle-aged males and may give rise to change in bowel habit, rectal bleeding due to cyst rupture and pneumoperitoneum.

Macroscopically, the cysts cause gross irregularity of the mucosal surface and may project from the serosal surface. Histologically, the cyst linings characteristically contain macrophages and multinucleated giant cells. A positive diagnosis can therefore be made by rectal biopsy.

Malakoplakia

Malakoplakia of the urinary tract is discussed on p. 233. The condition occasionally affects the colon and may present as a tumour-like lesion or as multiple polypoid lesions. The histology is similar to malakoplakia of the urinary tract.

Pseudo-obstruction

This term is used when there are symptoms and signs of intestinal obstruction without the presence of a lesion causing mechanical obstruction. The cause is abnormal motility in the small bowel, the colon or both.

Primary pseudo-obstruction is of unknown cause, although in some cases it is familial. There may be hypertrophy of the smooth muscle layer of the bowel wall and in others there are abnormalities of the myenteric plexus. The patient has recurrent symptoms of obstruction. Steatorrhoea due to the stagnant loop syndrome may be found.

Secondary pseudo-obstruction is associated with smooth muscle disorders such as occur with scleroderma, amyloid and diabetes mellitus. It may also be associated with various drugs.

Acute pseudo-obstruction of the colon (Ogilvie's syndrome) is commonly secondary to metabolic disorders and is usually transient.

Radiation enteropathy

This is a fairly common clinical problem, affecting about 15% of patients undergoing abdominal irradiation. The critical dose appears to be in the region of 4500 rads. The small bowel is more sensitive than the large bowel and the addition of chemotherapy may compound the damage.

Radiation initially damages the dividing cells in the intestinal crypts, reducing cell turnover, with subsequent villous atrophy and mucosal thinning. In the acute phase there is mucosal oedema and inflammation with crypt abscesses. This may lead to ulceration. Vascular changes include endothelial cell swelling, thrombosis and endarteritis obliterans. The consequent ischaemia produces persistent ulceration and replacement of the intestinal smooth muscle by fibrosis. Eventually, submucosal telangiectasia and bizarre ('radiation') fibroblasts are seen.

Acute symptoms include pain, diarrhoea, bleeding and mucoid discharge. Later (after 6–12 months) patients may develop intestinal obstruction, due to stricture formation, fistulas and malabsorption.

Isolated small bowel ulceration

A proportion of small bowel ulcers do not fit into the recognized inflammatory, vascular and neoplastic categories and are termed 'non-specific'. Some of these were due to ingestion of enteric coated potassium, but a few remain of unknown aetiology.

Clinical presentations include intermittent intestinal obstruction, bleeding and peritonitis due to perforation.

The majority of non-specific small bowel ulcers occur in the ileum where they start as small well defined ulcers. Eventually they may involve the entire circumference of the bowel wall producing a napkin-ring constriction. The histological features are those of non-specific ulceration.

Solitary non-specific colonic ulcer

Non-specific ulcers may occur in any part of the colon, but are most common in the caecum (solitary caecal ulcer), ascending colon and sigmoid colon. The condition is to be distinguished from solitary rectal ulcer which is probably a different entity (see p. 106).

The aetiology is unknown, although some may be associated with drugs or ischaemia. Other cases are associated with diverticulitis. Symptoms include bleeding, pain and constipation. Some present as an acute inflammatory condition, similar to appendicitis and they occasionally perforate.

The ulcer is usually solitary but may be multiple, and is most commonly situated on the antimesenteric wall of the bowel. Histological examination shows an ulcerated area of colon with no special features.

THE APPENDIX

Normal Structure

The normal adult appendix is on average 7 cm long. In children it arises from the distal end of the caecum whereas in adults it arises from the medial wall of the caecum, below the ileocaecal valve. The appendix normally lies behind the caecum and ascending colon although it may also lie anterior or posterior to the terminal ileum or on the psoas muscle or hang down over the brim of the pelvis. The blood supply is by a branch of the caecal artery and the lymphatic drainage is to the ileocaecal nodes and the right paracolic nodes.

Histologically, the structure is similar to that of the large bowel. The most prominent feature is the presence of many lymphoid follicles in the lamina propria.

Appendicitis

Acute appendicitis is the most common abdominal surgical emergency. The highest incidence is during the second and third decade at a time when the amount of lymphoid tissue in the appendix is maximal. The sex ratio before puberty is one to one but after puberty the M : F ratio is 2 : 1. There is evidence that the incidence of appendicitis in the UK and the USA is decreasing.

Aetiology
Burkitt (1971) has drawn attention to the geographical epidemiology of

appendicitis. The condition is rare in rural communities and in Third World countries, and the incidence rises with increasing economic development. He suggested that a low residue diet and increased sugar intake leads to an altered pattern of intestinal function which in some way predisposes to appendicitis.

It is known from animal experiments that neither bacteria nor obstruction of the appendix lumen acting individually will cause appendicitis, whereas a combination of both is a potent cause. The obstruction may be caused by a faecolith, food debris, hypertrophy of lymphoid tissue or kinking. When obstruction occurs, epithelial mucus secretion continues and causes a rise in intraluminal pressure. When intraluminal pressure exceeds venous pressure, engorgement occurs and the appendix wall becomes ischaemic with consequent secondary bacterial invasion of the wall. As pressure increases still further, arterial blood flow ceases and infarction, gangrene and perforation occur.

Morphology

The appearance depends on the stage of the inflammation. Initially there is hyperaemia of the serosa and a fibrino-purulent exudate. When gangrene occurs the wall becomes green or black and perforation is often seen. The lumen may contain an obstructing faecolith, distal to which pus is present. In these cases, the inflammation is often confined to the distal appendix.

Histologically, the typical specimen shows a transmural infiltrate of polymorphs, associated in the later stages with tissue necrosis (*see Fig.* 4.21). The finding of minimal changes, such as small collections of pus in the lumen and some polymorphs and crypt abscesses in the lamina propria, is more difficult to interpret. Morson and Dawson (1979) consider these changes to be significant whereas

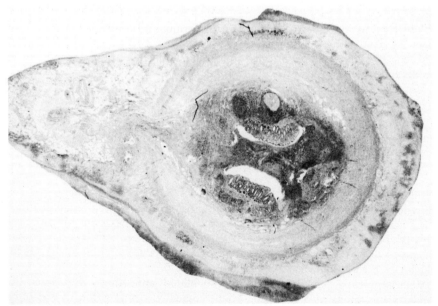

Fig. 4.21. Acute appendicitis. The mucosa is ulcerated and the lumen is filled with pus. A serosal reaction can be seen. (H and E × 8)

Lee and Toner (1983) point out that they occur in up to 30% of specimens resected electively.

The presence of submucosal or subserosal fibrosis may give an indication of previous appendicitis. There is little evidence that these changes can cause the symptoms of 'chronic' or 'grumbling' appendicitis which is now believed to be a manifestation of the irritable bowel syndrome.

Complications

Although some cases of acute appendicitis undergo resolution and fibrosis, many will perforate if not treated. Perforation most often causes a palpable mass of inflamed omentum and loops of bowel as the amount of pus liberated is usually small and because the inflamed appendix is already walled off by omentum. In some cases, progressive suppuration leads to a peri-appendiceal abscess. If the initial perforation is not walled off, or if a peri-appendiceal abscess ruptures, generalized peritonitis results. Alternatively, pus may track downwards to the pelvis or upwards to the right subhepatic space forming either a pelvic or a subphrenic abscess. Occasionally, portal pyaemia leads to an intrahepatic abscess.

Perforation occurs at an earlier stage in young children and often causes generalized peritonitis because the underdeveloped omentum is less able to wall off the developing inflammation.

Simple Mucocoele of the Appendix

When the appendix becomes distended with mucus it is termed a mucocoele. This may be a simple mucocoele or one associated with an adenoma (cystadenoma) or a carcinoma (cystadenocarcinoma). A simple mucocoele can develop after appendicitis if the lumen becomes obstructed by fibrosis. The epithelium distal to the obstruction continues to secrete mucus forming a thin walled grossly dilated appendix. This is often symptomless.

Mucocoeles may become infected to form an empyema of the appendix or may rupture to form one type of pseudomyxoma peritoneii.

Tumours of the Appendix

Tumours of the appendix are adenomas, carcinomas and carcinoids. The last are the most common, whereas adenomas and carcinomas are rare.

Adenomas

The adenoma is identical to those occurring in the large bowel. Small adenomas, particularly of the tubular type, may occur without a coexistent mucocoele but most of the rest are associated with a mucocoele and are termed cystadenomas. The mucocoele arises partly as a result of copious mucus secretion by the adenoma and partly as a consequence of luminal obstruction.

Macroscopically, some have a multiloculated appearance and some show papillary infoldings into the wall. Microscopically, compression of the tumour makes interpretation difficult. The adenomas show the usual features of colonic adenomas with associated epithelial dysplasia.

Adenocarcinomas

These may occur as ordinary adenocarcinomas or as mucinous cystadenocarcinomas. Their behaviour is similar to colorectal adenocarcinomas and the prognosis depends on the depth of invasion and histological grade. Spread occurs to the mesoappendiceal and ileocolic nodes. A four year survival rate of 66% after hemicolectomy has been quoted. Cystadenocarcinomas appear to have a better prognosis than the non-cystic type.

Carcinoids

Eighty-five per cent of all appendiceal tumours are carcinoids (McNeal 1971). They are found in approximately 0·32% of all appendicectomy specimens.

Histologically, they are similar to small bowel carcinoids. The tumours tend to expand in the submucosa and infiltrate muscle and serosa. Even in these areas, however, metastases and the carcinoid syndrome are rare.

Mucus secreting carcinoid

Recently this tumour has been recognized as a separate entity. It is a tumour which has similarities to both carcinoids and carcinomas in that the cells contain granules (like carcinoids) and secrete mucus (like adenocarcinomas). The cell of origin is debatable although they may arise from crypt stem cells which have the capacity to differentiate into both epithelial and endocrine cells.

They are more often symptomatic than ordinary carcinoids and may present as appendicitis or with secondary deposits. Macroscopically, they appear small in size

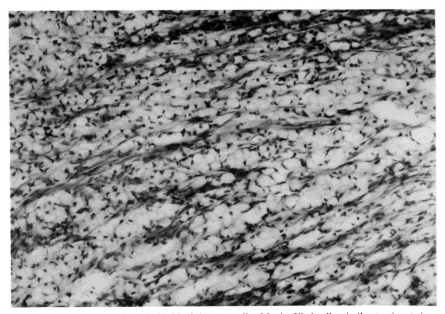

Fig. 4.22. Mucus secreting carcinoid of the appendix. Mucin filled cells, similar to signet ring cells, infiltrating the muscle coat of the appendix. (H and E × 75)

and widespread infiltration may not be appreciated by simple palpation. Histologically, the tumour arises from the crypt bases of the epithelial glands. The cells are distended with mucus and form nests of goblet cells and tubulo-glandular structures (*Fig.* 4.22).

These tumours have a prognosis somewhere between appendiceal carcinoids and carcinomas (Edmonds *et al.* 1984).

References

Anderson J. R., Lee D. (1981) The management of acute sigmoid volvulus. *Br. J. Surg.* **68**, 117–20.

Anderson J. R., Lee D., Taylor T. V., Ross A. H. (1981) Volvulus of the transverse colon. *Br. J. Surg.* **68**, 179–81.

Arminski T. C., McLean D. W. (1964) Incidence and distribution of adenomatous polyps of the colon and rectum based on 1000 autopsy examinations. *Dis. Colon. Rectum.* **7**, 249–61.

Astler V. B., Coller F. A. (1954) The prognostic significance of direct extension of carcinoma of the colon and rectum. *Ann. Surg.* **139**, 846–52.

Boley S. J., Sammartano R., Adams A., DiBiase A., Kleinhaus S., Srayregen S. (1977) On the nature and etiology of vascular ectasias of the colon. Degenerative lesions of aging. *Gastroenterology* **72**, 650–60.

Burkitt D. P. (1971) The aetiology of appendicitis. *Br. J. Surg.* **58**, 695–9.

Burnham W. R., Lennard-Jones J. E., Stanford J. L., Bird R. G. (1978) Mycobacteria as a possible cause of inflammatory bowel disease. *Lancet* **2**, 693–6.

Civetta J. M., Kolodny M. (1970) Mesenteric venous thrombosis associated with oral contraceptives. *Gastroenterology* **58**, 713–6.

Croft R. J., Menon G. P., Marston A. (1981) Does 'intestinal angina' exist? A critical study of obstructed visceral arteries. *Br. J. Surg.* **68**, 316–18.

Edmonds P., Merino M. J., Livolski V. A., Duray P. H. (1984) Adenocarcinoid (mucinous carcinoid) of the appendix. *Gastroenterology* **86**, 302–9.

Ford M. J., Anderson J. R., Gilmour H. M., Holt S., Sircus W., Heading R. C. (1983) Clinical spectrum of 'solitary ulcer' of the rectum. *Gastroenterology* **84**, 1533–40.

Gardner P. S., Knox E. G., Court S. D., Green C. A. (1962) Virus infection and intussusception in childhood. *Br. Med. J.* **2**, 697–700.

Gear J. S., Ware A., Fursdon P. *et al.* (1979) Symptomless diverticular disease and intake of dietary fibre. *Lancet* **1**, 511–14.

Gillespie P. E., Chambers T. J., Chan K. W., Doronzo F., Morson B. C., Williams C. B. (1979) Colonic adenomas—a colonoscopy survey. *Gut* **20**, 240–5.

Golden T., Stout A. P. (1941) Smooth muscle tumours of gastrointestinal tract and retroperitoneal tissues. *Surg. Gynaecol. Obstet.* **73**, 784–810.

Goligher J. C. (1984) *Surgery of the Anus, Rectum and Colon*, 5th ed. London, Baillière Tindall.

Greenstein A. J., Sachar D. B. (1983) Cancer in Crohn's disease. In: Alan R. N., Keighley M. R. B., Alexander-Williams J., Hawkins C. (eds.) *Inflammatory Bowel Diseases*, pp. 332–7. Edinburgh, Churchill Livingstone.

Heuman R., Boeryd B., Bolin T., Sjodahl R. (1983) The influence of disease at the margin of resection on the outcome of Crohn's disease. *Br. J. Surg.* **70**, 519–21.

Hill M. J., Morson B. C., Bussey H. J. R. (1978) Aetiology of adenoma–carcinoma sequence in large bowel. *Lancet* **1**, 245–7.

Irving M. (1983) Assessment and management of external fistulas in Crohn's disease. *Br. J. Surg.* **70**, 233–6.

Jarvinen H. J., Peltokallio P., Landtman M., Wolf J. (1982) Gardner's stigmas in patients with familial adenomatosis coli. *Br. J. Surg.* **69**, 718–21.

Jewell D. P. (1980) Aetiology (of ulcerative colitis). In: Truelove S. C., Kennedy H. J. (eds.) *Topics in Gastroenterology 8*, pp. 157–68. Oxford, Blackwell Scientific Publications.

Kirsner J. B., Shorter R. G. (1982) Recent developments in 'non-specific' inflammatory bowel disease. *N. Engl. J. Med.* **306**, 775–85.

Lake B. D. (1983) Acetylcholinesterase in the diagnosis of Hirschsprung's disease and other gastrointestinal disorders. In: Filipe M. I., Lake B. D. (eds.) *Histochemistry in Pathology*, pp. 145–50. Edinburgh, Churchill Livingstone.

Lee F. D., Toner P. G. (1983) Non-neoplastic diseases of the small and large bowel. In: Silverberg S. G. (ed.) *Principles and Practice of Surgical Pathology*, Vol. 2, pp. 845–98. New York, John Wiley and Sons.

Lennard-Jones J. E., Morson B. C., Ritchie J. K., Shove D. C., Williams C. B. (1977) Cancer in colitis: assessment of the individual risk by clinical and histological criteria. *Gastroenterology* **73**, 1280–9.

Lewi H., Blumgart L. H., Carter D. C. *et al.* (1984) Preoperative carcino-embryonic antigen and survival in patients with colorectal cancer. *Br. J. Surg.* **71**, 206–8.

Logan R. F., Edmond M., Somerville K. W., Langman M. J. (1984) Smoking and ulcerative colitis. *Br. Med. J.* **288**, 751–3.

McDermott F. T., Hughes E. S., Pihl E. A., Milne B. J., Price A. B. (1981) Prognosis in relation to symptom duration in colon cancer. *Br. J. Surg.* **68**, 846–9.

McNeal J. E. (1971) Mechanism of obstruction in carcinoid tumours of the small intestine. *Am. J. Clin. Pathol.* **56**, 452–8.

Marks C. G., Ritchie J. K., Lockhart-Mummery H. E. (1981) Anal fistulas in Crohn's disease. *Br. J. Surg.* **68**, 525–7.

Marston A. (1977) *Intestinal Ischaemia.* London, Edward Arnold.

Martin C. J., Parks T. G., Biggart J. D. (1981) Solitary rectal ulcer syndrome in Northern Ireland 1971–1980. *Br. J. Surg.* **68**, 744–7.

Martin C. J., Parks T. G., Biggart J. D. (1982) Management of the solitary rectal ulcer syndrome. In: Heberer G., Denecke H. (eds.) *Colorectal Surgery.* Berlin, Springer-Verlag.

Modan B., Barell V., Lubin F., Modan M., Greenberg R. A., Graham S. (1975) Low-fibre intake as an etiological factor in cancer of the colon. *J. Natl. Cancer Inst.* **55**, 15–18.

Morson B. C., Dawson I. M. P (1979) *Gastrointestinal Pathology.* Oxford, Blackwell Scientific Publications.

Moses W. R. (1947) Meckel's diverticulum. Report of two unusual cases. *N. Engl. J. Med.* **237**, 118–22.

Perzin K. H., Bridge M. F. (1981) Adenomas of the small intestine: a clinicopathologic review of 51 cases and a study of their relationship to carcinoma. *Cancer* **48**, 799–819.

Perzin K. H., Fenoglio C. M., Pascal R. R. (1983) Neoplastic diseases of the small and large intestine. In: Silverberg S. G. (ed.) *Principles and Practice of Surgical Pathology*, Vol. II, pp. 899–937. New York, John Wiley and Sons.

Phillips R. K. S., Hittinger R., Blesovsky L., Fry J. S., Fielding L. P. (1984) Large bowel cancer: surgical pathology and its relationship to survival. *Br. J. Surg.* **71**, 604–10.

Phillpotts R. J., Hermon-Taylor J., Brooke B. N. (1979) Virus isolation studies in Crohn's disease: a negative report. *Gut* **20**, 1057–62.

Rees H. C., Wright N. A. (1984) Angiodysplasia of the colon. In: Anthony P. P., MacSween N. M. (eds.) *Recent Advances in Histopathology 12*, pp. 178–88. Edinburgh, Churchill Livingstone.

Rhodes J. M. (1981) Aetiology of Crohn's disease. In: Jewell D. P., Lee E. (eds.) *Topics in Gastroenterology 9*, pp. 21–35. Oxford, Blackwell Scientific Publications.

Soltero M. J., Bill A. H. (1976) The natural history of Meckel's diverticulum and its relation to incidental removal. A study of 202 cases of diseased Meckel's diverticulum found in King County, Washington, over a 15 year period. *Am. J. Surg.* **132**, 168–73.

Somerville K. W., Logan R. E. A., Edmond M., Langman M. J. S. (1984) Smoking and Crohn's disease. *Br. Med. J.* **289**, 954–6.

Strickland R. G., McLaren L. C. (1981) Studies of the *in vitro* cytopathic effect of inflammatory bowel disease tissue preparations. In: Pena A. S., Weterman I. T., Booth C. C., Strober W. (eds.) *Recent Advances in Crohn's Disease*, pp. 246–51. The Hague, Martinus Nijhoff.

Stubbs R. S. (1983) The aetiology of colorectal cancer. *Br. J. Surg.* **70**, 313–16.

Talbot I. C., Ritchie S., Leighton M. H., Hughes A. O., Bussey H. J., Morson B. C. (1980) The clinical significance of invasion of veins by rectal cancer. *Br. J. Surg.* **67**, 439–42.

Thompson P. M., Hill J. T., Packham D. A. (1979) Colonic carcinoma at the site of ureterosigmoidostomy: what is the risk? *Br. J. Surg.* **66**, 809.

Thornton J. R., Emmett P. M., Heaton K. W. (1980) Diet and ulcerative colitis. *Br. Med. J.* **1**, 293–4.

Turnbull P. R., Smith A. H., Isbister W. H. (1981) Cholecystectomy and cancer of the large bowel. *Br. J. Surg.* **68**, 551–3.

Williams N. S. (1984) The rationale for preservation of the anal sphincter in patients with low rectal cancer. *Br. J. Surg.* **71**, 575–81.

Wolfer J. A., Beaton L. E., Anson B. J. (1942) Volvulus of the caecum. Anatomical factors in its aetiology: report of a case. *Surg. Gynecol. Obstet.* **74**, 882–94.

Wood C. B., Gillis C. R., Hole D., Malcolm A. J., Blumgart L. H. (1981) Local tumour invasion as a prognostic factor in colorectal cancer. *Br. J. Surg.* **68**, 326–8.

Wright D. H., Isaacson P. G. (1983) *Biopsy Pathology of the Lymphoreticular System.* London, Chapman and Hall.

Chapter 5

The Anal Region

Normal Structure

The anal canal is approximately 3·5 cm long and is surrounded by an internal and an external sphincter. Embryologically, the upper anal canal is derived from endoderm and the lower anal canal from ectoderm. The junction is marked in fetal life by the anal membrane and in adult life by the anal valves which form a line known as the dentate or pectinate line. The anal mucosa is plum coloured above the dentate line and pale and opaque below, where it is composed of squamous epithelium which lacks hair follicles, and sweat and sebaceous glands. At the lower border of the internal sphincter, the perianal skin, which contains normal adnexal structures, starts.

At the junction of the endoderm and ectoderm is the transitional or cloacogenic zone which extends for about 1 cm above the dentate line (*see Fig.* 5.1). It joins the rectal mucosa above to the squamous epithelium below and is interpreted as being a remnant of the cloacal endoderm. Microscopically, various types of epithelium are seen in this transition zone, including squamous, transitional (similar to the urinary tract), stratified columnar and columnar types. The ducts of the anal glands arise in the transitional zone behind the anal valves and pass into the submucosa. They are lined by stratified columnar epithelium.

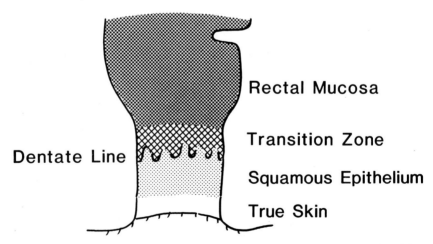

Fig. 5.1. Schematic diagram of the different types of mucosa in the anal region. (Adapted from Morson and Dawson 1979.)

The internal sphincter consists of smooth muscle and is a combination of the muscle coats of the rectum. The external sphincter is divided into subcutaneous, superficial and deep parts and is composed of voluntary muscle.

Congenital Anorectal Abnormalities

Early in embryological life the urinary and gastrointestinal tracts empty into a common cavity known as the cloaca, which is bound ventrally by the cloacal membrane. A urogenital septum then forms and grows down between the urogenital and gastrointestinal parts of the cloaca and it eventually reaches the cloacal membrane. Anal tubercles form behind the urogenital septum and fuse with it to form a proctodaeum. This is surrounded by mesoderm which forms the external sphincter. The proctodaeum and its mesoderm then migrate backwards and grow towards the rectum and eventually fuse with it to form the anal canal.

Anorectal abnormalities are divided into high, intermediate and low (Santulli *et al.* 1970). In high lesions the abnormality occurs proximal to the levator ani and therefore incontinence results. In low lesions, the abnormality occurs distal to the levator ani and continence is maintained. Intermediate varieties occur in the region of the levator ani.

LOW ABNORMALITIES: If the anus fails to migrate backwards it may open into the vulva or perineum forming an ectopic anus. If the lateral genital folds which form the labia or scrotum fuse posteriorly, they cause a covered anus. This is usually associated with a track running forwards into the perineum. The fusion may not be complete, leaving a 'microscopic anus'.

INTERMEDIATE ABNORMALITIES: The anorectal membrane which lies at the upper end of the proctodaeum may remain intact (imperforate anal membrane). It may eventually rupture spontaneously and give rise to anal stenosis.

HIGH ABNORMALITIES: In these cases the rectum extends down to the pelvic floor but the anus (which should pass through the pelvic floor to meet it) is absent and therefore no sphincter mechanism is present. In the male, the commonest form is anorectal agenesis with recto-urethral fistula (i.e. the rectum enters the prostatic urethra). In the female, the rectum may enter the posterior vagina. Some females retain a primitive cloaca, into which the urogenital and gastrointestinal tracts both open.

Haemorrhoids

Haemorrhoids have been classified into internal and external, the former arising in the upper two-thirds of the anal canal (lined by columnar epithelium) and the latter in the skin covered lower one-third of the anal canal.

In most patients, two internal piles are found on the right side of the anal canal (right anterior and right posterior) and the third forms the left lateral pile. Additional secondary piles may be found between these primary sites.

As well as dilated venous plexuses, haemorrhoids comprise small arterial branches of the superior haemorrhoidal artery and loose submucous and subcutaneous areolar tissue.

Classically, internal piles have been regarded as varicosities of the venous plexuses in the wall of the anal canal and lower rectum. These are chiefly tributaries of the internal haemorrhoidal plexus and drain to the superior haemorrhoidal vein.

The traditional view of haemorrhoids has been altered in recent years with the development of the concept of anal cushions which are believed to play a role in the continence of flatus. Thomson (1975) injected the superior rectal vein in cadavers and showed that fusiform and saccular dilatations of the submucous venous plexus of the anal canal were part of normal anatomy. The theory of anal cushions with arterio-venous connections in the area of the 'haemorrhoid' is supported by the fact that bleeding from haemorrhoids is bright red and not dark in colour. Current theory is that internal piles are due to prolapse of normal mucosal cushions, although it is difficult to explain those haemorrhoids which bleed and do not prolapse on this basis.

Internal haemorrhoids are occasionally associated with organic obstruction to the venous return from the superior haemorrhoidal veins. Although patients with portal hypertension may have life-threatening rectal bleeding from haemorrhoids, this is an exceedingly rare complication and the incidence of haemorrhoids in these patients is probably similar to that of the general population.

Haemorrhoids are extremely common in pregnancy as there is venous obstruction in the latter stages as well as increased laxity and vascularity of the pelvic tissues. Cancer of the middle third of the rectum may obstruct venous return.

The majority of patients with symptomatic haemorrhoids have no obvious cause but a number of precipitating factors may play a role.

1. *Heredity*: Certain families seem predisposed to haemorrhoids, especially at a young age, suggesting there may be a structural defect in the venous wall.
2. *Constipation and straining at stool*: This increases the portal venous pressure and as the system is without valves, the pressure is transmitted to the haemorrhoidal plexus. In addition, hard stool may mechanically compress the superior haemorrhoidal veins in the lower rectum.
3. *Diet*: Haemorrhoids are exceedingly rare in Africa. The low roughage diet common in the West and the associated delay in faecal transit and high incidence of chronic constipation are probably major factors in the development of haemorrhoids.
4. *Alteration in sphincter tone*: Several studies have shown that increased anal canal pressure is present in patients with haemorrhoids compared with age/sex matched controls. It is unclear whether increased anal tone plays a primary role in the pathogenesis of haemorrhoids.

External piles

These are covered with skin, have cutaneous sensation and may be painful. There are two groups: (1) thrombosed external piles or anal haematomas which occur in the veins of the external haemorrhoidal plexus and are caused by spontaneous rupture of one of the external veins. They are extremely painful. (2) Anal skin tags which are common and often multiple. Idiopathic skin tags are soft and pliable whereas skin tags associated with an infected fissure-in-ano are stiff with oedema.

Anal Fissure

This is an ulcer in the skin-lined part of the anal canal. It is most commonly sited in the midline of the posterior wall of the anal canal, but sometimes it occurs in the anterior midline and very rarely elsewhere in the anal circumference. Anterior fissures are more common in women than men. The fissure lies vertically in the cutaneous part of the anal lining between the anal valves and the anal orifice. It is superficial to the lower one-third of the internal sphincter muscle which may be seen in the base of the fissure. Although it begins as a simple ulcer in the skin of the canal, secondary changes occur. An oedematous skin tag, a so-called 'sentinel pile', develops distal to the end of the fissure; the anal papilla immediately proximal to the fissure hypertrophies and this may lead to the development of a fibrous polyp; and the edges of the fissure become indurated.

There is associated tight spasm of the internal sphincter which causes considerable discomfort.

The cause of most fissures is thought to be the passage of a hard stool but occasionally secondary fissures form after haemorrhoidectomy or operation for low anal fistula, or in association with ulcerative colitis. Crohn's disease may present with an anal fissure: squamous carcinoma of the anus, syphilis and tuberculosis may masquerade as a fissure. If doubt exists then biopsy should be performed.

Anorectal Abscess

This is a common clinical problem. Whitehead et al. (1982) have shown that 'gut organisms' such as Bacteroides fragilis, E. coli and Streptococcus faecalis are frequently cultured from anorectal abscesses. Staph. aureus is relatively unusual but anaerobes such as Clostridium welchii are commonly found. The isolation of 'gut organisms' from a perianal or ischiorectal abscess suggests the presence of an associated fistula.

Occasionally, there is an obvious precipitating cause such as fissure, an infected perianal haematoma or a recent haemorrhoidectomy, but most cases have no obvious cause.

Parks (1961) suggested that the first event was the formation of an inter-sphincteric abscess in relation to an anal gland lying between the internal and external sphincters. If pus then spreads downwards in the inter-sphincteric plane, a perianal abscess forms, but if lateral spread occurs by the trans-sphincteric route, an ischiorectal abscess forms.

Rarely, septicaemic patients with diabetes or leukaemia have blood-borne associated sepsis in the anal region.

Other important conditions associated with anorectal sepsis and fistula are Crohn's disease and tuberculosis.

The classification of anorectal abscesses based on Parks' theory of pathogenesis is: (1) perianal, (2) ischiorectal, (3) submucosal, (4) intersphincteric, (5) high intermuscular (see Fig. 5.2). Pelvi-rectal abscesses tend to arise from a source of pelvic sepsis.

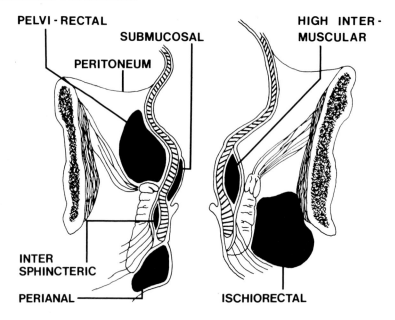

Fig. 5.2. Different anatomical types of abscess in the anal region. (From Goligher 1984; reproduced with permission.)

Fistula-in-Ano

The term fistula is defined as a chronic granulating track between two epithelial lined surfaces which may be either cutaneous or mucosal.

Aetiology

Pyogenic anorectal abscess is by far the most common predisposing factor, especially if there has been inadequate treatment. Occasionally, a foreign body may be lodged in the abscess cavity provoking chronicity. Some cases occur after anorectal surgery.

Crohn's disease and tuberculosis account for a number of cases and, if these diseases are suspected, material should be sent for histology and culture at the time of operation. Other rare causes include ulcerative colitis, colorectal cancer, lymphogranuloma venereum and actinomycosis.

Classification and morphology

The classification of fistula-in-ano is confusing due to the different terminologies used by different authors. In this section, the terminology of Parks *et al.* (1976) will be used. These authors divided fistulas into four main groups. Most belong to the first group.

1. INTERSPHINCTERIC FISTULA: In this case, the fistula lies in the intersphincteric plane and gains entrance to the anal canal by crossing the internal sphincter. It

does not cross the external sphincter at any point. The external sphincter and anorectal ring do not have to be cut during treatment and incontinence is not a problem. Several types are recognized:

i. Simple intersphincteric, as illustrated in *Fig. 5.3a*.
ii. Intersphincteric fistula with a high blind tract in which a blind extension occurs upwards in the intersphincteric plane.
iii. Intersphincteric fistula with a high tract opening into the rectum (*see Fig. 5.3b*).
iv. High intersphincteric fistula without a perineal opening in which infection commences in the intersphincteric zone of the mid-anal canal. The fistula crosses the internal sphincter and enters the anal canal and an extension passes upwards in the intersphincteric plane where there may be a secondary entrance into the rectum. There is no downward extension and therefore no external opening (*see Fig. 5.3c*).
v. High intersphincteric fistula with a pelvic extension in which infection spreads from the intersphincteric plane into the pelvic cavity.
vi. Intersphincteric fistula from pelvic disease in which a pelvic focus of infection spreads downwards through the intersphincteric plane to the anal verge.

2. TRANS-SPHINCTERIC FISTULA: In this type, the track passes from the intersphincteric plane through the external sphincter (*see Fig. 5.3d*). Some cases are complicated by a high blind track which extends upwards in the ischiorectal fossa and may pierce the levator muscle, although rupture into the rectum is rare (*see Fig. 5.3e*).

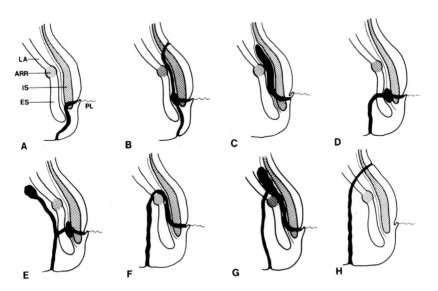

Fig. 5.3. Fistula-in-ano (LA—levator ani; ARR—anorectal ring; IS—internal sphincter; ES—external sphincter; PL—pectinate line): *a.* intersphincteric; *b.* intersphincteric with a track passing upwards and entering rectum; *c.* intersphincteric in which the track passes upwards without a perineal opening; *d.* trans-sphincteric; *e.* trans-sphincteric with a secondary track which reaches the apex of the ischiorectal fossa; *f.* suprasphincteric; *g.* suprasphincteric with a supralevator abscess; *h.* extrasphincteric.

3. SUPRASPHINCTERIC FISTULA: The track passes in the intersphincteric plane over the top of the anorectal ring and then downwards through the levator muscle to the ischiorectal fossa and finally the skin (*see Fig. 5.3f*). There may be a blind upward extension (*see Fig. 5.3g*).

4. EXTRASPHINCTERIC FISTULA: The track passes from the perineal skin through the ischiorectal fat and levator muscles into the rectum. It is outside the external sphincter complex (*see Fig. 5.3h*). There may be a side arm which passes through the internal and external sphincters into the anal canal.

Rectal Prolapse

Rectal prolapse may be complete, when the full thickness of the rectal wall prolapses, or partial, when only the mucosa prolapses. Internal prolapse refers to prolapse of the upper rectum into the middle or lower rectum without reaching the anal canal.

Partial prolapse

This is the most common type of rectal prolapse in children. The absence of the sacral hollow in children is a possible anatomical predisposing factor; diarrhoea, prolonged straining and severe chronic cough are other factors. In adults, some mucosal prolapse often accompanies third degree haemorrhoids. In the elderly, laxity of the anal sphincter is the main predisposing factor; this is usually idiopathic, although, rarely, cauda equina lesions may be the cause.

Complete prolapse

Complete rectal prolapse usually occurs in adults; 85% of patients are females, of which more than half are nulliparous. It used to be believed that complete rectal prolapse represented a sliding hernia involving the pouch of Douglas which pushed the anterior wall of the rectum into the rectal lumen and then out through the anus. The more recent view, based on cineradiographic studies (Brodén and Snellman 1968) is that rectal prolapse is an intussusception of the rectum, starting about 6 cm from the anal verge. The cause of the intussusception is unknown. Rectal prolapse is frequently associated with anal incontinence and laxity of the anal sphincter. In these cases, Parks *et al.* (1977) have demonstrated histological evidence of denervation of the external anal sphincter muscle and to a lesser extent the levator ani muscles. They suggest that this may be due to stretch injury of the pudendal or perineal nerves which may occur during straining at stool or childbirth. The relationship between complete rectal prolapse and these findings is uncertain. Complications of complete rectal prolapse include proctitis, rectal ulceration, bleeding and, rarely, gangrene.

Descending Perineal Syndrome

Parks *et al.* (1966) described this syndrome in which a loss of the normal tone of the pelvic floor muscles leads to descent of the pelvic floor with the result that the anterior rectal wall protrudes into the bowel lumen and impedes emptying of the rectum. Symptoms include a sensation of rectal obstruction and concomitant excessive straining at stool. On examination, the perineum descends when the patient is asked to strain and digital examination reveals a lax anal sphincter. EMG studies show that the muscle tone is abnormal.

Tumours and Tumour-like Conditions of the Anal Margin

Condylomata accuminata

Viral warts or condylomata accuminata are papillary growths of viral origin with a predilection for warm, moist surfaces. The majority are sexually transmitted (in both sexes) and they appear as pink or red soft papillary growths which are often multiple. Microscopically, there is acanthosis and hyperplasia of the epidermis and the reti ridges are elongated and broad. However, the maturation of the epithelium is normal and the demarcation from normal epithelium is sharp. The human papilloma virus can be detected on electron microscopy.

The pathologist should be informed in cases where there was prior treatment with podophyllin as this may increase the mitotic rate and lead to a mistaken diagnosis of malignancy.

Bowen's disease

Bowen's disease rarely occurs in the perianal skin. It appears as a red plaque which may be erythematous, scaly or nodular. Microscopically, the changes of epithelial dysplasia are similar to Bowen's disease elsewhere (*see* p. 50).

Paget's disease of the perianal skin

Very rarely, extramammary Paget's disease is found in areas such as the axilla or the perianal region where there are abundant apocrine glands. The patient has erythematous skin changes, sometimes with crusting and ulceration. Microscopically, Paget's cells are seen in the epithelium, especially at the tips of reti pegs. They are large cells with abundant often vacuolated cytoplasm and a pale staining nucleus. Serial sections may often show intraduct carcinoma or adenocarcinoma of an apocrine gland. Some cases appear to be associated with rectal carcinoma or with a concurrent breast carcinoma although the reason for these associations is unclear.

Squamous carcinoma of the anal margin

Squamous carcinoma of the anal margin is similar to other squamous carcinomas of the skin and should therefore be distinguished from carcinoma of the anal canal which has a different natural history (*see* p. 140). It occurs in elderly patients and is more common in men than women. It presents as a typical ulcerating squamous carcinoma or as a protuberant growth. Microscopically, it is usually a well differentiated squamous carcinoma with epithelial nests and keratin pearls. It spreads to the inguinal nodes. Most cases can be treated by wide local excision. The five year survival rate (about 50%) is better than for carcinoma of the anal canal.

Basal cell carcinoma of the anal margin

This is a rare tumour. In a large series of 34 cases (Neilson and Jenson 1981) most presented as chronic indurated growths with raised borders and central ulceration. Most patients underwent wide local excision. Prognosis is good with a 70% five year survival.

Tumours of the Anal Canal

Squamous cell carcinoma

Squamous cell carcinoma of the anal canal may arise *de novo* or following a history of various anorectal lesions, such as fistula, leukoplakia or lymphogranuloma venereum. They occur more commonly in countries where the population has poor personal hygiene.

The common presenting symptoms are anorectal bleeding and anal pain. The associated mass is usually ulcerating but may be polypoidal (*see Fig.* 5.4).

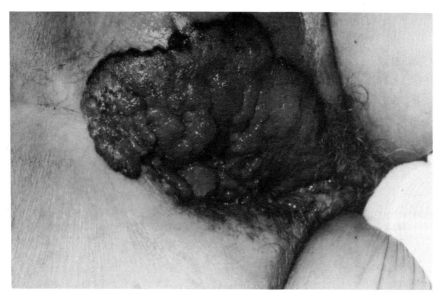

Fig. 5.4. Fungating squamous carcinoma of anal canal.

The majority of anal canal carcinomas arise from the area above the dentate line known as the transition zone. Here, the histological picture ranges from typically squamous to those showing a pattern similar to basal cell carcinomas of the skin. The latter are termed basaloid or cloacogenic tumours. The minority which arise from below the dentate line are all squamous in type.

Well differentiated cloacogenic tumours show clumps of basaloid cells with peripheral palisading, very similar to the pattern seen in the basal cell carcinoma of skin (*see Fig.* 5.5). Less well differentiated cloacogenic tumours appear as invasive, finger-like projections of malignant, transitional cell epithelium.

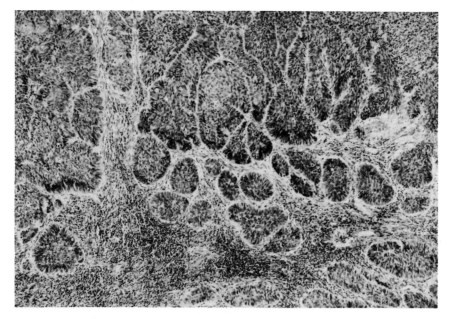

Fig. 5.5. Basaloid carcinoma of anal canal. (H and E × 30)

The dentate line is adherent to the underlying internal sphincter and obliterates the lamina propria at this point, thus forming a barrier to downward spread. Local spread is, therefore, preferentially upwards and lymph node metastases may be found both within the pelvis and in the inguinal nodes. The latter site is more common with tumours arising below the dentate line.

Carcinomas of the anal ducts and glands are similar to cloacogenic tumours since the anal ducts arise from the cloacogenic transition zone. In destructive lesions, it may be impossible to establish whether a particular tumour arose from the anal glands or from the anal canal itself.

The prognosis of anal canal carcinoma depends on the presence or absence of lymph node metastases and the histological grade of the tumour. These are inter-related since the poorly differentiated tumours tend to have lymph node metastases at presentation. The tumour pattern (i.e. squamous or basaloid) does not appear to influence prognosis independent of the histological grade. Morson and Dawson (1979) quote five year survival rates of 80%, 50% and 30% respectively for well, moderately and poorly differentiated anal canal tumours.

Carcinoma in anorectal fistula

This condition presents as a perianal fistula or abscess which sometimes contains mucinous material. It is thought that, at least in some cases, the tumour arises in a fistula which is in fact a duplication of the lower hindgut, as it is possible to demonstrate normal rectal mucosa lining the fistula tract in areas adjacent to the carcinoma. Histologically, the tumour is a mucin secreting adenocarcinoma.

Malignant melanoma

The anal canal is the third most common site of malignant melanoma, after the skin and eye. It is, however, rare and only one-eighth as common as squamous carcinoma of the anus. It most commonly arises from the transitional zone of the anal canal.

It characteristically presents as a polypoid anal mass, rather than an ulcer. It may be pigmented and can therefore sometimes be confused with a thrombosed pile. Microscopically, the pattern seen depends on the amount of differentiation which may range from sheeting of cells on the one hand to well formed cell nests on the other hand. Giant cells are frequently seen and help to distinguish this tumour from other poorly differentiated anal canal tumours.

Malignant melanomas of the anal canal are aggressive tumours and lymphatic and vascular spread are common. The five year survival rate approaches zero.

References

Brodén B., Snellman B. (1968) Procidentia of the rectum studied with cineradiography: a contribution to the discussion of causative mechanisms. *Dis. Colon Rectum*, **11**, 330–5.

Goligher J. C. (1984) *Surgery of the Anus, Rectum and Colon.* London, Baillière Tindall.

Morson B. C., Dawson I. M. P. (1979) *Gastrointestinal Pathology.* Oxford, Blackwell Scientific Publications.

Nielsen O. V., Jensen S. L. (1981) Basal cell carcinoma of the anus—a clinical study of 34 cases. *Br. J. Surg.* **68**, 856–7.

Parks A. G. (1961) Pathogenesis and treatment of fistula-in-ano. *Br. Med. J.* **1**, 463–9.

Parks A. G., Gordon P. H., Hardcastle J. D. (1976) A classification of fistulae-in-ano. *Br. J. Surg.* **63**, 1–12.

Parks A. G., Porter N. H., Hardcastle J. D. (1966) The syndrome of the descending perineum. *Proc. Roy. Soc. Med.* **59**, 477–82.

Parks A. G., Swash M., Urich H. (1977) Sphincter denervation in anorectal incontinence and rectal prolapse. *Gut* **18**, 656–65.

Santulli T. V., Kiesewetter W. B., Bill A. H. (1970) Anorectal anomalies: A suggested international classification. *J. Pediat. Surg.* **5**, 281–7.

Thomson W. H. (1975) The nature of haemorrhoids. *Br. J. Surg.* **62**, 542–52.

Whitehead S. M., Leach R. D., Eykyn S. J., Phillips I. (1982) The aetiology of perirectal sepsis. *Br. J. Surg.* **69**, 166–8.

Chapter 6

The Liver

Normal Structure and Function

The liver develops as a diverticulum from the foregut. It connects with the vitelline veins of the yolk sac during the third week in utero, and these eventually form the portal and hepatic veins in adult life. The left umbilical vein persists as the ductus venosus and after birth the remnant runs in the free edge of the falciform ligament. It may recanalize in portal hypertension and can be used for angiography. Traditionally the right and left lobes of the liver are divided by the falciform ligament. The functional separation of the two major lobes is, however, along a plane from the gallbladder fossa to a position just to the left of the vena cava. This is the practical surgical division, based on the left and right branches of the portal vein and biliary tree. The lobes are further divided into segments, numbering eight in total, based on further vascular and biliary branching. Knowledge of these divisions allows an anatomical resection for tumour or trauma.

There is much variation in the anatomy of the extrahepatic blood vessels and angiography is important to delineate the anatomy before resection or infusion of cytotoxic agents. The hepatic artery, which usually arises from the coeliac axis, may arise instead from the aorta, the superior mesenteric artery, or the left gastric artery, and accessory hepatic arteries are not uncommon. Total liver blood flow is about 1500 ml/min and most (75%) comes from the portal vein at low pressure (3–5 mmHg). Some authorities consider that there is streaming of blood so that mesenteric blood reaches the right lobe and splenic blood passes to the left lobe.

Hepatic lymph is formed in the space of Disse and most drains to the porta hepatis via lymphatics which run with the portal tracts. Some drains to the nodes around the hepatic veins via lymphatics which run with the hepatic vein branches.

Microscopically, the liver cells are arranged into hexagonal lobules, each of which consists of a central vein and plates of hepatocytes. The plates of liver cells are normally one cell thick and radiate away from the central vein towards the periphery of the lobule. They are separated from each other by the hepatic sinusoids which are lined by fenestrated endothelial cells and Kupffer cells; the latter act as macrophages and are part of the reticuloendothelial system. Between the endothelium and the liver cells is the space of Disse. The portal tracts are at the peripheries of the lobules and contain bile ducts, branches of the hepatic artery and branches of the portal vein. The blood supply of the liver passes from the portal tracts, through the sinusoids, to the central vein.

Liver cell damage may be classified as centrilobular (around the central vein), peripheral lobular and mid-zonal. A more functional view of microscopic liver structure, based on blood supply, is to consider the portal tract as the central focus and the centrilobular vein to be at the periphery of a functional unit of the liver known as the 'acinus'. This is divided into zone 1 (surrounding the portal tract), zone 3 (adjacent to the centrilobular vein) and zone 2 (between zone 1 and 3). Thus hypoxic damage, as happens for example in cardiac failure, causes necrosis of liver cells which have the poorest blood supply, i.e. acinar zone 3 (centrilobular necrosis in lobular terminology). Certain toxins (e.g. phosphorus) cause necrosis of zone 1 of the acinus where the concentration is at its highest (in lobular terminology this would be peripheral lobular necrosis) (*see Fig. 6.1*).

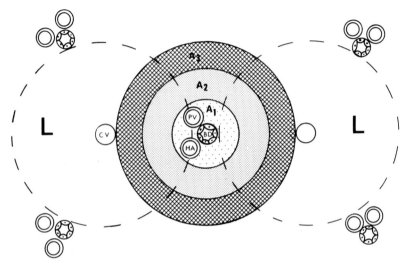

Fig 6.1. Simplified schematic diagram to show the relationship between the liver lobule L and the three zones of the liver acinus A_1, A_2, A_3. (CV—central vein; PV—portal vein; BD—bile duct; HA—hepatic artery.)

The biliary system starts as minute bile canaliculi which are situated between adjacent hepatocytes. The walls of the canaliculi therefore consist only of the plasma membranes of the hepatocytes. Where the plasma membranes form canalicular walls they contain actin microfilaments which are important in the transport of bile along the drainage system. The bile canaliculi drain via the canals of Hering, which are lined partly by hepatocytes and partly by bile duct epithelium, into the interlobular bile ducts, which are completely lined by cuboidal epithelium. The interlobular ducts drain via septal ducts into the main right and left hepatic ducts.

As well as the formation and secretion of bile, the liver is involved in the synthesis of albumin, globulins, clotting factors (I, II, V, VII, IX, X), urea, glucose, cholesterol, lipoproteins, phospholipids and many other substances.

The liver also removes from the circulation and destroys toxins, ammonia and other products of the gut, fibrin degradation products, plasminogen activators, certain hormones and many other substances.

Storage of glycogen is a further major function and hypoglycaemia is a sequela of major hepatic resection.

Liver Biopsy

Liver biopsy can be obtained percutaneously, at laparoscopy, at laparotomy or by using a transjugular catheter.

Percutaneous biopsy can be carried out with the Menghini or Tru-cut needle and ultrasound or CT scan can be used to guide the needle into a focal lesion. Ultrasound will also detect dilated bile ducts due to biliary obstruction; this is a contraindication to biopsy as puncture of the obstructed ducts may cause bile peritonitis. Other contraindications are poor patient co-operation, defective haemostasis, hydatid disease, vascular tumours and marked ascites. Other complications include bleeding, pneumothorax, haemobilia, perforation of the gallbladder and tumour seeding along the needle tract. The incidence of major complications is about 0·3%. If bleeding occurs, laparotomy may be required and therefore the patient must be fit for laparotomy before a biopsy is carried out.

The normal biopsy is a chocolate colour; pale yellow indicates fatty change and fragmentation suggests cirrhosis. In obstructive jaundice, the specimen may be green; it is dark brown in haemochromatosis, white in secondary carcinoma and black in the Dubin–Johnson syndrome.

Transjugular biopsy is useful in patients who have ascites or a bleeding problem; an adequate biopsy can be obtained in 95% of patients. The method also permits simultaneous hepatic venography and measurement of free and wedge hepatic venous pressure.

Jaundice

Jaundice is a yellow pigmentation of the skin caused by hyperbilirubinaemia. It becomes clinically apparent when the serum bilirubin reaches 35 μmol/l (2 mg per 100 ml).

Bilirubin is derived mainly from the haem part of the haemoglobin molecule which in turn is derived from the breakdown of senescent red blood cells; some does come from other haem pigments such as myoglobin. The haem is converted into biliverdin and then to bilirubin within phagocytes of the reticuloendothelial system. The bilirubin then enters the plasma where the majority of it is bound to albumin as unconjugated bilirubin. This bilirubin/albumin complex is not water-soluble and therefore does not pass through the glomeruli into the urine. The bilirubin is taken up by hepatocytes where it is conjugated by the enzyme glucuronyl transferase, first to bilirubin monoglucuronide and then to bilirubin diglucuronide, both of which are water soluble. The conjugated bilirubin is excreted into the bile canaliculi where it forms one of the constituents of bile. Bile flow in the canaliculi is maintained by (1) osmotic forces created by membrane pumps which actively secrete bile acid and sodium into the bile canaliculi, and possibly by (2) contractile tone caused by the actin microfilaments within the walls of the bile canaliculi. When bilirubin enters the gut it is converted by gut bacteria into urobilinogen which is reabsorbed and re-excreted by the liver thus forming an enterohepatic circulation. Excess urobilinogen is excreted in the urine.

Jaundice occurs if this system breaks down or is overloaded. Hyperbilirubinaemia is clinically divided into predominantly unconjugated and predominantly conjugated. In unconjugated hyperbilirubinaemia the albumin–bilirubin complex does not pass into the urine (acholuric jaundice). In conjugated hyperbilirubinaemia the urine is bile stained.

Unconjugated hyperbilirubinaemia

The major causes of unconjugated hyperbilirubinaemia are as follows.

1. Haemolysis

This may be intravascular in the case of haemolytic anaemia or extra-vascular in the case of reabsorption from a haematoma, infarction or gastrointestinal haemorrhage. In either case there is an increase in bilirubin production.

2. Impaired hepatic uptake of bilirubin

This may occur in cases of severe sepsis and physiological stress.

3. Congenital unconjugated hyperbilirubinaemia

Gilbert's syndrome (probably autosomal dominant) is caused by a defect in hepatic uptake of unconjugated bilirubin which is combined with mild haemolysis in about half the cases. It is the most common anomaly of bilirubin transport and it causes jaundice in otherwise well patients. The condition is entirely benign. The Crigler–Najjar syndrome occurs as two types. In type 1 (autosomal recessive) there is virtual absence of the enzyme glucuronyl transferase, causing severe jaundice, kernicterus and death in infancy. In type 2 (autosomal dominant) there is a mild reduction in glucuronyl transferase activity and normal survival is possible.

4. Other causes

Impaired conjugation of bilirubin also occurs in jaundice of the newborn and in advanced hepatocellular disease, such as cirrhosis.

Conjugated hyperbilirubinaemia

Besides hereditary conjugated hyperbilirubinaemia, the majority of these cases are due to obstruction of bile flow (cholestasis). Cholestasis is characterized chemically by conjugated hyperbilirubinaemia, bilirubinuria, increased levels of serum bile acids, and increased serum alkaline phosphatase. The major causes of conjugated hyperbilirubinaemia are as follows.

1. Impaired secretion of bilirubin

The Dubin–Johnson syndrome and Rotor syndrome are rare inherited disorders (autosomal recessive) in which there is a defect in excretion of bilirubin by hepatocytes and consequently a conjugated hyperbilirubinaemia. In the Rotor syndrome the liver is of normal appearance, whereas in the Dubin–Johnson syndrome it is black due to deposition of pigment, the nature of which is unknown.

2. Intrahepatic cholestasis

Intrahepatic cholestasis may be associated with hepatocellular disease (e.g. viral hepatitis, alcoholic hepatitis and cirrhosis), or it may occur independently of hepatocellular disease (pure cholestasis). Examples of the latter are: (1) congenital atresia of the intrahepatic bile ducts; (2) administration of sex hormones, such as oestrogens, the contraceptive pill and anabolic steroids; (3) primary biliary cirrhosis (in the early stages); (4) benign, familial recurrent cholestasis (possibly due to an inherited abnormality of bile canaliculi); and (5) recurrent jaundice of pregnancy (jaundice occurs in the last trimester, clears after delivery and may be due to increased levels of oestrogen).

It is possible that some of these types of intrahepatic cholestasis are due to an abnormality of one of the factors which cause bile flow in the bile canaliculi, i.e. a defect in the sodium or bile acid pumps or in the actin microfilaments which are found in the bile canalicular walls (*see* above).

3. Obstruction of the main bile ducts

This is due most commonly to one of the following conditions: (1) gallstones, (2) carcinoma of the head of the pancreas, (3) other malignant obstructions including cancer of the bile ducts and lymph nodes in the porta hepatis, (4) pancreatitis, (5) benign stricture of the bile ducts, (6) atresia of the bile ducts, (7) sclerosing cholangitis. These are all discussed elsewhere.

Liver changes in jaundice

In many cases of unconjugated hyperbilirubinaemia the liver appears normal or almost normal.

In intrahepatic cholestasis there may be features of the underlying disease (e.g. viral hepatitis or primary biliary cirrhosis) which are discussed elsewhere. The distinctive histological feature of intrahepatic cholestasis of any aetiology is the presence of brown bile plugs which are seen in the bile canaliculi (i.e. between hepatocytes) in the centres of the hepatic lobules (acinar zone 3).

In obstruction of major bile ducts, portal tract changes are seen as well as bile plugs. These include oedema, an inflammatory cell infiltration and marginal bile duct proliferation. The latter results from an increased tortuosity of the bile ducts and is seen as an apparent increased number of bile ducts at the margins of the portal tracts. A further feature of large duct obstruction is the presence of bile infarcts which appear as circumscribed areas of necrotic liver cells adjacent to portal tracts.

Systemic effects of jaundice

Many biochemical and metabolic abnormalities are found in patients with jaundice. Some of these are a direct consequence of the jaundice and some are the result of associated hepatic dysfunction, such as failure to produce clotting factors or failure to deal with endotoxins.

Pruritus may be due to retained bile salts, although this is not proven. Cardiovascular changes include bradycardia and a reduced peripheral vascular resistance, both of which may impair the response to haemorrhage during surgery. Vascular changes in the kidney may be partly responsible for the renal complications which are discussed on p. 158. Coagulation abnormalities are not entirely due to failure to synthesize coagulation factors since, although the administration of vitamin K corrects the prothrombin time, excess bleeding may still occur during surgery. There appears to be a low grade disseminated intravascular coagulation as indicated by a raised level of serum fibrin degradation products. The endotoxaemia may be responsible.

Most reports indicate that wound healing is impaired in obstructive jaundice, both in experimental animals and in man, as shown by the development of wound dehiscence and incisional hernia.

Sepsis causes considerable morbidity and mortality after surgery for obstructive jaundice. In vitro experiments show that unconjugated bilirubin and bile salts impair antibacterial defence mechanisms, including phagocytosis. The function of the reticuloendothelial system is also impaired. The perioperative administration of antibiotics reduces the incidence of sepsis.

Viral Hepatitis

Hepatitis may occur as a result of several different viral infections, including yellow fever, infectious mononucleosis and occasionally adenovirus and enterovirus. The term viral hepatitis, when used without qualification, refers to infection by the hepatitis A virus (HAV), the hepatitis B virus (HBV), or the non-A non-B (NANB) agent(s).

Hepatitis A

This is due to a 27 nm RNA virus which is spread by the faecal–oral route in conditions of poor hygiene. The incubation period is 15–45 days and the disease is relatively mild and self-limiting. It can be diagnosed by the presence of serum IgM anti-HAV during the acute illness. IgG anti-HAV occurs during convalescence, remains elevated for life and confers life-long immunity.

Hepatitis A differs from hepatitis B in three important respects: (1) it very rarely causes fulminant hepatitis; (2) it does not produce chronic active hepatitis; and (3) it does not give rise to a carrier state.

Hepatitis B

This is caused by a 42 nm DNA virus consisting of an inner 27 nm core (synthesized in the hepatocyte nucleus), surrounded by an outer coat (synthesized in the hepatocyte cytoplasm). The main modes of spread are (1) by blood or blood products, (2) vertically from mother to infant, and (3) as a sexually transmitted disease, especially in homosexuals. Infected blood can spread the disease by either injection or by contamination of the conjunctiva. The incubation period is one to six months. The core of the virus contains two main antigens, the core antigen (HBcAg) and the e antigen (HBeAg). The outer coat contains a surface antigen (HBsAg) which is also known as the Australia antigen. Each of these antigens stimulates production of a corresponding antibody. The complete virion is termed the Dane particle and can be demonstrated in hepatocytes and occasionally also in blood.

The HBsAg (Australia antigen) is synthesized in excess and circulates in the blood as spheres and tubules. Since these are incomplete viral particles they are not infective. The level of HBsAg in the blood rises before the onset of symptoms and usually disappears at the time of recovery. Anti-HBs appears sometime after the disappearance of HBsAg and therefore there is a lag phase or 'window' during which neither is found. During this time the diagnosis may be missed serologically if only HBsAg and anti-HBs are measured. Anti-HBs confers life-long immunity. Persistence of HBsAg indicates a risk of developing chronic liver disease. The HBcAg is found within hepatocytes and does not appear in the circulation. Anti-HBc does, however, appear at about the time of onset of symptoms and it remains present during the 'window' period noted above. HBeAg is found in the circulation, appearing after and disappearing before HBsAg. HBeAg is usually associated with circulating Dane particles (whole viruses) and, therefore, its presence indicates active infection and infectivity. Anti-HBe occurs at the time of recovery and is a marker of recent disease (*see Fig.* 6.2).

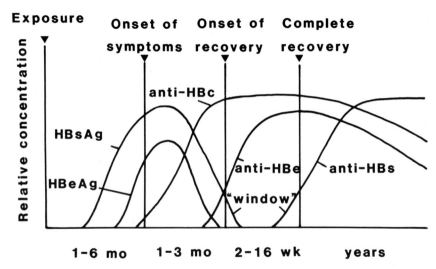

Fig 6.2. Graph to show the rises in antigen and antibodies with time in hepatitis B. (Reproduced with permission from Robbins *et al.* 1984.)

Hepatitis B may give rise to a carrier state. Healthy carriers are those who are HBsAg positive but who have no symptoms and no history of acute hepatitis. Liver disease carriers are those who are HBsAg positive and have chronic persistent or chronic active hepatitis, with or without a history of acute hepatitis. Carriers of HBsAg are common in Asia and Africa but less common in Western countries.

THE DELTA AGENT AND HEPATITIS B: The delta agent is thought to be an incomplete RNA virus which requires the presence of hepatitis B virus for replication. Therefore, the presence of the delta agent in the liver cells or serum is indicative also of the presence of hepatitis B. The delta agent may be important in the causation of fulminant hepatitis. It is also implicated in the progression of acute hepatitis B to chronic active hepatitis.

Non-A non-B (NANB) hepatitis

This is diagnosed when the other causes of hepatitis noted above and drug ingestion have been excluded. There are probably three agents involved although none has been conclusively identified. Non-A non-B hepatitis may follow blood transfusion and is not detected on routine screening of blood. It can also spread by non-percutaneous routes. The incubation period is 14–120 days.

NANB hepatitis can cause fulminant hepatitis, chronic hepatitis and probably also a carrier state.

Clinical features of viral hepatitis

Sporadic cases of viral hepatitis are due to hepatitis A in about half of the cases, hepatitis B in about one-third and non-A non-B in the remainder. In contrast, post-transfusion hepatitis is almost entirely (90%) due to non-A non-B because of the effectiveness of screening blood for hepatitis B.

Hepatitis A virus causes the mildest while hepatitis B virus causes the most severe symptoms.

The prodromal symptoms include nausea, vomiting, abdominal pain (due to swollen liver), pyrexia and a general flu-like illness. This is followed by the icteric phase which is accompanied by dark urine and pale faeces and return of the temperature to normal. The icteric phase lasts 1–4 weeks and is followed by recovery in most cases. The condition may be completely anicteric in some patients.

Fulminant hepatitis may rarely occur and in these cases the patient rapidly deteriorates and goes into acute liver failure; the liver function tests are grossly deranged and the prognosis is extremely poor.

Morphology

Grossly the liver is swollen and can be appreciated by palpation.

Histologically, the findings are similar in all three forms, although some distinguishing features have been described. The main findings are necrosis of individual hepatocytes (spotty necrosis) and inflammation, most severe in the centrilobular area (acinar zone 3). Kupffer cells are enlarged and some portal inflammation is seen. Areas of necrosis may be seen extending between the central veins and portal tracts (bridging necrosis), although this finding is not necessarily indicative of a poor prognosis. Necrosis of whole acini (panacinar necrosis) is seen in fulminant hepatitis.

Outcome of viral hepatitis

There are several possible outcomes after viral hepatitis.

RESOLUTION: This is the usual course.

MASSIVE OR SUBMASSIVE NECROSIS: This is frequently fatal. In those who survive, the liver cells may regenerate without scarring. Alternatively, if there is a prolonged course and repeated episodes of submassive necrosis, large scars of fibrous tissue are seen replacing the parenchyma. This is termed post-necrotic scarring rather than cirrhosis, since it does not have the nodularity of the latter.

POST-NECROTIC SCARRING: *See* above.

CHRONIC PERSISTENT HEPATITIS: *See* p. 152.

CHRONIC ACTIVE HEPATITIS: *See* p. 152.

CIRRHOSIS: This usually occurs in cases that have gone on to chronic active hepatitis and is termed post-necrotic cirrhosis. (*See* p. 155).

Precautions against viral hepatitis

The surgeon at risk from the patient

1. If a surgeon operating on a patient who is HBsAg positive gets blood inoculated into skin or conjunctiva, he should receive hepatitis B immunoglobulin immediately and repeated one month later. If the surgeon's skin is grossly contaminated without actual inoculation, the same procedure should apply.
2. If the patient is e antigen positive, he is highly infective and therefore maximum precautions are required, including restricting theatre access. All personnel in the theatre wear gloves and surgeons wear double gloves and eye protection. No equipment liable to produce an aerosol of the patient's blood should be used. Contaminated swabs and disposables are incinerated, contaminated linen should be autoclaved before washing, endoscopes should be treated with glutaraldehyde and the operating table washed with glutaraldehyde. Specimens are placed in formalin which kills all viruses.
3. Hepatitis A is transmitted by the faecal–oral route and there should be no major risk problem to the surgeon.
4. Non-A non-B hepatitis shows no evidence to date of hospital acquired infection.

The patient at risk from the surgeon

1. Hepatitis A has no carrier state and therefore there should be no significant risk problem.
2. Non-A non-B hepatitis—occasional carrier state has been reported but to date there is no instance of transmission from surgeon to patient.
3. Hepatitis B—Department of Health guidelines suggest that a surgeon who is HBsAg positive can work anywhere except in a renal unit. If there are clustered cases of hepatitis due to the surgeon, he should not operate.

The hepatitis B vaccine, available since 1982, is recommended for a wide variety of health workers who may be exposed to hepatitis B patients. Fears of possible transmission of acquired immune deficiency syndrome (AIDS) in this vaccine have so far proved groundless as the manufacturing process inactivates viruses such as human T-cell lymphotropic virus (HTLV III), recently implicated in the causation of AIDS.

Chronic Hepatitis

Chronic hepatitis refers to a chronic inflammatory condition of the liver which has lasted for a minimum of six months. The two types which are clinically recognized are chronic persistent and chronic active hepatitis.

Chronic persistent hepatitis

Following hepatitis B or non-A non-B hepatitis, clinical and/or biochemical changes may last for several years before the patient is completely recovered. During this time, liver function tests are abnormal, although there is no progressive liver damage. In many cases there is no history of clinical hepatitis. Histologically there is a mild chronic inflammatory infiltrate confined to the portal tracts. Significant hepatocyte necrosis is not seen.

Chronic active hepatitis

Cases of chronic active hepatitis may be divided into those which are HBsAg positive (following hepatitis B infection) and those which are HBsAg negative, which may be idiopathic or associated with drug toxicity, Wilson's disease or alpha-1-antitrypsin deficiency. A proportion of the HBsAg negative cases may follow non-A non-B hepatitis, although this is not entirely proven.

Clinically, the symptoms such as general malaise, anorexia, etc., are vague. Liver function tests are abnormal. The condition is progressive towards cirrhosis although this may take ten or more years to develop and may be prevented by immunosuppressive therapy.

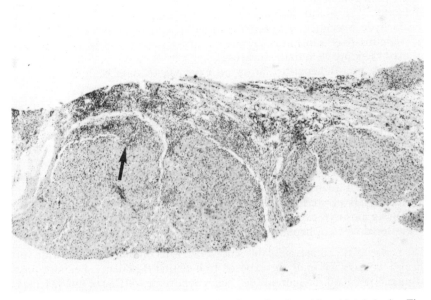

Fig 6.3. Needle biopsy of liver showing chronic active hepatitis with cirrhosis. The inflammatory cells appear to be invading the liver parenchyma giving it a 'moth-eaten' appearance (arrow). (H and E × 35)

Histologically the inflammatory infiltrate involves not only the portal triad, but also the surrounding parenchyma. Characteristically there is necrosis of individual hepatocytes, situated at the limiting plate of the hepatic lobule, i.e. the layer of hepatocytes next to the portal tract, giving it a moth-eaten appearance. This is termed piecemeal necrosis. Areas of necrosis may join the central vein to the portal triad (bridging necrosis). Eventually there is fibrosis and the liver becomes cirrhotic (*see Fig.* 6.3).

Alcoholic Liver Disease

Alcoholic liver disease occurs in three forms: (1) fatty liver, (2) alcoholic hepatitis, and (3) liver cirrhosis. The relationship between these is not clear. Fatty change probably has no role in the production of cirrhosis. Some cases of alcohol related cirrhosis develop after alcoholic hepatitis, whereas other cases develop without a hepatitis phase.

Epidemiology and aetiology

The epidemiological pattern of alcoholic liver cirrhosis in different countries is directly related to the quantity of alcohol consumed. In France the *per capita* alcohol consumption per year is 16·4 litres of absolute alcohol and mortality from cirrhosis is 57·2 per 100 000 persons over 25 years old. The respective figures for the UK are 6·2 litres and 5·7 per 100 000 (Sherlock 1981). Although consumption of 160 g of alcohol per day used to be considered safe, it has more recently been established from various reports that a chronic consumption of 80 g per day in men and 60 g per day in women over many years can lead to cirrhosis.

There is good evidence that alcohol itself is the cause of liver damage rather than the associated nutritional deficiency.

Alcohol is metabolized in the liver to acetaldehyde by the enzyme alcohol dehydrogenase with the concomitant production of NADH. The NADH can be used as an alternative fuel source, leading to an accumulation of fat.

Fleming and McGee (1984) have recently reviewed the mechanisms of damage which occur in alcoholic hepatitis and cirrhosis. They suggested that alcohol causes damage to the cytoskeleton of the hepatocyte. The cytoskeleton which maintains the cell structure has three components—microfilaments, microtubules and intermediate filaments. It appears that alcohol, in some unknown way, damages a particular type of intermediate filament and that these damaged intermediate filaments appear in the cell cytoplasm as eosinophilic material known as Mallory's hyaline (*see* below). The integrity of intermediate filaments appears to be necessary for the translation of messenger RNA. Therefore, alcohol may cause cell death by damaging certain intermediate filaments and this in turn interferes with the translation of mRNA.

The cell death causes an inflammatory response either directly or by an immunological mechanism. Mallory's hyaline may act antigenically and therefore it may be involved in the immunological reaction. The resultant inflammatory reaction causes hepatitis. Various factors released by lymphocytes (lymphokines) and macrophages stimulate fibroblasts to produce collagen and this fibrosis plus the regeneration of liver cells leads to liver cirrhosis.

Clinical features

Patients with a fatty liver are often asymptomatic although the liver may be palpable. Alcoholic hepatitis presents as an acute disease, similar to infective hepatitis, with pyrexia, jaundice, tender hepatosplenomegaly and abnormal liver function tests. In severe cases there is hepatic failure and encephalopathy. Alcoholic cirrhosis presents with the various features of advanced liver disease and portal hypertension.

Morphology

In a fatty liver, cut section shows it to be pale and greasy. Histologically, fat accumulates within hepatocytes so that they become vacuolated with the nucleus pushed to one side. In some cases, a pericellular fibrosis occurs in the vicinity of the central vein and this is said to be highly characteristic of an alcoholic aetiology. Alcoholic hepatitis may occur in pre-cirrhotic and in cirrhotic livers. There is invariably an accumulation of fat and the hepatitic process is characterized by necrosis of individual hepatocytes and an infiltrate of inflammatory cells including polymorphs (*see Fig.* 6.4). Cirrhosis is described later.

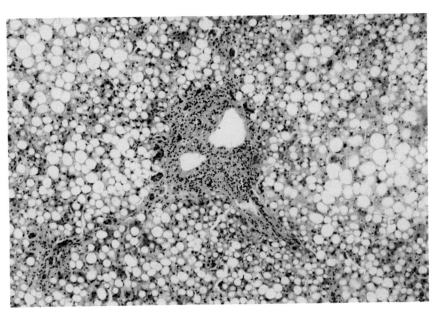

Fig 6.4. Alcoholic hepatitis with fatty change of liver. Note the inflammatory cells in the portal tract and scattered in the liver parenchyma. (H and E × 75)

Prognosis

The prognosis for an acute bout of alcoholic hepatitis depends on the severity. In severe cases the mortality is up to 20%. The long-term outlook depends on the degree of liver disease and whether or not the patient stops drinking.

Liver Cirrhosis

Cirrhosis is a diffuse condition of the liver characterized by fibrosis and the conversion of normal liver architecture into structurally abnormal nodules.

Aetiology

ALCOHOL: This is discussed above.

VIRAL HEPATITIS: Hepatitis B virus and probably also non-A non-B viruses (but not hepatitis A virus) can lead to cirrhosis. There is usually an evolution through chronic active hepatitis to a macronodular type of cirrhosis termed post-necrotic cirrhosis.

PRIMARY BILIARY CIRRHOSIS: This condition occurs most commonly in middle-aged women. They often have other autoimmune diseases such as rheumatoid arthritis; antimitochondrial antibodies are present in 90% of cases. There appears to be an immunological attack on the bile duct epithelium which is associated histologically with a granulomatous inflammatory reaction centred on the bile ducts in the portal tract.

SECONDARY BILIARY CIRRHOSIS: Extrahepatic obstruction of the biliary tree may eventually lead to secondary biliary cirrhosis. The intrahepatic bile ducts are damaged causing inflammation and scarring. Ascending cholangitis adds to the damage.

HAEMOCHROMATOSIS: This may be primary or secondary. Primary haemochromatosis is an inherited (probably autosomal recessive) condition in which there is excessive absorption of iron by the gastrointestinal tract. There is probably a defect in the control of iron absorption actually within the gut mucosal cells, although this may be associated with abnormal iron metabolism in the liver. Secondary haemochromatosis occurs in states of iron overload, such as certain anaemias, e.g. thalassaemia, and in states of high iron intake (multiple transfusions and ingestion of alcoholic beverages rich in iron). In both cases iron is deposited (in the form of ferritin and haemosiderin) in the liver, pancreas, heart, skin and synovial membranes.

The mechanism of cell damage is unclear. One possibility is that an increase in iron deposition overloads the liver's mechanism for storing iron in the harmless ferritin form. Excess free iron undergoes reduction from the ferric state to the ferrous state with concomitant formation of toxic free radicals from oxygen.

Haemosiderosis of liver refers to iron deposition without parenchymal damage as opposed to haemochromatosis in which there is parenchymal damage.

Clinically, primary haemochromatosis presents mainly in males aged between 40 and 60 years (male : female ratio 10 : 1; females are protected by menstruation). The clinical features are those of liver disease, diabetes mellitus, skin pigmentation, heart disease and joint disease. The serum iron is raised to a variable degree and the serum transferrin is 90% saturated (normally 30% saturated). The disease can be prevented by venesection therapy prior to the onset of cirrhosis and thus the unexpected finding of raised serum iron merits investigation.

WILSON'S DISEASE (HEPATOLENTICULAR DEGENERATION): This is an autosomal recessive disorder of copper metabolism in which excessive copper is laid down in the liver, basal ganglia (causing chorea and athetosis), cerebellum and the eye (producing a Kayser-Fleischer ring).

Copper is normally transported to the liver where it is bound to a carrier protein before being either excreted in the bile or bound to caeruloplasmin and released into the plasma. In Wilson's disease both biliary copper and plasma caeruloplasmin concentrations are low. Therefore, some as yet unidentified defect(s) in copper excretion by the liver has been postulated. The mechanism of cell damage is unclear, although it may be due to production of free radicals by free copper within the cells.

Clinically, the presentation is with hepatic or neuropsychiatric symptoms between the ages of 5 and 30 years. The hepatic form may appear as fulminant hepatitis, chronic active hepatitis or cirrhosis.

ALPHA-1-ANTITRYPSIN DEFICIENCY: Alpha-1-antitrypsin is a protease inhibitor which is synthesized in the liver and released into the plasma. Alpha-1-antitrypsin deficiency is a genetically determined disease in which there is accumulation of intracytoplasmic globules of alpha-1-antitrypsin in hepatocytes. This is associated with a type of neonatal hepatitis which is followed by the development of cirrhosis in childhood or adult life. The mechanism of cell injury is unknown.

OTHER METABOLIC DISORDERS: Galactosaemia and congenital tyrosinosis are associated with the development of hepatic cirrhosis.

DRUGS: Methotrexate and methyldopa administration have been associated with cirrhosis.

INTESTINAL BYPASS: In patients who undergo jejuno-ileal or jejuno-colic bypass for morbid obesity, there may follow a series of liver conditions ranging from fatty change (often present prior to surgery) to a condition resembling alcoholic hepatitis and finally cirrhosis. The cause may be metabolic rather than due to nutritional deficiency. One possibility is that the primary bile salt, chenodeoxy-cholate (which would normally be absorbed in the terminal ileum), passes directly into the large bowel where it is metabolized by bacteria to lithocholate, which is absorbed and can cause hepatocellular damage.

INDIAN CHILDHOOD CIRRHOSIS: This occurs mainly in India, South-East Asia and the Middle East. It affects children aged 1–3 years old and is usually followed by death within a year. The cause is unknown.

CRYPTOGENIC: In the UK the cause of cirrhosis is unknown in up to 30% of cases.

Pathogenesis of liver cirrhosis

The pathogenesis of alcoholic liver cirrhosis has been mentioned above. It is likely that when the liver is injured by any of the factors noted above, its response is similar in most cases; cell necrosis leads to fibrosis, possibly due to stimulation of fibroblasts by factors released by macrophages and lymphocytes. The fibrosis disrupts the liver architecture and vascular pattern and cell regeneration in response to the necrosis produces nodularity. However, this process does not explain all cases as in some forms (e.g. haemochromatosis and methotrexate toxicity) necrosis is rarely seen.

Morphology

Cirrhosis is classically divided into macronodular and micronodular forms. The micronodular form is characterized by thick fibrous septa, separating small nodules of regenerating liver cells which are about 3 mm in diameter (*see Fig.* 6.5). In macronodular cirrhosis, fibrous septa separate nodules of various sizes up to several centimetres in diameter.

In many cases, such as alcoholic cirrhosis and Wilson's disease, a micronodular form is seen in the early stage of the disease and this progresses to a macronodular pattern in the later stages. A micronodular pattern is typical in haemochromatosis and primary biliary cirrhosis, while a macronodular pattern is typical in the cirrhosis following HBsAg positive chronic active hepatitis. The liver may be greasy due to fat accumulation in alcoholic cirrhosis; in haemochromatosis, the liver is a dark brown colour.

The diagnosis of cirrhosis is suspected at the time of biopsy if the liver is tough to penetrate. On histological examination, rounded nodules of liver cells are seen, surrounded by fibrous tissue. Micronodular cirrhosis is readily apparent, since the nodules are small enough to be seen *in toto* on a needle biopsy. Macronodular cirrhosis is more difficult since a sample from the centre of a large nodule may appear as relatively normal liver tissue. A false negative rate of up to 10% has been quoted in the diagnosis of macronodular cirrhosis on needle biopsy.

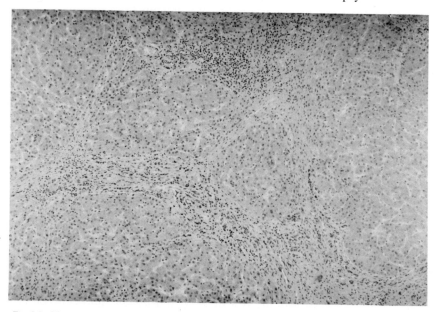

Fig 6.5. Liver cirrhosis. (H and E × 30)

The aetiology of the cirrhosis is often not apparent on microscopic examination. In some cases, however, the cause may be seen or certain features may point towards a specific aetiology.

In alcoholic cirrhosis, the aetiology may be suspected if there is fatty change or if Mallory's hyaline is present (although both features are non-specific). Mallory's hyaline is seen as deeply eosinophilic material around the hepatocyte nucleus. There may also be the superimposed features of an alcoholic hepatitis, in which case there is an associated inflammatory reaction which includes many polymorphs. Chronic active hepatitis due to hepatitis B infection is suspected if HBsAg can be demonstrated by immunohistochemistry. Primary biliary cirrhosis characteristically shows a lymphocytic infiltrate of the portal tracts together with a paucity of bile ducts and the presence of granulomas in some cases. In secondary biliary cirrhosis, the portal tracts are oedematous and somewhat inflamed while the bile plugs indicative of cholestasis are seen. The presence of ascending cholangitis is denoted by the finding of pus within the bile ducts. In haemochromatosis, Wilson's disease and alpha-1-antitrypsin deficiency, special stains will demonstrate the presence of iron, copper and alpha-1-antitrypsin respectively in the hepatocytes.

Complications of Advanced Liver Disease

Portal hypertension and ascites are major complications of liver cirrhosis and are discussed later. Other complications of liver disease include the following.

Hepatic failure

Liver cirrhosis is a progressive disease which eventually leads to hepatic failure if the patient does not succumb to one of the other complications in the meantime. Jaundice occurs due to both conjugated and unconjugated hyperbilirubinaemia. Failure to manufacture protein leads to hypoalbuminaemia and bleeding disorders. Foetor hepaticus appears. Failure to degrade oestrogen leads to gynaecomastia, testicular atrophy, palmar erythema and spider angiomas of the skin. Renal failure (due to several different mechanisms) and hepatic encephalopathy may occur and these are discussed below.

Renal complications

Functional renal failure (hepatorenal syndrome)

Renal failure may occur in the course of liver disease without obvious structural changes in the kidney. In the UK and Europe this is termed 'functional renal failure' (FRF), although in the USA it is sometimes called 'hepatorenal syndrome'. It may occur in cirrhosis or in other forms of liver failure.

The patient has a rising blood urea and hyponatraemia. The renal tubules, however, act appropriately and reabsorb sodium, resulting in a low urinary sodium concentration.

Kidneys from patients with the syndrome are functionally normal when transplanted into other patients and renal function returns to normal in affected patients who have undergone liver transplantation. It seems, therefore, that there is little or no intrinsic abnormality of renal structure and that normal liver function is somehow necessary for normal renal function.

The cardiac output in these patients is normal and the actual plasma volume is normal. There is, however, diversion of blood away from the kidney due to a raised renal vascular resistance in the presence of a normal vascular resistance elsewhere; in some cases total renal plasma flow is normal and there is diversion of renal blood flow from the cortex to the medulla. There may also be a reduction in effective blood plasma volume, i.e. the volume of plasma involved in organ perfusion. The cause of the renal vasoconstriction is unknown. Several possibilities have been suggested: (1) patients with liver failure have a decreased ability to produce bradykinin, which is a powerful vasodilator; (2) the main renal prostaglandin (E2) is a potent vasodilator and its production is stimulated by the kallikrein–kinin system which is defective in liver failure; (3) endotoxins are powerful renal vasoconstrictors and endotoxaemia may be due to failure of the liver to filter bacterial endotoxin from the gut.

FRF carries a poor prognosis.

Acute tubular necrosis

Patients who have obstructive jaundice (as opposed to cirrhosis) have an increased risk of developing post-operative renal failure due to acute tubular necrosis. It may be due to endotoxaemia or to the effect of bilirubin on the renal tubules.

When patients with obstructive jaundice undergo surgery, the risk of acute tubular necrosis may be reduced by maintaining good hydration and by maintaining renal output with mannitol. Cahill (1983) has shown that pre-operative administration of oral sodium deoxycholate prevents renal failure in patients with obstructed jaundice, probably due to its detergent effect on bacterial endotoxins in the gut.

Hepatic encephalopathy

Hepatic encephalopathy often has a precipitating cause such as uraemia, certain drugs (e.g. tranquillizers), gastrointestinal haemorrhage, excessive protein intake or hypokalaemic alkalosis.

The clinical features are changes in personality, intellect and emotional behaviour and an alteration in the level of consciousness. Characteristically the patient has a flapping tremor and constructional apraxia.

It is likely that the encephalopathy is due to a toxic agent produced in the gut which is not filtered by the damaged liver. The agent is probably a bacterial product of protein metabolism since a protein load (e.g. gastrointestinal haemorrhage) often precipitates the condition and antibiotics help in the treatment of it. Several possible agents have been implicated.

1. Ammonia is produced from bacterial protein metabolism in the gut and is usually converted to urea in the liver. If this fails to happen, serum ammonia rises and it is converted in the brain to glutamine. Serum ammonia concentration does not correlate well with the degree of encephalopathy but CSF glutamine does. It is possible that glutamine acts as a false neurotransmitter, replacing the normal neuro-transmitter glutamate.

2. Amino-acids are metabolized in the liver; in liver failure there is an increase in the serum concentration of aromatic amino-acids and since aromatic amino-acids are precursors of several cerebral neuro-transmitters, it is possible that a change in amino-acid metabolism might interfere with neuro-transmitter production.

The false neuro-transmitters which may result from these abnormalities of ammonia and amino-acid metabolism are similar to normal neuro-transmitters. They are taken up by neurones and, when stimulated, the neurone releases the false neuro-transmitter which functions poorly or not at all, thus interfering with normal neuro-transmission.

Histological changes occur in the brain after long-standing hepatic encephalopathy. There is hyperplasia of astrocytes in cerebral cortex to form cells with large nuclei which typically contain a 'glycogen dot'.

Portal Hypertension

Normal portal pressure is 5–7 mmHg. This is raised if the portal venous flow is obstructed or occasionally if portal flow is greatly increased as happens in massive splenomegaly.

Portal hypertension has been classified according to the presumed site of obstruction into presinusoidal, sinusoidal and postsinusoidal. Since in many cases the site of the obstruction is mixed or unknown, Silk and Williams (1979) regard the simpler classification into extrahepatic, intrahepatic and suprahepatic as more satisfactory (see Table 6.1).

Table 6.1 Causes of portal hypertension

Extrahepatic (prehepatic):	— Portal vein thrombosis
Intrahepatic:	— Cirrhosis
	— Hepatitis
	— Congenital hepatic fibrosis
	— Partial nodular transformation
	— Schistosomiasis
	— Portal tract infiltration (e.g. lymphoproliferative disease)
	— Sarcoidosis
	— Idiopathic portal hypertension
	— Veno-occlusive disease
Suprahepatic:	— Budd–Chiari syndrome
	— Constrictive pericarditis
	— Right sided heart failure
Increased hepatic blood flow:	— Massive splenomegaly
	— Hepatoportal arteriovenous fistulas

Extrahepatic portal hypertension

The main cause is portal vein thrombosis. In children there may be a history of umbilical or other neonatal infection or of umbilical vein catheterization. In adults, predisposing factors for portal vein thrombosis include trauma, sepsis, malignant invasion and pancreatitis. No aetiological factor can be found in over half the cases.

Intrahepatic portal hypertension

Cirrhosis is the most important cause. In cirrhotic livers the hepatic vasculature is diminished and distorted and the regenerating nodules compress the sinusoids and hepatic veins. In some cases, especially in alcoholic liver disease, portal hypertension occurs before the development of regenerative nodules and is due to perivenular intrasinusoidal collagen deposition. The presence of intrahepatic arteriovenous anastomoses with resultant transmission of hepatic artery pressure to the portal vein is a further factor. In cirrhotic livers, the obstruction to flow occurs at presinusoidal, sinusoidal and postsinusoidal levels. Other causes of this 'mixed' pattern of obstruction include chronic active hepatitis, partial nodular transformation of the liver and cystic disease of the liver.

The classical cause of intrahepatic presinusoidal portal hypertension is schistosomiasis. The life cycle of the organism is described on p. 233. The ova penetrate and obstruct the portal vein branches and produce a fibrosis of the portal tracts (pipe stem fibrosis), although a true cirrhosis does not develop. Idiopathic portal hypertension is a condition in which intrahepatic portal hypertension arises without obvious cause. The obstruction appears to be mainly presinusoidal and some studies have shown an obliteration of small portal vein branches by thrombosis, in association with perivenular fibrosis. Other causes of intrahepatic presinusoidal portal hypertension include congenital hepatic fibrosis and infiltration of the portal tracts by lymphoproliferative disorders.

Postsinusoidal intrahepatic portal hypertension may be caused by veno-occlusive disease, in which there is widespread obstruction of the centrilobular and small collecting hepatic veins. The obliteration of the veins is most often due to ingestion of pyrrolizidine alkaloids which are present in bush teas. Other causes of veno-occlusive disease include radiotherapy and chemotherapy. In the long term it may give rise to cirrhosis.

Suprahepatic portal hypertension

The Budd–Chiari syndrome is defined as an occlusion of the main hepatic veins or their ostia; it is generally the result of thrombosis. This is in contrast to veno-occlusive disease which affects the small hepatic vein branches. Thrombosis of the hepatic veins may be associated with myeloproliferative disease, paroxysmal nocturnal haemoglobinuria and occasionally the oral contraceptive pill. The hepatic veins may be obstructed by tumour (e.g. HCC) alone or in company with thrombosis, and the syndrome may be caused by a web at or just above the entrance of the left and middle hepatic veins into the inferior vena cava. This last cause is important to recognize as it may be surgically treated.

Suprahepatic portal hypertension may also be due to constrictive pericarditis.

Portal hypertension due to increased portal blood flow

Massive splenomegaly may increase the portal blood flow to the extent that portal hypertension arises. Hepatoportal arteriovenous fistulas may cause portal hypertension on a similar basis.

Complications of portal hypertension

Bleeding varices
See p. 40.

Ascites

Ascites commonly develops in patients with intrahepatic and suprahepatic portal hypertension, but only rarely in patients with portal vein thrombosis. Several factors contribute to the formation of ascites.

Patients with liver disease tend to have hypoalbuminaemia due to poor hepatic synthesis. This reduces plasma colloid oncotic pressure and predisposes to ascites.

Cirrhotic patients have an increased hepatic lymph flow due to the increase in portal hydrostatic pressure. A contributory factor is the hypoalbuminaemia.

Disordered salt and water metabolism have been implicated in the formation of ascites. Traditionally, it is said that there is increased aldosterone activity (due to overproduction and reduced hepatic breakdown) which causes salt retention by the kidneys. However, about two-thirds of patients who have cirrhosis and ascites do not have increased aldosterone activity (Wilkinson and Williams 1980). An alternative view is that the accumulation of ascites leads to a reduced effective circulatory volume which in turn leads to conservation of sodium by the kidneys. Also, a decrease in effective central blood volume could activate baro-receptors, which in turn would inhibit the vagus, increase sympathetic activity and activate the renin–angiotensin–aldosterone axis as secondary phenomena.

Other proposed factors include failure to produce a natriuretic factor, failure of prostaglandin production by the liver and excess antidiuretic hormone activity.

Patients with ascites are subject to the condition of spontaneous bacterial peritonitis. This presents as general clinical deterioration without the classical signs of peritonitis and diagnosis is by the demonstration of increased white blood cells in the ascitic fluid. Infection is with a single organism, usually a Gram-negative bacillus such as *E. coli* (Crossley and Williams 1985).

Liver Cysts

Non-parasitic

Simple liver cysts are usually small solitary lesions, although they can enlarge to involve a segment or lobe. They contain dark brown fluid and are lined by cuboidal epithelium surrounding which is a layer of connective tissue.

Traumatic cysts are bile filled, solitary and have no epithelial lining.

Polycystic disease of the liver is associated with polycystic renal disease and congenital anomalies such as spina bifida and gastrointestinal malrotation. Most cysts are asymptomatic and only exert pressure effects when large. Occasionally, rupture and haemorrhage occur.

Hydatid liver cysts

These are due to the larval or cyst stage of the tapeworm Echinococcus. The life cycle of this organism usually has a larval or cystic stage in sheep (intermediate host) and an adult stage in dogs (definite host). The adult worm produces ova which are excreted in the dog's faeces and are ingested by sheep. Within the sheep they form liver cysts. Dogs are then infected by eating the viscera of sheep. Man may ingest the ova and act as an intermediate host instead of sheep.

The ovum burrows through the intestinal wall and is carried in the portal blood to the liver where it encysts. Some pass through the hepatic sinusoids to form cysts in brain, bone, spleen, etc. The cysts grow very slowly. Structurally they consist of an inner nucleated germinal layer and an outer laminated non-nucleated layer (*see* *Fig*. 6.6). Outside this is a dense fibrous capsule formed by the host. Budding of the germinal layer takes place and the buds develop central vesicles to become 'brood cysts'. Within the brood cysts the scolices of the worm develop. These scolices, which have characteristic hooks, rupture through the walls of the brood cysts and lie on the bottom of the hydatid cyst as 'hydatid sand'. When ingested by dogs the cycle begins again.

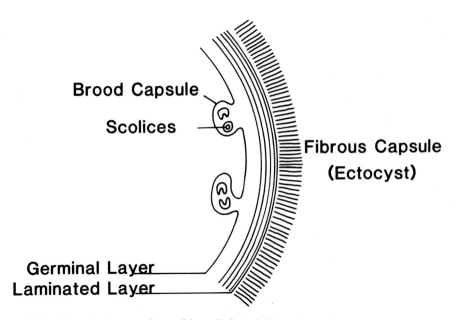

Fig 6.6. Schematic diagram of part of the wall of a hydatid cyst (*see* text).

Two main varieties of the Echinococcus infest man. The more common is *E. granulosus* which forms unilocular cysts, and the less common is *E. multilocularis* which forms multilocular cysts; the latter invade the liver substance and clinically mimic a liver tumour. Rupture of the cyst may cause peritoneal seeding; other complications include secondary infection, biliary obstruction and portal hypertension. Blood eosinophilia and the Casoni reaction aid the diagnosis.

Treatment is by surgical excision. The cyst contents are usually under pressure and this can cause spillage at the time of surgery. The risk of dissemination is reduced by injecting the cyst with formalin.

Liver Abscess

The two main types of liver abscess are pyogenic and amoebic; both are relatively uncommon in the West.

Pyogenic abscess

Pyogenic abscesses are most common in the elderly with 20% occurring in patients over 70 years old. The causes of pyogenic abscesses include (1) biliary obstruction from stones, tumour or stricture; (2) portal pyaemia from appendicitis or diverticulitis; (3) septicaemia via the hepatic artery; (4) direct extension from cholecystitis or perihepatic abscess; (5) infection of a liver lesion such as a tumour; and (6) trauma. Ascending cholangitis secondary to choledocholithiasis is the most common cause today. In 20% of cases no cause can be found. Liver abscesses in young persons are usually due to trauma when areas of liver tissue become devitalized. Abscesses in young children are usually due to systemic spread of infection associated with leukaemia or immunosuppression.

The usual presenting features of a liver abscess are pain and the systemic signs of infection; rigors are common.

The commonest organisms found are Gram-negative bacilli, *E. coli*, Klebsiella, Proteus and rarely Pseudomonas. Staphylococcal and streptococcal abscesses are usually blood borne. More recently anaerobic organisms such as Clostridia, Actinomyces and Bacteroides have been found in approximately half of all liver abscesses. Thirty per cent are due to multiple organisms and in 20% no organism can be isolated.

The abscesses, which vary in size, may be single or multiple. Biliary obstruction causes multiple abscesses in the distribution of the biliary tree, whereas most other sources of abscesses cause a single lesion. Chronic abscesses have a surrounding fibrous capsule with an inner wall of granulation tissue containing acute and chronic inflammatory cells. The cavity contains pus and occasionally gas. Local extension may cause subphrenic or pleural collections and occasionally perforation causes peritonitis. Metastatic abscesses may occur to lung or brain.

Ultrasound is the most useful diagnostic aid and treatment is with drainage and appropriate antibodies. Percutaneous catheter drainage with ultrasound guidance may be useful in the ill patient. Mortality is high, ranging from 40–80%. A clinical misdiagnosis of malignancy is not uncommon (Northover *et al.* 1982).

Amoebic abscess

This results from intestinal amoebiasis which has spread to the liver via the portal vein from a bowel ulcer. Invasion of the portal tracts causes cell necrosis and eventually an abscess. Characteristically, the pus is said to look like anchovy sauce. Amoebic abscesses cause progressive painful hepatomegaly with adjacent pleural and lung signs. Sweating and swinging temperatures are common. The differential diagnosis is from a pyogenic abscess and hepatocellular carcinoma. Aspiration under ultrasound guidance aids diagnosis. Complications include pleural effusion (35%), pneumonia (45%) and rupture of the abscess into pleural space, lung, peritoneal cavity or pericardium.

Drainage, percutaneous or operative, combined with metronidazole therapy is usually required.

Benign Epithelial Liver Tumours and Tumour-like Conditions

Liver adenomas

Liver adenomas occur most commonly in women during their reproductive years. There are two main clinical presentations.

1. As a mass which is associated with pain and which may be confused with primary or secondary malignancy, either on liver scan or at laparotomy.
2. As an acute abdominal emergency due to rupture of the tumour. This latter presentation is more likely to occur in patients who have been using oral contraceptives.

Many patients who develop hepatic adenomas have been using the oral contraceptive pill, although occasional cases have been reported in diabetics and in patients with iron overload.

Macroscopically most are single nodules which can vary between 2 and 15 cm in diameter. They arise in otherwise normal livers and do not have a capsule although they are well demarcated from the rest of the liver. Necrosis may be seen in the centre.

Histologically the tumour is composed of plates of liver cells, 2–3 cells thick, which are not arranged in the normal liver lobules. Normal portal tracts with bile ducts are absent. The cells closely resemble normal hepatocytes.

Local resection of the tumour may be necessary for the complications of rupture and haemoperitoneum. However, in asymptomatic cases, regression has been described after stopping the contraceptive pill and Sherlock (1981) therefore advocates withdrawal of contraceptives and follow-up with ultrasound.

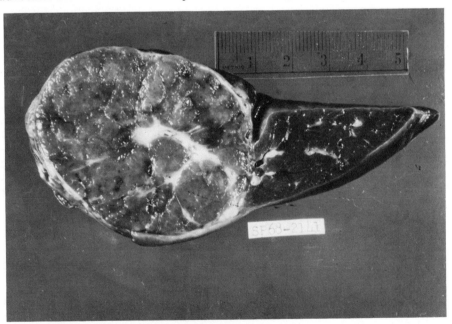

Fig 6.7. Focal nodular hyperplasia of liver showing the characteristic central scar. (Photograph kindly supplied by Dr B. H. Ruebner and reproduced with the permission of John Wiley & Sons.)

Focal nodular hyperplasia

This is a nodular lesion found in an otherwise normal liver. Knowles and Wolff (1976) reported 20 cases which were all asymptomatic incidental findings. Other cases have been reported which have caused pain and very rarely they rupture and cause intraperitoneal haemorrhage. The male : female ratio is 1 : 2; the age range of 20–50 years is greater than for adenoma. Cases have been described in women who have been on the contraceptive pill but the association is less strong than for hepatic adenoma.

The gross features are characteristic. There is a large nodular mass, yellow-brown in colour, which on cross section typically shows a central stellate scar with the limbs radiating out towards the periphery (*see Fig.* 6.7).

Microscopically they consist of nodules of cytologically normal liver cells with interlacing fibrous septa which contain proliferating bile ducts. Large vascular channels are often seen.

The condition appears to be completely benign. Knowles and Wolff (1976) advocate no treatment while the patient is asymptomatic. If patients are on the contraceptive pill, it should be withdrawn.

Partial nodular transformation of the liver

This is a rare condition in which nodules are found in the region of the liver hilum. Portal hypertension may result but liver function is excellent. The cause is unknown.

Malignant Epithelial Liver Tumours
Hepatocellular carcinoma

Epidemiology

In Western countries the annual incidence of hepatocellular carcinoma (HCC) is 2–3 per 100 000 and it occurs predominantly in elderly males (male : female ratio 9 : 1). In China, South-East Asia and Africa, it is much more common with an incidence of almost 100 per 100 000 in Mozambique (where it is the commonest form of cancer) and 17 per 100 000 in China. The male : female ratio in these countries is approximately 3 : 1 and the disease occurs commonly in patients under 40 years of age, as well as in the elderly.

Aetiology

HEPATITIS B: There is strong evidence that the hepatitis B virus is important in the development of HCC. The evidence can be summarized as follows.

1. There is a strong positive correlation between the incidence of hepatocellular carcinoma in any one area and the proportion of patients who are carriers for HBsAg in the same area. In the high incidence areas of Africa and Asia, 10% of the population are HBsAg positive, whereas in Europe and the USA, only 1% or less are HBsAg positive.

2. Patients with HCC more frequently have circulating HBsAg than controls from the same area. In the UK, 25% of patients with hepatocellular carcinoma are HBsAg positive, compared with only approximately 1% of the normal population.
3. An important prospective study of 22 707 Chinese males in Taiwan showed that 50 cases of primary HCC occurred on follow-up and, of these, 49 arose in a subset of 3500 people who were HBsAg carriers (Beasley *et al.* 1981).

It is not clear exactly how the hepatitis B virus actually causes HCC. There is evidence that the DNA of the virus becomes integrated into the hepatocyte DNA. It is possible that this viral DNA acts directly as a viral oncogene or, more likely, that it promotes an oncogene already in the hepatocyte DNA. In either case, the cell would undergo malignant transformation.

Recently, the importance of the hepatitis B virus in the pathogenesis of HCC has been challenged by a prospective study in England, in which seropositivity for hepatitis B surface antigen was not related to the development of cirrhosis into HCC (Zaman 1985).

CIRRHOSIS: In Western countries, between 80 and 90% of HCC arises in cirrhotic livers and about 5–15% of all cases of cirrhosis go on to develop cancer. In the high risk areas of Africa and Asia, up to 50% of patients with cirrhosis develop cancer, although HCC is also common in non-cirrhotic livers.

There is a particularly high incidence of HCC in cases of HBsAg positive chronic active hepatitis which have gone on to develop cirrhosis. In haemochromatosis, about 30% of the affected patients will develop HCC. HCC occurs in 3–5% of cases of alcoholic cirrhosis, being particularly common in those patients who are also HBsAg positive. It has been suggested that the virus acts as an initiator and the alcohol as a promoter. Malignant transformation is rare in Wilson's disease, in primary biliary cirrhosis and in HBsAg negative chronic active hepatitis. In general terms, cirrhosis may predispose to HCC, either because: (1) carcinogens are more likely to act upon regenerating cells (i.e. cells which are actively dividing), and/or (2) damaged liver may be less resistant to carcinogens.

MYCOTOXINS: Aspergillus is a fungus which contaminates human food supplies, especially improperly stored grain in tropical parts of the world. Certain strains of this fungus produce aflatoxins which are known carcinogens in certain mammals. Ingestion of aflatoxin correlates with both the incidence of HCC in a particular area and also with the incidence of HBsAg positivity. Aflatoxins may act synergistically with hepatitis B virus to cause HCC or alternatively they may suppress cell-mediated immunity, thereby predisposing to hepatitis B infection.

ORAL STEROID CONTRACEPTIVES: HCC has occasionally been described in patients using the oral contraceptive pill, but the association is exceedingly rare.

Clinical features
HCC usually arises in the clinical background of cirrhosis and may be suspected in a patient who has had a sudden unexplained deterioration or who has had a rapid increase in liver size. Weight loss and abdominal pain are common. Monitoring of

serum alpha fetoprotein level is a useful method of detecting early cases of HCC in at-risk patients. Alpha fetoprotein is an alpha-1 globulin found in the normal fetus. Its reappearance in adults in high concentrations is highly suggestive of the development of HCC, although it also rises in some tumours of the gonads. It is positive in up to 90% of patients with HCC. Low levels can be found in other liver diseases and in some cases of gastrointestinal carcinoma.

Morphology

HCC appears as massive, nodular and diffuse forms. The massive form is a solitary tumour which occurs most commonly in non-cirrhotic livers of young patients. Nodular forms occur in cirrhotic livers and it is not known whether they represent multifocal origin or intrahepatic spread (*see Fig.* 6.8). The diffuse form occurs as widespread small nodules of tumour interspersed with the cirrhotic nodules. The tumours are often soft due to lack of fibrous tissue and may show necrosis.

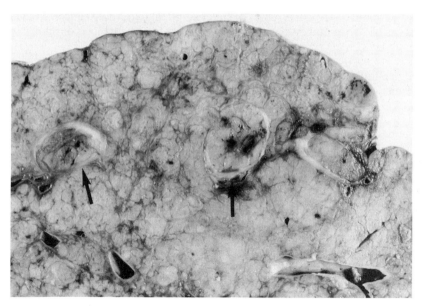

Fig 6.8. Liver cirrhosis with a nodular hepatocellular carcinoma (arrows).

Microscopically the cells resemble normal hepatocytes. The normal lobular architecture of the liver is, however, lost and replaced by plates of neoplastic hepatocytes, three or more cells thick, forming a trabecular pattern which is characteristic. The trabeculae may, however, be so close together that a solid pattern is seen. Gland-like structures are commonly found (pseudoglandular pattern) as are papillary areas (*see Fig.* 6.9). The histological pattern of HCC does not appear to affect prognosis, except in the fibrolamellar variant (*see below*).

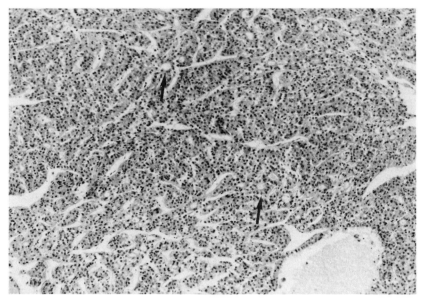

Fig 6.9. Hepatocellular carcinoma. A pseudoglandular pattern is seen in some areas (arrows). (H and E × 30)

Although the individual cells resemble hepatocytes, they are atypical and show nuclear pleomorphism and hyperchromasia. Tumour giant cells may also be seen and occasionally clear cell varieties are encountered. In some tumours the cells contain Mallory's hyaline.

Immunohistochemical studies may demonstrate HBsAg in the tumour or, more likely, in the surrounding non-neoplastic cirrhotic liver, and this gives a clue as to the aetiology.

Spread and prognosis

The tumour has a predilection to spread via the hepatic veins and may cause venous thrombosis and the Budd–Chiari syndrome. Metastases occur only in about 50% of cases. Peritoneal dissemination is rare. Ninety per cent of patients are unsuitable for curative resection either because of the extent of the tumour or because of the severity of the underlying cirrhosis. Only non-cirrhotic cases are suitable for surgery since cirrhotic cases are usually multifocal. Hepatic artery embolization and intra-arterial chemotherapy may provide some palliation.

The prognosis is exceedingly poor with a survival of more than two years after diagnosis being rare. Patients who are HBsAg positive and/or cirrhotic do particularly badly.

Prevention

There is some optimism that mass immunization programmes for hepatitis B will reduce the worldwide incidence of HCC.

Fibrolamellar variant of HCC

This is a pathologically distinct form of HCC which generally occurs in young patients (mean age approximately 25 years old) without pre-existing liver disease. The tumour is usually a well defined large firm nodule, often with an area of central scar resembling focal nodular hyperplasia. Occasionally, several nodules are noted. Histologically, the cardinal features are trabeculae of large deeply eosinophilic malignant hepatocytes, separated by abundant fibrous stroma. Fibrolamellar HCC is operable in up to 50% of cases and has a better prognosis than other forms of HCC.

Hepatoblastomas

These are rare tumours of childhood occurring most frequently under the age of two years and very rarely in adults. They present as an expanding abdominal mass and failure to thrive. Occasionally they rupture causing haemoperitoneum. Serum alpha fetoprotein is virtually always raised and occasionally they produce gonadotrophin which causes precocious puberty. Associated congenital abnormalities, such as hemihypertrophy and cardiac anomalies, occur in a proportion of patients.

Grossly, the tumour is usually a single circumscribed mass showing necrosis and haemorrhage.

Histologically, the tumour is either epithelial or mixed. In the mixed type there is, in addition to the malignant epithelial cells, a benign mesenchymal portion consisting of fibromyxoid, osteoid and chondroid areas.

Non-epithelial Tumours of the Liver

Benign

Haemangiomas are the commonest benign non-epithelial tumours of the liver. They often occur as an incidental finding at autopsy. In females they may enlarge during pregnancy, causing pain, and rarely they rupture.

Hepatic lipomas, leiomyomas and other benign tumours are exceedingly rare.

Uncertain malignant potential

Infantile haemangioendothelioma presents before the age of 4 years as an abdominal mass and/or cardiac failure due to the arterio-venous shunting present in the tumour mass. It may rupture to give a haemoperitoneum. Grossly, the tumour may be solitary or multifocal and it is always haemorrhagic. Histologically, numerous vascular channels are seen with intervening bile ducts. The condition may be infiltrative locally and in rare cases metastases have been described.

Malignant

Haemangiosarcoma (Kupffer cell sarcoma) is rare although it may occur in the following situations: (1) after thorotrast injections (thorium dioxide injected for X-ray purposes). This substance is taken up by the Kupffer cells and emits radioactivity. It was used in the mid-1950s and cases of haemangiosarcoma on this basis still occur. (2) Exposure to vinylchloride monomer, a substance used in the manufacture of PVC. (3) Exposure to arsenic (e.g. in insecticides). (4) Possibly after use of the contraceptive pill or androgens.

The patient presents with hepatomegaly, ascites, pain and jaundice. Grossly, the lesions are usually multicentric and on cut section show numerous blood filled cavities.

Histologically the typical finding is of neoplastic sinusoidal cells spreading along the surface of preserved liver cell plates. Solid areas and blood filled spaces are also seen. The tumour cells are pleomorphic and hyperchromatic. In thorium cases the material can be seen as brown granules in the Kupffer cells.

Secondary liver tumours

These are the commonest tumours of the liver in the West. Most secondary deposits reach the liver via the blood, either by portal vein or hepatic artery. Lymphatic spread also occurs, as does direct invasion. Pancreas, large bowel, stomach, lung and breast are the most common sites of the primary lesion.

At surgery the lesions appear as well defined spheres, usually multiple and white with yellow central areas of necrosis (*see Fig.* 6.10). Often the tumours are anaplastic and give no indication of the site of origin.

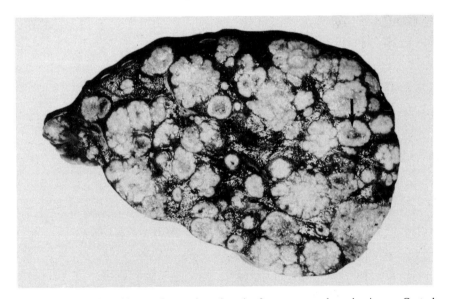

Fig 6.10. Liver with widespread secondary deposits from an oesophageal primary. Central necrosis can be seen in some of the tumour nodules (arrow).

Attempts may be made to resect single secondary deposits in the liver. Intrahepatic artery chemotherapy or embolization can be used for palliation of widespread deposits. This may have a greater effect than expected since, despite the fact that most secondary deposits arrive via the portal system, they appear to derive their blood supply from the hepatic artery. The long-term prognosis is, however, poor with median survivals of 3–11 months. Secondary deposits from endocrine tumours are, however, especially sensitive to chemotherapy.

References

Beasley R. P., Hwang L. Y., Lin C. C., Chein C. S. (1981) Hepatocellular carcinoma and hepatitis B virus. A prospective study of 22 707 men in Taiwan. *Lancet* **2**, 1129–33.

Cahill C. J. (1983) Prevention of postoperative renal failure in patients with obstructive jaundice—the role of bile salts. *Br. J. Surg.* **70**, 590–5.

Crossley I. R., Williams R. (1985) Spontaneous bacterial peritonitis. *Gut* **26**, 325–31

Fleming K. A., McGee J. O'D. (1984) Alcohol induced liver disease. *J. Clin. Pathol.* **37**, 721–33.

Knowles D. M., Wolff M. (1976) Focal nodular hyperplasia of the liver. A clinicopathologic study and review of the literature. *Human Pathol.* **7**, 533–45.

Northover J. M. A., Jones B. J. M., Dawson J. L., Williams R. (1982) Difficulties in the diagnosis and management of pyogenic liver abscess. *Br. J. Surg.* **69**, 48–51.

Robbins S. L., Cotran R. S., Kumar V. (1984) *Pathologic Basis of Disease*, 3rd ed. Philadelphia, W. B. Saunders.

Sherlock S. (1981) *Diseases of the Liver and Biliary System*, 5th ed. Oxford, Blackwell Scientific Publications.

Silk D. B., Williams R. (1979) Acute liver failure. *Br. J. Hosp. Med.* **22**, 437–46.

Wilkinson S. P., Williams R. (1980) Renin–angiotensin–aldosterone system in cirrhosis. *Gut* **21**, 545–54.

Zaman S. N., Melia W. M., Johnson R. D., Portmann B. C., Johnson P. J., Williams R. (1985) Risk factors in development of hepatocellular carcinoma in cirrhosis: prospective study of 613 patients. *Lancet* **1**, 1357–9.

Chapter 7

The Biliary System

Normal Structure

The extrahepatic biliary system consists of the right and left hepatic ducts, the common hepatic duct, the common bile duct, the cystic duct and the gallbladder. The left and right hepatic ducts unite outside the liver to form the common hepatic duct. The confluence is therefore accessible at surgery. The common hepatic duct descends in the free edge of the lesser omentum and is joined by the cystic duct to form the common bile duct. Variations of the normal anatomy are commonly seen and a knowledge of these is essential in order to avoid iatrogenic damage at the time of surgery.

The lower 2 cm of the common bile duct is surrounded by the choledochal sphincter. Its relationship to the termination of the pancreatic duct is variable. The narrowest portion of the common bile duct is at the entrance to the duodenal wall and the most common site for impaction of a stone is just proximal to the transduodenal segment.

The arterial supply of the gallbladder is via the cystic artery and in 20% of cases there is an accessory artery present. Venous drainage is via vessels running directly into the liver and via a pericholedochal venous plexus. The fundus has the poorest blood supply especially when distended. Cholecystohepatic ducts passing directly into the liver are unusual but may produce troublesome bile leakage after cholecystectomy.

Recent studies on the blood supply of the common bile duct have shown an axial supply along the duct from the retroduodenal artery (below) and the right hepatic and cystic arteries (above). The most constant vessels appear to be along the lateral borders at 3 and 9 o'clock (Northover and Terblanche 1979) and therefore a vertical incision in the common duct interferes least with blood supply and hence healing. Transverse sectioning from operative incision during liver transplantation or at a choledochoenteric anastomosis is prone to fibrous stricture. Excessive dissection round the duct will also interfere with its blood supply.

Histologically the gallbladder has a folded mucous membrane lined with columnar epithelial cells. There is no muscularis mucosa but there is a thick wall with interlacing muscle fibres and connective tissue. On the outer aspect is the serosa. The bile ducts have a flat mucosa with many mucous glands. The proximal ducts have thin walls with little muscle while distally there is the powerful choledochal sphincter.

The choledochal sphincter shows peristaltic activity with pulses of contraction and relaxation which vary the amount of bile reaching the duodenum. Narcotic drugs are thought to increase sphincter tone. While fasting, most bile enters the gallbladder because sphincter tone exceeds gallbladder pressure. In the gallbladder, reabsorption of sodium chloride along with passive diffusion of water and potassium occurs and the bile becomes concentrated. Cholecystokinin released by the duodenum in response to food causes gallbladder contraction and relaxation of the choledochal sphincter. Vagal activity may be important in maintaining gallbladder tone, as the gallbladder distends after vagotomy.

Congenital and Neonatal Conditions of the Biliary Tree

Congenital anomalies of the gallbladder

The gallbladder may be absent (agenesis) or small (hypoplasia). Occasionally there may be total duplication to form a double gallbladder or partial duplication to create a bilobed gallbladder. A constriction of the body of the gallbladder may give rise to an expanded fundus termed a Phrygian cap. The gallbladder may rarely be totally within the liver (intrahepatic) or it may have a long mesentery (floating gallbladder). The latter may predispose to torsion.

Cysts and dilatations of the bile ducts

These are divided into four types (Olbourne 1975; *see Fig.* 7.1).

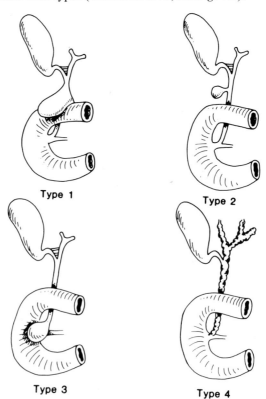

Type 1

Type 2

Type 3

Type 4

Fig. 7.1. Cysts and dilatations of the bile ducts: 1. choledochal cyst; 2. diverticulum of the bile duct; 3. choledochocoele; 4. Caroli's disease. (Reproduced with permission from Olbourne 1975.)

Type 1 (choledochal cyst)

This is a dilatation of the extrahepatic bile ducts, most commonly starting distally, i.e. at the duodenal end and extending proximally. The commonest site is, therefore, the lower third of the common bile duct. It may present as neonatal jaundice but more frequently it presents in childhood between the ages of five and ten years. Females are more commonly affected than males. It is common in the Japanese.

The aetiology is unknown. Muscular weakness and neuromuscular incoordination have been implicated. It has also been proposed that these patients have a long common channel between the distal part of the pancreatic duct and the bile duct and that this allows reflux of pancreatic juice into the latter. This may cause weakness of the wall and subsequent dilatation. This theory would explain the common position of choledochal cysts in the lower third of the biliary tree.

Clinically the classical triad is abdominal pain, jaundice and a palpable mass. Ultrasound confirms the diagnosis.

The cyst wall may be very large and contain up to 5 litres of bile. The wall is thickened by inflammation. Microscopically the epithelium is largely lost although islands remain.

Complications include perforation, pancreatitis, abscesses, cholangitis, secondary biliary cirrhosis and malignant change (usually adenocarcinoma).

Malignant change is avoided by removal; if gross fibrosis prevents complete removal, malignant change may be avoided by excision of the cyst lining at the time of drainage.

Type 2

This is a diverticulum of the extrahepatic bile ducts. It may be completely excised.

Type 3 (choledochocoele)

This is a dilatation of that part of the common bile duct within the duodenal wall. It can cause duodenal obstruction and can be incised to allow free drainage or excised with an accompanying reconstruction.

Type 4 (Caroli's disease)

This consists of multiple dilatations of intrahepatic and extrahepatic bile ducts. Cholangitis and septicaemia are common complications. The lesion may be solely intrahepatic and may occasionally affect just one lobe. Cholangiography shows sacculations of the affected ducts. Localized intrahepatic disease may be treated by resection but in generalized disease, prognosis is poor due to the complications of cholangitis or the onset of cholangiocarcinoma.

Biliary atresia

This condition presents as jaundice in the neonatal period and can easily be confused with neonatal hepatitis. The incidence is approximately one per 10 000 live births.

The aetiology is unknown. The fact that the jaundice does not occur in the immediate period after birth suggests that the condition is acquired rather than congenital. It appears to be the result of an inflammatory process of the biliary tree, the cause of which is unknown, although both viruses and bacteria have been implicated. It appears that the obliterative process starts as an extrahepatic lesion and proceeds to destruction of the whole duct system.

Pathologically there is fibrous obliteration of the bile ducts. The liver parenchyma shows the features of cholestatic jaundice and giant cells are present, making distinction from neonatal hepatitis difficult. The site of the obliteration is variable. The older terminology divided biliary atresia into 'correctable' and 'uncorrectable' forms. In the correctable form there is a communication between the extrahepatic and intrahepatic ducts whereas in the uncorrectable form there is no such communication. However, with the introduction of the Kasai operation (Kasai et al. 1975), the uncorrectable form may now be amenable to treatment, although the old terminology still persists.

Liver biopsy can be difficult to interpret due to the similarity to neonatal hepatitis. Several serial biopsies, at two-weekly intervals, may be useful.

In the correctable form (approximately 10% of cases) a Roux-en-Y loop may be anastomosed to an extrahepatic duct to allow drainage. Results have, however, been disappointing and the Kasai operation (see below) may be preferable for both the 'correctable' and 'uncorrectable' forms. In the uncorrectable form the Kasai operation (porto-enterostomy) is the treatment of choice. The basis of this operation is that the 'fibrous mass' which replaces the left and right bile ducts at the porta hepatis contains many minute bile ducts which communicate with the intrahepatic ducts. These minute ducts within the fibrous mass only persist for about 2 months after birth and, therefore, it is essential that surgery be carried out early (within 60 days of birth). At surgery a frozen section of liver may be carried out to exclude neonatal hepatitis if this could not be done by needle biopsy preoperatively the fibrous mass is transected and a Roux-en-Y loop is anastomosed to the cut surface. The resected piece of fibrous tissue is sent for histology since the number of minute bile ducts found in it and their size influence the prognosis.

Complications after surgery include cholangitis, stenosis of the anastomosis and cirrhosis. Recent long-term results from Japan are good with 85% being asymptomatic at 5 years, although the alkaline phosphatase remains high. In the long-term liver transplantation may provide an alternative approach in those children who fail to respond to other procedures, although current results are not encouraging (Howard 1983).

Gallstones

Gallstones may be composed purely of cholesterol or of pigment or they may be mixed. Chemical analysis shows that the majority are mixed; mixed stones are usually considered to be variants of cholesterol stones.

Epidemiology

CHOLESTEROL AND MIXED STONES: These are common in Europe and North America where about 20% of women and 8% of men are affected. They are much less common in Africa and Asia. They occur 2–3 times more commonly in women than men and the incidence increases with age, especially for men. The high incidence in women, especially those taking exogenous oestrogen and possibly also the contraceptive pill, is thought to be related to hormonal factors which influence cholesterol metabolism. Obesity and a high calorie diet also predispose to cholesterol stones.

Conditions associated with the presence of gallstones include gallbladder cancer, pancreatitis, cirrhosis (especially alcoholic), cystic fibrosis, diabetes mellitus, ileal resection or ileal disease and total parenteral nutrition.

BILIRUBIN (PIGMENT) STONES: These are relatively more common in the Far East, especially in rural areas, where they are associated with infected bile, liver cirrhosis and haemolytic anaemias.

Pathogenesis

CHOLESTEROL AND MIXED STONES: The formation of gallstones requires firstly that the bile be supersaturated with cholesterol, secondly that some factor initiates crystallization of cholesterol and thirdly that the stone should enlarge. The gallbladder plays a role by providing a suitable environment.

1. *Supersaturation of bile.* Cholesterol is insoluble in water and is kept in solution in bile by bile salts and phospholipids (especially lecithin) which form micelles. Bile becomes lithogenic, therefore, either by an increased formation of cholesterol or by a reduced bile salt pool. The rate limiting enzyme for cholesterol production in the liver is 3-hydroxy-3-methylglutaryl coenzyme A and an increased activity of this enzyme is found in obese patients. Oestrogen and progesterone also increase the secretion of cholesterol by the liver.

   A reduced bile salt pool occurs in patients with ileal disease (e.g. Crohn's disease) or ileal resection. The ileum normally reabsorbs bile salts and is therefore an integral part of the enterohepatic circulation. If it fails, therefore, bile salts are lost in the faeces. In some patients with gallstones, a reduced bile salt pool, due to overactivity of a negative feedback inhibition system for the control of bile salt formation, has been found (Mok *et al.* 1977).

2. *Crystallization.* Since gallstones do not form in all supersaturated bile, some factor must be responsible for the initiation of crystallization. The most probable factors are particles such as bacteria, parasites and epithelial cells, any of which may serve as a nidus for crystallization. Calcium crystals may also be important in the process of nidation (Williamson and Percy-Robb 1980). Mucin may have a prime role as most gallstones contain a core of mucin and the lattice of the stone is bound with mucin glycoproteins.

3. *Growth.* Once a nidus has formed, growth appears to occur provided the bile remains supersaturated with cholesterol.

4. *The role of the gallbladder.* Nidation and growth appear to occur more rapidly in the gallbladder than in hepatic bile. This is particularly so if there is stasis or reduced emptying as occurs in pregnancy, or due to the contraceptive pill. Activity of enzymes, such as glucuronidase and alkaline phosphatase, in the wall of the gallbladder may affect lithogenesis (Bouchier 1984).

PIGMENT STONES: Most bilirubin in bile is in the water soluble conjugated form. For bilirubin (pigment) stones to form, the bile must become supersaturated with the insoluble unconjugated form. This supersaturation can occur if the bile is overloaded with bilirubin as in haemolytic anaemias. It can also occur by the action of the enzyme beta-glucuronidase, which deconjugates bilirubin in bile, and this enzyme may be released by bacteria such as *E. coli*. The high incidence of bilirubin stones in the Far East may be related to infection by liver flukes such as *Clonorchis sinensis*. Pigment stones in these areas are found in intrahepatic bile ducts where the parasite also resides.

Morphology

Stones which are composed purely or almost entirely of cholesterol tend to be large (about 2 cm), round, pale, smooth and solitary. Pigment stones are small, black and multiple. Mixed stones vary in colour and tend to be multiple and faceted. They are laminated on cross section suggesting repeated episodes of lithogenesis. Between 10% and 20% of gallstones contain sufficient calcium to be radio-opaque.

X-ray diffraction techniques on gallstones from 152 patients showed that no pure stones were found. Eighty per cent consisted of a mixture of cholesterol, bile salts, bilirubin and inorganic calcium salts. The remaining 20% were composed of minerals such as calcium salts and oxides of silicone and aluminium (Arnaud *et al.* 1979).

Complications of gallstones within the gallbladder

Biliary colic

This is presumably due to temporary impaction of a gallstone in the cystic duct. The patient develops a continuous non-colicky pain in the right hypochondrium. If acute cholecystitis does not supervene the pain subsides in a few hours and no constitutional symptoms occur.

Acute cholecystitis

The common cause of acute cholecystitis is impaction of a stone in Hartmann's pouch with consequent obstruction of the cystic duct and inflammatory reaction in the gallbladder. Rarely, obstruction to the cystic duct may be caused by tumour. The inflammatory reaction is considered to be chemical, at least initially, since bacteria are not always found in the early stages. The exact nature of the chemical irritation is unknown. One possibility is that lecithin is converted to the cytotoxic compound, lysolecithin, by the action of lysosomal enzymes released by damaged epithelial cells and bacteria. Increasing luminal pressure in the gallbladder with subsequent reduction in blood supply may potentiate the inflammation.

Clinically, acute cholecystitis may start as biliary colic. When inflammation occurs the pain becomes prolonged, lasting several days instead of hours, and constitutional symptoms and signs, such as pyrexia and leucocytosis, are found.

Macroscopically, the gallbladder is enlarged and may be palpable. The surface is hyperaemic and may be covered by a layer of fibrin or pus. Opening the gallbladder shows a grossly thickened and oedematous wall. The mucosa is hyperaemic and ulcerated. In the later stages the gallbladder may be black or blue (gangrenous cholecystitis).

Eighty per cent of patients coming to emergency surgery for acute cholecystitis have positive bile cultures. Organisms cultured include *E. coli*, *Strep. faecalis*, *Klebsiella aerogenes*, *Clostridium welchii*, Bacteroides and occasionally, other aerobes and anaerobes. Patients undergoing surgery for resolving acute cholecystitis have a 48% incidence of positive bile culture, whereas bile at elective cholecystectomy is positive for organisms in less than 20% of cases.

Currently, early cholecystectomy for acute cholecystitis is favoured. In view of the high incidence of infected bile, perioperative antibiotic cover is advised.

Emphysematous cholecystitis

This is caused by gas forming bacteria and presents as a severe cholecystitis. Diabetics are commonly affected. The diagnosis can be made by the presence of gas in the gallbladder wall on a plain X-ray film.

Empyema of the gallbladder

When acute cholecystitis does not resolve it may progress to empyema, i.e. the lumen becomes filled with pus. The patient has the signs and symptoms of an abscess.

Perforation of the gallbladder

The good vascular supply and thickened wall due to previous episodes of inflammation make this complication rare. When perforation does occur, the abdominal signs spread to include all four quadrants of the abdomen and the condition of the patient deteriorates. The fundus has the poorest blood supply and is usually the site of perforation.

Mucocoele of the gallbladder

Occasionally, obstruction of the cystic duct does not produce acute symptoms but rather the gallbladder secretes mucus into its lumen and eventually it becomes a mucocoele (*see Fig. 7.2*). This is often asymptomatic and may present as a right hypochondrial mass which can be confused with an HCC or a colonic or renal neoplasm. Histological examination shows that the gallbladder has usually lost its epithelial lining and is lined only by connective tissue. Bile cultured from a mucocoele is positive for organisms in approximately 30% of cases.

Chronic cholecystitis

Clinically, chronic cholecystitis refers to patients with either chronic low-grade symptoms or recurrent attacks of biliary colic or both.

The condition may or may not be preceded by acute cholecystitis. Gallstones are virtually always present. It is possible that the chemical abnormalities which lead to gallstone formation also cause chronic inflammation of the gallbladder wall and that gallstones do not directly cause the disease. The inflammation is likely to be on a chemical rather than a bacterial basis since organisms are not always found. Grossly, the gallbladder wall is thickened to a variable degree by fibrous tissue and

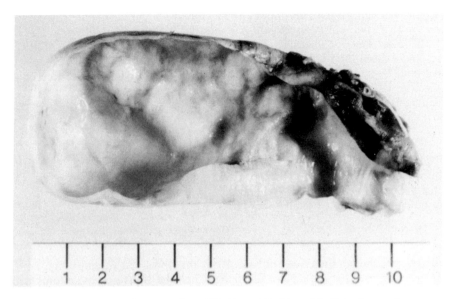

Fig. 7.2. Mucocoele of gallbladder. The gallbladder wall is thin and the lining is smooth.

the mucosa is usually intact. Histologically, the inflammatory reaction may be very mild. Some fibrosis is seen and this may replace the smooth muscle of the gallbladder wall. Rokitansky-Aschoff sinuses are characteristic. These are herniations of the epithelium through the muscle coat of the gallbladder wall (*see Fig.* 7.3).

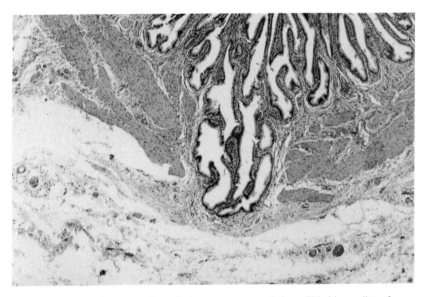

Fig. 7.3. Herniation of mucosa through the muscle coat of the gallbladder wall to form a Rokitansky–Aschoff sinus. (H and E × 30)

Porcelain gallbladder

Dystrophic calcification after acute cholecystitis or, in some cases, chronic cholecystitis, leads to a hard, radio-opaque 'porcelain' gallbladder. It has a high risk of malignant change.

Carcinoma of the gallbladder

This is discussed on p. 186.

Complications of gallstones in the biliary tree

Obstructive jaundice

Most bile duct stones migrate from the gallbladder and increase in size in the ducts. Some, however, arise in the ducts in association with strictures. At operation, primary duct stones are soft and disintegrate easily. Impaction of a gallstone in the biliary tree is the commonest form of obstructive jaundice as has been discussed previously. Bile cultured from these patients is positive in 84% of cases and perioperative antibiotic therapy is required before manipulation of the common bile duct either at operation or ERCP.

Secondary biliary cirrhosis

Long-standing obstruction of the biliary tree may lead to secondary biliary cirrhosis. This has been discussed previously.

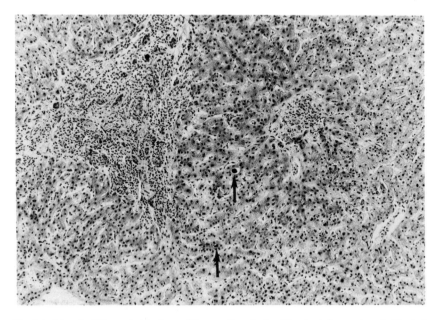

Fig. 7.4. Liver in biliary obstruction with ascending cholangitis. An inflammatory infiltrate is present in the portal tract and bile plugs are seen (arrows). (H and E × 30)

Ascending cholangitis (see Fig. 7.4)

Obstruction of the biliary tree due to stone or stricture with subsequent stasis may lead to infection and ascending cholangitis. The classical symptoms are pain, swinging temperature and jaundice (Charcot's triad). Liver biopsy shows a polymorph infiltration and oedema of the portal tracts with pus in the bile duct lumina. Surgical drainage of the biliary tree may be required. The organisms probably reach the liver and hence the biliary tree from the gut via the portal blood.

Liver abscess

Progression of ascending cholangitis will eventually lead to intrahepatic abscesses if untreated. This has been discussed previously.

Pancreatitis

The role of gallstones in pancreatitis is discussed on p. 197.

Complications of gallstones in the gastrointestinal tract

Gallstone ileus

Biliary–enteric fistulas may occur between the gallbladder and duodenum or less commonly the stomach or colon. Occasionally fistulas occur between the common bile duct and duodenum. Passage of a large gallstone through the fistula may cause obstruction at a narrow point of the gastrointestinal tract (usually in the ileum, 25–50 cm from the ileocaecal valve or proximal to an area of diverticular disease). Straight X-ray of the abdomen will show gas in the biliary tree.

The patients are often elderly females who are subject to intermittent small bowel obstruction as the gallstone frees itself and then re-impacts.

Acalculous Cholecystitis

Acute

Acute cholecystitis may occur in the absence of gallstones but does so only in about 10% of cases. Pathological features in the gallbladder wall are similar to calculous cholecystitis. The condition is associated with diabetes (possibly due to predisposition to infection), burns, arteritis and trauma. Histologically, a necrotizing vasculitis of the gallbladder wall is seen in those cases in which vasculitis is the cause.

Chronic

This presents with the typical symptoms of chronic cholecystitis in the absence of stones. The reason may be a failure to detect stones by routine methods and in these cases, if bile is aspirated from the duodenum and examined, it shows the presence of cholesterol crystals which are strongly suggestive of coexistent gallstones. It does, however, appear that fibrosis and inflammation of the gallbladder can occur in the absence of gallstones although some authorities remain sceptical.

Keddie *et al.* (1976) operated on 62 patients with acalculous cholecystitis and found chronic inflammation in 39%. The other findings were adenomyosis (48%), cholesterolosis (10%) and acute inflammation (3%). Ninety per cent were completely symptom-free after surgery.

Cholesterolosis

Cholesterolosis or strawberry gallbladder is a frequent incidental finding, occurring in about 10% of autopsies. In most cases it probably does not cause any symptoms. The pathogenesis may be absorption of cholesterol from supersaturated bile and in support of this theory is the frequent coexistence of cholesterol stones.

Grossly, the gallbladder mucosa has multiple yellow flecks giving a strawberry-like appearance (*see Fig.* 7.5). Histologically, the mucosal folds are blunted due to the accumulation of many lipid-filled foamy histiocytes beneath the epithelium.

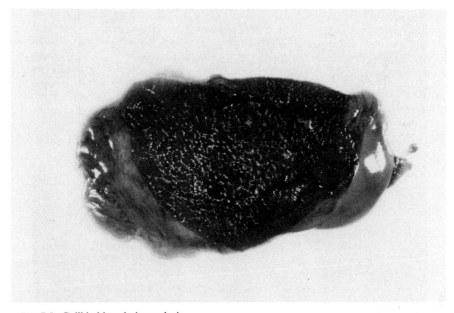

Fig. 7.5. Gallbladder: cholesterolosis.

Primary Sclerosing Cholangitis

This is a rare condition in which progressive obliteration of the extrahepatic and often also the intrahepatic bile ducts occurs. The disease usually presents between the ages of 25 and 45; the male to female ratio is 2 : 1. The aetiology is unknown. A disturbance of immunity has been suggested and in support of this view is the strong association with ulcerative colitis which is present in between half and three-quarters of patients. One possible explanation for this is the presence of excessive bacteria in the portal blood. There is also a less strong association with Crohn's disease, Riedel's thyroiditis, hypothyroidism and retroperitoneal fibrosis.

Clinically the patients present with jaundice, abdominal pain and cholangitis. The criteria for diagnosis are: (1) a diffuse generalized involvement of the intra or extrahepatic ducts; (2) absence of previous biliary surgery; (3) absence of gallstones; and (4) exclusion of carcinoma of the bile ducts by reasonably long follow-up.

The gross features are seen on the cholangiogram (*see Fig.* 7.6). These are areas of irregular strictures and dilatations giving a typical 'beaded' appearance. The disease can be diffuse or segmented and the extrahepatic ducts and intrahepatic ducts can be involved together or alone.

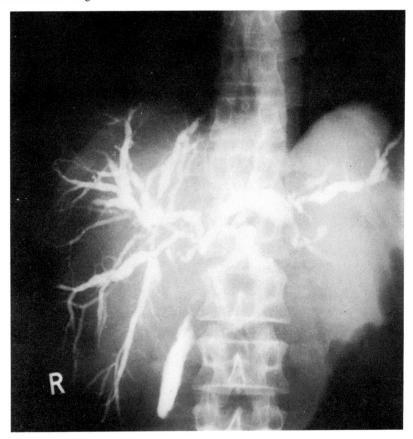

Fig. 7.6. Sclerosing cholangitis.

At surgery, the extrahepatic ducts show thickened walls and narrowed lumina. The gallbladder is also affected by chronic fibrosis. Adjacent lymph nodes are markedly enlarged. Histologically there is fibrous thickening of the submucosal and subserosal layers of the bile duct walls. An infiltrate of acute and chronic inflammatory cells is seen and areas of epithelial cell proliferation in the duct walls can make the distinction between sclerosing cholangitis and cholangiocarcinoma exceedingly difficult on biopsy.

Liver biopsy shows an inflammatory infiltrate in the duct walls and, in the later stages, circumductal fibrosis.

Complications include bleeding varices, liver failure and the onset of cholangiocarcinoma (Sherlock 1981). Corticosteroid and penicillamine therapy are under investigation but not established. Some centres in the United States advocate an aggressive surgical policy (Pitt *et al.* 1982).

Bile Duct Strictures

Cholangiocarcinoma and primary sclerosing cholangitis are discussed elsewhere. Other causes include—

Stenosis of the papilla

Narrowing of the papilla at the termination of the common bile duct has been described following recurrent papillitis. The aetiology is often unknown although in some cases there is a history of common bile duct exploration at the time of cholecystectomy.

At surgery, there is a dilated duct system with narrowing at the papilla. Histology shows an increase in subepithelial fibrous tissue and a decrease in muscle.

Post-inflammatory strictures

These are uncommon. They are associated with gallstones, chronic pancreatitis and duodenal ulcer. In the latter cases, the retropancreatic part of the common bile duct is affected. Biopsy may be necessary to distinguish inflammatory strictures from malignant strictures.

Traumatic strictures

The vast majority of biliary strictures are due to iatrogenic damage at the time of surgery, usually cholecystectomy. The operative circumstances include blind application of clips to control bleeding, traction on the gallbladder which causes tenting of the common bile duct and inadequate knowledge of the variations in anatomy. Some traumatic strictures are due to penetrating abdominal injuries.

The presentation is with obstructive jaundice, bile peritonitis or biliary fistulas occurring postoperatively. Occasionally, presentation is late with cholangitis.

Following the injury there is a marked inflammatory reaction causing fibrosis in the region of the damage, both proximally and distally.

Bismuth (1982) has classified postoperative strictures into five types:

1. low common hepatic duct stricture: hepatic duct stump more than 2 cm;
2. middle common hepatic duct stricture: hepatic duct stump less than 2 cm;
3. high stricture preserving the biliary confluence (i.e. the junction of left and right hepatic ducts);

4. hilar stricture interrupting the confluence;
5. stricture involving an anomalous distribution of the right segmental branches of the biliary tree.

Complications of biliary strictures include cholangitis, secondary biliary cirrhosis, oesophageal varices and liver failure.

Most patients require restoration of biliary–enteric continuity by surgery, although there may be a role for endoscopic dilatation of certain strictures. A poor prognosis is indicated by a long history of a high stricture involving the hepatic ducts, multiple previous attempts at repair, infection, secondary biliary cirrhosis, portal hypertension and a low serum albumin.

Tumours of the Gallbladder

Benign

Adenomas and papillomas

These are both rare. The papilloma is a pedunculated branching structure and the adenoma forms a sessile mass. Microscopically, the papilloma consists of a papillary structure with finger-like projections which are covered with well differentiated columnar epithelium. In adenomas the same type of epithelium forms glands. They are not thought to predispose to cancer but they may cause acute cholecystitis and produce filling defects in the gallbladder on ultrasound or oral cholecystography.

Adenomyoma and adenomyomatosis

An adenomyoma is a localized collection of cystic or gland-like spaces lying in the gallbladder wall. The spaces are lined by gallbladder epithelium and surrounded by hyperplastic smooth muscle. The spaces, therefore, resemble Rokitansky–Aschoff sinuses and may be an extreme example of them. Some authors, however, believe them to be hamartomas. Grossly, the lesion is a nodule which is seen to contain microcysts on cut section.

When the condition affects a large area of the gallbladder, or all of the gallbladder, it is termed adenomyomatosis. This may be seen at oral cholecystography as a halo of dye around the normal gallbladder outline.

Carcinoma of the gallbladder

Carcinoma of the gallbladder presents either symptomatically (usually at a late stage) or as an incidental finding in a gallbladder removed at the time of cholecystectomy for either acute or chronic cholescystitis (often at an early stage).

Carcinoma is found in approximately 1% of cholecystectomy specimens if carefully searched for. The tumour is between 3 and 6 times more common in females than in males and mainly affects the age group 60–80 years. Whites are more commonly affected than blacks.

The tumour is associated with gallstones in over 80% of cases. No proven causal relationship has been established although chronic damage to the gallbladder by stones may potentiate carcinogens in bile. Patients who have a porcelain gall-bladder have a particularly high risk (up to 20% of cases develop cancer).

When confined to the gallbladder, there may be no symptoms. When the disease spreads, however, symptoms may arise, especially when involvement of the cystic duct lymph node causes obstructive jaundice.

Morphology

The tumour may be infiltrating (more common) or fungating (less common). The infiltrating type contains much fibrous tissue and is, therefore, hard or scirrhous. Widespread areas of the gallbladder wall may be affected and the liver bed may be infiltrated. On cutting the gallbladder, the wall is hard and gritty. Some cases may be mistaken for chronic cholecystitis.

The fungating form grows as a cauliflower-like mass into the lumen; it may also invade the liver.

The common histological type is an adenocarcinoma (at least 80% of cases) (*see Fig.* 7.7). This can be well differentiated (good gland formation), poorly differ-entiated (poor gland formation), or may show a papillary pattern. The papillary type invariably occurs as a fungating tumour. Squamous and adenosquamous types are less frequent (about 10%). Rare variants include giant cell and oat cell types.

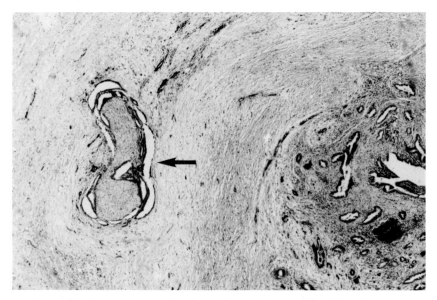

Fig. 7.7. Gallbladder carcinoma with perineural invasion (arrow). (H and E × 30)

Staging, spread and prognosis

Lymphatic spread is to the cystic duct node and then to the supraduodenal nodes. Venous spread takes place via the gallbladder bed directly into the liver where the spread is often extensive. Nevin *et al.* (1976) divided gallbladder carcinoma into five stages as follows: I—intramucosal; II—involvement of mucosa and muscularis; III—involvement of all layers; IV—involvement of all layers plus the cystic duct lymph node; V—involvement of liver and/or the presence of distant metastases.

The commonest patient with gallbladder cancer has advanced disease (Stage V) and does not survive more than one year. Nevin *et al.*, however, found that patients with Stage I and II were cured by cholecystectomy.

It appears from Nevin *et al.*'s study that the incidental finding of early carcinoma in a cholecystectomy specimen (Stage I or II) requires no further treatment and that Stage V requires only palliative treatment. Treatment of Stages III and IV is controversial for two reasons:

1. The stage of the lesion may not be fully realized until after cholecystectomy and in these cases further radical surgery will involve another laparotomy.
2. The gallbladder lies across the plane of the left and right lobes of the liver and, therefore, if lobectomy is carried out, it should be an extended right hepatic lobectomy (i.e. removal of the right lobe and medial segment of the left lobe). Many surgeons compromise by treating these patients with the so-called radical cholecystectomy (i.e. removal of the gallbladder along with a wedge of adjacent liver tissue and local lymph nodes).

A series of 100 patients from Hong Kong indicated that radical surgery has a high hospital mortality. The overall five year survival rate for advanced disease was 2% (Koo *et al.* 1981).

Tumours of the Bile Ducts

Benign
These are very rare. Sessile or pedunculated papillary adenomas have been described. Bile duct cystadenomas may occur and they are commonly intrahepatic and present with an abdominal mass. They have a good prognosis after resection. Intrahepatic biliary papillomatosis is an extremely rare condition which, although benign, has a high recurrence rate following local excision and therefore radical excision may be required (Gouma *et al.* 1984).

Carcinoma of the bile ducts
Carcinoma of the bile ducts (cholangiocarcinoma) can affect any part of the intra- or extrahepatic biliary tree. The tumour is histologically the same, but clinically different at different sites. In contrast to gallbladder cancer, males are affected as often as females. It tends to be a disease of older patients.

Epidemiology and aetiology
Intrahepatic cholangiocarcinoma is common in South-East Asia and in these areas it is related to infestation by the liver flukes, *Clonorchis sinensis* and *Opisthorchis viverrini*. These flukes are confined to the lumina of the larger intrahepatic bile ducts where they excite an inflammatory reaction and are associated with adenomatous hyperplasia of the bile duct lining (Belamaric 1973). The inflammatory

reaction may potentiate carcinogenic agents secreted in bile. Cholangiocarcinomas have also been reported in typhoid carriers.

Cholangiocarcinoma arises in about 4% of cases of choledochal cyst and 7% of cases of congenital cystic dilatation of the bile ducts (Caroli's disease).

The tumour occurs ten times more frequently in patients with ulcerative colitis than in the general population (Ritchie et al. 1974). Colectomy does not appear to prevent the occurrence of biliary cancer.

The hepatitis virus and liver cirrhosis do not predispose to cholangiocarcinoma. Gallstones are present in half of the cases.

Clinical features

Tumours proximal to the junction of the left and right hepatic ducts tend to present as space occupying lesions of the liver and can be confused with HCC. Jaundice is not present in the early stages. Tumours arising distal to the junction of the left and right hepatic ducts present as obstructive jaundice. Presentation is often late since the detergent properties of bile allow it to pass through very small lumina. Alpha fetoprotein is not elevated.

Morphology

Intrahepatic cholangiocarcinoma commonly appears as a single mass although, like HCC, it may form multiple nodules or be diffuse. They tend to be firmer than hepatocellular carcinoma due to the associated fibrous stroma. Subcapsular lesions tend to be umbilicated.

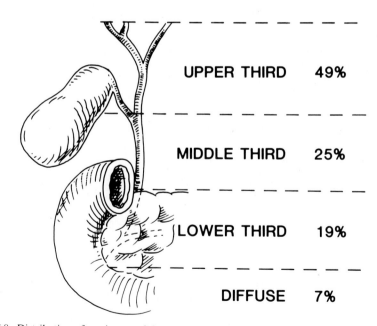

UPPER THIRD   49%

MIDDLE THIRD   25%

LOWER THIRD   19%

DIFFUSE   7%

Fig. 7.8. Distribution of carcinoma of the extrahepatic biliary system. (From Tompkins *et al.* 1981; reproduced with permission.)

The extrahepatic lesion may be seen as a hard fibrous cuff, constricting the bile ducts and possibly invading the liver substance, or else as a spongy mass within the bile ducts. The latter have a better prognosis. The distribution of extrahepatic cholangiocarcinomas in one study is shown in *Fig.* 7.8. The commonest site is in the upper third which is surgically the most difficult area. Cystic biliary carcinomas (cystadenocarcinomas) have been reported but this variant of the tumour appears to be rare.

Histologically the most common pattern is a proliferation of tubular structures surrounded by much fibrous tissue which makes them hard or scirrhous (*see Fig.* 7.9). The tubules are lined by columnar or cuboidal cells which are often well differentiated. In the case of an intrahepatic mass, it can be impossible on a histological basis to distinguish between a primary cholangiocarcinoma and a metastatic deposit from a carcinoma of the pancreas, gallbladder or elsewhere. The presence of *in situ* carcinoma in surrounding non-neoplastic bile ducts does, however, strongly point towards a primary lesion. Papillary and solid patterns are less common. Some tumours show a cholangiocarcinoma pattern in one area and an HCC in other areas.

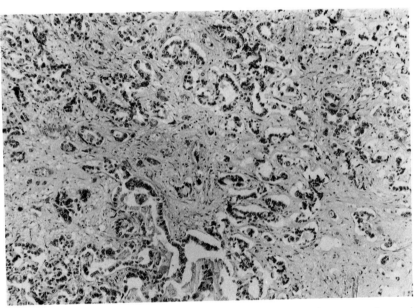

Fig. 7.9. Cholangiocarcinoma showing the marked desmoplastic reaction commonly seen in these tumours. (H and E × 75)

A histological variant of intrahepatic cholangiocarcinoma is sometimes termed a cholangiolocarcinoma. The tumour consists of a proliferation of very small ductules, resembling cholangioles (ductules of Hering). In the cystadenocarcinoma variant, areas of benign epithelium may occur in some of the cysts, suggesting that they arise in pre-existing benign cystadenomas.

Since bile duct carcinomas tend to be well differentiated the diagnosis by frozen section may be exceedingly difficult. At the time of surgery, biopsy may be taken by curettage of the lesion after opening the bile duct. However, biopsy directed by choledochoscopy may give a better sample.

Spread and prognosis

Direct spread may occur along the bile ducts. Compared with hepatocellular carcinoma, cholangiocarcinoma spreads more commonly to lymph nodes and less commonly by blood.

The prognosis is generally poor. One study reported an average survival of 16·5 months and 7 months for resectable and non-resectable lesions respectively (Beazley *et al.* 1984).

References

Arnaud J. P., Aprahamian M., Eloy R., Adloff M. (1979) Cristallographie de la lithiase biliaire. *Med. Chir. Dig.* **8**, 195–8.

Beazley R. M., Hadjis N., Benjamin I. S., Blumgart L. H. (1984) Clinicopathological aspects of high bile duct cancer. Experience with resection and bypass surgical treatments. *Ann. Surg.* **199**, 623–36.

Belamaric J. (1973) Intrahepatic bile duct carcinoma and *C. sinensis* infection in Hong Kong. *Cancer* **31**, 468–73.

Bismuth H. (1982) Postoperative strictures of the bile duct. In: Blumgart L. H. (ed.) *Clinical Surgery International 5: The Biliary Tract*, pp. 209–18. Edinburgh, Churchill Livingstone.

Bouchier I. A. D. (1984) Debits and credits: a current account of cholesterol gallstone disease. *Gut* **25**, 1021–8.

Gouma D. J., Mutum S. S., Benjamin I. S., Blumgart L. H. (1984) Intrahepatic biliary papillomatosis. *Br. J. Surg.* **71**, 72–4.

Howard E. R. (1983) Extrahepatic biliary atresia: a review of current management. *Br. J. Surg.* **70**, 193–7.

Kasai M., Watanabe I., Ohi R. (1975) Follow-up studies of long-term survivors after hepatic portoenterostomy for 'non-correctable' biliary atresia. *J. Pediatr. Surg.* **10**, 173–82.

Keddie N. C., Gough A. L., Galland R. B. (1976) Acalculous gallbladder disease: a prospective study. *Br. J. Surg.* **63**, 797–8.

Koo J., Wong J., Cheng F. C. Y., Ong G. B. (1981) Carcinoma of the gallbladder. *Br. J. Surg.* **68**, 161–5.

Mok H. Y., Von Bergman K., Grundy S. M. (1977) Regulation of pool size of bile acids in man. *Gastroenterology* **73**, 684–90.

Nevin J. E., Moran T. J., Kay S., King R. (1976) Carcinoma of the gallbladder. Staging, treatment and prognosis. *Cancer* **37**, 141–8.

Northover J. M. A., Terblanche J. (1979) A new look at the arterial supply of the bile duct in man and its surgical implications. *Br. J. Surg.* **66**, 379–84.

Olbourne N. A. (1975) Choledochal cysts: a review of the cystic anomalies of the biliary tree. *Ann. R. Coll. Surg. Engl.* **56**, 26–32.

Pitt H. A., Thompson H. H., Tompkins R. K., Longmire W. P. (1982) Primary sclerosing cholangitis: results of an aggressive surgical approach. *Ann. Surg.* **196**, 259–68.

Ritchie J. K., Allan R. N., Macartney J., Thompson H., Hawley P. R., Cooke W. T. (1974) Biliary tract carcinoma associated with ulcerative colitis. *Quart. J. Med.* **170**, 263–79.

Sherlock S. (1981) *Diseases of the Liver and Biliary System*, 5th ed. Oxford, Blackwell Scientific Publications.

Tompkins R. K., Thomas D., Wile A., Longmire W. P. (1981) Prognostic factors in bile duct carcinoma. *Ann. Surg.* **194**, 447–57.

Williamson B. W. A., Percy-Robb I. W. (1980) Contribution of biliary lipids to calcium binding in bile. *Gastroenterology* **78**, 696–702.

Chapter 8

The Pancreas

Normal Development, Structure and Function

The pancreas develops from ventral and dorsal outpouchings of the foregut (*see Fig.* 8.1). The ventral part is bilobed and arises from the lateral aspect of the hepatic duct. The larger dorsal pancreas drains directly into the gut. One lobe of the ventral pancreatic bud disappears and the remaining lobe, together with the hepatic duct, migrates around the gut to its dorsal aspect. The ventral bud then lies below the dorsal bud and the two fuse. The ventral bud gives rise to the lower part of the head and the uncinate process. The dorsal bud gives rise to the body, neck, tail and the upper part of the head. The duct systems fuse, so that the secretion from the body and tail is diverted into the duct of the ventral bud which becomes the main draining duct of the pancreas and is termed the duct of Wirsung. The remainder of the duct of the dorsal pancreatic bud becomes the accessory duct of Santorini, which may drain directly into the duodenum or may form a branch of the duct of Wirsung.

The commonest variations are: (1) both ducts open into the duodenum; (2) the duct of Wirsung carries the entire secretion, while the duct of Santorini ends blindly; and (3) the duct of Santorini carries the entire secretion and the duct of Wirsung is small or absent. The remaining configurations are rare.

The adult pancreas is 15 cm long, consisting of a head, neck, body and tail. The head and tail lie in the right and left paravertebral gutters respectively, while the neck and body curve over the inferior vena cava and aorta, in front of the first lumbar vertebra. The head fills the concavity of the duodenum and lies over the renal veins and cava. It has an uncinate process inferiorly which lies between the aorta (behind) and the superior mesenteric artery and vein (in front). The neck lies in front of the point where the superior mesenteric vein and splenic vein coalesce to form the portal vein. The body lies behind the lesser sac, stomach and transverse mesocolon and in front of the aorta, left adrenal, left renal vessels and left kidney. The tail rises to the level of T12 and its tip reaches the hilum of the spleen.

The head of the pancreas is supplied by the superior and inferior pancreatico-duodenal arteries. The neck, body and tail are chiefly supplied by the splenic artery. The head drains via the superior and inferior pancreatico-duodenal veins into the portal and superior mesenteric veins respectively. The rest of the gland drains via numerous small veins into the splenic vein.

Lymphatic drainage to the left of the neck is to the adjacent retroperitoneal nodes. The head drains to the coeliac group, while the uncinate process drains to the superior mesenteric group of pre-aortic nodes.

The pancreas is divided into many lobules which are separated from each other

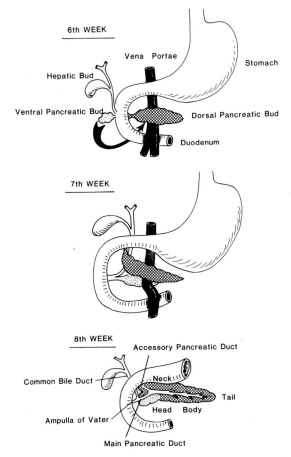

Fig. 8.1. Diagram to show the normal development of the pancreas. (After Stark 1965.)

by interlobular septa. The lobules are composed of acini (the exocrine pancreas) and the islets of Langerhans (the endocrine pancreas).

The acini are formed by clusters of pyramidal shaped cells, the bases of which are situated on a basement membrane and the apices of which point towards a central lumen. The cells have a basally situated nucleus and the cytoplasm appears granular, especially near the apex, due to the enzyme containing cytoplasmic granules (zymogen granules).

The duct system of the exocrine pancreas originates within the lumina of the acini. The smallest ducts are called intercalated ducts and the intra-acinar portions of these ducts are lined by clear cells called centro-acinar cells. The intercalated ducts drain into the intralobular ducts, then into the interlobular ducts (which run in the interlobular septa) and finally into the main pancreatic duct.

The main pancreatic duct fuses with the common bile duct to form the ampulla of Vater. The common channel is sufficiently long to allow reflux of bile from the common bile duct into the pancreatic duct in many cases (50–65%). This may be important in the pathogenesis of gallstone-associated pancreatitis (*see* p. 197).

The blood supply courses through the interlobular septa and individual arterial branches enter the lobules. Foulis (1984) considers these intralobular arteries to be end arteries which run into the lobules with the pancreatic ducts. The periphery of the lobule has the most tenuous blood supply and is the first part to become ischaemic if the blood supply is reduced or if the intralobular artery is damaged. He believes that these anatomical points are important in determining the pattern of damage in the various types of pancreatitis (see p. 202).

The intralobular arteries first supply the islets of Langerhans and then the exocrine acini. The acini therefore get a blood supply rich in islet hormones and these may influence their function.

The islets of Langerhans are equally distributed throughout the gland, except in the posterior part of the head and the tail where they are more numerous. They contain α cells, β cells, δ cells and PP cells. α cells produce glucagon and are sited at the periphery of the islets; β cells produce insulin and are centrally located; δ cells produce somatostatin and tend to be sited between α and β cells. PP cells produce pancreatic polypeptide and are sited at the islet periphery. There are no gastrin producing G-cells normally present in the adult.

The exocrine pancreas produces digestive enzymes (from the acinar cells) and electrolytes including bicarbonate (from the ductal cells). The enzymes are mainly produced as inactive 'pro' forms which are activated in the duodenum. The enzymes digest protein (trypsin, chymotrypsin, elastase and carboxypeptidase A and B), fat (lipase and phospholipase), starch (amylase) and nucleic acids (ribonuclease and deoxyribonuclease). Trypsinogen (the inactive form of trypsin) is converted into trypsin by the enzyme enterokinase which is present in the brush border of the duodenal epithelium. Trypsin, in turn, converts other pro-enzymes into active forms, thus starting a cascade of activation.

Control of exocrine pancreatic secretion is divided into a cephalic phase (mediated by the vagus nerve), a gastric phase (mediated by the vagus nerve and by gastrin) and an intestinal phase. Entry of acid into the duodenum causes release of secretin and entry of amino acids or fatty acids causes the release of cholecystokinin. Secretin increases pancreatic bicarbonate secretion and cholecystokinin causes secretion of enzymes.

Pancreatic Biopsy

Tissue diagnosis is often necessary to distinguish carcinoma from chronic pancreatitis since they may mimic each other both clinically and at laparotomy. Biopsy may be preoperative (by cytology) or intraoperative (by cytology or histology).

Preoperative biopsy

Pancreatic juice for cytology can be obtained by endoscopic retrograde cholangio-pancreatography (ERCP) and aspiration after secretin stimulation. The combination of ERCP, radiographic appearance and cytology has an accuracy rate of up to 90%.

Ultrasound or CT scan guided percutaneous fine needle aspiration cytology is also accurate in up to 90% of cases. False-negative results may be due to sampling error, especially if the lesion is less than 2 cm in diameter. Complications are rare, even though other organs are penetrated in the procedure, and seeding of the track with malignant cells does not seem to occur. There were no instances reported in one large series of over 3000 cases (Kline and Neal 1978).

Intraoperative biopsy

Aspiration cytology can also be used intraoperatively and rapid results are possible.

Wedge and needle biopsy both give sufficient tissue for histological diagnosis. Wedge biopsies are preferable if frozen tissue section diagnosis is required. False-negative results occur due to sampling error especially in the case of needle biopsy of a deep seated lesion. False positive results can rarely occur with some cases of chronic pancreatitis which can grossly and histologically mimic malignancy. A review of the literature by Reuben and Cotton (1978) showed that complications of bleeding, fistula and pancreatitis occur in about 7% after needle biopsy and in about 3% after wedge biopsy. Presumably wedge biopsy is safer as it is used for superficial lesions and is done under direct vision. A transduodenal approach to needle biopsy of lesions of the head of the pancreas may be used so that any resultant fistula drains into the duodenum. This method, which is preferred by many surgeons, does not, however, appear to substantially reduce the overall complication rate (Lightwood et al. 1976).

Congenital Abnormalities

Pancreas divisum

This is a congenital abnormality of the duct system in which the ventral and dorsal parts fail to fuse or else fuse incompletely. The duct of Santorini, therefore, remains as the main duct draining the tail, body and most of the head into the duodenum. The duct of Wirsung drains only that part of the pancreas derived from the ventral bud, i.e. the lower head and uncinate process.

The abnormality may be seen at ERCP in up to 6% of patients. Dye injected into the duct of Wirsung shows a tree-like appearance and this may simulate carcinoma. The main duct system can therefore only be demonstrated by cannulating the accessory duct, but this is often unsuccessful. There is some evidence that the condition predisposes to acute and chronic pancreatitis. The reason may be that the duct of Santorini is inadequate to drain the major part of the pancreatic secretion and there is therefore a functional obstruction. Recent attempts at treating the condition either endoscopically or surgically have been disappointing.

Annular pancreas

In this condition the ventral pancreatic bud fails to rotate round the gut, resulting in a ring of pancreatic tissue around the circumference of the duodenum. Other congenital malformations of the gastrointestinal tract are commonly present. Many cases present as vomiting in the first year of life, most commonly in the first week. The remaining symptomatic cases present in adult life with duodenal obstruction caused by recurrent chronic inflammation of the pancreas. Symptoms therefore mimic those of pyloric stenosis. Since the pancreatic tissue is very closely applied to the duodenum, it cannot be resected and a bypass procedure is usually performed.

Ectopic pancreas

Nodules of ectopic pancreas are seen most commonly in the submucosa of the stomach and duodenal wall, although they can occur at other sites. They are seen endoscopically as nodules, sometimes with a central dimple where a duct opens onto the mucosal surface. They may be ulcerated and they can cause bleeding. Occasionally they may cause pyloric obstruction. Most cases found during upper gastrointestinal tract investigation are incidental and are not the cause of the patient's symptoms.

Pancreatitis

Classification

In 1963, a symposium in Marseille led to the Marseille classification of pancreatitis (Sarles 1965) in which four groups are recognized.

1. *Acute pancreatitis*: an acute inflammatory condition of the pancreas, after which there is complete clinical, functional and pathological restitution of the gland (i.e. there is no residual damage).
2. *Relapsing acute pancreatitis*: recurrent episodes of acute pancreatitis.
3. *Chronic pancreatitis*: a chronic inflammatory condition of the pancreas in which there is anatomical and/or functional residual damage to the gland.
4. *Chronic relapsing pancreatitis*: chronic pancreatitis with acute exacerbations.

The problem with this classification is the distinction between relapsing acute pancreatitis and chronic relapsing pancreatitis. Clinically, these two groups are very similar, that is, patients with recurrent acute episodes of upper abdominal pain and raised serum amylase. In theory, the distinction can only be made by demonstrating the presence or absence of structural/functional changes by ERCP, pancreatic function tests, etc., which are not done in all cases. Furthermore, pathological changes may still exist even in the absence of abnormalities as demonstrated by these tests.

In order to clarify this problem, an International Workshop was held in Cambridge (Sarner and Cotton 1984). This Workshop simplified the classification into two groups.

1. *Acute pancreatitis*: this is defined as an acute condition typically presenting with abdominal pain and usually associated with raised pancreatic enzymes in blood or urine due to inflammatory disease of the pancreas.
2. *Chronic pancreatitis*: this is defined as a continuing inflammatory disease of the pancreas, characterized by irreversible morphological change and typically causing pain and/or permanent loss of function.

This Workshop added that 'acute pancreatitis may recur' and that 'many patients with chronic pancreatitis may have acute exacerbations'. According to this classification, the diagnosis of chronic pancreatitis can only be made after the demonstration of 'irreversible morphological change' on ERCP or pancreatic function tests, although the term 'probable chronic pancreatitis' can be used where necessary. A subgroup of obstructive chronic pancreatitis is also recognized.

The Workshop therefore concluded that, clinically, pancreatitis need only be divided into acute or chronic, but that in each case, a statement should be made on aetiology and on functional and morphological damage as defined by exocrine pancreatic function tests and ERCP respectively.

Acute pancreatitis

The incidence of acute pancreatitis appears to be increasing. Imrie (1981) reported an increase in incidence from 90 new patients per million of the population in 1960 to 200 new cases per million of the population during the 1970s.

Aetiology

Many cases of acute pancreatitis are associated with biliary disease. Gallstones are found in the gallbladder in up to 70% of these patients and in the bile ducts in up to 20%. Eight per cent of patients with biliary disease associated with pancreatitis have cholecystitis without gallstones.

Although some authorities consider that alcohol always causes irreversible pancreatic damage (i.e. chronic pancreatitis), it is now appreciated that alcohol-induced pancreatitis may present acutely and that alcohol-induced disease is not inevitably progressive (Sarner and Cotton 1984).

Pancreatic trauma may cause rupture of the pancreatic ducts and lead to acute pancreatitis as a complication of the pancreatic juice leak. Other mechanical causes include ERCP, obstruction from a pancreatic carcinoma and perhaps the presence of a pancreas divisum. Pancreatitis may occur on an ischaemic basis, particularly in the elderly, and in cases of hypothermia. Infectious agents, such as mumps virus, Coxsackie B virus and Campylobacter may be associated with pancreatitis, as may several drugs, such as steroids, thiazide diuretics, tetracyclines and azathioprine. Hyperlipidaemia, hyperparathyroidism and haemochromatosis are also occasionally associated with acute pancreatitis. Many cases are idiopathic with no clear aetiological factor. Finally, a hereditary form of pancreatitis is recognized.

Acute pancreatitis in children is being recognized with increasing frequency. The aetiological factors differ greatly from adults and many are due to viral infections such as mumps. Blunt abdominal trauma, frequently from a minor abdominal injury, is a not uncommon cause. Some cases are due to pigment gallstones associated with congenital spherocytosis, and occasionally congenital abnormalities, such as an annular pancreas, are implicated. Ascaris infestation is a common cause of pancreatitis in children in certain countries.

Pathogenesis

It is generally accepted that acute pancreatitis results from an initiating event which causes activation of pancreatic enzymes followed by autodigestion of the pancreatic substance (see Fig. 8.2).

THE INITIATING EVENT: The exact pathogenesis of gallstone associated pancreatitis is controversial. A common channel theory was proposed by Opie (1901) who suggested that impaction of a gallstone at the ampulla could lead to reflux of bile into the pancreatic duct by virtue of the fact that the biliary and pancreatic ducts terminated in a common channel. Doubt was cast on this theory because some authorities did not believe that a common channel existed and because obstruction

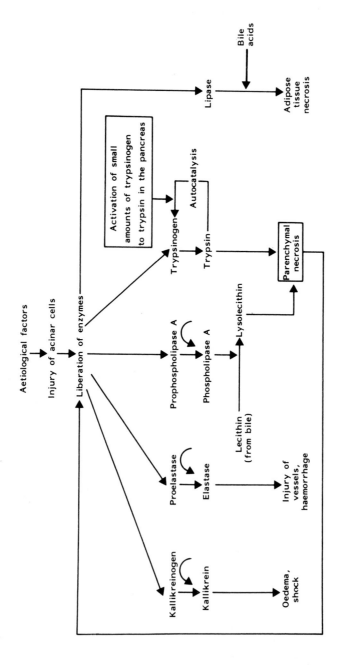

Fig. 8.2. Diagram to show the pathogenesis of acute pancreatitis. (Adapted from Lankisch and Creutzfelot 1981.)

of the ampulla could only be demonstrated at autopsy in a few patients with pancreatitis. However, these doubts have been repudiated by studies which have:

(i) demonstrated that reflux of contrast medium into the pancreatic duct during operative cholangiography is common (Kelly 1976);
(ii) demonstrated that gallstones are found in the faeces of the majority of patients with gallstone associated pancreatitis, but not in those with uncomplicated cholecystitis. This indicates that gallstones pass down the bile duct and may cause a transient obstruction of the ampulla in those patients who have gallstone associated pancreatitis (Acosta and Ledesma 1974).

Exactly how bile in the pancreatic duct initiates pancreatitis is unclear, although there are several possibilities: (1) bile under high pressure may cause duct rupture; (2) in bile which is infected by *E. coli* (this being common in gallstone patients) primary bile acids are metabolized to secondary bile acids which can damage the mucosal barrier of the pancreatic ducts; (3) bile salts may be able to liberate the tiny amounts of trypsin necessary to activate the pancreatic pro-enzymes and initiate the cascade of activation (Shearman and Finlayson 1982). A further factor may be an incompetent ampulla, secondary to passage of a stone, allowing reflux of duodenal content.

Hyperparathyroidism may be associated with pancreatic duct obstruction, possibly caused by precipitation of calcium salts. The mechanism by which most of the other aetiological factors cause pancreatitis is unknown. The role of alcohol is discussed on p. 204.

THE AUTODIGESTION: It is likely that the initiating events lead to pancreatitis via a final common pathway in which a rise of trypsin activity within the pancreas causes a cascade of activation of pancreatic enzymes. The concentration of trypsin within the pancreas depends on the amount formed from its precursor, trypsinogen, and the amount destroyed by trypsin inactivators. An imbalance of these factors may cause a rise in trypsin activity which, in turn, can activate further trypsinogen by autocatalysis and also activate other enzymes including elastase, phospholipase A and kallikrein. Kallikrein is capable of producing the polypeptides kallidin and bradykinin from kininogens which are alpha-2-globulins found in plasma and lymph. Bradykinin and kallidin are vasoactive and cause vasodilatation and increased vascular permeability. Locally, they cause inflammation and pain, and systemically, they cause shock.

Lipase causes fat necrosis while phospholipase A causes destruction of cell membranes and converts the lecithin in bile to lysolecithin which is cytotoxic to the pancreatic duct cells.

Clinical features

Upper abdominal pain is present in nearly all patients and radiates into the back in about 50%. Vomiting and pyrexia are also commonly present. In this clinical setting, a serum amylase greater than 1200 iu/l is strongly suggestive of acute pancreatitis. Difficulty in diagnosis may arise in patients with other causes of hyperamylasaemia (especially perforated duodenal ulcer and mesenteric vascular occlusion), in patients who arrive in hospital late, in those who have hyperlipidaemia (this interferes with amylase measurement) and in macroamylasaemia.

Occasionally, the serum amylase is not elevated in severe haemorrhagic pancreatitis.

It is of importance to recognize those patients likely to develop severe pancreatitis so that they can have intensive treatment. Ranson and Pasternack (1977) described eleven indicators of prognosis. These have been modified by Imrie *et al.* (1978) who use the nine prognostic indicators listed in *Table* 8.1. These factors accurately predict severity in 72% of cases (Blamey *et al.* 1984). Others have used the physical characteristics of peritoneal lavage fluid to determine the severity of acute pancreatitis (McMahon *et al.* 1980).

Table 8.1 Prognostic factors in patients with acute pancreatitis (Imrie 1981)*

WBC	>	15×10^9/l
Glucose	>	10 mmol/l (no diabetic history)
Urea	>	16 mmol/l (no response to IV fluids)
Pao_2	<	60 mmHg
Calcium	<	2.0 mmol/l
Albumin	<	32 g/l
LDH	>	600 units/l
GOT/GPT	>	100 units/l
Age	>	55 years

* If three or more adverse prognostic factors are present within 48 hours of hospital admission, then severe acute pancreatitis is confirmed. All other cases are classified as mild.

Morphology

Acute pancreatitis is often divided into oedematous and haemorrhagic types, although these are degrees of severity rather than distinct entities. In the oedematous phase, the pancreas is swollen with minimal or no necrosis. The more severe forms are characterized by varying degrees of necrotic softening, interspaced with areas of haemorrhage giving a map-like appearance. The areas of haemorrhage may coalesce to give the gland a blue or black appearance. Chalky white areas of fat necrosis are seen on the pancreas (*see Fig.* 8.3) and elsewhere in the abdomen where fat is found, especially the mesentery and greater omentum. Fat necrosis may occasionally occur outside the abdomen in various sites including the subcutaneous tissues.

Histologically, in the early phase, there is only oedema of the interstitial tissue. Later the four characteristic features of acute pancreatitis are seen.

1. Proteolytic destruction of pancreatic parenchyma is seen as areas of cell breakdown (*see Fig.* 8.4).
2. Necrosis of blood vessels is associated with inflammation of the vessel walls, thrombosis of the lumina and pancreatic haemorrhage.
3. Fat necrosis occurs in the peripancreatic fat and in the interstitial fat in the pancreas. Fat cells become shadowy in outline and are filled with a pink precipitate. Basophilic foci of calcification may be seen (*see Fig.* 8.5).
4. An inflammatory reaction is seen surrounding the areas of pancreatic necrosis (*see Fig.* 8.4).

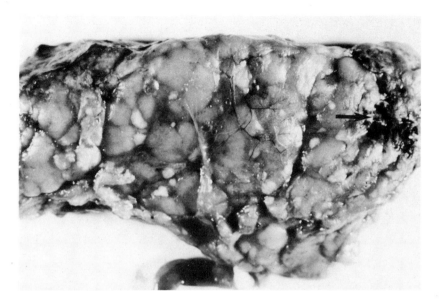

Fig. 8.3. Acute pancreatitis showing foci of fat necrosis and an area of haemorrhagic necrosis (arrow).

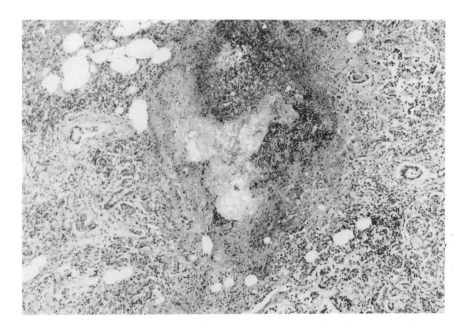

Fig. 8.4. Acute pancreatitis. An area of necrosis with a surrounding acute inflammatory response. (H and E × 30)

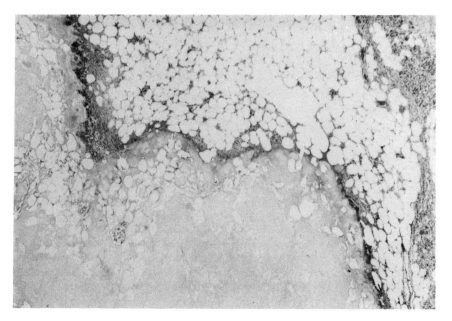

Fig. 8.5. Fat necrosis in peripancreatic fat. The fat in the lower part of the picture has undergone necrosis and is surrounded by a rim of acute inflammation. (H and E × 30)

Foulis (1984) considers that the pattern of necrosis within the pancreatic lobule gives a clue as to aetiology. In gallstone associated and alcohol associated acute pancreatitis the damaging agents come from the pancreatic ducts and therefore the necrosis is in the area surrounding the duct (periductal necrosis). In ischaemic pancreatitis, the necrosis tends to affect the periphery of the lobule which is furthermost from the arterial supply (perilobular necrosis).

Complications

PULMONARY: Hypoxia with an arterial Po_2 less than 60 mmHg occurs in about half of all patients with acute pancreatitis (Imrie *et al.* 1978) but the signs on the chest X-ray may be minimal. At least two factors have been suggested to explain this and they may occur in combination: (1) right to left shunting as a result of subclinical diffuse intravascular coagulation in which microthrombi block the pulmonary microvasculature; (2) diffuse alveolar damage with hyaline membrane formation, causing a type of adult respiratory distress syndrome (*see* p. 397). This may be caused by phospholipase A which is known to damage pulmonary surfactant.

SHOCK: Several mechanisms may cause shock in pancreatitis. The exudation of oedema fluid into the pancreas and adjacent tissue causes hypovolaemia. Kinins cause vasodilatation and increased vascular permeability. A myocardial depressant factor (MDF) may be produced by the pancreas and cause myocardial dysfunction. Haemorrhage into the pancreas causes further hypovolaemia.

RENAL: Renal dysfunction is often the result of shock. It can, however, occur in the absence of shock and is accompanied by an increase in renal vascular resistance. This may be due to fibrin deposits in glomerular capillaries.

HYPOCALCAEMIA: Hypocalcaemia is explained in most cases by a fall in serum albumin and therefore in protein-bound calcium. In more severe cases the sequestration of calcium into areas of fat necrosis may be an additional factor. Another theory is that magnesium is also lowered in acute pancreatitis and the hypomagnesaemia might reduce the responsiveness of bone to parathormone, preventing mobilization of calcium. However, there is little evidence of any disturbance in parathormone release or responsiveness. Currently, a shift of calcium from extra- to intracellular compartments is considered important in the pathogenesis of the hypocalcaemia.

HYPERGLYCAEMIA: Hyperglycaemia appears to be due to a relative excess secretion of glucagon over insulin, rather than a defect of insulin secretion. Rarely does permanent diabetes ensue.

GASTROINTESTINAL HAEMORRHAGE: This is commonly due to gastric or duodenal stress-related erosions or ulcers or may be part of a diffuse intravascular coagulation problem. It may also be due to direct involvement of the duodenal wall in the inflammatory process or, rarely, due to gastric varices which can occur in cases of splenic vein thrombosis. Finally, a false aneurysm of the splenic artery can occur and rupture into the stomach.

SKIN AND BONE COMPLICATIONS: Subcutaneous fat necrosis occasionally results in subcutaneous nodules in the limbs and trunk. Intramedullary fat necrosis in the long bones can cause painful osteolytic lesions.

PANCREATIC PSEUDOCYST: *See* p. 207.

PANCREATIC ABSCESS: This is an uncommon condition and complicates about 4% of patients with acute pancreatitis of average severity, although the incidence after very severe acute pancreatitis may approach 25%. It should be distinguished from a localized collection of pus in the lesser sac which is an infected pseudocyst. Most authors understand a pancreatic abscess to imply pancreatic necrosis with secondary infection, usually occurring in the second week after an attack of acute pancreatitis. There is a high fever and leucocytosis. Without early and adequate external drainage, the mortality is high. The recurrence rate is also high at about 30%. One study of 34 patients found that the abscesses tended to follow alcohol or gallstone associated pancreatitis and only two followed blunt trauma (Shi *et al.* 1984). The abscesses were frequently multilocular and some were retropancreatic. Eight patients had major bleeding into the abscess cavity. Twelve patients (35%) died, most deaths being due to sepsis or major bleeding.

Prognosis
The overall survival for acute pancreatitis is up to 90%. If, however, cases are divided into mild and severe, as defined in *Table* 8.1 (*see* p. 200), then the mortality

for the former is minimal, whereas up to 20% of patients with severe pancreatitis die during the acute attack.

Chronic pancreatitis

When pancreatic inflammation leads to permanent structural or functional damage, the term chronic pancreatitis is used.

In Western countries, the incidence depends upon the pattern of alcohol consumption. Chronic pancreatitis is found in less than 1% of all autopsies and males account for at least two-thirds of patients. Patients are usually over 40 years old, although in the Afro-Asian type (*see* below) the age of onset is usually less than 20 years.

Aetiology

ALCOHOL: Chronic pancreatitis occurs after some years of alcohol abuse (usually 10–20 years). It is unclear why some alcoholics develop chronic pancreatitis while others do not. Alcohol excess is responsible for about 75% of cases of chronic pancreatitis in Europe and up to 90% of those cases of chronic pancreatitis in which there is significant calcification.

GALLSTONES: Pancreatitis associated with gallstones is usually acute, that is, without residual damage. Some cases of chronic pancreatitis, however, may be associated with a benign stenosis of the distal common bile duct occurring after surgical operation or passage of a calculus.

HYPERPARATHYROIDISM: Hyperparathyroidism may be associated with acute or chronic pancreatitis. Hypercalcaemia causes an increase in pancreatic protein secretion and protein plugs may therefore occur in the duct system.

IDIOPATHIC: In many cases of chronic pancreatitis, no cause is found.

AFRO-ASIAN: The Afro-Asian form is of obscure aetiology and occurs in young people who have no history of alcohol abuse or biliary disease. The pancreatic ducts become blocked by mucous plugs which later calcify. Diabetes occurs at an early stage. Protein malnutrition may be an important factor in these patients, although other additional factors such as dehydration may also be necessary.

RARE CAUSES: Hereditary chronic relapsing pancreatitis has been described and is autosomal dominant. Haemochromatosis may also cause chronic pancreatitis.

Pathogenesis

The exact mechanism by which alcohol causes pancreatitis is unknown. However, pancreatic juice obtained at ERCP has a higher protein concentration in alcoholics (with or without pancreatitis) than controls (Sahel and Sarles 1979). The raised concentration of protein leads to precipitation and stone formation with subsequent duct obstruction and pancreatitis. One group has implicated a particular protein, known as 'stone protein' which may have a particular affinity for calcium

(De Caro *et al.* 1979). An individual susceptibility factor must exist as not all chronic alcoholics develop pancreatitis. This susceptibility factor is not the same as that which exists for liver cirrhosis, as only a minority of patients with liver cirrhosis develop chronic pancreatitis and vice-versa.

Clinical features

Clinical features include abdominal pain which typically radiates to the back and may be persistent. Severe diabetes mellitus has been reported in 75% of patients with calcific pancreatitis and it usually requires control with insulin. Steatorrhoea, weight loss and mild jaundice may also occur. Acute exacerbations have the same clinical features as acute pancreatitis.

Morphology

The gland is usually increased in size (although it may be atrophic later in the disease process) and firm. The surface loses its normal lobulation. Plain radiographs may show diffuse calcification, particularly in those cases associated with alcohol. During acute exacerbations, the gross findings of acute pancreatitis are superimposed on the background of fibrosis. The ductal changes are seen at ERCP. The side ducts become stubby and the main duct may be dilated to over 1 cm and may have many points of narrowing, giving a 'chain of lakes' appearance. Calculi in the ducts and cysts are also commonly seen.

Histologically, chronic calcific pancreatitis characteristically involves the pancreas in a lobular fashion (i.e. affected lobules may be adjacent to unaffected

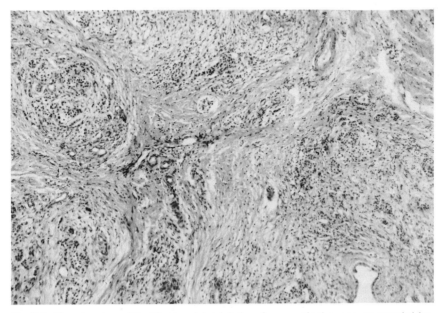

Fig. 8.6. Chronic pancreatitis. The remaining lobules of pancreatic tissue are surrounded by much fibrous tissue. (H and E × 30)

ones). Within the affected lobules the ducts tend to be dilated and contain calculi or protein plugs. In some areas the epithelium of the ducts is destroyed and periductal fibrous tissue forms strictures. There is general atrophy of the pancreatic paren-chyma with fibrosis and possibly a chronic inflammatory cell infiltrate (*see Fig. 8.6*). During acute exacerbations, the changes of acute pancreatitis are super-imposed. The pancreatic islets tend to be preserved until late in the course of the disease.

Complications

ACUTE EXACERBATIONS: Acute exacerbations occurring in the course of chronic pancreatitis may be clinically identical to acute pancreatitis and are subject to the same complications (*see* p. 202).

EXOCRINE DYSFUNCTION: Steatorrhoea occurs late in the course of the disease and is seen in about one-third of patients. Occasionally, chronic pancreatitis is painless and steatorrhoea may be the presenting symptom.

ENDOCRINE DYSFUNCTION: This is common in the late stages of the disease and serum levels of insulin and glucagon are both reduced.

OBSTRUCTIVE JAUNDICE: This occurs if the distal end of the common bile duct becomes involved in an inflammatory process and is seen in 5–10% of cases. Only a minority of such patients require treatment for the jaundice.

SPLENIC VEIN THROMBOSIS: This may occur if the splenic vein becomes involved in the inflammatory process. There is a sudden increase in the size of the spleen with resultant hypersplenism. Varices may arise and, if so, are limited to the gas-troepiploic veins. This so-called 'sectorial portal hypertension' may be diagnosed by splenoportography and can cause severe bleeding from gastric varices. The portal vein pressure is normal and therefore shunting procedures are not indicated. Splenectomy is curative.

Cysts of the Pancreas

These are divided into true cysts which have an epithelial lining and pseudocysts which have no epithelial lining.

Epithelial cysts

Congenital cysts

Congenital pancreatic cysts are rare and are usually associated with inherited polycystic disease of kidney, liver or spleen. The cysts are usually multiple but can be solitary. Usually they have a thin fibrous capsule which is lined by a smooth membrane; the fluid is turbid, unless there has been previous haemorrhage. Microscopically, the lining is of flattened epithelial cells which may be absent in some places. They rarely cause symptoms.

Retention cysts

These arise behind a duct obstruction which may be due to a tumour or calculus. They are, therefore, associated with malignant disease and chronic pancreatitis.

Neoplastic cysts

Serous cystadenomas and mucinous cystic tumours are the commonest forms of neoplastic pancreatic cysts and are discussed on p. 208.

Non-epithelial cysts (pseudocysts)

A pseudocyst is an encapsulated collection of fluid which contains a high concentration of pancreatic enzymes. Unlike a true cyst, it has no epithelial lining. Pseudocysts may occur after trauma but are more commonly associated with pancreatitis. They may develop after acute pancreatitis or after an acute exacerbation of chronic pancreatitis when the inflammatory exudate becomes walled off by adjacent serosal and peritoneal surfaces. They are found most commonly in the lesser sac and tend to expand along lines of least resistance. The cyst wall is initially thin but later it becomes thick and fibrous. Alternatively, pseudocysts may arise during the course of chronic pancreatitis unrelated to an acute episode. In these cases, they result from dilatation of the ducts, secondary to an obstruction. The epithelium atrophies, bringing them within the definition of pseudocyst. This type may remain within or grow beyond the confines of the pancreas.

Clinically, a pseudocyst develops 3–4 weeks after an acute episode of pancreatitis. The patient either fails to improve or symptoms return after a period of improvement. Pain is common and persistent with low grade fever, nausea and vomiting. Jaundice may result from pressure on the common bile duct or gastric outlet obstruction may occur. An epigastric mass is palpable and this may be differentiated from a phlegmon (a mass of inflamed and oedematous tissue) by ultrasound.

Microscopically, the cyst wall has no epithelial lining. The capsule consists of fibrous tissue which may be inflamed. Organized blood clot and calcification may be seen in the cyst wall.

The major complications are as follows.

1. Infection is usually caused by enteric organisms and may follow ERCP. Gas may be seen in the cyst on a plain abdominal radiograph. Percutaneous needle aspiration will give samples which can be cultured.
2. Rupture into the peritoneal cavity causes pancreatic ascites which may have an acute or chronic onset. Perforation into the stomach or colon may result in spontaneous resolution or in complications such as abscess formation or gastrointestinal haemorrhage.
3. Haemorrhage may occur into the cyst as a result of erosion of a vessel in the cyst wall. Haemorrhage into the peritoneal cavity is due to erosion of the cyst into a major vessel such as the splenic artery. Haemorrhage into the gastrointestinal tract may also occur.

The natural history is such that most authorities suggest conservative monitoring (clinically and by ultrasound) for 6 weeks. This has two advantages: (1) the cyst may resolve in this period; (2) surgery is easier and has a lower morbidity and mortality later in the disease process when the wall is well defined.

There has been a recent trend for ultrasound guided percutaneous drainage of pancreatic pseudocysts, although repeated drainage is often required (Colhoun *et al.* 1984).

A follow-up of one series of 54 pancreatic pseudocysts showed that they are unlikely to resolve if present for more than 6 weeks and also that complications are more common in persistent cases (Bradley *et al.* 1979).

Tumours of the Exocrine Pancreas (Duct Cell Origin)

Classification of pancreatic tumours is complex. In this section the classification used by Kloppel (1984), which is based on that of Cubilla and Fitzgerald (1979), is used. This classification divides tumours histologically into those derived from duct cells and those from acinar cells. It includes a separate section for those of uncertain histogenesis.

Benign

SEROUS CYSTADENOMA: These tumours occur as well circumscribed tumours, most commonly in the tail of the pancreas in elderly patients. The lesion is usually an incidental finding at autopsy, although if it is located in the head of the pancreas, it may cause biliary obstruction. Cut section shows multiple cysts filled with serous fluid. Histologically the cysts are lined by cuboidal cells. Some normal pancreatic tissue may be trapped within the stroma. They may require excision if causing pressure symptoms.

Intraduct papilloma

These are rare and occur as a papillary mass confined to a pancreatic duct. They may cause duct obstruction and the patients present with intermittent pain.

Uncertain malignant potential

Mucinous cystic neoplasm

Although these tumours have, in the past, been divided into mucinous cystadenomas and mucinous cystadenocarcinomas, Kloppel (1984) believes that no clear distinction can be made, since all have malignant potential and the capacity to recur. Foci of carcinomatous transformation are seen in virtually all cases on detailed histological examination.

They occur mainly in middle-aged women, most commonly in the tail of the pancreas. A radiating 'sun burst' calcification, as seen on X-ray, is considered pathognomonic of the lesion.

Grossly, the tumour is unilocular or there may be a few daughter cysts present. The cyst contains viscous mucus and papillary growths are seen on the inner surface. Histologically the epithelial lining is composed of mucus secreting cells. Foci of dysplastic epithelium or invasive carcinoma are frequently seen.

The tumours can usually be resected and if resection is complete, the prognosis is good.

Malignant tumours

Carcinoma of ductal cell origin is the most common type of malignancy in the pancreas and the general term 'carcinoma of the pancreas' refers to this tumour.

Epidemiology and aetiology

The incidence of carcinoma of the pancreas in Western countries is approximately 9 per 100 000 annually. The incidence is increasing but this may be partly due to the increased average age of the population. The male to female ratio is about 1·5 : 1 and the tumour generally occurs in patients who are over the age of 55 years.

Cigarette smokers have twice the incidence when compared with non-smokers. Aetiological links between pancreatic cancer and a high fat diet, a high coffee intake (Benarde and Weiss 1982) and biliary disease have been suggested but not proven. Exposure to industrial carcinogens such as benzidine have been documented in some patients.

Diabetes mellitus may be a risk factor, although in many cases the finding of diabetes in a patient with pancreatic carcinoma is due to fibrosis of the distal pancreas and islet destruction caused by obstructing tumour.

There is no strong evidence that chronic pancreatitis predisposes to pancreatic carcinoma, with the possible exception of the hereditary variety (see p. 204).

Clinical features

Carcinoma of the head of the pancreas often presents with pain (often in the back), jaundice, weight loss, malaise and vomiting. Eventually, 90% of patients become jaundiced: The vomiting is due to obstruction of the pylorus or duodenum. Some authors have stressed the development of unstable diabetes in patients over 60 years of age as an early sign of cancer of the pancreas. Thrombophlebitis and psychiatric symptoms are less common. Physical findings may include a palpable gallbladder (Courvoisier's sign), hepatomegaly and jaundice.

In patients with carcinoma of the body or tail, pain, weight loss and nausea are more common. If jaundice occurs it is more likely to be due to liver metastases. If vomiting occurs, it is due to obstruction of the duodenojejunal flexure.

Morphology

Pancreatic carcinoma may involve the head (70%), body (15%), or tail (10%), or may extensively involve several parts of the gland (5%). Grossly, the tumours are hard and infiltrating and white or grey on cut section with little necrosis or haemorrhage. Tumours of the body and tail are large at the time of presentation and may have already spread to the retroperitoneal fat, the splenic hilum, the left adrenal or stomach. Tumours confined to the pancreas are often difficult to distinguish from chronic pancreatitis. As a guide, a hard mass in the head, associated with obstructive jaundice and dilatation of the common bile duct and pancreatic duct, is usually a carcinoma. Conversely, a mass that includes most of the gland and is unassociated with jaundice or biliary dilatation is usually chronic pancreatitis. The distinction is further complicated by the common occurrence of pancreatitis surrounding a carcinoma.

The common histological pattern of pancreatic carcinoma is the well differentiated type with good formation of ducts and a characteristic dense fibrous stroma (*see Fig.* 8.7). The ducts are irregular in shape and the cells show atypia. In the poorly differentiated type, anaplastic epithelial cells are seen with necrosis and little stroma. Several histological variants are described.

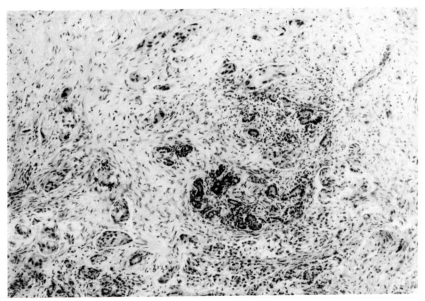

Fig. 8.7. Carcinoma of pancreas. The malignant glands are set in fibrous tissue and this can be difficult to distinguish from chronic pancreatitis (*see Fig.* 8.6).

1. Mucinous adenocarcinomas are gelatinous on gross appearance. Histologically, mucin production is seen as signet ring type cells, often floating in lakes of the mucus.
2. Adenosquamous carcinomas are characterized histologically by having areas of both adenocarcinoma showing tubule formation and islands of atypical squamous cells.
3. Pleomorphic carcinomas are divided into giant cell types and small cell types. The pleomorphic carcinoma with giant cells is a large tumour with necrosis and haemorrhage. Histologically, numerous bizarre multinucleated giant cells are seen. Some of these tumours contain, in addition to the bizarre giant cells, osteoclast-like giant cells and this feature indicates a better prognosis. Pleomorphic carcinomas of the small cell type also show necrosis. Microscopically, they consist of sheets of small basophilic cells and the condition can therefore be mistaken for lymphoma.

In many cases of pancreatic carcinoma, the remaining pancreas may show changes of fibrosis, atrophy and chronic pancreatitis due to obstruction of the pancreatic ducts.

Spread and prognosis

Within the pancreas, spread occurs along the interlobular septa and the tumour also tends to destroy the surrounding pancreatic parenchyma. There is a tendency to spread along the pancreatic duct. One study showed intraduct spread up to 3 cm from the main tumour mass in 30% of patients (Kloppel 1984). The tumour also spreads along perineural spaces and within lymphatics. Lymph nodes adjacent to the pancreas are first involved, followed by nodes at the porta hepatis. Blood-borne spread occurs later and is mainly to the liver.

The prognosis is poor, with five year survival rates in the region of 2–5%. This is partly due to the advanced stage of many tumours at the time of initial diagnosis. Tumours confined to the pancreas without histological lymph node involvement have a better prognosis than those which present at a later stage, but even these apparently early tumours are rarely cured. This may be due to failure to detect involved lymph nodes at the time of surgery or because of residual tumour in the pancreas (e.g. within the pancreatic duct).

The prognosis is worse with large tumours than with small ones and in tumours of the body and tail compared with those in the head. The poorly differentiated and pleomorphic types have a worse prognosis than the well differentiated type.

Tumours of the Exocrine Pancreas (Acinar Cell Origin)

Benign

Solid and cystic tumours

These tumours, which are also known as papillary cystic neoplasms, have several characteristic features. Almost all occur in young women or adolescent girls. They are usually large and cut section shows peripheral solid areas with central cystic areas filled with debris.

Microscopically, large areas of cystic necrosis and haemorrhage are confirmed. The solid areas consist of polygonal cells surrounding fibrovascular material. Electron microscopy studies show that these tumours are probably derived from the enzyme-secreting acinar cells.

Prognosis after resection is excellent and they are considered to be benign.

Malignant

Acinar cell carcinoma

These occur in elderly patients. Grossly, they are large, soft tumours with areas of necrosis. Microscopically, the cells form acini and tubular arrangements. The individual cells are similar to acinar cells in that they have a granular cytoplasm and electron microscopy shows that they contain zymogen granules. High serum lipase levels may be seen and this may cause subcutaneous fat necrosis. The prognosis is poor.

Tumours of Uncertain Histogenesis

Pancreaticoblastoma

This is an exceedingly rare tumour of the pancreas occurring in infants and children under seven years. Grossly, they show cystic change. Microscopically, the characteristic feature is a mixture of epithelial (tubular, acinar and squamous) and mesenchymal elements. The prognosis is good if resection is possible.

Other Tumours of the Exocrine Pancreas

Benign non-epithelial tumours of the pancreas are rare. Dermoid cysts and neurogenic tumours have been reported. Malignant non-epithelial tumours are also rare and include leiomyosarcoma and fibrosarcoma. Lymphomas of both the Hodgkin's and non-Hodgkin's type may occur. Secondary carcinoma is rare.

Endocrine Tumours of the Pancreas

All pancreatic islets contain the following cells: α cells (glucagon secreting); β cells (insulin secreting); δ cells (somatostatin secreting); and PP cells (pancreatic polypeptide secreting). There may also be cells which secrete vasoactive intestinal polypeptide (VIP), although this is not yet certain. Gastrin (G) cells are found in fetal life but disappear after birth. Corresponding tumours which predominantly secrete each of these hormones have been described in the pancreas.

Non-functional endocrine tumours also occur.

Clinical features

Symptoms may be related to either the tumour mass (e.g. pain and obstructive jaundice) or to hormone secretion. Even if several hormones are produced by one tumour, the symptoms are invariably due to one dominant hormone.

Morphology

Endocrine tumours are evenly distributed throughout the gland. They are usually encapsulated, firm and normally compress the surrounding tissue rather than infiltrate it. Malignant endocrine tumours, however, do invade the normal pancreatic tissue and may show lymph node metastases. Gross appearance is no guide as to the type of hormone produced, except that gastrinomas and glucagonomas are more likely to be malignant than insulinomas.

Endocrine tumours of the gut, pancreas and bronchus have been divided into histological groups by various authors, most of whom accept the four following basic categories.

TYPE A: This is the carcinoid pattern consisting of nests and cords of cells as described on p. 109. It is the same pattern as that seen in carcinoid tumours of the appendix.

TYPE B: These tumours show ribbons of cells, one or two cells thick, which form various interlacing patterns (*see Fig.* 8.8).

TYPE C: These are rare and appear histologically as cells in tubular and acinar formations.

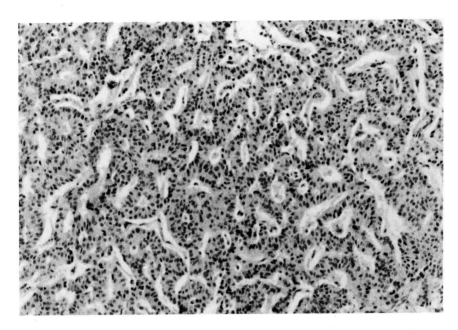

Fig. 8.8. Islet cell tumour of pancreas. Mainly of type B pattern (*see text*). (H and E × 75)

TYPE D: These are undifferentiated tumours which form sheets of cells with no characteristic pattern.

Many tumours show combinations of these histological types. Benign and malignant tumours are difficult to distinguish histologically, as the malignant forms may show little anaplasia whereas the benign form is not always encapsulated. The only absolute indicators of malignancy are invasion of the normal pancreatic substance and the presence of metastases.

The histological type of the tumour is not an absolute indicator of which hormone (if any) it produces, although some hormones have an association with certain histological types.

Hormone production by tumours can be demonstrated by immunohistochemistry (i.e. antibodies specific to each individual hormone are incorporated into special stains). A battery of stains can be used, each member of which shows up a different hormone-producing cell. This technique shows that many tumours stain for more than one hormone, although the predominant staining is for the dominant hormone being produced. The technique is therefore useful for diagnosis.

Insulinomas

Seventy-five per cent of pancreatic endocrine tumours are insulinomas. They cause episodes of hypoglycaemia as the cells have a complete or partial loss of control of secretion.

They usually occur in middle-aged patients and have only very rarely been described outside the pancreas. The presence of Whipple's triad of (1) symptoms produced by fasting, (2) hypoglycaemia during an attack and (3) correction of symptoms by ingestion of glucose, strongly suggests the presence of an insulinoma. The hypoglycaemia often causes cerebral symptoms. Modern immunoassays of insulin are helpful in the diagnosis (Le Quesne *et al.* 1979).

Insulinomas are usually solitary, except when associated with the multiple endocrine adenomatosis (MEA) type 1 syndrome (*see Fig.* 8.9 and p. 475). The tumours are usually small (less than 1·5 cm in diameter), red-brown in colour and may be completely embedded in the gland. About 90% are benign and the majority show histological pattern type **B**.

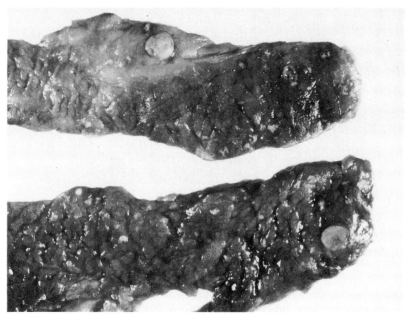

Fig. 8.9. Multiple insulinomas of pancreas in a case of multiple endocrine adenomatosis type 1 (same patient as *Fig.* 20.24).

If an insulinoma is malignant, objective tumour regression has been shown by the use of streptozotocin. This agent selectively destroys the pancreatic β cells by inhibition of DNA synthesis. Persistent hypoglycaemia due to either a benign or malignant insulinoma can be controlled by diazoxide therapy. This drug accumulates in the β cells and inhibits the release of insulin.

Gastrinomas

Gastrin is not produced in the normal pancreas and these tumours are therefore examples of inappropriate hormone secretion. They account for 20–25% of endocrine tumours of the pancreas and give rise clinically to the Zollinger–Ellison (Z–E) syndrome. Apart from the type of hormone production, they differ from insulinomas in several important respects: (1) they are more often multiple (60%); (2) they are more often malignant (60–90%); (3) they are frequently found outside the pancreas in the duodenal and gastric walls. Like insulinomas, they can be associated with the MEA type 1 syndrome (*see* p. 475).

Histologically, they are most commonly of type B and less commonly of type A pattern.

The Z–E syndrome is slightly more common in men than in women. Most cases occur in the age group 30–50 years. Ulcer pain, usually resistant to medical therapy, is the most frequent symptom. The ulcers, which frequently bleed, often occur in atypical sites such as the jejunum or second part of the duodenum. Diarrhoea occurs in about 30% of cases, partly due to the low pH in the duodenum and jejunum which inactivates pancreatic lipase. Increased intestinal motility also occurs.

The diagnosis of the Z–E syndrome is suggested by intractable ulcer symptoms, early ulcer recurrence after operation, large gastric folds on endoscopy and multiple or atypical ulcers. Many cases do, however, present in a similar fashion to 'normal' duodenal ulceration. Acid studies show high basal secretion and as the parietal cells are already under maximal stimulation, there is little increase with pentagastrin. The key to the diagnosis is the radioimmunoassay of serum gastrin and levels of 1000 pg/ml are not uncommon.

The differential diagnosis of an elevated serum gastrin includes retained gastric antrum after previous gastrectomy, antral G-cell hyperplasia and gastric outlet obstruction. Also, patients with acid hyposecretion, such as occurs in pernicious anaemia, atrophic gastritis and gastric carcinoma, all may have an elevated serum gastrin.

Glucagonomas

These are much less common than insulinomas or gastrinomas, accounting for only 1% of pancreatic endocrine tumours. They cause a characteristic clinical syndrome, the main features of which are a skin rash, diabetes mellitus and anaemia. The skin rash is a migrating necrotizing erythema.

Glucagonomas occur in middle-aged patients and about 60% are malignant. They are usually single and virtually all occur in the pancreas. Histologically, most are of type B pattern.

Somatostatinomas

These are exceedingly rare with only a few examples having been described. The patients present with diabetes, steatorrhoea and hypochlorhydria. Most are solitary and malignant, and nearly all occur in the pancreas.

Pancreatic polypeptidomas (PP-omas)

PP is frequently identified by immunohistochemistry in many types of endocrine tumours. Pure PP-omas have, however, been described. They do not appear to cause symptoms referable to hormone production. Most are benign and are located in the pancreas.

Vipomas

Less than 5% of pancreatic endocrine tumours secrete vasoactive intestinal polypeptide. The Verner–Morrison syndrome or WDHA·(watery diarrhoea, hypokalaemia, achlorhydria) syndrome are the names given to the clinical symptoms.

Vipomas tend to be larger than the other pancreatic endocrine tumours and occur both in the pancreas and in the gut. The syndrome may also be caused by ganglioneuromas, ganglioneuroblastomas and oat cell carcinomas of the lung.

Fifty to seventy-five per cent of vipomas are malignant. They are usually solitary. Histologically, they show a type A or type B pattern.

Ectopic hormone production

Gastrin is an ectopic hormone in the pancreas. Other pancreatic endocrine tumours have been described which secrete ACTH, parathormone or calcitonin.

References

Acosta J. M., Ledesma C. L. (1974) Gallstone migration as a cause of acute pancreatitis. *N. Engl. J. Med.* **290**, 484–7.

Benarde M. A., Weiss W. (1982) Coffee consumption and pancreatic cancer: temporal and spatial correlation. *Br. Med. J.* **284**, 400–2.

Blamey S. L., Imrie C. W., O'Neill J., Gilmour W. H., Carter D. C. (1984) Prognostic factors in acute pancreatitis. *Gut* **25**, 1340–6.

Bradley E. L., Clements J. L., Gonzalez A. C. (1979) The natural history of pancreatic pseudocysts: a unified concept of management. *Am. J. Surg.* **137**, 135–41.

Colhoun E., Murphy J. J., MacErlean D. P. (1984) Percutaneous drainage of pancreatic pseudocysts. *Br. J. Surg.* **71**, 131–2.

Cubilla A. L., Fitzgerald P. J. (1979) Classification of pancreatic cancer (nonendocrine). *Mayo Clin. Proc.* **54**, 449–58.

De Caro A., Lohse J., Sarles H. (1979) Characterization of a protein isolated from pancreatic calculi of men suffering from chronic calcifying pancreatitis. *Biochem. Biophys. Res. Com.* **87**, 1176–82.

Foulis A. K. (1984) Acute pancreatitis. In: Anthony P. P., MacSween R. N. M. (eds.) *Recent Advances in Histopathology 12*, pp. 188–96. Edinburgh, Churchill Livingstone.

Imrie C. W. (1981) The treatment of acute pancreatitis. In: Jewell D. P., Lee E. (eds.) *Topics in Gastroenterology 9*, pp. 245–62. Oxford, Blackwell Scientific Publications.

Imrie C. W., Benjamin I. S., Ferguson J. C. *et al.* (1978) A single-centre double-blind trial of Trasylol therapy in primary acute pancreatitis. *Br. J. Surg.* **65**, 337–41.

Kelly T. R. (1976) Gallstone pancreatitis: pathophysiology. *Surgery* **80**, 488–92.

Kline T. S., Neal H. S. (1978) Needle aspiration biopsy: a critical appraisal. Eight years and 3267 specimens later. *J.A.M.A.* **239**, 36–9.

Kloppel G. (1984) Pancreatic nonendocrine tumours. In: Kloppel G., Heitz P. (eds.) *Pancreatic Pathology*, pp. 79–113. Edinburgh, Churchill Livingstone.

Lankisch P. G., Creutzfelot W. (1981) Akute und akut rezidivierende pankreatitis. In: Allgower M., Harder F., Hollender L. F., Peiper H. J., Siewert J. R. (eds.) *Chirurgiscae Gastroenterologie 2.* Berlin, Springer-Verlag.

Le Quesne L. P., Nabarro J. D. N., Kurtz A., Zweig S. (1979) The management of insulin tumours of the pancreas. *Br. J. Surg.* **66**, 373–8.

Lightwood R., Reber H. A., Way L. W. (1976) The risk and accuracy of pancreatic biopsy. *Am. J. Surg.* **132**, 189–94.

McMahon M. J., Playforth M. J., Pickford I. R. (1980) A comparative study of methods for the prediction of severity of attacks of acute pancreatitis. *Br. J. Surg.* **67**, 22–5.

Opie E. L. (1901) The etiology of acute haemorrhagic pancreatitis. *Johns Hopkins Hospital Bulletin* **12**, 182–8.

Ranson J. H. C., Pasternack B. S. (1977) Statistical methods for quantifying the severity of clinical acute pancreatitis. *J. Surg. Res.* **22**, 79–91.

Reuben A., Cotton P. B. (1978) Operative pancreatic biopsy: a survey of current practice. *Ann. R. Coll. Surg. Engl.* **60**, 53–7.

Sahel J., Sarles H. (1979) Modifications of pure human pancreatic juice induced by chronic alcoholic consumption. *Dig. Dis. Sci.* **24**, 897–905.

Sarles H. (1965) Pancreatitis. Symposium Marseille 1963. Basel, S. Karger.

Sarner M., Cotton P. B. (1984) Classification of pancreatitis. *Gut* **25**, 756–9.

Shearman D. J. C., Finlayson N. D. C. (eds.) (1982) *Diseases of the Gastrointestinal Tract and Liver.* Edinburgh, Churchill Livingstone.

Shi E. C. P., Yeo B. W., Ham J. M. (1984) Pancreatic abscesses. *Br. J. Surg.* **71**, 689–91.

Stark D. (1965) *Embryologie. Ein Lehrbuch auf allgemein biologischar Grundlage*, 2nd ed. Stuttgart, Georg Thieme.

Chapter 9

The Kidney, Ureter and Bladder

Normal Development, Structure and Function

Kidney

The development of the kidney is complex. A condensation of mesoderm known as the intermediate cell mass gives rise to the pronephros, mesonephros and metanephros from its lateral side, and the adrenal and gonads from its medial side.

The pronephros disappears but its duct persists to join with the mesonephric tubules, thus forming the mesonephric duct (Wolffian duct). The mesonephros disappears, but the mesonephric duct forms the epididymis, vas and ejaculatory duct in the male; in the female it becomes vestigial. Caudal to the mesonephros, the intermediate cell mass produces many excretory tubules (the metanephros) which induce a bud to grow from the caudal end of the mesonephric duct. This bud forms the ureter, the calyces of the renal pelvis and the collecting tubules of the pyramids; it joins with the distal convoluted tubules of the metanephros. This definitive kidney forms in the pelvis, and is supplied by the median sacral artery. It migrates superiorly with a successive series of new arteries from the iliac vessels and aorta. Failure to ascend may occur resulting in a pelvic kidney.

The normal adult kidney measures $12 \times 6 \times 3$ cm and weighs about 120 g. Posteriorly the kidneys are related to the diaphragm, quadratus lumborum and psoas muscles and the posterior recess of the pleura which may be opened during exposure of the kidney. Anterior is the second part of the duodenum on the right and tail of pancreas on the left. The hepatic and splenic flexures of the colon are also anterior relations and may be involved by a renal cell carcinoma. The kidneys are surrounded by perinephric fat which is within a perinephric fascia; this tends to restrain a perinephric abscess. The fascia is attached to the hilum of the kidney at the renal vessels and this prevents spread of pus across the midline.

The renal artery divides into three branches at the hilum, usually two in front and one behind the renal pelvis. The posterior branch usually passes to the upper pole. The presence of a posterior branch to the lower pole is associated with hydronephrosis. The veins of the kidney tend to form venous arcades along the bases of the medullary pyramids and about five main veins unite beyond the hilum to form the renal vein. The lymphatics drain to para-aortic nodes at L2. Accessory renal arteries from the aorta are common, representing normal fetal arteries and are associated with a lobulated kidney. The kidney receives both a sympathetic and parasympathetic nerve supply, the former having a vasomotor function.

The renal cortex is red in colour and extends towards the pelvis between the darker striated pyramids of the medulla. Several pyramids open into a renal papilla, each of which projects into a minor calyx. The cortex contains the glomeruli and convoluted tubules while the medulla contains the loops of Henle and collecting tubules.

Histologically the kidney is composed of nephrons. Each nephron consists of a glomerulus, a proximal convoluted tubule, a loop of Henle, a distal convoluted tubule and a collecting duct. The glomerulus is a network of capillaries invaginated into Bowman's capsule. It is supplied by an afferent and drained by an efferent arteriole. The loop of Henle has a thick limb which descends from the cortex into the medulla and a thin ascending limb which joins the distal convoluted tubule. The distal convoluted tubule comes in contact with the afferent arteriole of the same glomerulus, and at this point its wall forms part of the juxtaglomerular apparatus.

A proportion of the cardiac output is filtered by the glomerulus into Bowman's space and hence into the proximal convoluted tubule where about 80% of the filtrate is reabsorbed. Glucose, sodium chloride and sodium bicarbonate are actively reabsorbed, followed by passive reabsorption of water. The U-shaped loop of Henle is responsible for a 'countercurrent multiplier system' which generates a high osmotic pressure in the extracellular fluid. This allows the urine to be concentrated. In the distal convoluted tubule, water is reabsorbed, depending on the level of circulating antidiuretic hormone. The juxtaglomerular apparatus secretes renin in response to a fall in afferent arteriolar pressure. This initiates the renin-angiotensin system (*see* p. 478).

Ureter

The ureter is 25 cm long. It lies medial to the tips of the transverse processes of the lumbar vertebrae, crosses the bifurcation of the common iliac artery and the sacroiliac joint, passes to the ischial spine and then runs anteromedially above the levators to the base of the bladder. The narrowest points where stones will lodge are at the pelvi-ureteric junction, where it crosses the pelvic brim, and at its termination in the bladder. In the male the ureter is crossed by the vas in the pelvis; in the female it is crossed by the uterine artery and is related to the cervix where it is in danger during hysterectomy.

The ureters are supplied by vessels from the renal arteries, gonadal arteries, common iliac arteries and uterine or vesical vessels and there are good anastomoses between these vessels. Veins drain to renal, gonadal and internal iliac veins. Lymphatics run with the arteries; the abdominal ureter drains to the para-aortic nodes and the pelvic ureter drains to the nodes along the internal iliac vessels.

The ureteric muscle lies in three layers, inner and outer circular and intermediate longitudinal. These layers are in fact gradual spirals of smooth muscle. The mucous membrane consists of lax areolar tissue lined by transitional epithelium (the urothelium).

Bladder

The bladder develops from the urogenital sinus which in turn originates from the embryonic cloaca. The urogenital sinus continues cranially into the urachus which may remain patent after birth. The upper urogenital sinus forms the bladder and incorporates the terminal portions of the mesonephric ducts and the embryonic budding ureters. The mucous membrane between the prostatic ejaculatory ducts and the ureteric orifices (i.e. the trigone in adult life) is therefore derived from the mesonephric ducts.

The bladder wall contains the detrusor smooth muscle which runs in spirals to give a trabeculated appearance. It has a loose mucous membrane lined by transitional epithelium. The trigone which lies between the internal urethral orifice and ureteric orifices is fixed and relatively indistensible. In contrast the fundus is mobile and distensible. The ureters pierce the wall of the bladder obliquely and this tends to prevent vesico-ureteric reflux. The bladder has a good blood supply from the superior and inferior vesical arteries. The veins drain to a vesical plexus at the bladder base and eventually to the internal iliac veins. Lymph drainage follows the arteries, usually to the side walls of the pelvis.

The function of the bladder is to store urine. The sympathetic nerve supply is inhibitory to the bladder wall and motor to the sphincter, and thus it facilitates storage. The parasympathetic system is motor to the wall and inhibitory to the sphincter and therefore it mediates emptying.

Biopsy of Kidney and Bladder

Percutaneous needle biopsy of the kidney provides about 15–30 glomeruli and therefore is of little value in conditions with patchy changes. It is of value in severe proteinuria, in the nephrotic syndrome, in recurrent haematuria when other investigations are negative, and in acute renal failure with no obvious cause after exclusion of obstructive and major vascular lesions. It is occasionally required in chronic renal failure. Needle aspiration under ultrasound control is useful for renal cysts. Needle biopsy is contraindicated if the opposite kidney is absent or if the patient has a bleeding tendency; in these cases open surgical biopsy is used.

Punch biopsy forceps passed through the endoscope obtain mucosal biopsies of the bladder. If a patient has a bladder tumour, multiple biopsies should be taken from other areas of the bladder to determine if dysplasia or carcinoma-in-situ are present. Biopsy of a bladder tumour is best done with the resectoscope so that underlying muscle may be obtained in order to aid staging.

Congenital Anomalies

Kidney

Abnormalities of size and number

BILATERAL RENAL AGENESIS (POTTER'S SYNDROME): This is rare and most cases are stillborn. It is associated with oligohydramnios and other congenital defects. The cause may be failure of development of the ureteric bud and hence the metanephrogenic cap is not stimulated to develop.

UNILATERAL RENAL AGENESIS: This occurs in approximately one in 1000 live births. It is more frequent in males and usually affects the left kidney. Other congenital malformations are common, especially congenital heart disease. The cause is probably failure of the ureteric bud to develop. If no other defects are present the condition is compatible with adult life. Care must be taken during nephrectomy for trauma to ensure that there is a functioning contralateral kidney. Occasionally the entire mesonephric duct fails to develop so that the kidney, ureter, half of the trigone, testis and vas may be absent.

RENAL HYPOPLASIA: This is a significant reduction of renal mass without evidence of parenchymal malformation. It occurs when the metanephrogenic cap fails to develop properly, either due to an intrinsic defect in the mesoderm or to a ureteric bud abnormality. The affected kidney is susceptible to infection and hypertension is a complication. Other congenital and cardiovascular abnormalities may be present. In bilateral hypoplasia the child presents with failure to thrive, polyuria and renal rickets.

If one kidney is hypoplastic the other becomes large due to both hypertrophy and hyperplasia. If, however, a kidney is removed after birth the remaining kidney can only hypertrophy.

FREE SUPERNUMERARY KIDNEY: While duplex kidneys are common, a free third kidney is very rare. Six separate kidneys in one patient have been reported.

Abnormalities of structure
The most important abnormality of structure is cyst formation which is discussed on p. 241.

Abnormalities of form
CONTRALATERAL FUSION: The kidneys are joined usually at the lower poles to form a horseshoe kidney. The 'joined' area or isthmus is either fibrous or composed of renal tissue. The ureters cross the isthmus anteriorly and may be partially obstructed. In addition, the kidneys fail to rotate so that the pelvi-ureteric junctions lie anteriorly. The incidence of horseshoe kidney is about one in 500 live births and it affects males more often than females. One-third of the cases are symptom-free. The remaining two-thirds have abdominal pain or fainting due to pressure on the inferior vena cava. The kidney is more prone to trauma, infection, stone formation and hydronephrosis. Tumours may be more common than in normal kidneys (Castro and Green 1975).

IPSILATERAL FUSION: In this case both kidneys lie on the same side of the vertebrae, the upper pole of one being fused to the lower pole of the other.

Abnormalities of location
An ectopic kidney fails to ascend and remains medially in the iliac fossa or pelvis. It may present as a puzzling pelvic mass clinically or at laparotomy. The cause is failure of the ureteric bud to lengthen. Blood supply is from adjacent vessels.

Ureter

Duplication of the ureter, ectopic ureter and ureterocoele
The ureteric bud which grows from the mesonephric duct (Wolffian duct) towards the metanephros (definitive kidney) may divide at some point along its path (sim-

ple partial duplication) or two ureteric buds may grow from the mesonephric duct (simple complete duplication). In some cases the duplication is not simple, but is complicated by an ectopic ureter or an ectopic ureterocoele. Ectopic ureters and ureterocoeles may also be seen in isolation without other abnormalities.

SIMPLE PARTIAL DUPLICATION (*see Fig.* 9.1*a*): The ureter can become double at any point along its length and usually this is an incidental finding and gives rise to no symptoms. Occasionally there is movement of urine from one stem of the ureter to the other. This 'see-saw' uretero-ureteral reflux predisposes to stasis and infection. The two hemi-kidneys are usually fused. At the point of fusion, there may be a bulge seen on the intravenous urogram (IVU) (so-called 'pseudotumour').

SIMPLE COMPLETE DUPLICATION (*see Fig.* 9.1*b*): In this case the entire ureter is duplicated. Both ureteric buds grow from that part of the mesonephric duct which becomes incorporated into the bladder. Since this part of the mesonephric duct

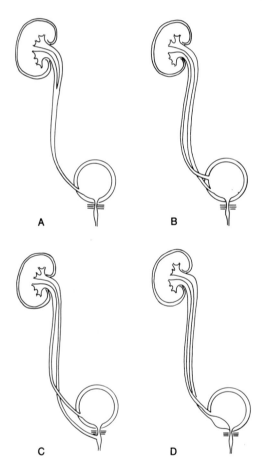

Fig. 9.1. *a.* Partial duplication of ureter. *b.* Complete duplication of ureter. *c.* Complete duplication of ureter with ectopic ureter. *d.* Complete duplication of ureter with ectopic ureterocoele.

loops sharply downwards (i.e. caudal) prior to being incorporated into the bladder, the positions of the ureteric buds become inverted relative to each other. Therefore, the ureter draining the upper pole of the kidney always enters the bladder below and medial to the lower pole ureter. Complete duplication often gives no symptoms. The lower pole ureter does tend to have a direct course through the bladder wall and this predisposes to vesico-ureteric reflux.

DUPLICATION WITH ECTOPIC URETER (*see Fig.* 9.1*c*): The ureteric bud to the upper pole of the kidney may arise some distance away from the other ureteric bud. This gives rise to an upper pole ureter which opens considerably lower than the normally situated lower pole ureter. It is therefore ectopic. This ectopic ureter may show reflux on voiding or it may be obstructed and, in either case, it becomes infected and dilated. There is massive dilatation of the upper pole renal pelvis which is seen on a ureterogram as a 'drooping flower' appearance.

Common points of entry for the ectopic ureter are the lower trigone and bladder neck. In boys, the ectopic ureter may enter the urethra as far down as the ejaculatory ducts which mark the ends of the mesonephric ducts. Since the ejaculatory ducts are above the external sphincter, boys do not develop continuous dribbling incontinence. Alternatively, the ectopic ureter may enter the ejaculatory ducts themselves, the vas or the seminal vesicles. This can give rise to a multiloculated mass in the region of the seminal vesicles (felt per rectum) and can present as epididymitis which is otherwise rare in prepubertal boys.

In girls, the ectopic ureter can enter the urethra distal to the sphincter and this does cause continuous dribbling incontinence. Alternatively, the ureter may enter the vagina.

DUPLICATION WITH ECTOPIC URETEROCOELE (*see Fig.* 9.1*d*): The end of an ectopic ureter may end in a ballooned segment which lies within the bladder wall. The ureteric opening may be narrowed, thus giving rise to stasis and infection or it may be subject to vesico-ureteric reflux. The condition is seen on a cystogram as a filling defect.

Duplication of the ureter, ectopic ureters and ureterocoeles may be unilateral or bilateral and can occur in any combination. Ectopic ureters and ureterocoeles can occur in the absence of duplications. Symptoms often start in childhood with frequent urinary tract infections. Incontinence may be spurious (due to infection) or true (due to an ectopic ureter opening below the urethral sphincter).

These conditions require contrast radiology to delineate the exact anatomy. Treatment includes reimplantation of a ureter (in cases of vesico-ureteric reflux) and upper pole nephroureterectomy (when the upper pole is damaged to the extent that there is no function).

Postcaval ureter

The right ureter passes behind the inferior vena cava where it is partially obstructed between spine and cava; surgery may be required.

Congenital ureteral valves

These are folds of redundant mucosa; they occasionally persist and cause obstruction.

Diverticula of the ureter

These are rare. They represent accessory ureteral buds and are found near the bladder. Occasionally they obstruct the ureter or cause reflux.

Congenital megaureter

This is congenital dilatation of the ureter without obvious obstruction and without reflux. The cause is probably a lower segment which does not transmit peristalsis. The condition is discussed on p. 240

Bladder

Congenital diverticula
These are discussed on p. 241.

Ectopia vesicae

This is a congenital abnormality in which there is a defect in the anterior abdominal wall and bladder wall. The symphysis is also frequently absent. The bladder mucosa is exposed, resulting in a chronic inflammation. The mucosa may be replaced by granulation tissue and adenocarcinoma may develop if the patient survives into adult life.

Persistent urachus

Total persistence of the urachus produces a vesico-umbilical fistula. Middle segment persistence gives an urachal cyst while persistence of the cloacal segment gives rise to a vesicle diverticulum.

Acute Renal Failure

Acute renal failure may be due to pre-renal causes (e.g. severe hypotension), post-renal causes (obstruction from stones, pelvic carcinoma, enlarged prostate, etc.) or renal disease. The renal diseases include acute glomerulonephritis, acute pyelonephritis, papillary necrosis, malignant hypertension, diffuse intravascular coagulation, eclampsia, arteritis, acute tubular necrosis, etc. In addition, if pre-renal or post-renal causes are prolonged, they will lead to renal damage as a secondary phenomenon. Thus prolonged hypotension will cause acute tubular necrosis. Of the many causes of acute renal failure, only acute tubular necrosis will be discussed here.

Acute tubular necrosis

Aetiology

The two main forms of acute tubular necrosis are: (1) ischaemic and (2) nephrotoxic. Ischaemic tubular necrosis occurs after an episode of hypotension which may be associated with trauma, surgery, bacterial infection, burns, severe vomiting and diarrhoea, myocardial infarction, etc. Nephrotoxic acute tubular necrosis is due to a variety of substances including heavy metals (mercury and *cis*-platinum), solvents (carbon tetrachloride), drugs (aminoglycosides, cephalosporins, cotrimoxazole, paracetamol) and poisons (Paraquat).

Pathogenesis

Exactly why necrosis of tubular cells causes acute renal failure is not clear. There are several possibilities: (1) tubular obstruction due either to casts or to compression by interstitial oedema; (2) leakage of filtrate through the tubules; (3) suppression of glomerular filtration due to a reduction in blood flow. The reduction in blood flow could be mediated by (i) direct vascular damage or (ii) stimulation of the renin–angiotensin system to produce the vasoconstrictor angiotensin II or (iii) inhibition of the synthesis of prostaglandins, most of which act as renal vasodilators.

There is some evidence that in nephrotoxic acute tubular necrosis, each of these three main factors contributes a different amount depending on the toxin. In ischaemic injury the main problem appears to be obstruction of the tubules and leakage of the filtrate through the damaged tubules.

Clinical features

Acute tubular necrosis is classically characterized by a series of phases. After the initiating event the patient enters an oliguric phase during which time the urine output is less than 400 ml per day; the blood urea level rises. After one to two weeks the patient enters the diuretic phase. In the early diuretic phase there is polyuria and loss of electrolytes, including sodium and potassium. In the late diuretic phase urinary output gradually returns to normal as the concentrating ability of the kidneys returns. Some cases of acute tubular necrosis, however, do not have an oliguric phase. The presence of a good urinary output in these cases may mask the clinical diagnosis even in the presence of severe functional impairment.

Morphology

Grossly, the kidneys may be pale and swollen. Histologically, in the early stages of ischaemic acute tubular necrosis, there is a patchy necrosis of the epithelial lining of the proximal convoluted tubules. The cell nuclei become pyknotic and eventually disappear leaving only cell outlines. Rupture of the basement membrane of the tubule (tubulorrhexis) is characteristic of ischaemic acute tubular necrosis. Eosinophilic casts are seen in the distal tubules and collecting ducts and these add to tubular obstruction. In patients who have received severe crushing injuries to the limbs with muscle damage, the acute renal failure may be aggravated by the presence of myoglobin casts in the renal tubules. When recovery occurs the epithelial cells regenerate. This is seen histologically as epithelium consisting of flattened cells with hyperchromatic nuclei and some mitotic figures; binucleate cells are seen. The patchy nature of ischaemic acute tubular necrosis was shown by Oliver *et al.* (1951) in microdissection experiments in which it was shown that the necrosis affected only short segments of the proximal convoluted tubules, leaving the intervening parts relatively normal.

In nephrotoxic acute tubular necrosis the findings are similar, although tubulorrhexis is rare and microdissection experiments show that the whole of the proximal convoluted tubule tends to be involved in continuity.

Due to the patchy nature of the findings in ischaemic acute tubular necrosis, very little may be seen on a needle biopsy. The diagnosis may rely in these cases on subtle abnormalities such as loss of the brush border of the epithelial cells of the proximal convoluted tubules and on electron microscopic findings.

Prognosis

Since renal tubules have the ability to regenerate the prognosis is good if treatment is adequate. The treatment is aimed at maintaining electrolyte balance until recovery occurs. During the oliguric phase, the tubules are obstructed and the filtrate leaks back into the circulation. Fluid replacement is limited to insensible losses plus the urine output. Hyperkalaemia may require a glucose/insulin infusion or oral calcium resonium and severe electrolyte derangement will require dialysis. During the early diuretic phase, tubular obstruction and leaking cease but the tubules have a poor concentrating ability. This may result in electrolyte loss and it is therefore necessary to measure the exact urine output and urinary electrolyte concentration daily and give adequate replacement.

Urinary Tract Infection

After the first year of life up to middle age, urinary tract infections are much more common in females than males (male to female ratio is about 1 : 8). In the neonatal period boys are more commonly affected than girls. This may partly be due to the higher incidence of congenital urogenital abnormalities in boys. However, in some cases the systemic evidence of infection occurs several days before the onset of bacteriuria and in these cases it is postulated that organisms enter the blood stream at birth and spread to the kidneys via the haematogenous route. This may result in overt infection more commonly in boys than girls on account of the more mature immunological competence of the latter. The sex distribution becomes more even again in old age due to the common finding of obstruction of the bladder neck by benign nodular hyperplasia of the prostate in men.

Aetiology

E. coli accounts for about three-quarters of non-hospital and up to one-half of hospital urinary tract infections. Less common pathogens are Proteus, *Staphylococcus saprophyticus*, Klebsiella, Streptococcus and Candida. Proteus is a common pathogen in all ages. *Staphylococcus saprophyticus* occurs predominantly in young women. These organisms invariably infect the urinary tract by the ascending route.

Some organisms also infect the urinary tract by the haematogenous route. These include certain bacteria (Mycobacterium and Salmonella), fungi (e.g. *Histoplasma duboisii*), certain viruses (cytomegalovirus and adenovirus) and parasites (*Schistosoma haematobium*).

Pathogenesis (host factors)

It is generally agreed that the vast majority of organisms reach the urinary tract by the ascending route. The initiation of infection depends on a balance between the defence mechanisms of the host and the virulence of the organism. The important host factors are as follows.

1. ANATOMICAL: The higher incidence of urinary tract infection in females when compared with males may be due to the shorter urethra in the former and to prostatic secretions in the latter.

2. MECHANICAL WASHOUT: Bladder urine is normally sterile and is protected from contamination by micturition which has a 'washing out' effect. Interference with this 'washing' will predispose to urinary tract infection. Catheterization and instrumentation may overwhelm the washout mechanism and the washout system becomes inadequate if there is residual urine after voiding. Residual urine occurs in patients with obstructive conditions such as prostatic hypertrophy and urethral strictures, and also in patients with vesico-ureteric reflux (*see* below), bladder diverticula and neurological impairment of bladder function.

3. VESICO-URETERIC REFLUX: Normally the distal part of the ureter runs obliquely in the bladder wall prior to opening into the bladder lumen. When bladder pressure rises the intramural part of the ureter is compressed. This system therefore acts as a valve and vesico-ureteric reflux is prevented. In children with primary vesico-ureteric reflux, the intramural position of the ureter is short and this gives rise to an incompetent vesico-ureteric valve. Vesico-ureteric reflux is known to occur in up to half of children with recurrent urinary tract infection. It is an important cause of chronic pyelonephritis and therefore of hypertensive renal failure in children and young adults.

Secondary vesico-ureteric reflux may occur in adults as well as children and is due to other factors such as obstruction to the bladder outflow, neuropathic bladder and bladder diverticulum.

Vesico-ureteric reflux predisposes to urinary tract infection because, after each micturition, the urine which has entered the ureters returns to the bladder forming a residuum. The washout mechanism is therefore disturbed and proliferating organisms can easily ascend during the time of reflux. Of considerable importance is the fact that high intravesical pressures occurring at the time of voiding are transmitted to the renal calyces thus predisposing to intrarenal reflux (*see* below).

Vesico-ureteric reflux has been graded radiologically (Blowers *et al.* 1979) as follows: Grade I (mild)—contrast flows into the ureter but does not reach the kidney; Grade II (moderate)—contrast flows into the ureter and reaches the kidney without distension of calyces or ureter; Grade III (severe)—contrast distends the calyces, ureter or renal pelvis. The relationship between the degree of reflux and renal damage is, however, imperfect (*see* below).

The natural history of vesico-ureteric reflux is for it to gradually improve through childhood. It will completely disappear in 77% of all cases and in 90% of mild cases (Edwards *et al.* 1977).

4. INTRARENAL REFLUX: In cases of vesico-ureteric reflux the high intravesical pressure is transmitted to the renal pelvis where it reverses the normal pressure

gradient between the renal tubules and the pelvi-calyceal system. There is therefore a tendency to force urine backwards through the renal papillae into the collecting system.

Whether or not this intrarenal reflux actually occurs depends on the anatomy of the renal papillae. Ransley and Risdon (1975) have identified two types of renal papillae in young children (*see Fig.* 9.2).

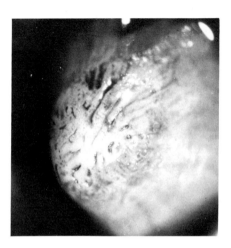

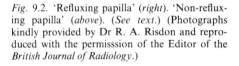

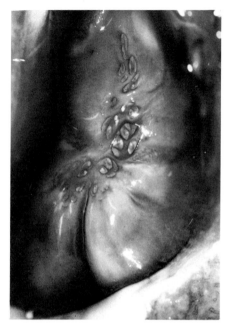

Fig. 9.2. 'Refluxing papilla' (*right*). 'Non-refluxing papilla' (*above*). (*See text.*) (Photographs kindly provided by Dr R. A. Risdon and reproduced with the permisssion of the Editor of the *British Journal of Radiology*.)

1. The non-refluxing papilla which is conical in shape; its papillary ducts are slit-like and pass obliquely through the convex tip of the papilla in such a way that they close when pressure rises in the renal pelvis.
2. The refluxing papilla has a concave surface and the papillary ducts open directly onto the surface so that they do not close and cannot prevent reflux when pressure rises in the renal pelvis.

The refluxing papillae are more commonly situated in the upper and lower poles of the kidneys and this is where scarring occurs most frequently in the non-obstructive variety of pyelonephritis. It seems likely that those children who have vesico-ureteric reflux and urinary tract infection without renal scarring are protected by having non-refluxing papillae. This may explain the imperfect relationship between the degree of reflux on the one hand and the amount of renal damage on the other.

There is controversy as to whether or not intrarenal reflux of noninfected urine will cause renal scarring *per se*. Some authorities suggest that it does whereas others claim that infection must also be present.

5. IMMUNOLOGICAL FACTORS: IgG and IgA are both present in the urine. IgA is secreted in the urethra and may prevent the establishment of infection. IgA is also produced in the lamina propria of the bladder near the surface of the mucosa and may prevent penetration of the mucous membrane by bacteria.

Pathogenesis (bacterial factors)

The majority of cases of urinary tract infection are caused by bacteria which are present in the patients' own faecal flora. In females with recurrent urinary tract infection there appears to be colonization of the vagina and distal urethra by these organisms prior to the onset of infection. Bacteria adhere to the urothelium by means of pili which interact with epithelial cell membrane receptors. The adhesiveness of a particular strain is one determinant of its virulence which has recently been recognized.

Clinical features

Urinary tract infection may present as cystitis, acute pyelonephritis or chronic pyelonephritis. Cystitis causes frequency of micturition, dysuria and lower abdominal pain. In acute pyelonephritis, loin pain occurs in addition to the symptoms of cystitis. Acute pyelonephritis may be complicated by pyonephrosis or perinephric abscess. Chronic pyelonephritis may have an insidious onset or may present as recurrent attacks of acute pyelonephritis. It eventually gives rise to the clinical features of chronic renal failure.

Morphology

CYSTITIS: The bladder mucosa initially becomes hyperaemic and later haemorrhage occurs and the mucosa beccmes friable. Pus may be visible on the mucosal surface. If the entire bladder lining is haemorrhagic, the condition is termed haemorrhagic cystitis. If actual necrosis of the bladder wall occurs, the mucosal surface becomes blue or black in appearance and this is termed gangrenous cystitis. In cases of chronic cystitis, the patients have frequent recurrent urinary tract infections. They tend to develop aggregates of submucosal lymphocytes which can be seen as tiny yellow dots at cystoscopy (follicular cystitis).

ACUTE PYELONEPHRITIS: Grossly, the kidneys are swollen and cortical abscesses may be seen on the external surfaces. On sectioning the kidney, yellow areas of abscess formation are seen. These may radiate outwards from the renal pelvis through the medulla to the cortex. In some patients, particularly diabetics, papillary necrosis occurs, that is, the tips of the renal pyramids become infarcted. They appear white or grey and are sharply defined by a hyperaemic border. Sloughing of the papilla may give rise to renal colic and the loss of the papillae gives rise to a very characteristic finding on contrast radiology.

If the ureter is obstructed, pus cannot escape. The pelvi-calyceal system therefore becomes filled with pus and the renal substance is destroyed. The renal pelvis and kidney are transformed into a bag of pus or pyonephrosis. In some patients, the infection bursts through the renal capsule into the perirenal space to form a perinephric abscess.

Histologically (*see Fig.* 9.3), the presence of an acute inflammatory reaction is confirmed by the presence of neutrophils. These initially spread throughout the interstitial tissue and later they form abscesses as tubules are destroyed. Glomeruli tend to be resistant to the inflammatory process. Areas of papillary necrosis show preservation of the tubular outline, although the tubular cells are necrotic, and an inflammatory response is seen at the interface between the necrotic and viable tissue.

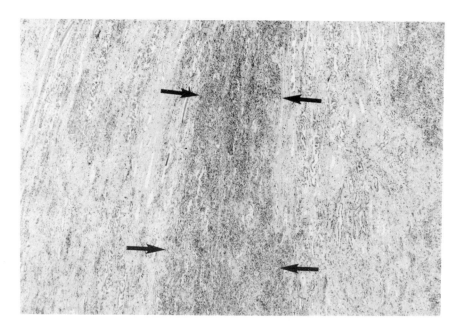

Fig. 9.3. Acute pyelonephritis. Note the inflammatory infiltrate forming a streak of inflammatory cells in the renal medulla (arrowed). (H and E × 7)

CHRONIC PYELONEPHRITIS: The classical gross feature of chronic pyelonephritis is the presence of coarse cortico-medullary scars overlying distorted calyces, i.e. both the renal substance and the pelvi-calyceal system are involved. In most other causes of scarred kidneys the calyceal system is not affected. The scars are irregular and if bilateral they are asymmetrical. Two forms of chronic pyelonephritis are recognized.

1. Chronic obstructive pyelonephritis is due to obstruction with superadded infection. Pyelonephritis may be bilateral if obstruction is in the urethra, e.g. due to benign nodular hyperplasia of the prostate, or unilateral if the obstruction is in the ureter, e.g. a stone. In these cases, scarring is irregularly placed throughout the kidney.

2. Reflux nephropathy is due to vesico-ureteric reflux. The scarring tends to be at the upper and lower poles where the refluxing papillae, which allow intrarenal reflux, are found (*see Fig.* 9.4).

Histologically, in all cases of chronic pyelonephritis there is atrophy of tubules with replacement by fibrous tissue. A residual inflammatory infiltrate, mainly of lymphocytes, is present. The glomeruli tend to be resistant to damage although periglomerular fibrosis is seen. Dilated tubules characteristically fill with eosinophilic casts and resemble thyroid tissue (thyroidization). In some cases islands of foamy macrophages are found in the inflammatory tissue, usually in cases of Proteus infection. Grossly these areas form yellow nodules which can be confused with renal cell carcinoma in radiological investigations. This variant is termed xanthogranulomatous pyelonephritis.

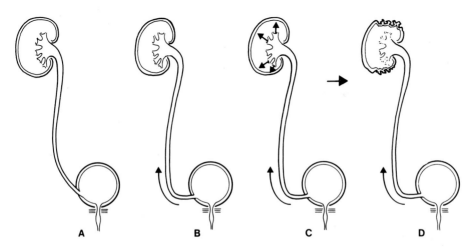

Fig. 9.4. Reflux nephropathy: *a.* normal; *b.* a straight passage of the ureter through the bladder wall allows reflux which, by itself, causes little damage; *c.* vesico-ureteric reflux plus intrarenal reflux predisposes to *d.* chronic pyelonephritis with the scarring mainly in the upper and lower poles.

Genitourinary Tuberculosis

Nearly all genitourinary tuberculosis is blood-borne, usually from a focus in the lung or, less commonly, the pharynx, intestines or bone. Tuberculosis of the urogenital tract usually appears 5–20 years after the primary lesion in the lung. Associated conditions include malnutrition, diabetes, measles and steroid administration. Most cases are due to the human variety of *Mycobacterium tuberculosis*. The blood-borne organisms lodge in the kidneys (or less commonly in the epididymis) and from here they spread to the ureters, bladder, prostate, etc. Clinically the diagnosis is suspected in patients who have a 'sterile pyuria'.

Initially, a granuloma forms in the kidney and it may heal or progress. Progression leads to destruction of renal parenchyma by caseous necrosis as the granulomata become confluent. Renal involvement may be unilateral or bilateral.

Spread may occur through the collecting system to form ulcers at the tips of the papillae. From here, spread occurs downwards so that at first the ureter and then the bladder become lined with tuberculous granulation tissue. Cystoscopy at this time shows a grossly oedematous and red bladder mucosa, sometimes resembling tumour; actual tubercles are rarely seen. In the late stages, the kidney is replaced by calcified caseous debris. Stones are found in about 10% of cases.

Healing by fibrosis (under the influence of antituberculous drugs) may lead to stricture formation. This may occur at a calyceal neck to give a dilated calyx upstream. Fibrosis at the pelvi-ureteric junction causes obstruction and hydronephrosis. Fibrosis of the ureter causes strictures and shortening. The ureteric orifice is pulled upwards, giving a 'golf-hole' appearance at cystoscopy. The bladder becomes contracted by fibrosis, thus causing severe frequency of micturition.

Histologically, the hallmark is the tuberculous granuloma, consisting of a central area of caseation surrounded by epithelioid macrophages within a mantle of lymphocytes (see Fig. 9.5). Multinucleate Langhans' giant cells may be present within the granulomas. Tubercle bacilli may be difficult to find, even with a Ziehl–Neelsen stain. In the late stages, much tissue destruction, fibrosis and calcification are seen.

Treatment is with antituberculous drugs. Since this may cause fibrosis, with consequent stricture formation, it is necessary to follow up the patients with an IVU about six weeks after the start of treatment. The finding of a progressive stricture which is causing obstruction may require surgical intervention if it does not respond to steroids. In the later stages of the disease, the surgeon may be required to remove a non-functioning kidney or to increase bladder capacity by cystoplasty.

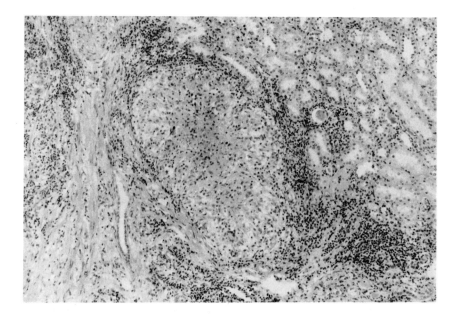

Fig. 9.5. Renal tuberculosis with granuloma showing central caseous necrosis. (H and E × 75)

Schistosomiasis

Schistosomiasis is caused by infestation with one of the species of trematode flukes. The three principal species to infest humans are *Schistosoma haematobium*, *S. mansoni* and *S. japonicum*. *S. haematobium*, which is found extensively in Africa and the Near East, has a predilection for the pelvic veins. The other two species reside in the portal vein tributaries and cause hepatic schistosomiasis. Patients with urinary schistosomiasis complain of vague general malaise, pyrexia and haematuria.

The adult worms attach themselves to the endothelium of veins by a sucker. Here, the female fluke becomes enveloped within the gynaecophoric canal of the male and starts to produce eggs. These eggs work their way through the bladder wall and urothelium into the urine. When voided, each egg hatches out and produces a miracidium which swims around in water until it enters a snail. Within the snail, the asexual part of the cycle takes place and the parasites are eventually released as cercariae. The cercariae penetrate the human skin, enter lymphatics and then the blood-stream. They are converted into young worms which are disseminated throughout the body. Within the pelvic veins, the *S. haematobium* species matures into the adult worms and the cycle repeats.

The damage within the bladder is caused by the eggs which release a soluble antigen which causes an inflammatory reaction. The eggs become surrounded by granulomas and inflammatory cells. Inflammatory (bilharzial) polyps, sand patches (due to massed deposits of eggs) and ulceration are seen at cystoscopy. Later, as fibrosis occurs, the bladder contracts and calcification occurs. The fibrosis causes ischaemia and further chronic ulcers of the mucosa. The entire bladder mucosa may become surrounded by a calcified layer of dead eggs which can be seen on X-ray. The process invades the ureteric wall, causing fibrosis with obstructive uropathy, hydronephrosis and eventually, in severe cases, renal failure. The bladder mucosa frequently undergoes metaplasia to squamous epithelium and if malignant change occurs, the tumour is a squamous carcinoma (although the exact relationship between schistosomiasis and bladder cancer is unclear—see p. 253). Other common complications include secondary infection with stone formation.

The condition may be treated by various drugs including antimony preparations. The surgeon may be involved in the treatment of ureteric strictures, stones and bladder cancer.

Unusual Inflammatory Conditions of the Bladder

Malakoplakia

This is a rare condition in which patients who usually have a long history of urinary tract infection develop yellow plaques in the bladder, ureter and renal pelvis. These may bleed and cause haematuria. Although the condition runs a benign course, in some cases there may be obstruction of the urinary tract. Malakoplakia can also affect other organs such as the gastrointestinal tract and testes.

Malakoplakia is seen at cystoscopy as yellow plaques up to 4 cm in diameter on the bladder mucosa; the surrounding mucosa is inflamed. Histologically, these plaques are very characteristic. They consist of sheets of large macrophages with granular cytoplasm, together with other interspersed inflammatory cells. The most specific feature is the presence of Michaelis–Gutmann bodies which are small, round, laminated bodies present within and between the macrophages.

Normally macrophages engulf bacteria by phagocytosis and the phagosomes coalesce with lysosomes so that the lysosomal enzymes digest and destroy the phagocytozed material. In malakoplakia there is thought to be a defect in the movement of lysosomes so that they cannot coalesce with phagosomes. The granular cytoplasm is due to the accumulation of these phagosomes and the Michaelis–Gutmann bodies are due to calcification of phagosomes.

Hunner's ulcer (ulcerative interstitial cystitis)

This specific form of cystitis presents with frequency, dysuria and lower abdominal pain. Both women and men may be affected and symptoms may be severe. At cystoscopy an ulcerated lesion, several centimetres across, is seen anywhere in the bladder mucosa, although the trigone is not commonly affected. Histologically, the features are ulceration and involvement of the entire thickness of the bladder wall by an inflammatory process in which mast cells are present. Treatment is difficult. Fulguration or excision may be required (Smith and Dehner 1972).

Proliferative and Metaplastic Conditions of the Bladder

Brunn's nests are nodular thickenings of the bladder epithelium which result in nests of transitional epithelium in the lamina propria. They are very common. If these nests develop lumina they appear as cyst-like spaces lined by transitional epithelium within the lamina propria. This is termed 'cystitis cystica'. Metaplasia of the cyst lining to mucus secreting columnar cells gives rise to 'cystitis glandularis'. The aetiology of these lesions is controversial although they may be related to long-standing inflammation. The relationship to urothelial cancer is also unknown and Pugh (1982) regards them as not being pre-malignant, but as 'an indicator of unstable mucosa'.

Squamous metaplasia may result from long-standing chronic inflammation and since squamous carcinoma may develop, close follow-up is advised. In women of reproductive age, the trigone of the bladder can become lined with vaginal-type epithelium and this may cause confusion as to the site of a biopsy.

Urinary Stones

Epidemiology

It is estimated that the annual incidence of urinary stones is 7 per 10 000 of the population and that the prevalence is 3–4% of the population. Calcium and uric acid stones are commoner in males than females. Stones formed on an infective basis are more common in females than males. Cystine stones are equally distributed between the sexes.

In countries which undergo industrialization there is a gradual decrease in the incidence of bladder stones occurring in young boys and a rise in the incidence of renal stones in adults. This change occurred in the United Kingdom during the last century and it was possibly related to the change in diet. Bladder stones are still common in poor countries, such as Thailand, where they have a peak incidence at age three years and are associated with shortage of drinking water and recurrent gastroenteritis of infancy.

In the USA and UK, chemical analysis of stones shows that 75% are composed of calcium salts, usually a mixture of calcium oxalate and calcium phosphate. Mixed phosphate stones which have formed in an infected urine count for 15%, uric acid stones for 7%, cystine and other rare stones for 3%.

Aetiology

Calcium stones

Approximately 10% of patients with calcium stones have hypercalciuria due to hypercalcaemia; 45% have 'idiopathic hypercalciuria'; 20% have hyperuricosuria; 5% have hyperoxaluria and 20% have no identifiable abnormality. Although most standard texts quote figures of this order, some authorities have, however, not identified differences in urinary calcium concentrations between stone formers and controls and they consequently put a larger proportion of patients into the 'no identifiable abnormality' category (Welshman and McGeown 1975).

Rare causes of calcium stones are: (1) renal tubular acidosis in which there is a defect in the acidification of urine which becomes alkaline and predisposes to stone formation, and (2) medullary sponge kidney which is often associated with renal tubular acidosis.

HYPERCALCAEMIA: Primary hyperparathyroidism is the most important condition in this category and is found more frequently in females than males. A high (alkaline) urinary pH predisposes to calcium stones and this also occurs in hyperparathyroidism due to the action of parathormone on tubular reabsorption of bicarbonate. Other causes of hypercalcaemia include sarcoidosis, active Paget's disease, vitamin D intoxication, Cushing's syndrome and malignant tumours.

IDIOPATHIC HYPERCALCIURIA: This refers to a condition in which there is an increased urinary calcium in the presence of a normal serum calcium. It occurs in males more commonly than females and appears to have a hereditary basis. Two forms are recognized: (1) absorptive, due to an increase in intestinal absorption of calcium, and (2) renal, due to a defect in calcium reabsorption by the renal tubules.

HYPERURICOSURIA: The causes of this are discussed below. As well as causing uric acid stones, the uricosuria produces uric acid crystals and these may act as nuclei for calcium stones.

HYPEROXALURIA: This leads to stones which are rich in calcium oxalate. The causes may be : (1) primary hyperoxaluria which is due to a hereditary disorder of oxalate metabolism in which oxalate crystals form in the renal tubules, or (2) secondary hyperoxaluria in which oxalate absorption is increased due to gastrointestinal disease (see p. 96).

Uric acid stones

These may be due to the various causes of hyperuricosuria such as gout, high dietary protein intake and uricosuric drugs. In many cases there is no increase in urinary uric acid concentration and in these patients there is an unexplained low urinary pH. At low pH uric acid becomes insoluble and stone formation may occur.

Infective stones

These are composed of magnesium ammonium phosphate and calcium carbonate. They occur in urine which is infected by urea splitting organisms (Proteus and some Staphylococci). These split urea into ammonia (NH_3) and carbon dioxide (CO_2) thus causing an alkaline urine. The NH_3 and CO_2 react with water to form NH_4^+, H_2CO_3 and hydroxyl ions (OH^-). The OH^- reacts with HCO_3^- and HPO_4^{2-} to produce water and CO_3^{2-} and PO_4^{3-}. These latter then react with magnesium, ammonium and calcium to form magnesium ammonium phosphate ($MgNH_4PO_4$) and calcium carbonate ($CaCO_3$) which crystallize to form stones. The stones formed are usually of the staghorn type. (*See Fig.* 9.6.)

Cystine stones

These occur in the autosomal recessive condition of cystinuria which is characterized by a defect of the tubular reabsorption of cystine and other amino acids. Cystine stones occur at an alkaline pH.

Pathogenesis

Supersaturation theory

This theory suggests that stones form when the urine becomes supersaturated with one of the substances described above. In a simple chemistry experiment, solids can be added to water until no more will dissolve; the solution is then saturated. Below this saturation point the solid will always stay in solution and will not crystallize out. If the supernatant is removed from a saturated solution and carefully evaporated, the concentration of the solute rises above the saturation level but it still remains in solution; the solution is then supersaturated. This is an unstable situation since if particulate matter is added, crystallization of solute will occur. In urine, supersaturation may occur and various particles such as epithelial cells and other debris may act as nuclei for crystallization. Urine is also thought to contain certain inhibitors of crystallization such as polypeptides, citrate, urea and pyrophosphate. Stone formation, therefore, will depend on the presence of a supersaturated solution of urine, particles within the urine and a low concentration of inhibitors. However, some authorities consider that these basic laws of physical chemistry cannot be directly applied to urine because of its complex nature.

Matrix theory

It is known that approximately 1–5% of the content of urinary stones is composed of a matrix of mucoproteins which may be derived from uromucoid. Hallson and Rose (1979) ultrafiltered urine in order to remove macromolecules and then evaporated it. They observed (1) that the calcium oxalate crystallization was reduced or abolished and (2) that calcium phosphate crystals formed but remained dispersed and did not clump in the usual way. These changes were reversed by adding uromucoid. Since an increase in urinary osmolality causes aggregation of protein, these authors suggested that the critical stage of stone formation is precipitation of uromucoid in the renal tubules (caused by urine of high osmolality) followed by deposition of calcium salts to form a microlith. Since this aggregate is relatively large, it lodges in the upper renal tract and therefore has the opportunity to grow and form a urinary stone.

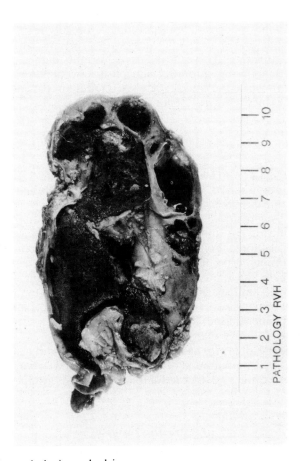

Fig. 9.6. Staghorn calculus in renal pelvis.

Morphology

Within the collecting ducts of the renal papillae, tiny concretions may be seen (Carr's concretions) and these may be the earliest stage of stone formation. An accumulation of concretions may be visible under the epithelium of the renal papillae (Randall's plaques) and these may break off to form nuclei for stones. Most urinary stones consist of a scaffolding of mucoprotein material which supports concentric rings of crystalline material.

The majority of renal stones are radio-opaque, either because they contain calcium or sulphate (e.g. cystine stones). Pure uric acid stones are radiolucent. Stones with a high calcium oxalate content may be jagged whereas uric acid stones are smooth. Cystine stones are soft. Staghorn calculi are large and take up the shape of the renal pelvis and calyceal system (*see Fig.* 9.6).

Complications of renal stones

When a renal stone enters the ureter the patient experiences ureteric colic. The stones are commonly associated with infection, especially if they are larger than 10 mm in diameter and if they are causing obstruction (hydroureter, hydro-nephrosis and hydrocalyx). This can lead to the various complications of infection such as acute pyelonephritis, chronic pyelonephritis, pyonephrosis and perinephric abscess. Ureteric obstruction causes acute renal failure in patients who have only one functioning kidney. Bilateral stones have also been reported as a cause of acute renal failure.

Prognosis

Blandy and Marshall (1976) have shown that stones less than 5 mm in diameter are likely either to pass spontaneously or to require only Dormia basket removal. Stones over 10 mm are likely to require surgery. However, increasing numbers of stones are being removed by percutaneous nephrolithotomy which may be combined with ultrasound stone disintegration (Wickham and Kellet 1981).

Detection of metabolic defects and their treatment reduces the incidence of recurrence. Screening procedures include measurement of serum and urinary calcium, phosphate and urate. Urinary oxalate measurement will detect hyper-oxaluria and urinary amino acid chromatography will detect cystinuria.

Recurrence of urinary stones is very common. In Sweden, Ljunghall (1977) fol-lowed up 17 145 patients aged 35–63. The cumulative recurrence rate rose to 77% for those followed for more than 25 years.

Blandy and Marshall (1976) have shown that patients with a stone greater than 10 mm in size at first presentation are more likely to have recurrence than those with small stones and they advise careful follow-up of this group.

Obstructive Uropathy

Obstruction of the urinary tract may be due to lesions in the prepuce (phimosis), urethra, bladder or ureters. The effect on the kidneys depends on the complications and duration of the obstruction. When obstruction occurs the glomerula filtration rate falls, although even with complete obstruction some filtration still takes place and duration of the obstruction. When obstruction occurs the glomerular filtration lar function is damaged and in partial obstruction there is an impaired ability to concentrate and acidify urine. This may lead to the paradoxical situation of the partially obstructed patient presenting with polyuria and polydipsia or with acquired renal tubular acidosis.

The ureter proximal to an obstruction becomes dilated (hydroureter) as does the renal pelvis (hydronephrosis). The stasis predisposes to infection which may go on to pyonephrosis. With persistent obstruction, there is atrophy of the renal papillae and fibrosis which is followed by progressive loss of the renal medulla and cortex. Eventually the hydronephrosis consists of a dilated renal pelvis and a thin rim of renal tissue.

When the obstruction is in the urethra or bladder neck, changes are also seen in the bladder. At first, the bladder muscle undergoes hypertrophy in an attempt to overcome the obstruction and this is seen as a coarsely trabeculated bladder at cystoscopy. Eventually the muscle is overwhelmed and the bladder becomes distended with urine as renal failure develops.

Renal effects of obstructive uropathy

Complete obstruction due, for example, to a stone, will cause irreversible damage to the kidney within three weeks and the timing of relief of obstruction must be considered in this light. The degree of urgency to relieve asymptomatic partial obstruction is unclear and depends on whether or not the damage is progressive. If infection is present, relief of obstruction is urgent.

After relief of obstruction a massive diuresis may occur and cause severe electrolyte disturbances. The diuresis is due to a combination of tubular damage (with impaired concentrating ability) and urea acting as an osmotic diuretic. There may also be a reduced renal response to anti-diuretic hormone.

Many of the conditions which obstruct the urinary tract are discussed elsewhere. Three are discussed here in more detail.

Idiopathic hydronephrosis

This is defined as a dilatation of the renal pelvis and calyces associated with a normal calibre ureter. In some cases the cause may be an abnormal renal vascular supply, especially the presence of an artery to the lower pole. The renal pelvis tends to protrude forward through the vascular window between the main renal and the polar renal arteries with consequent kinking of the ureter. This situation pertains in only a small number of cases. More recently, light and electron microscopy studies have shown an increase in collagen in the ureteric wall at the site of obstruction. This collagen replaces the smooth muscle of the ureteric wall and it is thought likely that it prevents the normal distension of the ureter, thereby causing an obstruction. Gosling and Dixon (1978) found this abnormality, not only in the area immediately below the obstruction, but also throughout the distended segment. They proposed two theories to explain this finding: (1) that idiopathic hydronephrosis is due to a primary abnormality of the ureter and renal pelvis in which the smooth muscle is replaced by excessive connective tissue, and (2) that the changes seen are secondary to the obstruction. Which of these theories is correct is unclear.

In idiopathic hydronephrosis the renal pelvis and calyces are dilated and the calyces show 'clubbing' on intravenous urogram. The kidney shows atrophy of the parenchyma which starts with cupping of the renal pyramids. The atrophy is progressive and if obstruction is not relieved the kidney eventually becomes a thin-walled sac (see Fig. 9.7).

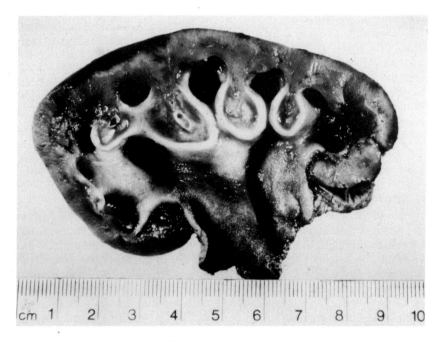

Fig. 9.7. Hydronephrosis showing dilatation of the renal pelvis and calyceal system.

Primary obstructive megaureter

This is defined as an obstruction of the entire ureter except for the terminal segment, without obvious cause and without vesico-ureteric reflux. It presents in childhood or occasionally during adult life. The same histological abnormalities of the ureter which were described by Gosling and Dixon (1978) in the case of idiopathic hydronephrosis are seen in the lower narrowed segment and in the proximal dilated segment. The condition is thought to represent the same disease process as idiopathic hydronephrosis but at a different location. The morphological changes are similar to those seen in idiopathic hydronephrosis except that almost the entire ureter is dilated.

Retroperitoneal fibrosis (*see* also p. 526)

In this condition, dense plaques of fibrous tissue form in the retroperitoneal space. There may be associated mediastinal fibrosis, sclerosing cholangitis, Riedel's struma or fibromatoses (*see* p. 524). Some cases are associated with a neoplasm.

If the ureters become obstructed, this leads to obstructive uropathy and finally to renal failure. The obstruction is often intermittent at first. Intravenous urography characteristically shows the ureters drawn in towards the midline.

Treatment may require surgery, at which time the ureters may be wrapped in tunnels of omentum in order to prevent recurrence.

Bladder Diverticula

A congenital bladder diverticulum may be due to obstruction of the bladder out-flow during intrauterine life (e.g. due to a posterior urethral valve) or to a developmental abnormality at the point where the mesonephric ducts fuse with the cloaca. Those seen in the vault represent a persistent urachus. These congenital diverticula have muscle in their walls and therefore contract during micturition. This prevents urinary stasis and consequently there is less risk of infection than in acquired diverticula.

The bladder musculature is arranged in criss-crossing bundles which form a net-like pattern. In cases of acquired bladder neck obstruction, most commonly due to benign nodular hyperplasia of the prostate, the bladder muscle hypertrophies to form a trabeculated pattern. Saccules of mucosa form in the intervening spaces. The saccules enlarge and eventually protrude through the bladder wall to form diverticula which are composed of mucosa with little or no muscle. These diverticula do not contract during micturition but rather tend to distend and become larger. At cystoscopy the diverticula are seen as 'black holes' against a background of coarse trabeculated bladder mucosa. They are most commonly situated in the region of the ureteric orifices.

Diverticula may obstruct the ureter causing hydronephrosis. Urinary stasis within the diverticula may cause infection and stone formation and the epithelium tends to undergo metaplasia to a squamous type. Carcinoma develops in up to 4% of cases; about a third of these are primary squamous cell carcinomas and the remainder are transitional cell tumours.

Bladder Fistulas

Vesicovaginal fistulas are caused by prolonged second stage of labour, hyster-ectomy, malignancy of the bladder, especially following radiotherapy, and trauma. Vesico-uterine fistulas are rare and causes include neoplasia, radiation and uterine surgery. Vesico-enteric fistulas are produced by diverticular disease, sigmoid carci-noma, Crohn's disease, tuberculosis and perforating injury. The commonest cause of a vesico-cutaneous fistula is bladder surgery.

Cystic Disease of the Kidney

Cystic dysplasia

Renal dysplasia is an abnormality of development almost invariably associated with cyst formation. The condition may be unilateral or bilateral and each kidney may be completely or segmentally affected. Congenital abnormalities of the lower urinary tract are frequently present and are usually obstructive in nature (e.g. posterior urethral valves, ectopic ureter and ureterocoele). It is considered likely that the maldevelopment is due to either vesico-ureteric reflux or ureteric obstruc-tion occurring in utero.

Clinically, cases of total involvement of both kidneys present as stillbirths or die shortly after birth. Unilateral involvement commonly presents in infancy as a loin mass. These cases are easily confused with Wilms' tumour or with congenital hydronephrosis. If left *in situ*, the dysplastic kidney may produce hypertension.

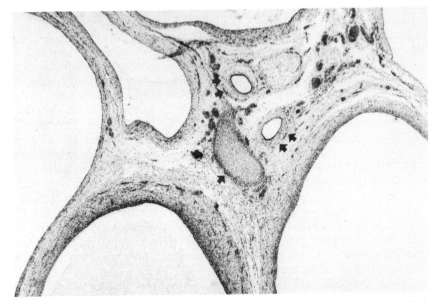

Fig. 9.8. Cystic dysplasia. Note the area of cartilage (single arrow) and the tubules surrounded by mesenchyme (double arrows). (H and E × 30)

Other cases of renal dysplasia commonly present during investigation of a congenital abnormality of the lower urinary tract.

Grossly the kidney is enlarged, cystic and irregular in outline. Histological examination confirms the cystic change. Between the cysts abnormal differentiation of the renal tissue is seen as primitive tubules surrounded by primitive mesenchyme. Immature glomeruli are seen and foci of cartilage are characteristic (*see Fig.* 9.8).

Polycystic disease of the kidneys

Infantile form

The clinical presentation of this condition is a baby with very large kidneys. In the classical case the infant is either stillborn or dies within a few weeks of birth. It is inherited in an autosomal recessive fashion. It is now, however, realized that some patients survive into infancy or even childhood. Consequently, four types are now recognized—perinatal, neonatal, infantile and juvenile. The condition is always associated with some degree of hepatic fibrosis. The perinatal cases present as described above. The neonatal cases present in the first month and die within one year from renal failure. The infantile form presents at 3–6 months with large kidneys and hepatosplenomegaly. These patients die in childhood with systemic and portal hypertension and renal failure. The juvenile group presents in childhood and patients die in their teens from portal hypertension and its complications. Thus, with late presentation, the renal features become less prominent. Grossly, both kidneys are always affected and their reniform shape is preserved. On the surface, small uniform cysts are seen. On cut section the kidney has a sponge-like appearance due to fusiform shaped cysts running radially through the cortex and medulla. Microscopically, the cysts are dilated collecting tubules between which are normal glomeruli and tubules.

In the liver, fibrosis of the portal tracts with proliferation of bile ducts is seen. Bile ducts may become cystically dilated in some areas.

Adult polycystic kidneys

This is inherited as an autosomal dominant trait. Although the common age of presentation is between 20–50 years, cases have been reported presenting in infancy and in old age.

The pathogenesis of the condition is unclear. The cystic dilatation can occur anywhere in the nephron and the cysts consequently can be lined with any form of tubular epithelium. Possible causes are a developmental defect or an inherited metabolic defect producing cyst formation (Editorial 1979).

Presentation is with hypertension, slowly progressive renal failure and haematuria. Pain or dragging sensation in the loin may be the main symptoms and some patients have urinary infections. Adult polycystic disease accounts for 8% of patients in the European Dialysis and Transplantation Registry (Editorial 1979).

Polycystic disease of the kidney is associated with liver cysts in 30% of cases. These may become infected but they do not cause cirrhosis or portal hypertension. Cysts are less frequently seen in the lung and pancreas. Berry aneurysms are also associated with polycystic kidneys and death from subarachnoid haemorrhage occurs in 10% of cases.

Grossly, both kidneys are affected. They are greatly enlarged, weighing up to 4 kg each. The renal outline is grossly disrupted due to the cysts and the reniform shape is obliterated. On cut section the kidney is seen to be a mass of cysts, usually without apparent intervening parenchymal tissue. The calyceal system is distorted (see Fig. 9.9).

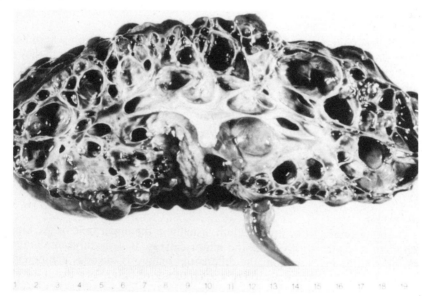

Fig. 9.9. Polycystic kidney, adult type.

Microscopically the cysts either have no epithelial lining or else a lining of flattened cells. The intervening tissue is atrophic due to pressure from the cysts, although a few glomeruli and tubules may be seen. There is frequently evidence of haemorrhage and previous infection within the cyst walls. The only effective treatment is renal transplantation.

Medullary cysts

Medullary sponge kidney

This occurs sporadically and usually presents as a finding on intravenous urography in which dilated collecting ducts are demonstrated in one or more papillae. The walls of the dilated ducts may become calcified. The condition itself does not give rise to symptoms although the complications of stone formation and infection may occur.

Gross inspection of the cut surface shows dilated ducts in the renal papillae, possibly with cyst formation. Histologically, the cysts are lined with attenuated epithelium.

Medullary cystic kidney

Medullary cystic kidney is also known as nephronophthisis. It is inherited as an autosomal recessive trait and presents in childhood or early adult life with polyuria and polydipsia, due to a severe tubular defect. Renal failure eventually occurs. The main pathological feature is the presence of cysts of the renal medulla along with tubular atrophy and interstitial fibrosis.

Simple cysts

These are very common in elderly patients and are thought to be present in half of all people over 50 years old. They are commonly asymptomatic although they may present as an abdominal mass or as an incidental finding during investigation of the urinary tract. They are likely to be due to distension of nephrons which have become blocked by scarring.

Grossly, they may be single or multiple to the extent that they may be confused with polycystic kidney. On cut section, they have a smooth inner wall which on histological examination is seen to be composed of flattened epithelial cells. Commonly, they require no treatment, although the possibility of a cystic renal carcinoma must be excluded.

Calyceal cyst

This is a congenital cyst or diverticulum, usually in the upper pole of the kidney, which communicates with one of the minor calyces. It is asymptomatic and, if found on routine investigation, the differential diagnosis includes a tuberculous cavity. It may be due to obstruction of a renal tubule or failure of a distal tubule to unite with a collecting duct.

Renal Artery Stenosis

Renal artery stenosis is the cause of hypertension in less than 5% of cases. The cause of the hypertension is likely to be increased production of renin by the ischaemic kidney with the consequent stimulation of the renin–angiotensin–aldosterone system, although other theories such as reduced renal prostaglandin synthesis have been suggested. The two common causes of renal artery stenosis are atheroma and fibromuscular dysplasia.

Atheroma is the more common cause in the elderly, especially those with established risk factors (see p. 331). The plaque is usually situated at, or near, the ostium of the renal artery.

Fibromuscular dysplasia is the more common cause of renal artery stenosis in patients under 40 years old. Dysplasias are more often in the middle or distal renal artery. Several types are recognized, depending on the part of the arterial wall most affected. Intimal disease is a rare variety. Medial fibromuscular dysplasia is the most common type and this often appears as alternating ridges of stenosis with intervening thinned areas of arterial wall which form small aneurysms. These features give the typical 'string of beads' appearance on arteriography. Histologically, the thickened areas show a proliferation of fibrous tissue and smooth muscle cells. Adventitial lesions are rare; a cuff of collagen is seen replacing the adventitia.

The prognosis after surgery is better for fibromuscular dysplasia than for atheroma.

Renal Tumours

Renal cell adenoma

These occur as well defined cortical nodules which are found as an incidental finding in up to 15% of all autopsies. They rarely cause symptoms. On cut section, they are pale yellow and discrete. Histologically, the most common pattern is papillary, although other patterns which occur in renal cell carcinoma are also seen. The cells show no atypia.

Renal cell adenoma is exceedingly difficult, if not impossible, to distinguish from well differentiated renal cell carcinoma. Both tumours appear to be derived from the epithelial cells of the proximal convoluted tubule. An arbitrary distinction used to be made on the basis of size in that those tumours under 3 cm in diameter rarely metastasize and were considered adenomas whereas those over 3 cm were considered carcinomas. While this is largely true, it is now appreciated, however, that small tumours even less than 2 cm in diameter can metastasize. Bannayan and Lamm (1980), therefore, regard these small lesions as borderline renal tumours of unpredictable behaviour. The relationship between renal cell carcinoma and renal cell adenoma is, therefore, not clear. There are two possibilities: (1) all adenomas are low-grade carcinomas which will eventually enlarge and metastasize; (2) malignant change occurs in a proportion of benign adenomas. The fact that many are found at autopsy as incidental findings suggests that growth or malignant transformation is very slow.

If found in the course of routine investigation, many authorities suggest that they should be considered to be early cancers and resected.

Oncocytoma of the kidney

These are recently recognized tumours which arise from the cells of the proximal convoluted tubules. Early examples were probably diagnosed as renal cell carcinoma of granular cell type. The tumour has a male to female ratio of 3 : 1 with a mean age of presentation at about 60 years.

Clinically, they frequently produce no symptoms and are often detected as an incidental finding on urography or at autopsy. Distinction from renal cell carcinoma or renal cell adenoma on urography may be difficult. However, oncocytomas do have a typical angiogram finding in which the vessels form a 'spoked wheel pattern'.

Grossly, they are well circumscribed tumours showing no invasion (*see Fig. 9.10*). They are tan in colour on cross section, often with a central scar.

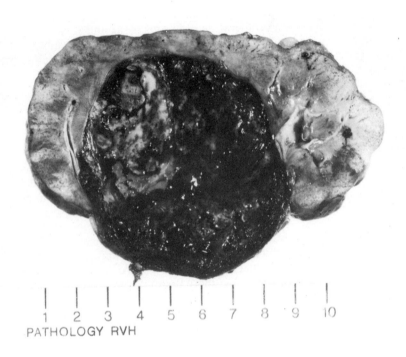

PATHOLOGY RVH

Fig. 9.10. Oncocytoma of kidney.

Histologically the cells are characteristically polygonal, with a deeply eosinophilic granular cytoplasm. The nuclei are small, round and central without pleomorphism. The pattern of cell growth can be tubular, trabecular or alveolar. On electron microscopy the cytoplasm is packed with mitochondria.

The prognosis is excellent and the tumour is considered benign.

Renal cell carcinoma

Epidemiology and aetiology

Renal cell carcinoma (Grawitz's tumour, hypernephroma) accounts for 3% of all cancers and for 85–90% of all malignant renal tumours in adults. The annual incidence is approximately four per 100 000 and it is 2–3 times more common in men than women. They are common in Scandinavia and rare in Asia.

There is evidence that smoking (especially pipes and cigars) doubles the risk of developing renal cell carcinoma and associations have also been noted with obesity and diabetes.

Little else is known of the aetiology. Certain carcinogens and viruses are known to cause renal cell carcinomas in animals but none has been proven to cause the tumour in humans.

Renal cell carcinomas develop in two-thirds of patients who have Von Hippel–Lindau disease. It also occurs slightly more commonly in horseshoe kidneys and polycystic kidneys than in otherwise normal kidneys. Patients with end-stage renal failure may develop cysts lined with tubular epithelium which can undergo malignant change.

Like renal cell adenomas, renal cell carcinomas arise from the cells of the proximal convoluted tubules. The relationship to renal cell adenoma has been discussed above.

Clinical features

The tumour may present as follows.

1. UROLOGICAL SYMPTOMS: These are the presenting features in 75% of cases and include haematuria (65%), flank pain (40%) and a palpable mass (32%). A small number present with an acute varicocoele, especially on the left, due to renal vein obstruction.

2. METASTATIC DEPOSITS: These include lung (haemoptysis), bone (pathological fracture) and brain (headache, hemiparesis).

3. NON-SPECIFIC SIGNS OF MALIGNANCY: These include anaemia (30%), pyrexia (possibly due to a tumour pyrogen), elevated ESR and gastrointestinal symptoms. The latter are so common (25% of cases) that a urogram is recommended in cases of X-ray negative gastrointestinal symptoms.

4. NON-METASTATIC EFFECTS OF MALIGNANCY: These are particularly characteristic of renal cell carcinoma. Examples include (1) hypertension which occurs in 20% of cases; in some it is due to elevated renin levels; (2) polycythaemia due to erythropoietin production; (3) hypercalcaemia (due to ectopic parathormone-like hormone production, although some cases are due to bone metastases); (4) neuromuscular abnormalities; (5) hepatic dysfunction (well described in renal cell carcinoma although the causative factor is unknown); (6) leukaemoid reaction; (7) ectopic hormone production including ACTH, human chorionic gonadotrophin, enteroglucagon and insulin (Editorial 1981).

Morphology

The early lesion is seen as a spherical mass (*see Fig.* 9.11), often at one pole (more commonly the upper pole) of the kidney. Initially it is confined by the renal capsule but later may invade through it into the perinephric fat and adrenal gland. At first it distorts and later invades the calyceal system to form a fungating mass within the renal pelvis. On sectioning the kidney, the mass may appear to be encapsulated due to surrounding compressed renal tissue. Satellite nodules are evidence of aggression. The cut surface has a variegated and lobulated appearance. Haemorrhage and necrotic areas are common, as are bands of fibrous tissue. The colour of the viable tissue depends on the cell type, being yellow or tan in the clear cell variety and grey or white in the granular or spindle cell varieties. Exploring the renal vein often shows a column of tumour cells which can extend into the inferior vena cava and in rare cases as far as the right atrium.

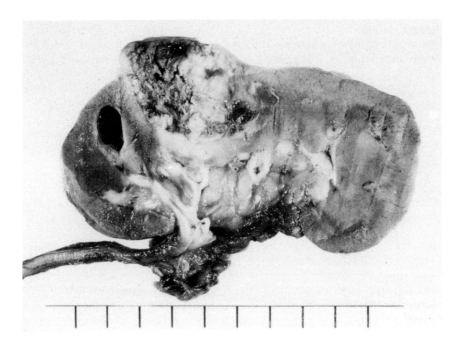

Fig. 9.11. Renal cell carcinoma.

The classic gross appearance is frequently not seen in resected specimens which, in many cases, have undergone therapeutic embolization prior to surgery, leaving only a haemorrhagic mass containing little or no viable tumour.

The histological appearance depends on : (1) the cell type, (2) the pattern of cell growth, and (3) the nuclear grading.

The commonest variety is the clear cell type (*see Fig.* 9.12). The cells are rounded with a central nucleus and clear cytoplasm. Clear cell tumours are usually of low histological grade (*see* below). Granular cell tumours consist of rounded cells with granular cytoplasm and are often of a high histological grade. Spindle cell types consist of spindle shaped cells, usually of high histological grade. Some tumours contain a mixture of cell types.

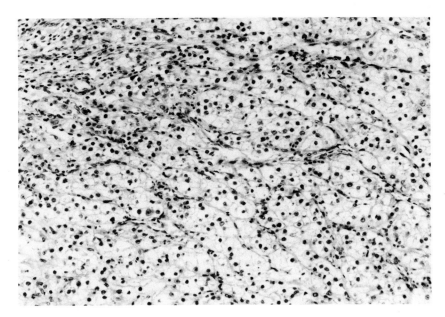

Fig. 9.12. Renal cell carcinoma. Clear cell type with alveolar pattern. (H and E × 30)

The various patterns include alveolar (packages of cells surrounded by a fine stroma), trabecular (plates of several cells separated by a fine stroma), tubular, papillary and solid. Clear cell tumours tend to be alveolar, granular cell tumours tend to be papillary and spindle cell tumours tend to be solid. Mixed patterns are very common.

The histological grade depends largely on nuclear characteristics. Low grade tumours (grade 1 and 2) have little pleomorphism or hyperchromasia. High grade tumours (grade 3 and 4) have marked pleomorphism and hyperchromasia with coarsely clumped chromatin and numerous mitotic figures.

Spread and staging

Spread may be directly through the renal capsule to the adrenal gland, colon, liver or spleen.

Approximately one-third of patients have metastases at the time of diagnosis and of these many have metastases limited to one organ. Between 2% and 3% of metastases are solitary.

Table 9.1. Comparison of TNM and Robson system of staging renal cell carcinoma*

TNM	Extent of disease	Robson Stage	Frequency at diagnosis (%)
T1	Tumour within capsule (small)	I	33
T2	Tumour within capsule (large)		
T3	Tumour in perinephric fat	II	12
N1–N3	Tumour in regional nodes	III	24
V1	Tumour in renal vein		
V2	Tumour in vena cava		
T4	Adjacent organ invasion	IV	31
M1	Distant metastases		
N4	Tumour in juxta-regional nodes		

* Adapted from Sufrin (1982).

Lymphatic spread to the local lymph nodes is seen in about one-half of autopsy cases. Blood-borne spread is to the lungs, bone, liver, opposite kidney, adrenal and brain in approximate order of frequency.

Staging is by the TNM or by the Robson system. These are given in *Table* 9.1.

Prognosis

Overall five year survival after nephrectomy is approximately 40%. The prognosis in any one patient depends on the following.

THE STAGE: After radical nephrectomy with lymphadenectomy the five year survival for Stage I is 70–80% and for Stage IV less than 30% (Sufrin 1982).

HISTOLOGICAL FEATURES: The clear cell types have a slightly better prognosis than the granular cell or spindle cell types. The pattern of growth *per se* does not appear to influence prognosis. Tumours of high histological grade (3 and 4) have a poor prognosis compared with those of low grade (1 and 2).

Regression

Spontaneous regression of renal cell carcinomas has been documented but is rare. Regression of metastases is also documented both before and after nephrectomy.

Wilms' tumour (nephroblastoma)

Nephroblastoma accounts for 90% of renal tumours in childhood. It is most common in children between the ages of one and four years and it is rarely seen in adults. Males and females are equally affected and the geographical distribution appears to be even. It accounts for 8% of childhood malignancy, the annual incidence being one in 50 000 of the general population.

Clinically the commonest presentation is with an abdominal mass or abdominal pain. Rarely, rupture of the tumour gives rise to an acute abdominal emergency.

Wilms' tumours are associated with a variety of congenital malformations. In one study of 482 cases, 51 children had a total of 72 malformations. Commonest among these were urinary tract abnormalities (ureteric duplication, horseshoe kidney, etc.), genital abnormalities (e.g. hypospadias), hemihypertrophy and aniridia (Schweisguth 1982).

Grossly, the tumours tend to be large. They are bilateral in 5–7% of cases. The tumour may have breached its capsule with associated invasion of the perirenal fat or adrenal and invasion of the renal vein is also commonly seen. On cut section there is a heterogeneous appearance which depends on the tissue types present. Haemorrhage and necrosis are exceedingly common.

Histologically three elements are seen: (1) sheets of mesenchymal cells which are small and darkly staining; (2) primitive imperfectly formed tubules and glomeruli; (3) connective tissue which includes skeletal muscle, cartilage and occasionally bone. There is a great variation in the histological appearance with some tumours being composed almost entirely of sheets of undifferentiated cells while others show marked glomerular differentiation (*see Fig.* 9.13).

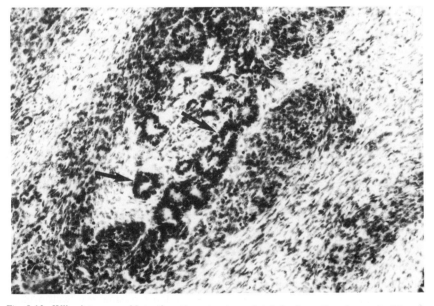

Fig. 9.13. Wilms' tumour. Note the attempts at renal tubule formation (arrows). (H and E × 30)

Spread and staging

Local spread to neighbouring organs and into the renal veins is common. Spread to lymph nodes is much less common than blood-borne spread. Metastases mostly

Table 9.2. Staging of Wilms' Tumour (Medical Research Council's Working Party 1978)

Stage I	Tumour confined to kidney and completely resected.
Stage II	Tumour extending beyond the capsule of the kidney either by local infiltration or extension along the renal vein or involvement of the para-aortic nodes but complete macroscopic removal achieved.
Stage III	Tumour extending beyond the capsule of the kidney and not completely resected or the operative field contaminated with tumour spilled at operation.
Stage IV	Haematogenous metastases.
Stage V	Bilateral renal involvement.

occur to the lungs and are often of the cannon ball type. The staging system used in the Medical Research Council trials is given in *Table* 9.2 (Medical Research Council's Working Party 1978).

Prognosis

The National Wilms' Tumour Studies (American) and the Medical Research Council work (British) have all shown the benefits of combined surgery, radiotherapy and chemotherapy (D'Angio *et al.* 1980; Medical Research Council's Working Party 1978).

Stage I children do not appear to require radiotherapy. Prognosis with surgery and chemotherapy is about 90% disease-free survival at two years. Stage II and III children receive postoperative radiotherapy and chemotherapy; they have a 75% disease-free survival at two years. Children with Stage IV disease receive postoperative radiotherapy and aggressive chemotherapy; 40% are disease-free survivors at two years.

Both the American and British studies have shown that the presence of anaplastic elements in the tumour and the involvement of lymph nodes are poor prognostic signs. Other studies have shown that a favourable prognosis is associated with tubular and glomerular differentiation and age less than two years at presentation (Lemerle *et al.* 1976).

Malignant and Pre-malignant Conditions of the Bladder

Transitional cell carcinoma

Urothelial tumours may be flat or papillary. A papillary lesion in which the fronds are covered with an epithelium indistinguishable from normal (i.e. well organized and not more than 4–5 cells thick) is termed a papilloma and is benign. These are very rare. Much more common are papillary lesions in which the epithelium is abnormal (i.e. more than 5–7 cells thick and/or atypical cells). By convention, these lesions are all termed papillary carcinomas and are subdivided into non-invasive and invasive, depending on whether or not there is invasion across the basement membrane into the lamina propria of the papillary cores.

Flat urothelial lesions may show varying degrees of cellular atypia (dysplasia) and when this is full thickness, the term carcinoma-in-situ is used. If the basement membrane is breached, the tumour becomes an invasive carcinoma.

Epidemiology

The majority of urothelial tumours occur in the bladder. Bladder cancer accounts for 7% of all cancers in men and 2·5% of all cancers in women. The male to female ratio is about 3 : 1. It is rare before the age of 50 years and then shows a steadily increasing incidence with increasing age. In general terms, the condition is more common in the Western industrialized nations than in the Third World, although there are exceptions to this, as in Egypt. In the course of this century there has been a gradual increase in the incidence of bladder cancer. The incidence rises with decreasing social class and is greater in urban than in rural areas.

Aetiology

There is much evidence to suggest that many bladder tumours are due to the concentration of carcinogens in urine. Several aetiological factors have been identified.

SMOKING: Several studies have shown that cigarette smoking predisposes to bladder cancer but that the latent period is longer than for lung cancer. Miller (1977) found the relative risk for smokers as opposed to non-smokers to be 3·9 for males and 2·6 for females.

INDUSTRIAL CARCINOGENS: Industrial exposure to certain aromatic amines is associated with a high incidence of bladder cancer. The most potent of these carcinogens are beta-naphthylamine and benzidine. These compounds are complexed to glucuronic acid to form glucuronides which are excreted in the urine. The bladder wall contains the enzyme beta-glucuronidase which is active at the pH of urine. This enzyme consequently splits the glucuronides, thereby releasing the pure carcinogens and this explains why these carcinogens act selectively in the bladder. The occupations which have a recognized risk (i.e. qualify the patient for financial compensation in the United Kingdom) include the manufacturing of dye stuffs, tyres, other rubber goods and coal gas. The latent period in these industries is in the region of 20 years and the increased incidence can be up to fifty-fold.

SCHISTOSOMIASIS: Cancer of the bladder is common in certain areas where infestation with S. haematobium is also common. It is not clear whether or not there is a causal relationship. The bladder cancer is usually of the squamous type.

ABNORMAL TRYPTOPHAN METABOLISM: Elevated levels of the amino acid tryptophan have been found in the urine of patients with bladder cancer. It is unclear whether these patients have a primary disorder of tryptophan metabolism which predisposes to bladder cancer or whether the excessive levels of tryptophan are due to impaired renal function as a result of ureteric obstruction by the tumour. Recurrences of tumour are more likely in those patients who have high urinary levels of tryptophan metabolites.

Clinical features

Painless haematuria is the commonest presentation. Superadded infection causes dysuria; obstruction of a ureteric orifice will cause loin pain.

Morphology

The commonest macroscopic appearance is a papillary growth with multiple fine or coarse fronds. Infiltrating tumours may appear nodular and ulcerated at cystoscopy. The papillary and infiltrating growth shows a papillary surface and thickening round the base, although the degree of infiltration may only be appreciated by bimanual palpation (*see Fig.* 9.14).

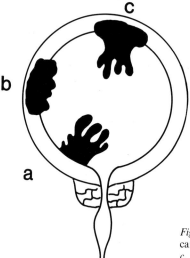

Fig. 9.14. Macroscopic types of transitional cell carcinoma of bladder: *a.* papillary, *b.* infiltrative, *c.* papillary and infiltrative.

In patients treated by radiotherapy, an inflammatory reaction occurs in the bladder and rectum. This may cause a contracted bladder and rectal stenosis. Fistula formation is rare.

In the histological assessment of bladder tumours, four features are noted: (1) the pattern of growth, (2) the cell type, (3) the degree of differentiation, and (4) the depth of invasion.

PATTERN OF GROWTH: Although the biopsy specimen taken by transurethral resection is fragmented, the pattern of growth can be assessed by the presence or absence of papillary fragments (*see Fig.* 9.15).

THE CELL TYPE: Approximately 90% of epithelial cell tumours of the urinary tract are of transitional cell type (i.e. they resemble the normal transitional cell lining of the urinary tract). The remainder are about equally distributed between squamous carcinomas and adenocarcinomas, each of which accounts for approximately 1–5% of epithelial tumours. Rarely spindle cell and giant cell variants have been reported.

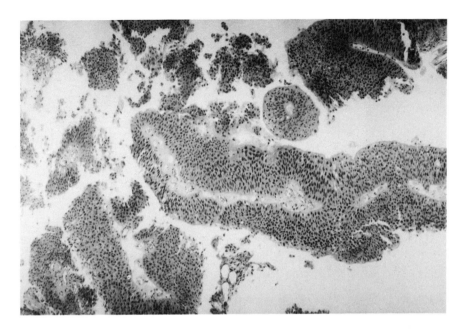

Fig. 9.15. Transitional papillary carcinoma of bladder. Typical fragments received after transurethral resection. (H and E × 30)

DEGREE OF DIFFERENTIATION (HISTOLOGICAL GRADING): Carcinomas of the urothelium are divided into three histological grades. In grade I tumours the epithelium is thicker than the 4–5 cells seen in normal transitional epithelium and there is some loss of polarity with hyperchromasia of nuclei. Grade II tumours show considerable loss of polarity although the cells can be recognized as transitional in type. Grade III tumours show considerable pleomorphism and hyperchromasia of nuclei and they are not easily recognizable as being of transitional cell type. Papillary lesions tend to be low grade (I–II) whereas invasive lesions tend to be high grade (III).

DEPTH OF GROWTH: The usual biopsy specimen taken at the time of transurethral resection is fragmented and the depth of invasion is difficult to assess histologically. However, invasion of the lamina propria or muscle may be seen in individual tumour fragments.

Staging
Staging of bladder cancer is essential before deciding on treatment. It may be carried out clinically and histologically. CT scan, ultrasound and bimanual palpation under anaesthesia at the time of cystoscopy help in the clinical staging. Histological staging is difficult in a fragmented biopsy as discussed above. The TNM system of staging is given in *Fig.* 9.16.

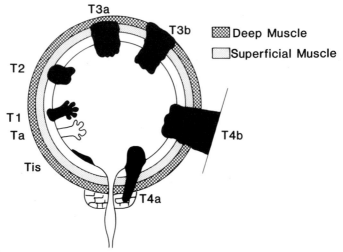

Fig. 9.16. T grading of the TNM staging system for bladder tumours: Tis is flat carcinoma-in-situ; Ta is papillary carcinoma which has not invaded across the basement membrane into the lamina propria of the papillary cores; T1 is a carcinoma which has invaded the lamina propria.

Spread, recurrence and prognosis

Spread occurs directly through the bladder wall and there is a positive correlation between the histological grade and the degree of local spread. Outside the bladder wall the tissue may infiltrate the side walls of the pelvis, the prostate, the uterus and vagina. The degree of lymphatic spread increases with both histological grade and depth of invasion. Spread is to the iliac and then to the para-aortic nodes. Blood-borne metastases may occur to the lungs and liver.

Bladder tumours have a great propensity to recur. Recurrence may be a true recurrence due to inadequate removal or, more likely, a second tumour elsewhere in the unstable urothelium. About 60–80% of grade I tumours recur and 80–90% of grade III tumours recur. The prognosis varies according to the stage, grade and treatment given. Approximate figures for five year survival are T1 70%, T2 50%, T3 20%, and T4 approaches zero.

The concept that papillary bladder tumours arise in a generally unstable urothelium dictates that even patients with early lesions must be extensively followed up by cystoscopy in order to detect recurrences.

Carcinoma-in-situ and dysplasia in the bladder

As previously mentioned, carcinoma-in-situ is a flat lesion of the bladder showing atypical cells throughout the mucosal thickness. Riddle *et al.* (1976) regard flat carcinoma-in-situ of the bladder as a distinct entity and exclude cases of carcinoma-in-situ found in the vicinity of an invasive carcinoma. The condition presents with dysuria associated with haematuria and pain (penile, perineal or suprapubic). Some cases present with painless haematuria. At endoscopy the mucosa usually shows colour changes and may appear to be inflamed or granular. In some cases the mucosa shows no abnormality.

The natural history of the condition is unclear. It appears to be unpredictable and different from the natural history of papillary lesions. Progression to invasive carcinoma is well documented (Riddle *et al.* 1976), although some cases appear to remain stable. The distinction between those lesions which become invasive and those which remain quiescent apparently cannot be made on histological grounds alone (Pugh 1982).

Riddle *et al.* (1976) suggested radical surgery for widespread flat carcinoma-in-situ of the bladder, and a conservative approach for small lesions.

Urothelial dysplasia implies an epithelium which shows less severe atypia than carcinoma-in-situ. Little is known of the natural history although current evidence suggests that it may be a precursor of malignancy in some patients (Murphy 1983).

Squamous carcinoma of the bladder

These account for less than 5% of epithelial tumours of the bladder. They are, however, more common in certain parts of the world such as Egypt, where they are probably related to the high incidence of chronic cystitis, bladder stones and *Schistosoma haematobium* infestation. Histologically, these tumours are composed entirely of squamous cells. Transitional cell tumours with areas of squamous differentiation are classified with transitional cell carcinomas.

Adenocarcinoma of the bladder

These tumours are also rare. They may arise from remnants of the urachus in the bladder wall, from areas of cystitis glandularis or from areas of glandular metaplasia. Glandular metaplasia is found in the bladder mucosa in cases of ectopic vesicae and accounts for the fact that malignancy developing in this condition tends to be of an adenocarcinoma pattern. Glandular metaplasia also occurs with schistosomiasis and patients with schistosomiasis may develop adenocarcinomas as well as squamous carcinomas.

Before accepting the diagnosis of a primary bladder adenocarcinoma, it is first essential to rule out the possibility of secondary spread from an adjacent organ such as the prostate or rectum. The prognosis of primary adenocarcinoma of the bladder depends on the stage.

Other Urothelial Tumours

Tumours of the renal pelvis

These account for less than 10% of renal tumours. They cause obstruction of a single calyx or of the whole pelvi-calyceal system, thereby causing hydronephrosis. Clot and tumour colic occur at an early stage. Tumours of the renal pelvis are associated with abuse of analgesics containing phenacetin, urinary stones and Balkan nephropathy. About 15% are associated with a bladder tumour.

Grossly, they are usually papillary. Histologically, they tend to be low grade transitional cell carcinomas. Adenocarcinoma and squamous carcinoma are exceedingly rare in this location. Invasion of the kidney may result in a lesion resembling renal cell carcinoma and, if the histology is not known at the time of surgery, a simple nephrectomy may be carried out instead of the recommended nephroureterectomy.

Tumours of the ureter

Transitional cell carcinoma of the ureter is commoner in its lower half and is pathologically identical to those arising in the renal pelvis and bladder. It can arise in the ureter left behind after simple nephrectomy (stump cancer). Multiple tumours in the ureter require a total nephroureterectomy, but in single tumours of the ureter conservative surgery gives good results. Long-term follow-up with clinical examination, urography and endoscopy is required in both renal pelvic and ureteric tumours (Mazeman 1976).

Tumours of the urethra

Primary tumours of the urethra are rare and tend to occur in elderly patients. The commonest histological type is squamous although adenocarcinomas and transitional cell carcinomas can also occur. Those arising posteriorly in the urethra have the worst prognosis as they spread to pelvic lymph nodes.

References

Bannayan G. A. and Lamm D. L. (1980) Renal cell tumours. *Pathol. Ann.* **15**, 271–308.

Blandy J. P., Marshall V. R. (1976) Size of renal calculi, recurrence rate and follow-up. *Br. J. Urol.* **48**, 525–30.

Blowers R., Asscher A. W., Brumfitt W. *et al.* (1979) Recommended terminology of urinary-tract infection. *Br. Med. J.* **2**, 717–19.

Castro J. E., Green N. A. (1975) Complications of horseshoe kidney. *Urology* **6**, 344–7.

D'Angio G. J., Beckwith J. B., Breslow N. E. *et al.* (1980) Wilms' tumour: an update. *Cancer* **45**, 1791–8.

Editorial (1979) Polycystic disease of the kidneys. *Br. Med. J.* **1**, 291–2.

Editorial (1981) Hypernephroma. *Br. Med. J.* **282**, 844–5.

Edwards D., Normand I. C., Prescod N., Smellie J. M. (1977) Disappearance of vesico-ureteric reflux during long-term prophylaxis of urinary tract infection in children. *Br. Med. J.* **2**, 285–8.

Gosling J. A., Dixon J. S. (1978) Functional obstruction of the ureter and renal pelvis. A histological and electron microscopic study. *Br. J. Urol.* **50**, 145–52.

Hallson P. C., Rose G. A. (1979) Uromucoids and urinary stone formation. *Lancet* **1**, 1000–2.

Lemerle J., Tournad M., Gerard-Merchant R. *et al.* (1976) Wilms' tumour: natural history and prognostic factors. *Cancer* **37**, 2557–66.

Ljunghall S. (1977) Renal stone disease. Studies of epidemiology and calcium metabolism. *Scand. J. Urol. Nephrol.* **41**, 1–96.

Mazeman E. (1976) Tumours of the upper urinary tract calyces, renal pelvis and ureter. *Eur. Urol.* **2**, 120–6.

Medical Research Council's Working Party on Embryonal Tumours in Childhood (1978) Management of nephroblastoma in childhood. Clinical study of two forms of maintenance chemotherapy. *Arch. Dis. Child.* **53**, 112–19.

Miller A. B. (1977) The aetiology of bladder cancer from the epidemiological viewpoint. *Cancer Res.* **37**, 2939–42.

Murphy W. M. (1983) Current topics in the pathology of bladder cancer. *Pathol. Ann.* **18**, 1–25.

Oliver J., MacDowell M., Tracy A. (1951) Pathogenesis of acute renal failure associated with traumatic and toxic injury. Renal ischaemia, nephrotoxic damage and ischaemuric episode. *J. Clin. Invest.* **30**, 1307–1439.

Pugh R. C. B. (1982) Histopathology. In: Chisholm G. D., Williams D. I. (eds.) *Scientific Foundations of Urology*, 2nd ed., pp. 701–11. London, Heinemann Medical.

Ransley P. G., Risdon R. A. (1975) Renal papillary morphology in infants and young children. *Urol. Res.* **3**, 111–13.

Riddle P. R., Chisholm G. D., Trott P. A., Pugh R. C. B. (1976) Flat carcinoma-in-situ of the bladder. *Br. J. Urol.* **47**, 829–33.

Schweisguth O. (1982) *Solid Tumours in Children*. New York, John Wiley and Sons.

Smith B. H., Dehner L. P. (1972) Chronic ulcerating interstitial cystitis (Hunner's ulcer). A study of 28 cases. *Arch. Pathol.* **93**, 76–81.

Sufrin G. (1982) The challenges of renal adenocarcinoma. In: Fair W. R. (ed.) *The Surgical Clinics of North America: Urological Surgery*, Vol. 2, No. 6, pp. 1101–18. Philadelphia, W. B. Saunders.

Welshman S. G., McGeown M. G. (1975) The relationship of the urinary cations, calcium, magnesium, sodium and potassium, in patients with renal calculi. *Br. J. Urol.* **47**, 237–42.

Wickham J. E. A., Kellet M. J. (1981) Percutaneous nephrolithotomy. *Br. J. Urol.* **53**, 297–9.

Chapter 10

The Male Genitalia

TESTIS AND EPIDIDYMIS

Normal Development and Structure

The primitive sex glands appear at six weeks in a region of the urogenital ridge. By the third month of fetal life the testis is located retroperitoneally and a fibromuscular band (the gubernaculum) extends from the lower pole of the testis through the anterior abdominal wall to end in the subcutaneous tissue of the scrotal swelling. Below the lower pole of the testis the peritoneum herniates as a diverticulum (processus vaginalis) along the anterior surface of the gubernaculum to reach the scrotal sac through the anterior abdominal wall muscles. The testis remains at the abdominal end of the inguinal canal until the seventh month. It then passes through the inguinal canal behind the processus vaginalis and invaginates it. It reaches the scrotal sac by the end of the eighth month in utero.

The average size of the adult testis is $4 \times 3 \times 2 \cdot 5$ cm. It is covered by dense fascia—the tunica albuginea, which posteriorly is thickened to form the mediastinum testis. Anteriorly and laterally is the visceral layer of the tunica vaginalis which is continuous with the parietal layer. Posterolaterally is the epididymis. Fibrous septa extend from the mediastinum into the testis to produce about 250 lobules. Each lobule consists of 1–4 convoluted seminiferous tubules which converge at the mediastinum. Here they connect with the efferent ducts which drain into the epididymis. Each seminiferous tubule has a basement membrane containing connective and elastic tissue. The seminiferous cells are of two types, Sertoli (supporting) cells and spermatogenic cells. The stroma between the seminiferous tubules contains connective tissue in which the interstitial (Leydig) cells are located.

The spermatic arteries arise from the aorta, just below the renal arteries, and are the main vessels supplying the testes. A smaller supply comes from the arteries of the vas. Venous drainage is via the pampiniform plexus of the cord. The right spermatic vein enters the vena cava just below the right renal vein while the left spermatic vein drains into the left renal vein. Lymphatics from the testes drain to the para-aortic nodes.

The upper portion of the epididymis (globus major) connects to the testis via numerous efferent ducts and the lower pole (globus minor) is continuous with the vas deferens. There is often a small cystic appendix of the epididymis present at the upper pole. The ducts of the epididymis are lined by pseudostratified columnar epithelium. Lymphatics drain to the external iliac and hypogastric nodes. Blood supply is from the internal spermatic artery and the artery of the vas.

Maldescended Testis

A maldescended testis is one which has failed to reach the normal low scrotal position. The testis may be found at some point along the line of normal descent and this is termed arrested descent or cryptorchidism. Less commonly, it may be in a position not on the normal line of descent, in which case it is termed an ectopic or deviated testis.

Scorer (1964) in a study of over 3600 infant boys showed that the incidence of undescended testis in full-term neonates was 2·7%. The figure was much higher in premature infants (21%) but, by nine months of age, only 0·8% had undescended testes. If descent has not occurred by one year, the testis is likely to remain undescended. In infancy, undescended testes are usually bilateral, but when the condition presents in children or young adults, it is usually unilateral. Scorer and Farrington (1971) found that 14·2% of affected boys had a family history of maldescent. In some cases, especially when the maldescent is bilateral, there is an associated chromosomal abnormality.

The aetiology of arrested descent is unclear. Possibilities include (1) mechanical factors, such as fascial bands, adhesions, gubernacular dysfunction and a short testicular artery; (2) endocrine factors, such as a relative lack of gonadotrophins or an insensitivity of the testis to gonadotrophins; and (3) an inherent abnormality in the testis.

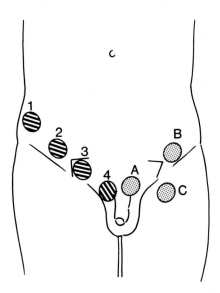

Fig. 10.1. Common positions for maldescended testes: arrested descent (on the left)—1. intra-abdominal, 2. inguinal canal, 3. superficial inguinal pouch, 4. high scrotum; ectopic testis (on the right)— A. penile, B. superficial inguinal, C. femoral.

The aetiology of deviated or ectopic testis is also unclear. Possibilities include (1) connections between the distal end of the gubernaculum (gubernacular tails) and an abnormal site, and (2) tethering of the testis to a fibrous adhesion which subsequently deviates it from its normal course.

In the majority of cases of arrested descent, the testis is found in the superficial inguinal pouch or high scrotum. In 20% of cases it is in the inguinal canal and in 10% it is intra-abdominal (*see Fig*. 10.1).

The most common site for an ectopic testis is the superficial inguinal position (superficial to the aponeurosis of external oblique). Other sites are (1) perineal, anterior to the anus, (2) femoral, in Scarpa's triangle, superficial to the femoral vessels, (3) penile, under the skin at the root of the penis and (4) pelvic (*see Fig*. 10.1).

By puberty, an undescended testis is significantly smaller than its fellow and the capsule is thickened and wrinkled. Histologically, before puberty, the undescended testis shows a delay in normal maturation. Tubular diameter is reduced and there is a reduction of spermatogonia content. At puberty, there is a progressive loss of spermatogonia and a persistence of undifferentiated cells in the tubules. Peritubular fibrosis is marked. The Leydig cells, however, are usually present in normal numbers.

Maldescent of the testis is associated with several important complications.

Impairment of testicular function is common in patients with maldescended testes. In cases of unilateral arrested descent, there is reduced fertility, suggesting that there is a bilateral testicular abnormality. Treatment of unilateral cryptorchidism by orchidopexy before puberty is associated with an impaired sperm count to less than 20×10^6/ml in one-third of cases (Lipshultz *et al.* 1976). If bilateral cryptorchidism is treated by orchidopexy before puberty, 40% of the patients will have azoospermia and 30% will have oligospermia (Werder *et al.* 1976). The prognosis for testicular function is best when the orchidopexy is carried out early.

Undescended testis is associated with a 20–50 times greater than average incidence of malignant testicular tumours. Abdominal testes are at greater risk than inguinal testes. In cases of unilateral undescended testis, both the normally and the abnormally placed testes are at increased risk. If orchidopexy is carried out before the age of six years, it protects against the development of malignancy, but if delayed until after puberty, there is no protection. The commonest malignant tumour to arise is a seminoma.

Other complications include hernia (present in 25%), torsion (occurs in about 2% and the diagnosis may be late) and trauma.

The current surgical management is early orchidopexy aided by microvascular surgery in difficult cases. Testicular venography and CT scanning may be helpful in localizing the impalpable undescended testis.

Inflammatory Conditions

Primary epididymitis and orchitis

This term implies an inflammation of the epididymis and/or testis which is not part of a generalized systemic infection. The condition commonly occurs in association with infection of the urinary tract such as cystitis, urethritis and prostatitis, or may follow trauma or instrumentation of the urinary tract. If the causative organism is neither *Neisseria gonococcus* or the tubercle bacillus, the term 'non-specific epididymitis/orchitis' is traditionally used. In patients aged over 35 years, *E. coli* and Pseudomonas are the commonest organisms, whereas in patients aged less than 35 years, sexually transmitted organisms (*N. gonococcus* and Chlamydia) are prominent.

The route of infection may be along the vas deferens or its associated lymphatics. There is some evidence that retrograde flow of urine can occur along the vas deferens and this phenomenon has been implicated in the pathogenesis (Pelouze 1931). Haematogenous spread may be the mechanism in tuberculosis and viral infections.

Grossly, the epididymis is injected, swollen and tense. The testis is frequently not involved although when it is affected it becomes swollen and tense with a fibrinous exudate on the surface. In tuberculous epididymitis, the epididymis is replaced by a caseous mass (*see Fig.* 10.2). Microscopically, the tail of the epididymis is most affected and often little change is seen in the head of the epididymis and in the testis itself. The tubules are filled with polymorphs and the interstitial tissue shows inflammation and vascular dilatation. If the condition becomes chronic, the tubules become obliterated with fibrous tissue, their linings undergo squamous metaplasia and an infiltrate of chronic inflammatory cells is seen in the interstitial area. In these cases, obstruction of the epididymis can result in sterility. In tuberculous epididymitis, characteristic caseating granulomas are seen.

Intravenous urography has been advised in patients with epididymitis over age 50 years and in children, in order to detect other abnormalities in the urinary tract (Bullock and Hunt 1981). Epididymectomy may be required for chronic or recurrent disease, epididymal abscess or for an infected hydrocoele.

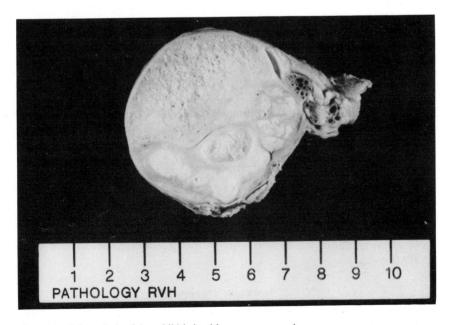

Fig. 10.2. Tuberculosis of the epididymis with caeseous necrosis.

Epididymitis and orchitis as part of a systemic infection

Epididymo-orchitis complicates 20% of cases of mumps occurring in adults. Unlike primary epididymo-orchitis, the testis is more affected than the epididymis. There is intense interstitial oedema and histologically, a mainly lymphocytic cell infiltrate is seen. This is accompanied by degeneration of the germinal epithelium, although the Leydig cells tend to survive. On follow-up, 76% of unilateral cases and 30% of bilateral cases eventually return to normospermia.

Epididymo-orchitis may also occur in patients suffering from brucellosis, enteric fever, infectious mononucleosis and malaria.

Sperm granuloma

This lesion occurs in the epididymis or spermatic cord. It may be symptomless or alternatively it may present as a painful nodule 1–3 cm in diameter. It may be due to extravasation of spermatozoa out of the epididymal tubules into the interstitial tissue. The condition often follows trauma or infection.

Grossly, the lesion is a white or yellow nodule. Microscopically, spermatozoa are seen in the interstitial tissue. They become phagocytosed by macrophages and clumps of spermatozoa and cell debris become surrounded by epithelioid cells to give a granulomatous appearance.

Granulomatous orchitis

This is a granulomatous condition of the testis which occurs in middle-aged to elderly men; it is often confused with malignancy. The aetiology is unknown although extravasation of spermatozoa out of the seminiferous tubules into the interstitial tissue has been suggested as a possibility. In support of this theory, many cases are associated with sperm granulomas of the epididymis. Clinically, the patient usually has a mild illness with pyrexia and testicular swelling which may be painful.

Grossly, the enlargement of the testis is mainly due to thickening of the tunica. On cut section, the testis has a rubbery consistency and is pale. Histologically, the testis is diffusely involved and spermatogenesis is absent from the affected seminiferous tubules. The tubules become filled with proliferating Sertoli cells and giant cells and so come to resemble granulomas. The symptoms may subside without treatment, although in many cases, the testis is removed to exclude malignancy.

Syphilitic orchitis

Syphilitic orchitis usually occurs in the tertiary stage of acquired syphilis. The affected testis may present as a painless, generalized enlargement which on histology shows interstitial inflammation and fibrosis with tubular atrophy. Alternatively, gummas form in the testis in which case the enlargement may be nodular. Histology of a gumma shows central necrosis with surrounding fibrosis and chronic inflammation.

Testicular Torsion

Torsion of the testis may be intravaginal or extravaginal.

In extravaginal torsion, which occurs in neonates and in patients with an undescended testis, the entire testis, including the tunica vaginalis, twists on the spermatic cord. In neonates, the testis is usually completely infarcted at the time of presentation; in these cases surgical fixation of the contralateral testis is advised.

In intravaginal torsion, which is the common type occurring in patients between 12 and 25 years old, the underlying defect is a high insertion of the tunica vaginalis on the cord. This leaves a length of cord free inside the tunica vaginalis and the testis may take up a horizontal lie. The abnormality is often bilateral. Contraction of the cremasteric muscle, which forms a spiral, may then initiate twisting of that part of the cord within the tunica (*see Fig.* 10.3). Usually the left testis twists anticlockwise and the right twists clockwise (i.e. away from the scrotal septum). Usually the testis and epididymis twist together, although occasionally the testis twists alone.

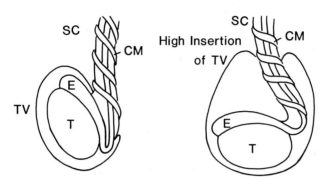

Fig. 10.3. Torsion of the testis (normal on the left). High insertion of tunica vaginalis (on the right) allows the testis to undergo torsion within the tunica. (SC—spermatic cord; CM—cremasteric muscle; T—testis; E—epididymis; TV—tunica vaginalis.)

By the age of 25, as many as 1 in 160 males have suffered testicular torsion.

Initially, the veins are occluded, causing the testis to be swollen and cyanotic; later arterial occlusion occurs and infarction ensues. After six hours, the seminiferous tubules become irreparably damaged although the interstitial cells can survive a few hours longer.

The clinical presentation is with sudden pain in the testis. In torsion there is often a history of several 'warning' attacks of pain and swelling (Chapman and Walton 1972) and this may help to distinguish the condition from epididymoorchitis.

Treatment is by surgical fixation as soon as possible. Since the anatomical abnormality of high insertion of the tunica vaginalis is usually bilateral, fixation of both testes is advised. Even after fixation, seminal analysis may be abnormal and a low motile sperm count occurs, especially in those who have had torsion of greater than eight hours' duration (Thomas *et al.* 1984). It appears that an acute ischaemic episode affecting one testis causes a bilateral impairment in exocrine function, although endocrine function is preserved. This bilateral damage may be on an immunological basis, although bilateral attacks of subclinical torsion may contribute.

Torsion of the hydatid of Morgagni occurs occasionally. This produces a tender cyst at the upper pole of the testis. It usually occurs before puberty.

Hydrocoele

A hydrocoele is a collection of serous fluid in the tunica vaginalis or in the processus vaginalis. It can be produced by defective absorption of fluid by the tunica vaginalis (often caused by chronic infection), excessive production of fluid (secondary hydrocoele), interference with the lymphatic vessels in the cord, or by a connection between the tunica vaginalis and the peritoneal cavity. The fluid is usually amber coloured. There are several anatomical types.

1. *Primary vaginal hydrocoele*—the tunica vaginalis becomes distended with fluid. This is common in middle-aged and elderly men. It may be associated with an ipsilateral inguinal hernia.
2. *Infantile*—the tunica vaginalis and processus vaginalis distend up to the internal ring but there is no connection with the abdominal cavity.
3. *Congenital*—the processus connects with the abdominal cavity and the hydrocoele may be emptied by gentle pressure.
4. *Encysted hydrocoele of the cord*—a segment of processus vaginalis persists and produces an ovoid swelling of the cord.

A secondary hydrocoele is usually associated with acute or chronic epididymo-orchitis. Occasionally, there is underlying syphilis or malignancy of the testis. Filariasis is a common cause in tropical areas.

Complications of hydrocoeles include rupture, herniation into the dartos muscle, haematocoele and calcification of the sac. These are all rare.

Haematocoele

Blood in the tunica vaginalis follows injury or tapping of a hydrocoele, although sometimes there is no clear history of trauma. Rarely, a testicular tumour presents in this fashion. In long-standing cases, the sac contains laminated clot which becomes organized. Late fibrosis and calcification may compress the testis.

Epididymal Cyst

These are common multilocular cysts occurring in middle-age. They contain clear fluid. The cause may be cystic degeneration of the paradidymis or the appendix of the epididymis. If uncomfortable, they require excision.

Spermatocoele

This is a unilocular retention cyst lying above and posterior to the testis. They probably arise from the vasa efferentia which connect the rete testis to the head of the epididymis. The contained fluid is white and cloudy.

Varicocoele

This is varicosity of the testicular veins. Most are found in young adults and 90% occur on the left side. Normally, the left testicular vein joins the renal vein in a vertical direction, while the right testicular vein joins the cava tangentially. This anatomical arrangement may explain the left-sided predominance, although Turner (1983) has suggested that incompetent or absent valves in the left testicular vein may be a factor in the pathogenesis. Very rarely, the left testicular vein may be obstructed by a renal tumour growing along the renal vein. The usual symptom of a varicocoele is dragging pain in the scrotum. The venous engorgement may raise the temperature and have an adverse effect on spermatogenesis.

Testicular Tumours

The complexity of testicular tumours has been clarified in the last ten years by the classification published by the British Testicular Tumour Panel (Pugh 1976). This classification, which is given in *Table* 10.1, is different from that used by American pathologists and by the World Health Organisation, but will be used in this section as it is widely accepted in the United Kingdom. A comparison of the various classifications has been given by Fraley *et al.* (1979).

Table 10.1. Classification of testicular tumours and the percentages seen in 2739 cases referred to the Testicular Tumour Panel (Pugh 1976)

	%
Seminoma	39.5
Teratoma	31.7
Combined tumour	13.5
Malignant lymphoma	6.7
Sertoli cell/mesenchyme	1.2
Interstitial (Leydig) cell	1.6
Yolk sac tumours	1.9
Metastases	0.9
Miscellaneous	0.8
Uncertain	2.2

Seminomas, teratomas and yolk sac tumours are all thought to arise from germ cells. There is little information on the aetiology of germ cell tumours. The most obvious association is with undescended testis which increases the risk by about 20–50 times for both seminoma and teratoma. Although associations with trauma, mumps orchitis, previous inguinal herniorraphy, herpes genitalis and exposure to the dye stuffs have all been reported, there is no controlled evidence for an increased incidence of testicular tumours in these conditions. One controlled study showed a higher incidence of testicular tumours in patients with venereal infection but this requires confirmation (Oliver 1984).

Most patients present with a hard, painless, enlarged testis, although presentation with a nodule, the symptoms of epididymo-orchitis or evidence of metastases have all been reported.

Elevated serum levels of certain tumour markers may be helpful in the diagnosis of testicular tumours and in the monitoring of treatment.

Alpha fetoprotein (AFP) is a product of the yolk sac and liver in fetal life. Elevated serum levels are found in yolk sac tumours and also in about 70% of patients with malignant teratomas. These teratomas sometimes, but not always, have a yolk sac component seen histologically. AFP is not found in patients with pure seminoma, although it may be elevated in patients who have hepatocellular carcinoma, ataxic telangiectasia or gastrointestinal malignancy.

Beta human chorionic gonadotrophin (BHCG) is produced by the normal placenta. Elevated levels are found in between 40% and 60% of patients with non-seminomatous tumours. Some, but not all, of these tumours have a trophoblastic element seen histologically. BHCG is also elevated in about 10% of patients who have seminomas. Elevated serum levels of BHCG may also be found in patients with carcinoma of the pancreas, stomach and bronchus.

There is some recent work which suggests that serum placental alkaline phosphatase may be a marker for seminomas.

Tumour markers may also be demonstrated in histological sections of the tumour tissue, by immunoperoxidase techniques, although the correlation between the presence of a particular marker in the tumour tissue and its presence in the serum is imperfect.

Seminoma

This is the commonest tumour of the testis. The incidence is about 1·5 per 100 000 males per year and it has become slightly more common in recent years. The peak age of presentation is between 30 and 40 years. As with other testicular tumours, it is more common in Caucasians than in non-Caucasians.

Seminomas occur more commonly in patients with maldescended testes than in normals. In patients with a unilateral maldescended testis, both testes are at risk of malignancy, suggesting a generalized abnormality of the reproductive system.

Morphology

The testis is symmetrically enlarged and may be associated with a hydrocoele. On the outer surface of the lesion there is typically a collection of large veins coursing towards the mediastinum. On cut section, the tumour is white with a few yellow areas of necrosis and bands of fibrous tissue may give a lobulated appearance to the cut surface (see Fig. 10.4). If any normal testis remains, the tumour is well demarcated from it.

Histologically, the tumour consists of sheets, clusters and trabeculae of seminoma cells, separated by bands of stroma (see Fig. 10.5). The cells are uniform in size and the cytoplasm is typically clear or finely granular. The stroma characteristically has a lymphocytic infiltrate and granulomas are seen in about one-third of cases. Necrosis is found in approximately half of all cases and tumour giant cells are occasionally present.

Spread

The tumour invades and destroys the surrounding normal testis, either directly or by permeating along the seminiferous tubules. The rete testis is involved in the majority of cases.

Distant metastatic spread is most commonly by lymphatics to the common iliac and para-aortic nodes. Later, thoracic nodes and supraclavicular nodes (especially on the left side at the termination of the thoracic duct) are involved. Finally, blood-borne metastases occur to the lungs, liver and bone.

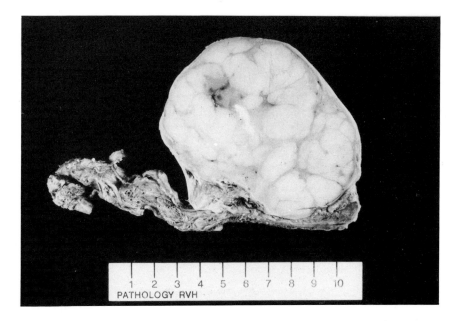

Fig. 10.4. Seminoma of testis.

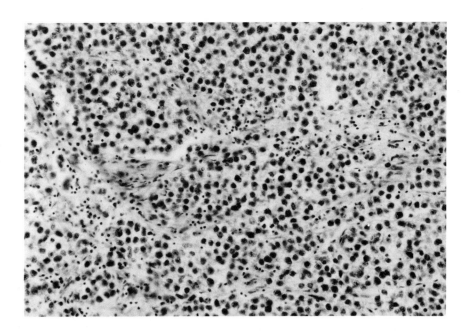

Fig. 10.5. Seminoma of testis. Between the seminoma cells is a scattering of lymphocytes. (H and E × 150)

Staging

Clinical staging of testicular tumours as used by the Royal Marsden Hospital is given in *Table* 10.2. The majority of patients (63%) present in Stage I and about 28% present in Stage II. The rest are about equally distributed between Stages III and IV.

Each orchidectomy specimen is also staged according to the amount of local spread as follows; P1, confined to the testis; P2, involvement of epididymis and/or lower cord; P3, involvement of the upper cord.

Table 10.2. Royal Marsden staging classification of testicular tumours (adapted from Peckham (1981))

I	No evidence of disease outside the testis

II	Infradiaphragmatic node involvement:
	  IIa Maximum diameter of metastases $< 2\,cm$
	  IIb Maximum diameter of metastases 2–5 cm
	  IIc Maximum diameter of metastases $> 5\,cm$

III	Supra- and infradiaphragmatic lymph node involvement:
	  a, b and c as for stage II
	  Mediastinal nodes noted M +
	  Neck nodes noted N +
	  0 = negative lymphogram

IV	Extension of tumour to extralymphatic sites:
	  a, b and c as for Stage II and III
	  Lung substage:
	    L_1 metastases < 3 in number
	    L_2 metastases > 3 in number, < 2 cm diameter
	    L_3 metastases > 3 in number, > 2 cm diameter

Prognosis

The prognosis for Stage I disease is excellent and very few of these patients die of their disease. In Stages IIa and IIb, 80% of patients are controlled. Prognosis gets worse with more extensive disease.

As well as stage, a good prognosis is indicated by a host reaction (that is, a lymphocytic infiltrate in the tumour tissue) and by a well differentiated histological grade (particularly if there is absence of mitotic figures).

Spermatocytic seminoma

The spermatocytic seminoma is now a well recognized variant of the classical seminoma. This tumour occurs in the older age group (peak incidence 45–50 years). Macroscopically, the lesion is soft and sometimes mucoid or cystic. Microscopically, the tumour consists of sheets of cells which show marked pleomorphism and a high mitotic rate. Giant cells are frequently seen but no lymphocytic infiltrate is present.

Although these tumours have an alarming histological appearance, the prognosis after orchidectomy is excellent.

Extrascrotal seminoma

Rarely, a seminoma may arise on the posterior abdominal wall. If the ipsilateral scrotum is empty, it is likely that the tumour has arisen in a maldescended testis. If both testes are in the scrotum and apparently normal, then either the tumour is a metastasis from an occult or regressed primary in one testis, or it has arisen from the testicular tissue which occasionally can be present on the posterior abdominal wall. Tumours histologically identical to a seminoma may arise in the mediastinum or in the hypothalamic region as primary lesions.

Teratoma

A teratoma is a tumour containing tissue derived from more than one germ layer. It is slightly less common than seminoma and occurs in a younger age group, the peak incidence being in the age group 20–30 years. They occur more commonly than normal in patients with maldescended testes. Other aetiological factors are obscure.

The majority of patients present with a testicular swelling. Rarely, presentation is with a metastasis. Testicular pain due to haemorrhage or necrosis occurs in about one-third of cases. In a small proportion of teratomas, gynaecomastia is present.

Terminology

Teratomas are divided by the British Testicular Tumour Panel into teratoma differentiated (TD); malignant teratoma intermediate (MTI); malignant teratoma undifferentiated (MTU); and malignant teratoma trophoblastic (MTT).

The TD is composed entirely of non-malignant differentiated tissue. The MTU is composed entirely of undifferentiated malignant tissue. An MTI is any combination of non-malignant differentiated and malignant undifferentiated tissue. An MTT is a teratoma which contains any amount of recognizable trophoblastic tissue.

Gross appearance

Like seminomas, large veins are often seen on the surface. Unlike seminomas, the testis is asymmetrically enlarged and the tumour is often nodular. The cut surface is typically haemorrhagic with necrotic areas and cysts (*see Fig.* 10.6).

Microscopic appearance

TERATOMA DIFFERENTIATED (TD) (4·9%)*: This is the most common teratoma found in children. No malignant tissue is seen. It is composed of different types of epithelium (for example, respiratory and gastrointestinal) interspersed with different types of connective tissue (for example, cartilage, bone and muscle). These may be arranged in an organoid form (that is, the various tissues may be arranged in a way that resembles a normal structure). Although no malignancy is seen, some immature tissue, which resembles tissue normally present in the embryo, is seen.

*Percentage of all teratomas.

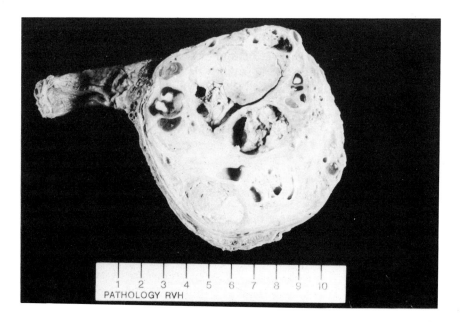

Fig. 10.6. Teratoma of testis.

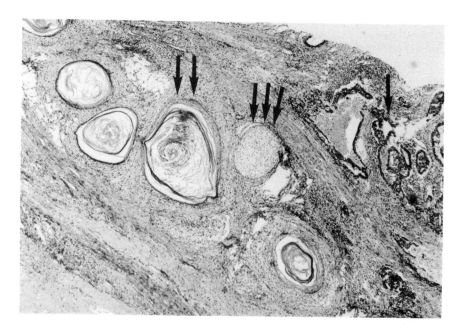

Fig. 10.7. Malignant teratoma intermediate. There are malignant areas (single arrow) and benign areas of squamous epithelium with keratin (double arrows) and cartilage (triple arrows). (H and E × 30)

In adults, especially, it is essential to section the tumour extensively to look for malignant areas which would bring the tumour into the MTI category. The British Testicular Tumour Panel consider that even though the prognosis is excellent, it is not justifiable to assume that TD is benign as metastases may rarely occur.

MALIGNANT TERATOMA INTERMEDIATE (MTI) (54·8%)*: This is the commonest type of teratoma. Differentiated tissues, sometimes showing an organoid arrangement similar to that described in TD, are present, together with unequivocally malignant areas. The malignant areas usually resemble carcinoma, although some malignant mesenchyme may also be present. Frequently, a yolk sac-like area is seen and this is associated with elevated serum AFP. As stressed earlier, a tiny area of malignant tissue in an otherwise TD makes the tumour MTI, whereas a tiny area of differentiated tumour in an otherwise MTU also makes it an MTI. Therefore, there is a wide spectrum of findings in MTI tumours and the prognosis in general gets worse with increasing amounts of malignant tissue (*see Fig.* 10.7).

MALIGNANT TERATOMA UNDIFFERENTIATED (MTU) (36·6%)*: There is a complete absence of differentiated tissue. The tumour consists of masses of cells usually resembling a carcinoma. There may be an adenocarcinoma-like pattern or it may consist of sheets of cells. Pleomorphism and mitoses are marked.

MALIGNANT TERATOMA TROPHOBLASTIC (MTT) (3·7%)*: This is the least common variety of teratoma. Grossly, it is characterized by the presence of much haemorrhage and necrosis. In order to make the diagnosis, it is essential to demonstrate that syncytiotrophoblast and cytotrophoblast are both present in a definite papillary pattern. This finding, even if present in a small proportion of a tumour which would otherwise be MTI or MTU, puts the tumour into the MTT category with its associated very poor prognosis.

Spread

Local spread is into the remaining part of the testis, epididymis and cord. Metastases occur most commonly via blood spread to the lung and liver. Metastases also occur to the abdominal and mediastinal lymph nodes.

Histologically, metastatic deposits are usually either of the same or of a worse degree of differentiation than the primary tumour, although after chemotherapy the metastases may become better differentiated.

Staging

Clinical and pathological staging is the same as that described for seminoma.

Prognosis

Accurate figures for prognosis are not readily available due to the multiple staging and treatment categories used for teratomas. Peckham, in 1981, reported on those patients treated in the Royal Marsden Hospital between 1976 and 1979. For Stage I and IIa, 95% were alive and disease-free and for Stages IIb, IIc and III, 76·5%

*Percentage of all teratomas.

were alive and disease-free. The results of the later stages were variable due to the small number in each group. A recent report showed that combination chemotherapy, especially with the addition of *cis*-platinum, gives a three year survival of 75% in patients with advanced teratomas (MRC Report 1985). With recent advances in therapy, histological typing is becoming less critical as an indicator of progress.

Combined seminoma and teratoma

Over 10% of testicular tumours are composed of a mixture of both seminoma and teratoma. In these combined tumours only the classical, as opposed to the spermatocytic, seminoma is seen, whereas any teratoma type may be found.

The peak incidence is between 30 and 34 years (i.e. between the seminoma and teratoma peaks).

Macroscopically, it is often possible to distinguish the seminoma and teratoma components which may be present in separate nodules. In other cases, the tumours are mutually infiltrating and no macroscopic demarcation can be made.

Histologically, the features are those of the classical seminoma and the various teratomas already described. The seminoma component is usually the smaller component and may be present as small nodules. It is usually separate from the teratoma component although they may be in contact. Less commonly, the two tissues are mixed together.

The behaviour and prognosis of these combined tumours tends towards that of the teratomatous component.

Sertoli cell/mesenchyme tumour

This tumour occurs at all ages but is commonest below the age of 40 years; it may occur in childhood and infancy. Presentation is with a testicular swelling and, occasionally, patients have gynaecomastia.

Macroscopically, they are well defined tumours, often with cystic areas. Histologically, the appearance depends on the relative amounts of Sertoli cells and stroma (the mesenchyme component). The Sertoli cells may be arranged in tubules, in sheets or in combinations of the two. The stromal component consists of spindle cells similar to those seen in a fibroma.

About 10% of cases behave in a malignant fashion. The remainder are benign with an excellent prognosis.

Lymphoma

Malignant lymphoma may involve the testis and is usually a manifestation of disseminated disease in an elderly patient. Primary lymphoma of the testis also occasionally occurs.

Clinically, the testis is symmetrically enlarged and very firm. The cut surface is homogenous and white or grey in colour. Histologically, there is a diffuse infiltrate of lymphoma cells forming sheets. A few residual seminiferous tubules may be seen. The histological subtype considerably affects prognosis (Turner *et al.* 1981).

Interstitial cell tumour (Leydig cell tumour)

Tumours which arise from the interstitial cells (Leydig cells) of the testis are rare. They occur at all age groups and are most prominent between 20 and 60 years of age.

The typical presentation is with a testicular mass, although endocrine effects are occasionally seen. In children, androgen production gives rise to precocious puberty; in adults, oestrogens tend to predominate and cause gynaecomastia.

Macroscopically, they form a well defined mass which is characteristically yellow/brown in colour. Microscopically, the tumour consists of sheets of plump, polygonal, strongly eosinophilic cells. Within the tumour, seminiferous tubules are absent and this distinguishes the tumour from interstitial cell hyperplasia.

About 10% of these tumours are malignant. The remainder are benign and have a good prognosis. The only conclusive evidence of malignancy is the presence of metastases, although large tumours with necrosis and a high mitotic rate tend to behave in a malignant fashion.

Yolk sac tumour (endodermal sinus tumour)

This is the commonest testicular tumour in childhood. The average age of presentation in the testicular tumour panel series was 17 months. The tumour rarely occurs in adults. Clinically, it presents as a testicular mass, associated with a raised serum level of AFP.

Macroscopically, the tumour is a white or yellow mass which may be cystic with haemorrhagic areas. Histologically, it is similar to an adenocarcinoma with tubular and papillary areas. Thin-walled microcysts are typically seen. A characteristic feature is the presence of Schiller–Duval bodies which are vascular tufts surrounded by cells. Mitotic figures may be numerous (*see Fig.* 10.8).

The tumour invades and destroys the surrounding testis and spreads locally to the epididymis and cord. It metastasizes to the para-aortic nodes.

The prognosis is dependent on the age of presentation. The three year survival rate is 76% for infants under two years of age and 58% for children over two years of age.

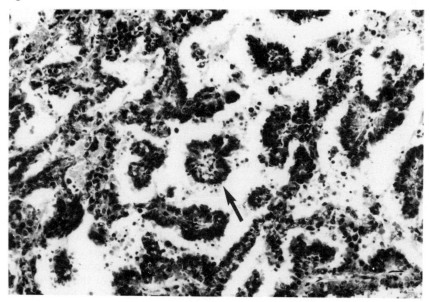

Fig. 10.8. Yolk sac tumour showing Schiller–Duval bodies (arrow). (H and E × 75)

Carcinoma-in-situ of the Testis

Carcinoma-in-situ is being increasingly recognized in testicular biopsies (Blandy and Oliver 1984). The management is controversial. About half of these patients subsequently develop invasive cancer and therefore orchidectomy has been proposed by some surgeons. However, others have pointed out that similar intratubular malignant cells can be found in undescended testes, in the contralateral testis of patients with testicular tumour and in the gonads of intersex patients; they advocate close surveillance rather than immediate orchidectomy. Carcinoma-in-situ has been found in men undergoing testicular biopsy for infertility and this poses a serious treatment problem.

Carcinoma-in-situ occurs commonly in the seminiferous tubules adjacent to both seminomas and non-seminomatous tumours (Jacobsen *et al.* 1981) and it has been suggested that it may be the precursor of malignant germ cell tumours.

Paratesticular Tumours

The adenomatoid tumour is a common benign tumour which presents as a nodule in the epididymis or cord. Grossly, they occasionally penetrate into the testis giving the false impression of malignancy. Histologically, the tumour consists of numerous slit-like spaces, lined by bland flat cells. They are probably of mesothelial origin and are cured by resection.

Malignant epithelial tumours may arise in the rete testis, epididymis or in vestigial structures. They are usually adenocarcinomas.

The commonest paratesticular sarcoma is the embryonal rhabdomyosarcoma which occurs in infants and children. Leiomyosarcomas, fibrosarcomas and other sarcomas occur in older patients.

THE PROSTATE

Normal Structure

The normal adult prostate weighs about 20 g and lies between the bladder neck and the perineal membrane. It contains the posterior urethra which is about 2·5 cm long and is perforated posteriorly by the ejaculatory ducts which enter the urethra at the verumontanum. The prostate is considered to have five lobes, anterior, posterior, median and left and right lateral. In practice, however, only three lobes can be distinguished, a median lobe which lies posteriorly between the urethra and ejaculatory ducts and two lateral lobes which are below and lateral to the median lobe.

McNeal (1972) has suggested that the prostate can be divided into zones as in *Fig.* 10.9. In this concept, the true prostate consists of a central and a peripheral zone. The central zone (of Wolffian origin) surrounds the ejaculatory ducts and the peripheral zone (of urogenital sinus origin) lies distal and peripheral to the central zone. The preprostatic sphincter surrounds the upper part of the urethra and is proximal to the verumontanum. The prostatic ducts develop from buds of urethral epithelium which sprout above and below the level of the verumontanum. Those

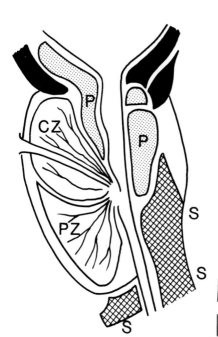

Fig. 10.9. Schematic diagram of prostate: P—pre-prostatic sphincter; CZ—central zone; PZ—peripheral zone; S—external sphincter (From Blacklock 1982; reproduced with permission of the publisher.)

above the verumontanum become the periurethral glands which are incorporated into the preprostatic sphincter. Prostatic ducts from the level of the verumontanum develop in close relationship to the ejaculatory ducts and become incorporated into the central zone. Those arising below the verumontanum become incorporated in the peripheral zone.

Benign nodular hyperplasia of the prostate develops in the periurethral glandular tissue, the central zone is relatively immune from disease and the peripheral zone is the site of origin of most prostatic cancers.

Histologically, the prostate consists of epithelial glands embedded in a fibromuscular stroma. The glands are lined by two layers of epithelium and drain into the excretory ducts which enter the floor of the urethra.

The prostate is supplied by the inferior vesical, internal pudendal and middle rectal arteries. Venous drainage is to the periprostatic venous bed and lymphatic drainage is to hypogastric, sacral, vesical and external iliac nodes.

Prostatic Biopsy

Open biopsy via the perineal or retropubic route is rarely used in the UK. Although it gives the greatest accuracy, the resulting fibrosis makes later surgery difficult.

The Franzen needle aspiration technique gives a sample for cytological diagnosis, but the services of an experienced cytologist are required. Most commonly, a needle biopsy is used and this gives a sample suitable for histological diagnosis. Either a perineal approach or a transrectal technique is used. The transrectal approach has the advantage that the operator can feel suspicious areas per rectum and direct the needle. Complications include bleeding and bacteraemic shock. Bacteraemia after transrectal biopsy occurs in up to 70% of cases and antibiotic cover is required (Thompson *et al.* 1980). Tumour implantation is rare but may occur in the perineal method (Rhind 1980).

At the time of transurethral resection, if tumour is suspected, the chips from the centre and periphery of the prostate should be sent to the laboratory in separate pots so that the adequacy of excision can be assessed (the two pot technique).

Prostatitis

Inflammation of the prostate is classified into acute bacterial prostatitis, chronic bacterial prostatitis, chronic non-bacterial prostatitis and granulomatous prostatitis.

Acute bacterial prostatitis

These patients have the systemic features of infection together with perineal pain and low back pain. Severe irritative and later obstructive urinary symptoms occur. On rectal examination, the prostate is swollen and tender.

The common causative organisms are those that cause urinary tract infections, i.e. *E. coli*, Proteus, Klebsiella, Enterobacteria, Pseudomonas and Serratia. The organism is cultured from a urine specimen as prostatic massage is dangerous in view of the possibility of bacteraemia.

The most likely route of infection is ascending from the urethra with subsequent reflux of urine into the prostatic ducts. Evidence for the latter comes from work which has shown that prostatic calculi contain debris normally found only in urine.

Pathologically, there is a cellulitis followed by the formation of small abscesses. If these coalesce, a prostatic abscess forms which may involve a lobe or the entire gland. Histologically, the gland lumina are filled with acute inflammatory cells and an inflammatory infiltrate is seen in the surrounding stroma.

Chronic bacterial prostatitis

This may follow acute prostatitis or it may arise insidiously. The importance of this condition is that it is the commonest cause of recurrent urinary tract infection in men. The prostate should always be suspected as the source of recurrent urinary tract infections, especially if the same pathogen is involved with each episode. Other than recurrent urinary tract infection, the patient may have referred pain in various areas (suprapubic, perineal, low back, scrotal, penile or inner thigh). On rectal examination, the prostate may be tender or hard like a carcinoma.

Several reasons have been suggested for the persistence of bacteria in the prostate: (1) prostatic calculi may act as foci of infection; (2) the prostatic fluid found in infected prostates is at a higher pH than normal, although this could be a secondary phenomenon; (3) antibiotics commonly used to eradicate urinary tract infections show poor diffusion into the prostatic tissue.

The following method of diagnosis is recommended by Meares (1980). A patient with a full bladder is asked to pass urine. The first 10 ml are collected and labelled 'voided bladder 1' (VB1). A further 200 ml are voided and discarded and then a mid-stream sample is taken and labelled VB2. The prostate is then systematically massaged and the secretions are collected and labelled 'expressed prostatic secre-tions' (EPS). Finally, a 10 ml sample of urine is collected after prostatic massage (VB3). The diagnosis is made by a significantly greater colony count on culturing EPS and VB3 compared with VB1 and VB2.

Histologically, there is an infiltrate of chronic inflammatory cells in the inter-stitium and in the prostatic tubules. Many prostates with simple benign nodular hyperplasia frequently show small foci of chronic inflammatory cells which are considered to be of no significance.

Chronic non-bacterial prostatitis

This has the same clinical features as chronic bacterial prostatitis and the sample collected after prostatic massage shows a high leucocyte count. However, the difference is that bacteria are not cultured. Possible causative agents include Chlamydia and other non-bacterial organisms.

Granulomatous prostatitis

This is divided into a specific type due to such conditions as tuberculosis and a non-specific granulomatous prostatitis which may be autoimmune in nature.

Benign Nodular Hyperplasia (BNH)

Epidemiology, aetiology and pathogenesis

Autopsy studies show that approximately half of all men aged between 40 and 59 years and 95% of those aged over 70 years have benign nodular hyperplasia of the prostate. However, less than 10% require treatment.

The aetiology and pathogenesis are thought to be related to changes in androgen and oestrogen metabolism with age. The main androgen in men is testosterone which is secreted by the testes. Some of the testosterone is metabolized into 5-alpha-dihydrotestosterone (DHT) by peripheral tissues. Plasma oestrogens in the male are derived from the peripheral conversion of testosterone to oestrogen and by direct secretion of oestrogens by the testis and adrenal glands. With advancing age, there is a slight decline in the plasma testosterone but oestrogen concentration either stays the same or rises slightly. Most studies have shown no difference in the plasma levels of testosterone or oestrogen in patients with benign nodular hyperplasia compared with controls. However, it is widely accepted that the concentration of DHT in the prostatic tissue of patients with BNH is markedly increased and this may be responsible for the hyperplasia. The reason for the increased DHT in prostatic tissue in the presence of normal serum levels is unknown, although it may be related to: (1) the relative elevation of plasma oes-trogen levels which increase the concentration of cytoplasmic androgen receptors in the prostate, or (2) a fall in the concentration of the enzymes which metabolize DHT.

Clinical features

The symptoms of frequency, poor stream and nocturia are well known. The sequelae of bladder outlet obstruction include bladder distension, trabeculation, sacculation, stasis and infection with the risk of stone formation. Hydroureter, hydronephrosis and renal failure may eventually occur.

Clinically, there is little correlation between the size of the prostate and the degree of symptomatology and urodynamic studies may be required to confirm that the prostate is the cause of symptoms.

Morphology

Benign nodular hyperplasia involves mainly the periurethral part of the gland and therefore it affects the prostatic urethra at an early stage. The urethra becomes compressed, slit-like and elongated. The surrounding prostatic tissue becomes compressed and forms a false capsule. On rectal examination, the size and consistency can be assessed. If the classical median lobe only is affected, rectal examination is normal. When the lateral lobes are affected, the prostate feels large and rubbery if hyperplasia of the glandular elements predominates, and small and firm if hyperplasia of the stroma predominates. At cysto-urethroscopy, inspection of the prostatic urethra at the level of the verumontanum reveals enlarged lateral lobes. With further advancement, an enlarged median lobe comes into view; it has characteristic vertical markings (the waterfall appearance). An enlarged median lobe may project upwards behind the urethra, in which case it can cause obstruction by a ball-valve effect.

Cut section of the prostatectomy specimen shows the presence of many nodules with surrounding compressed prostatic tissue. There may be a microcystic appearance if glandular proliferation predominates. If stromal proliferation predominates, the gland is firm and solid.

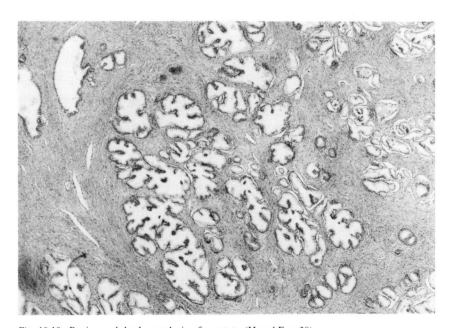

Fig. 10.10. Benign nodular hyperplasia of prostate. (H and E × 30)

Histological examination shows cystically dilated glands arranged in nodules (*see Fig.* 10.10). The glands are lined by two layers of regular cells (unlike malignant glands) and these layers are thrown up into folds. When hyperplasia of the stroma predominates, fibrous tissue and smooth muscle are seen with infrequent glands. Areas of squamous metaplasia, infarction and chronic inflammation are commonly seen.

Prognosis

It is estimated that 10% of men over the age of 40 years will require a prostatectomy. Over 90% of prostates can be resected transurethrally with a mortality of less than 0·5% (Habib and Luck 1983). Mortality from open prostatectomy rises from 1% to 3% if there is associated poor renal function or infection (Singh *et al.* 1973).

Prostatic Cancer

Terminology

A 'clinical' prostatic cancer is one which gives rise to prostatic symptoms. An 'occult' cancer is one in which only metastatic disease is symptomatic. A 'latent' cancer is an unsuspected one found at autopsy. An 'incidental' cancer is one found incidentally during histological examination of a prostate removed for BNH. The terms 'latent' and 'incidental' were formerly synonymous but now have different meanings.

Epidemiology

Cancer of the prostate is the fourth commonest cause of death from malignancy in UK males, accounting for approximately 4000 deaths annually. Latent prostatic cancer is very common and is found in up to 30% of cases at autopsy. The disease primarily affects males who are over 50 years of age. Prostatic cancer is less common in Orientals than Caucasians (Franks 1973). Native Japanese and Japanese immigrants in Hawaii have an equal incidence of latent prostatic cancer. The latter group, however, have a much higher mortality from prostatic cancer, approaching that of Caucasians in Hawaii. The reason may be that although latent cancer occurs in all races, environmental factors which promote its growth vary with location.

Aetiology

Workers in industries which use cadmium have a higher incidence of prostatic cancer than normal. Otherwise little is known of the aetiology. The relationship between androgen hormones and prostatic cancer is unclear. Eunuchs do not develop the disease and in normal men it can be controlled by castration or oestrogen therapy. This would suggest a role for androgens in the pathogenesis, although it appears likely that androgens merely maintain the prostatic epithelium so that sufficient cells are present for malignant change to occur.

A prospective study of 800 patients with benign nodular hyperplasia and a similar number of controls showed no association with prostatic carcinoma (Greenwald *et al.* 1974).

Clinical features

Since prostatic cancer arises in the peripheral zones of the prostate, it gives rise to urinary obstruction late in the disease process. Invasion through the rectal mucosa may cause confusion with a primary rectal carcinoma.

Normal and malignant prostatic epithelium both produce acid phosphatase. Using standard methods of assay, this is usually only elevated in the serum of patients in whom the tumour has extended beyond the capsule or has metastasized (although it may be raised in patients with very large benign glands). Prostatic acid phosphatase can be distinguished in the laboratory from other acid phosphatases (e.g. that present in red blood cells) by the fact that it is inhibited by L-tartrate.

New radioimmunoassays for prostatic acid phosphatase can detect smaller tumours localized to the prostate, although the use of this method for screening purposes has been criticized.

The use of digital examination is limited in the diagnosis of prostatic cancer since only about one-half of palpable nodules are cancers, the remainder being benign nodular hyperplasia, infarcts, calculi and prostatitis. Conversely, many palpably normal prostates do contain tumour. Rectal examination does not appear to affect serum acid phosphatase levels (Bannerjee *et al.* 1979).

Morphology

On sectioning the prostatectomy specimen (in the few cases in which open prostatectomy is carried out) the cancer is detected as an area which is firm and gritty compared with the surrounding tissue. It may be seen invading the prostatic capsule or surrounding tissues, such as the seminal vesicles, bladder or rectum.

Histologically, the majority of prostatic cancers are adenocarcinomas and arise from the acini of the peripheral zone of the gland. The better differentiated tumours are difficult to distinguish from normal prostatic tissue. However, in the tumour area, the regular acinar arrangement of prostatic glands is disturbed as malignant glands are distributed in a haphazard fashion. They tend to be close together with little intervening stroma (the so-called 'back-to-back' pattern). The diagnosis is confirmed if perineural invasion can be seen. A high power view of the malignant prostatic glands shows that the cells have larger than normal nuclei and that the normal regular double cell layer is replaced by a single cell layer. In less well differentiated cases (*see Fig.* 10.11), the acini are poorly formed and areas of sheeting of cells or areas showing a cribriform pattern are seen.

A small portion of prostatic carcinomas are transitional cell in type. They arise in the major prostatic ducts, the distal parts of which are lined by transitional epithelium. They may be confused with spread from a transitional cell tumour of the bladder. The main clinical implication is that they do not respond to hormonal treatment.

Endometrial carcinomas have been described in the prostate. They arise in Müllerian remnants and histologically resemble endometrial carcinomas of the female uterus. Usually they do not metastasize.

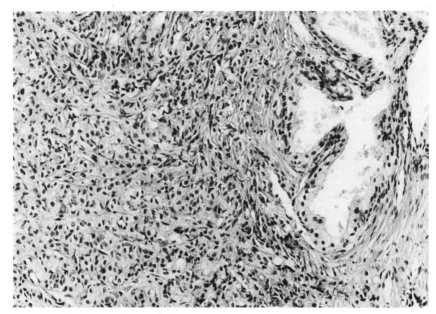

Fig. 10.11. Carcinoma of prostate. There are normal prostatic glands to the right and an area of poorly differentiated carcinoma to the left. (H and E × 75)

Spread

Direct spread outside the capsule occurs into the seminal vesicles, bladder or rectum. Involvement of the ureters may cause urinary obstruction. Lymphatic spread is to nodes along the internal and common iliac arteries and to the para-aortic nodes. Bony metastases are seen in the pelvis, lumbosacral spine and long bones. They are classically osteosclerotic in type.

Staging and prognosis

Staging in the UK is commonly by the TNM system. The T category is assessed by clinical examination, urography, endoscopy and bimanual palpation. CT scanning aids assessment of pelvic nodes and has largely superseded lymphangiography. The M status is assessed by serum acid phosphatase, chest X-ray and bone scan. The TNM system is shown in *Table* 10.3.

The prognosis depends on the histological grading as well as the stage. The Gleeson system of histological grading is commonly used. This divides prostatic cancers into five grades based on a spectrum ranging from small uniform glands (grade 1) to infiltrating anaplastic tumours (grade 5). The higher the grade, the worse the prognosis.

Few clinicians in the UK give any further treatment for an 'incidental' carcinoma found at transurethral resection. Several studies have shown that the life expectancy for patients with an incidental carcinoma found at transurethral resection is the same as for the general population of the same age, even if no treatment is given.

Table 10.3. TNM classification of prostatic cancer

Tis	—	Pre-invasive carcinoma (carcinoma-in-situ).
T0	—	No tumour palpable. Incidental finding at operation or biopsy.
T1	—	Intracapsular tumour surrounded by palpably normal gland.
T2	—	Tumour confined to gland. Smooth nodule deforming the gland contour but lateral sulci and seminal vesicles not involved.
T3	—	Tumour extending beyond the capsule with or without the involvement of the lateral sulci or seminal vesicles.
T4	—	Fixed tumour, or infiltration of adjacent structure.
N0	—	No evidence of regional node involvement.
N1	—	Single homolateral regional lymph node.
N2	—	Contralateral or bilateral node involvement or multiple regional nodes affected.
N3	—	Fixed regional nodes.
N4	—	Involved juxta-regional nodes.
M0	—	No distant metastases.
M1	—	Distant metastases.

For advanced disease, an attempt is made to control the disease by oestrogen therapy or orchidectomy. About 20% of patients will not respond to hormone manipulation and of the responders, half relapse within two years. Overall, for advanced disease treated by hormone manipulation, 10% survive for less than one year, 50% survive less than three years and very few are alive after ten years.

THE PENIS AND SCROTUM

Normal Structure

The penis consists of two corpora cavernosa and a corpus spongiosum which contains the urethra. The corpora are capped distally by the glans. Each corpus is enclosed in a fascial sheath (tunica albuginea) and all are surrounded by a fascial envelope—Buck's fascia. The proximal ends of the corpora cavernosa are attached to the pelvic bones while the corpus spongiosum is connected to the undersurface of the perineal membrane through which emerges the membranous urethra.

Histologically, the corpora and glans are composed of smooth muscle septa and erectile tissue enclosing vascular cavities. The urethral mucosa is formed of squamous epithelium distally and transitional epithelium proximally. The urethral submucosa contains connective tissue, elastic tissue, smooth muscle and numerous glands of Littré, the ducts of which drain into the urethral lumen. The penis and urethra are supplied by the internal pudendal arteries. Lymphatic drainage from the skin of the penis is to the superficial inguinal nodes while lymphatics from the glans pass to both inguinal and external iliac nodes.

The scrotum consists of skin, dartos muscle and three layers of fascia. Beneath these is the parietal layer of the tunica vaginalis. Lymphatics drain to the inguinal nodes.

Congenital and Developmental Abnormalities

Congenital absence is rare and in these cases the urethra opens on the perineum. Megalopenis is rare and occurs in boys suffering from an interstitial cell tumour of the testis or hyperplasia or tumour of the adrenal cortex. Micropenis is seen in male intersex and is associated with hypospadias.

Congenital stenosis of the external meatus, if severe, may cause dilatation of the entire proximal urinary tract and death from uraemia has been recorded. Congenital urethral stricture occasionally occurs in male infants. The two most common sites are the coronal region (fossa navicularis) and in the membranous urethra. Back pressure causes dilatation of the urethra, hypertrophy of bladder muscle and hydronephrosis. Symptoms arise from either obstruction or secondary infection. Rarely, congenital phimosis causes urinary obstruction.

Posterior urethral valves

A posterior urethral valve is a pair of mucosal folds attached to the verumontanum and anterior wall of the membranous urethra. They form an oblique diaphragm which acts as a one-way valve, similar to the valves in a vein. They are a common cause of urethral obstruction in young boys and, since they act as one-way valves, may be missed on endoscopy. Most present under one year (Williams *et al.* 1973) and diagnosis is made by voiding cystography. The posterior urethra dilates and elongates; the bladder is usually distended and hypertrophied with trabeculation; infection and chronic renal failure may ensue. Treatment requires resection of the valves.

Anterior urethral valves have been occasionally reported and may present with leakage of urine, enuresis and impairment of stream.

Urethral diverticulum

This can occur in either the posterior or anterior urethra. The former represents dilatation of the prostatic utricle while the latter occurs at the penoscrotal junction. The distal tip of the diverticulum may produce urinary obstruction as it fills during micturition.

Urethral duplication

This rare condition may be associated with two bladders and penises. When isolated, the abnormality occurs dorsal to the normal urethra and opens onto the dorsum of the glans. The proximal end may open into the bladder or end as a sinus. It is associated with chordee (*see* below).

Epispadias

This is rare (1 in 30 000 males); the urethra opens on the dorsum of the penis proximal to the glans, usually at the abdomino-penile junction. The condition is associated with dorsal chordee. There may be a defect in the urinary sphincters causing incontinence and the pubic bones may be separated.

Hypospadias

This occurs in one in 500 boys and is due to failure of development of the distal urethra which is replaced by fibrous tissue. The contraction of the latter causes bowing of the penis (chordee) and there is often associated meatal stenosis. Hypospadias is classified according to the site of the meatus into glandular, coronal, penile, penoscrotal and perineal. In severe forms, the scrotum is bifid. There is a high incidence of cryptorchidism and in these cases chromosomal sex should be determined.

Peyronie's Disease

In this condition, firm cords, nodules or plaques of dense fibrous tissue form in the corpora cavernosa, the midline septum or the fascia of the penis (plastic induration of the penis). The cause is unknown but it is related to Dupuytren's contracture and plantar fasciitis. Clinically, the patients complain of painful curvature of the penis on erection. Usually the dorsal surface is affected. Histologically, dense, acellular fibrous tissue is seen without an inflammatory infiltrate. Later, hyaline degeneration, calcification and ossification may occur. An autoimmune aetiology has been suggested and treatment with corticosteroids locally or systemically has been tried (Chesney 1975). However, progressive disease is uncommon and improvement or resolution occurs in some patients over several years (Mira 1980).

Priapism

This is persistent painful penile erection unrelated to sexual stimulation. Only the corpora cavernosa are involved and therefore urination is possible. Primary priapism occurs in young men and may be due to venous thrombosis. It may be secondary to obstruction of the dorsal vein of the penis which can occur as a result of muscle contraction in certain neurological disorders. Reflex muscle contraction also occurs in inflammatory or neoplastic lesions of the penis. Alternatively, venous drainage may be obstructed by thrombosis, in leukaemia or sickle cell disease, or by inflammatory or neoplastic lesions.

Fournier's Gangrene

Fournier's gangrene is a rare condition which most commonly affects men in the fourth and fifth decades. Clinically, there is a sudden onset of marked oedema of the scrotum which rapidly progresses to gangrene of the skin. The entire scrotum is soon involved and the patient is systemically ill.

The infection is usually caused by mixed organisms, particularly a combination of anaerobic Streptococci and *Bacteroides fragilis*. There is frequently a cutaneous vascular thrombosis and some authors have suggested that this is the primary aetiological event. One review of scrotal abscesses found that 90% contained anaerobic organisms, mainly types originating as commensals in the oropharynx and genital tract (Whitehead *et al.* 1982). Diabetes, local trauma, local surgical procedures, perianal abscesses and lower urinary tract infections have all been associated with Fournier's gangrene.

Histologically, there is active cellulitis with an inflammatory cell infiltrate. Coagulative necrosis, extensive thrombosis and obliterative endarteritis are typical. Appropriate antibiotic therapy with excision of dead tissue is required. Mortality is about 10% (Jones *et al.* 1979).

Cancer of the Penis

This is a rare disease in the USA and UK but is common in Uganda and Mexico. It occurs in the 40–70 year age group and more commonly in lower than upper social groups. Circumcision seems to be important in its prevention and the incidence is low among Jews. Retention of smegma beneath the prepuce is probably a factor. In animal studies, smegma can be shown to be carcinogenic and of interest is the fact that carcinoma of the cervix is significantly more common in the wives of uncircumcized men. Cancer of the penis is associated with poor penile hygiene (Hoppmann and Fraley 1978).

Several conditions predispose to carcinoma of the penis. Erythroplasia of Queyrat is seen clinically as a shiny red plaque on the glans or prepuce. Histologically, there is a dysplastic epithelium with an underlying dermal inflammatory infiltrate. The epithelial changes range from mild dysplasia to carcinoma-in-situ (which is difficult to distinguish from Bowen's disease). About 10–20% progress to squamous carcinoma. Bowen's disease may occur on the penis (*see* p. 501) and about 5% of cases develop squamous carcinoma. Some authorities maintain that there is an association with visceral malignancy. Multiple areas of Bowen's disease are termed Bowenoid papulosis (Wade *et al.* 1978) and appear as innocent looking papules. Leukoplakia similar to that seen in the mouth (*see* p. 4) may also occur on the penis.

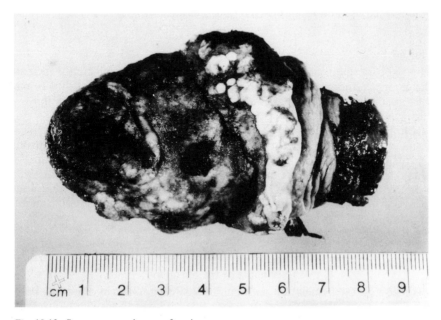

Fig. 10.12. Squamous carcinoma of penis.

Symptoms of carcinoma of the penis include foul discharge, pain and difficulty in micturition. Grossly, an infiltrating ulcerated or nodular lesion is situated most often on the glans (*see Fig.* 10.12). It rarely arises from the external surface of the shaft of the penis. Histologically, it is usually a moderately well differentiated squamous carcinoma. Local invasion into the corpora cavernosa occurs early but invasion of the corpus spongiosum and urethra occurs late. Inguinal lymph nodes are enlarged in 80% of cases due to infection and only about half of these contain tumour. Vascular spread is via the prostatic plexuses, pelvic veins and vertebral plexus. Four stages have been proposed (*see Table* 10.4).

Stage I disease has a median survival of 10 years; Stage II, 7 years; Stage III, 2–5 years; Stage IV, 2–5 months (Merrin 1980).

Table 10.4. Staging of carcinoma of the penis

I	— Tumour confined to the glans and/or prepuce.
II	— Tumour invasion of the shaft or corpora. No node or distant metastases.
III	— Tumour of the shaft with regional lymphatic spread.
IV	— Inoperable regional nodes and/or distant metastases.

Tumours of the Urethra

Papillomatosis

Solitary papillomas are rare but multiple lesions are not uncommon. Two types occur: (1) in association with papillary transitional cell tumours of the bladder, and (2) an extension of 'venereal warts' of the glans and prepuce. The latter are squamous in nature and probably viral in origin.

Carcinoma

Patients who develop carcinoma of the bladder have a significantly increased incidence of carcinoma of the urethra. The lesion is probably another primary tumour arising in unstable epithelium, although a secondary implantation from bladder cancer cannot always be excluded.

Carcinoma of the urethra may arise *de novo*, without bladder cancer, but it is rare. It occurs in patients over 50 years old; gonorrhoea and strictures may predispose. The growth is initially papillary but later it ulcerates. Histologically, most are squamous carcinomas. A few transitional carcinomas and adenocarcinomas occur.

Tumours in the anterior urethra spread by lymphatics to the inguinal nodes, while lesions in the posterior urethra spread to iliac nodes. Anterior lesions treated by amputation and block dissection of inguinal nodes have a better prognosis than posterior urethral lesions.

Carcinoma of the Scrotum

This is rare and the association with chimney sweeps noted by Percivall Pott in 1775 is well known. Soot adheres to greasy skin and its rugosity makes cleansing difficult. Lubricating oils used by male spinners and tar and pitch have also been implicated as aetiological factors. It is a disease of the elderly, although occupational cases occur in men in their sixth decade. The lesion may be ulcerated, nodular or papillary and becomes secondarily infected. It spreads locally to the inguinal nodes. Blood spread is rare. Histologically, most are moderately well differentiated squamous carcinomas.

References

Bannerjee S. K., Barker I. F., Waterworth T. A. (1979) Does rectal examination affect serum acid phosphatase levels? *Br. J. Surg.* **66**, 512–13.

Blacklock N. J. (1982) The prostate: surgical anatomy. In: Chisholm G. D., Williams D. I. (eds.), *Scientific Foundations of Urology,* 2nd ed. London, Heinemann Medical.

Blandy J. P., Oliver R. T. D. (1984) Cancer of the testis. *Br. J. Surg.* **71**, 962–3.

Bullock K. N., Hunt J. M. (1981) The intravenous urogram in acute epididymo-orchitis. *Br. J. Urol.* **53**, 47–9.

Chapman R. H., Walton A. J. (1972) Torsion of the testis and its appendages. *Br. Med. J.* **1**, 164–6.

Chesney J. (1975) Peyronie's disease. *Br. J. Urol.* **47**, 209–18.

Fraley E. E., Lange P. H., Kennedy B. J. (1979) Germ-cell testicular cancer in adults (Pt. 1). *N. Engl. J. Med.* **301**, 1370–7.

Franks L. M., (1973) Etiology, epidemiology, and pathology of prostatic cancer. *Cancer* **32**, 1092–5.

Greenwald P., Kirmss V., Polan A. K., Dick V. S. (1974) Cancer of the prostate among men with benign prostatic hyperplasia. *J. Natl. Cancer. Inst.* **53**, 335–40.

Habib N. A., Luck R. J. (1983) Results of transurethral resection of the benign prostate. *Br. J. Surg.* **70**, 218–19.

Hoppmann H. J., Fraley E. E. (1978) Squamous cell carcinoma of the penis. *J. Urol.* **120**, 393–8.

Jacobsen G. K., Henriksen O. B., Der Maase H. V. (1981) Carcinoma-in-situ of testicular tissue adjacent to malignant germ cell tumours: a study of 105 cases. *Cancer* **47**, 2660–2.

Jones R. B., Hirschmann J. V., Brown G. S., Tremann J. A. (1979) Fournier's syndrome: necrotizing subcutaneous infection of the male genitalia. *J. Urol.* **122**, 279–82.

Lipshultz L. I., Caminos-Torres R., Greenspan C. S., Snyder P. J. (1976) Testicular function after orchidopexy for unilaterally undescended testis. *N. Engl. J. Med.* **295**, 15–18.

McNeal J. E. (1972) The prostate and prostatic urethra: a morphologic synthesis. *J. Urol.* **107**, 1008–16.

Meares E. M. (1980) Prostatitis syndromes: new perspectives about old woes. *J. Urol.* **123**, 141–7.

Medical Research Council Working Party on Testicular Tumours (1985) Prognostic factors in advanced non-seminomatous germ-cell testicular tumours: results of a multicentric study. *Lancet* **1**, 8–11.

Merrin C. E. (1980) Cancer of the penis. *Cancer* **45**, 1973–9.

Mira J. G. (1980) Is it worthwhile to treat Peyronie's disease? *Urology* **16**, 1–6.

Oliver R. T. D. (1984) Testis cancer. *Br. J. Hosp. Med.* **1**, 23–35.

Peckham M. J. (1981) *The management of Testicular Tumours.* London, Edward Arnold.

Pelouze P. S. (1931) *Gonorrhoea in the Male and Female,* 2nd ed. Philadelphia, W. B. Saunders.

Pugh R. C. B. (ed.) (1976) *Pathology of the Testis.* Oxford, Blackwell Scientific Publications.

Rhind J. R. (1980) Prostatic biopsy. *Br. Med. J.* **281**, 722–3.

Scorer C. G. (1964) The descent of the testis. *Arch. Dis. Child.* **39**, 605–9.

Scorer C. G., Farrington G. H. (1971) *Congenital Deformities of the Testis and Epididymis.* London, Butterworth.

Singh M., Tresidder G. C., Blandy J. P. (1973) The evaluation of transurethral resection for benign enlargement of the prostate. *Br. J. Urol.* **45**, 93–102.

Thomas W. E. G., Cooper M. J., Crane G. A., Lee G., Williamson R. C. N. (1984) Testicular exocrine malfunction after torsion. *Lancet* **2**, 1357–9.

Thompson P. M., Talbot R. W., Packham D. A., Dulake C. (1980) Transrectal biopsy of the prostate and bacteraemia. *Br. J. Surg.* **67**, 127–8.

Turner R. R., Colby T. V., Mackintosh F. R. (1981) Testicular lymphomas: a clinicopathologic study of 35 cases. *Cancer* **48**, 2095–102.

Turner T. T. (1983) Varicocoele: still an enigma. *J. Urol.* **129**, 695–9.

Wade T. R., Kopf A. W., Ackerman A. B. (1978) Bowenoid papulosis of the penis. *Cancer* **42**, 1890–1903.

Werder E. A., Illig R., Torresani T. (1976) *et al.* Gonadal function in young adults after surgical treatment of cryptorchidism. *Br. Med. J.* **2**, 1357–9.

Whitehead S. M., Leach R. D., Eykyn S. J., Philips I. (1982) The aetiology of perirectal sepsis. *Br. J. Surg.* **69**, 166–8.

Williams D. I., Whitaker R. H., Barrat T. M., Keeton J. E. (1973) Urethral valves. *Br. J. Urol.* **45**, 200–10.

Chapter 11

The Breast

Normal Structure

The normal adult female breast consists of 10–15 segments. Distally each segment consists of a number of small lobules. These drain into ductules which, in turn, join subsegmental ducts at approximately right angles. The subsegmental ducts drain into segmental ducts which, just below the nipple, dilate to form lactiferous sinuses. The lactiferous sinuses open onto the nipple via the collecting ducts. Each lobule consists of a series of epithelial acini embedded in a specialized loose and vascular connective tissue. A lobule together with a draining ductule constitutes a terminal duct lobular unit (*see Fig.* 11.1).

A small part of the ductal system close to the nipple is lined by keratinizing stratified squamous epithelium and the remainder has a two cell type of lining. The inner (luminal) cell type is a cuboidal or columnar epithelial cell. Wedged between the inner layer and the basement membrane are the myoepithelial cells which are smaller and slightly spindle shaped. The identification of these two cell types in any lesion is an indicator that it is benign, whereas in malignant conditions only one cell type proliferates.

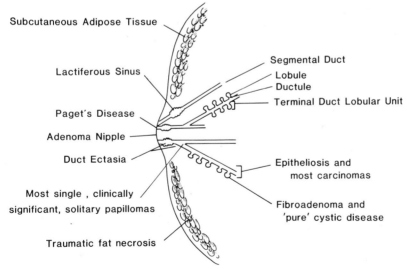

Fig. 11.1. General structure of female breast with the position of some pathological conditions. (Adapted from Azzopardi 1979.)

Before puberty the breast consists only of ducts without lobules. The lobules decline rapidly in number after the menopause.

Fibroadenomas and most cysts arise in the breast lobules. Epitheliosis and carcinomas commonly arise in the smaller ducts while papillary tumours arise in the larger ducts. Duct ectasia affects the large ducts (*see also Fig.* 11.1).

Breast Biopsy

A sample of tissue may be taken from a breast lump, either preoperatively or at the time of operation.

Preoperative biopsy

This may be carried out by aspiration cytology or by biopsy (e.g. Tru-cut needle biopsy or drill biopsy). It is essential that there should be no false positive diagnoses made, as this could lead to unnecessarily radical surgery. False negative results are more acceptable as it is essential to go on to open operative biopsy if a negative result is obtained.

Aspiration cytology may be carried out using a disposable 10 or 20 ml syringe and a fine needle (21–23 swg). After cleaning the skin, the lump is held by the finger and thumb of one hand and the needle is passed into the lump with the other. Local anaesthetic is not necessary. Negative pressure is created in the syringe by partially retracting the plunger. The tip of the needle is then passed back and forwards through the lump several times while, at the same time, rotating the needle. Cells are cut from the lesion by the rotating needle tip and sucked into the needle. The plunger is then gently released and the needle withdrawn. The syringe is disconnected from the needle, filled with air, reconnected and the contents of the needle gently squirted onto a microscope slide. If necessary, the tissue can be teased out or spread like a blood film to give a more even appearance. The slide is then waved in the air until dry and sent for staining.

The slide is only reported as malignant if there is complete certainty. All other slides are reported as negative or suspicious of malignancy, in which case excision biopsy is recommended. Gardecki *et al.* (1980) carried out aspiration cytology on 444 patients and were accurate in 80% to 90% of cases with no false positives. As in most other centres, they carried out definitive surgery if the report was positive and excision biopsy if the report was negative.

Trucut needle biopsy and drill biopsy, give an accuracy rate of 75–80% and false positives are rare. Small lesions are difficult to biopsy accurately and most false negatives are due to a failure to obtain a representative piece of tissue.

Operative biopsy

Operative biopsy is carried out in order to obtain a diagnosis, either intraoperatively (by frozen section) or postoperatively (by routine paraffin section). Frozen section diagnosis gives a very low false positive rate ($< 0.2\%$) but the false negative rate is up to 3% (Holaday and Assor 1974). For this reason, frozen section reports are normally followed up by a definitive diagnosis using routine paraffin sections, regardless of what action might be taken at the time of operation.

There is a growing fashion to perform excision biopsy with frozen section diagnosis, but without proceeding to definitive treatment at the time of the operation. This provides an opportunity for early discussion of the treatment options with the patient, on the basis of a definite diagnosis, and avoids the uncertainty of undergoing anaesthesia without knowledge of the outcome.

Congenital Abnormalities

Absence of the breast is termed amazia. This may be unilateral or bilateral and is sometimes associated with the absence of the sternal portion of the pectoralis major muscle. It is more common in males. Accessory breasts, or polymazia, most frequently occur in the axilla although they have been reported in the groin and thigh. They may function during lactation. Absence of a nipple is rare and usually associated with amazia. Supernumerary nipples may occur along the milk line from the anterior fold of the axilla to the fold of the groin.

Inflammatory Conditions

Breast abscess

These usually occur during the reproductive years, often as a complication of breast feeding. In the puerperium, milk engorgement becomes secondarily infected, through a cracked nipple, with skin organisms, usually a penicillin resistant *Staph. aureus*. Although, initially, there is a diffuse mastitis, a multiloculated abscess usually forms with pain, induration and fluctuation.

A breast abscess may also arise as a complication of mammary duct ectasia, probably as a result of blockage of the lactiferous ducts by debris (*see* p. 294).

Clinically, it is important to distinguish a breast abscess from inflammatory breast carcinoma (*see* p. 311). In all cases of breast abscess it is recommended that a biopsy be taken from the wall at the time of drainage. During the drainage of a breast abscess it is important that all loculi are broken down in order to provide complete drainage and prevent recurrence.

Retromammary abscess

This is a rare form of chronic abscess which occurs behind the deep fascia of the breast. Classically, it is due to empyema or tuberculosis of an underlying rib. It is usually drained through an incision which follows the junction of the inferior aspect of the breast with the chest wall.

Tuberculosis

Tuberculosis of the breast is exceedingly rare and may present as a breast lump or as multiple chronic abscesses with sinus formation. The condition is usually associated with pulmonary tuberculosis. Histologically, the classical caseating tuberculous granulomas are seen. Recently, increasing numbers of cases have been reported, mainly in Asian women. The condition may be confused with a carcinoma, especially when fibrosis is a significant feature, or with a simple breast abscess. Apps *et al.* (1984) recommended that specimens be sent for culture of tubercle bacilli in all cases of breast abscesses occurring in Asian women.

Actinomycosis

This is rare. Chronic abscesses, sinuses and a bluish discolouration of the skin are typical. It normally responds to penicillin.

Granulomatous mastitis

This is a condition of unknown aetiology in which granulomas confined to breast lobules occur. It affects parous women during childbearing age. Clinically, it presents as an extra-areolar breast lump which is often confused with a carcinoma. No infective agent has as yet been identified. Treatment with steroids has been used to good effect in some patients (De Hertogh *et al.* 1980).

Mammary duct ectasia

The two cardinal features of mammary duct ectasia are dilatation of ducts and periductal inflammation. Commonly the large ducts are involved.

Aetiology and pathogenesis

It is not clear whether the dilatation or the inflammation is the initiating event. Inflammation around the major ducts, possibly on an autoimmune basis, may be the first event leading eventually to ductal dilatation. Alternatively, the initial event may be duct blockage, which leads to inflammation as a result of the duct contents leaking through a duct wall which has been damaged at the time of suckling. Duct ectasia is more common in parous women who suckled their infants than in either nulliparous women or parous women who did not suckle their infants. An inverted nipple is commonly present and may contribute to duct blockage or may be the result of fibrosis beneath the nipple.

Clinical features

The condition may present with a yellow or green nipple discharge and is one of the two common benign causes of nipple discharge, the other being intraduct papilloma. In some cases, the presentation is as a breast abscess sited near the nipple. Other cases mimic carcinoma, even to the extent of tethering and *peau d'orange*. Recurrent abscesses and/or fistulas (mamillary fistulas) may form around the nipple and in the later stages, contraction of periductal fibrous tissue may cause nipple inversion. Although duct ectasia is common in older women, the more acute inflammatory lesions are often seen in younger women.

Pathology

A variable number of ducts in one or both breasts may be affected. The dilated ducts may be palpable as irregular cord-like structures. On sectioning, the ducts are dilated and contain a cheesy debris.

On microscopy, the dilatation of ducts is confirmed. They contain debris and, characteristically, foamy lipid-laden cells. The lining epithelium may only remain in small foci. Surrounding the ducts is periductal inflammation, the features of which depend on the stage of the disease. Plasma cells are often prominent (thus the alternative term of plasma cell mastitis). Eventually the ducts become filled with fibrous plugs and may become completely obliterated, although attempted recanalization is sometimes seen. If mamillary fistulas develop they lead from the lactiferous ducts to the margins of the areola.

Since the disease is confined to ducts and periductal tissue, Hadfield (1976) recommends treatment by excision of the major ductal system.

Mondor's disease

This is a self-limiting, superficial thrombophlebitis which affects the superficial veins of the breasts and lasts about 6–8 weeks. It usually affects the thoraco-epigastric vein which runs from the hypochondrium to the axilla. It presents as a tender palpable cord which typically grooves the skin when the arm is raised. Biopsy is unnecessary and treatment is symptomatic.

Trauma

Haematoma

Injury to the breast may give rise to a deep haematoma which causes a lump without overlying bruising. Clinically, differentiation from a carcinoma may be difficult, particularly in long-standing cases when calcification occurs and the lump becomes hard.

Fat necrosis

This condition typically occurs in obese middle-aged women, usually following direct injury but occasionally after vigorous contraction of the pectoralis major muscle. A painless lump appears which may be difficult to distinguish from carcinoma. Grossly, dimpling of the skin may be present and on sectioning the lump, chalky white necrotic fat is seen. The lesion excites an inflammatory response in which many giant cells are seen.

Fibrocystic Disease

Terminology

Fibrocystic disease is a condition in which cyst formation, fibrosis, adenosis and epitheliosis occur in various combinations. Azzopardi (1979) uses the term 'cystic disease' when cysts alone are present and 'cystic hyperplasia' when cysts occur in combination with epithelial hyperplasia (either adenosis, epitheliosis or both). Fibrosis is commonly seen but is not essential for the diagnosis. Fibroadenosis is an alternative and widely used name for the overall condition. Other names such as mazoplasia, mastopathy and mammary dysplasia are now considered unsatisfactory.

Aetiology

The cause of fibrocystic disease is uncertain but many authorities consider it to be due to a 'hormonal imbalance' because the disease occurs only between the menarche and menopause. Two possibilities have been suggested.

1. OESTROGEN PROGESTERONE IMBALANCE: During each menstrual cycle, oestrogen production prior to ovulation causes epithelial proliferation and progesterone production after ovulation causes stromal proliferation. An imbalance between these two hormones could result in structural changes, particularly if oestrogen activity is unopposed by progesterone. Such an event may arise during anovulatory cycles, in which case there is no progesterone production. Anovulatory cycles occur commonly at the time of the menarche and at the time of the menopause. Similarly, patients who have an inadequate corpus luteum may be unable to synthesize normal quantities of progesterone. However, no evidence is available that proves that patients with fibrocystic disease have reduced progesterone production.

2. HYPERPROLACTINAEMIA: Patients with hyperprolactinaemia are known to develop galactorrhoea due to stimulation of breast tissue and prolactin has been incriminated as a cause of fibrocystic disease. Again, no definite link has been proven.

Clinical features

Fibrocystic disease presents to the surgeon in three main ways; (1) a breast cyst which may seem on palpation to be single but which is in fact often associated with other smaller cysts; (2) a dominant solid lump in a nodular breast which on biopsy has various combinations of small cysts, fibrosis, adenosis and epitheliosis; (3) breast pain (mastalgia) which may be unilateral or bilateral.

Morphology

Breast cysts may be small but are sometimes 5 cm or more in diameter. Before opening, they appear brown or blue (blue-domed cyst of Bloodgood) due to the contained fluid. On opening, the presence of a smooth, glistening lining, devoid of outgrowth, confirms a simple cyst rather than a cystadenocarcinoma.

A dominant lump occurring in fibrocystic disease will vary in macroscopic appearance depending on its contents. On cut section, it does not show the long prolongations of infiltration seen at the edges of a carcinoma. If fibrous tissue is present, it may be hard but is not gritty on cutting, while areas of sclerosing adenosis (*see* below) are firm and rubbery. The presence of multiple small cysts in a breast lump is reassuring that it is benign (*see Fig.* 11.2). Close inspection of the cut surface may reveal small pink areas of epithelium but the chalky or yellow streaks which are characteristic of carcinoma do not occur.

Cysts, adenosis, epitheliosis and fibrosis are seen in varying proportions on histological examination.

CYSTS: The cyst lining is often of apocrine type (large cells with eosinophilic granular cytoplasm), although it may be attenuated or even absent. Sometimes the cyst ruptures causing first an inflammatory and, later, a fibrous reaction in the wall,

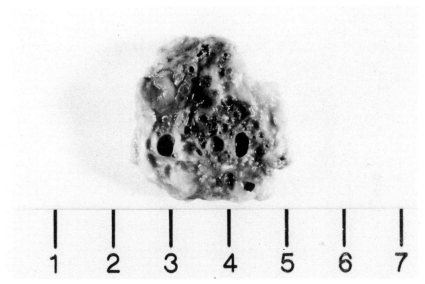

Fig. 11.2. Fibrocystic disease. The presence of many small cysts is reassuring that the lesion is benign.

making distinction from duct ectasia difficult. Cysts arise in breast lobules due to obstruction of the draining ductules. The obstruction may be due to epitheliosis or to kinking of ductules.

ADENOSIS: This refers to an increase in the size and/or number of lobular acini. Two main types are seen.

1. Blunt duct adenosis in which there is dilatation and increase in the size of the acini. The outlines of the acini are blunt as opposed to the angular irregularity seen in the glands of a carcinoma. The two cell layer comprising epithelial and myoepithelial cells is well preserved and thus the condition is benign. It usually does not give rise to palpable lumps.
2. Sclerosing adenosis in which there is proliferation of acini together with stromal proliferation and fibrosis. The fibrous tissue may compress the acini obliterating their lumina and giving an appearance similar to carcinoma. However, low power scanning of the section shows that, unlike carcinoma, the tissue is still arranged in lobules (*see Fig.* 11.3).

The so-called 'radial scar' is now recognized as an entity and is a variant of sclerosing adenosis. It consists of a central zone of dense fibrous tissue which is surrounded by radially distributed epithelial hyperplasia. On macroscopic examination it may appear similar to an infiltrating carcinoma. It is considered benign although it may have a pre-malignant potential.

EPITHELIOSIS: This is characterized by a proliferation of both epithelial and myoepithelial cells within the ductal system. Usually the small ducts are affected.

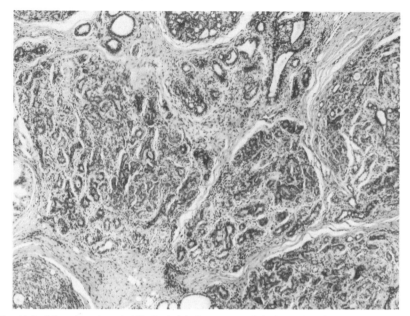

Fig. 11.3. Sclerosing adenosis. The basic lobular pattern of the breast is still discernible. (H and E × 30)

The lesion may partly or completely fill the duct lumina. The term 'papillomatosis' is used by American pathologists to describe this condition but in the United Kingdom, epitheliosis is preferred since true papillomas are not found. Since two cell types proliferate, the appearance can be variable with areas of spindle cells (probably of myoepithelial origin) and areas of rounded cells (epithelial cells). The condition may be difficult to distinguish from intraduct carcinoma (*see* p. 302).

A form of benign proliferation of cells may occur within the acini rather than the breast ducts and this condition is termed atypical lobular hyperplasia. It is difficult to distinguish from lobular carcinoma-in-situ (*see* p. 303).

FIBROSIS: Fibrocystic disease may occasionally consist almost entirely of fibrous tissue. The lump is firm and histological examination reveals proliferation of dense fibrous tissue between the epithelial structures.

Development of carcinoma in fibrocystic disease

Page *et al.* (1978) found that women with epitheliosis have double the risk of developing cancer if the lesion is diagnosed over the age of 45 years. Atypical lobular hyperplasia was associated with a three- to six-fold increased risk. Cysts, sclerosing adenosis and fibrosis were not associated with an increased risk of cancer development. A more recent report has broadly confirmed these findings (Dupont and Page 1985).

Other workers have studied the incidence of cancer development in fibrocystic disease without breaking it down into its individual component parts. These studies have, not surprisingly, given conflicting results leading to differences of opinion as to the true incidence.

Fibroadenoma

This is a benign neoplasm containing both epithelial and stromal components. It arises in breast lobules rather than breast ducts and is most common in young women at a time when the breast is undergoing physiological change. It may be caused by an increased sensitivity to oestrogen in a localized part of the breast. Clinically, it is extremely mobile (the breast mouse).

Macroscopically, fibroadenomas are encapsulated lesions. They may be spherical or lobular and on cut section are composed of white/grey fibrous tissue containing small pink areas of epithelium.

Microscopically, benign epithelial elements with both epithelial and myoepithelial layers and fibrous stroma are seen. There are two histological types. In the pericanalicular type the stroma surrounds but does not compress the epithelial tubules. In the intracanalicular type the stroma compresses and distorts the epithelial elements resulting in the formation of slit-like spaces (see Fig. 11.4). Both patterns may be seen in a single fibroadenoma. There is no increased risk of cancer development in patients with a fibroadenoma although it is unclear whether or not some cystosarcoma phyllodes tumours arise in a pre-existing fibroadenoma.

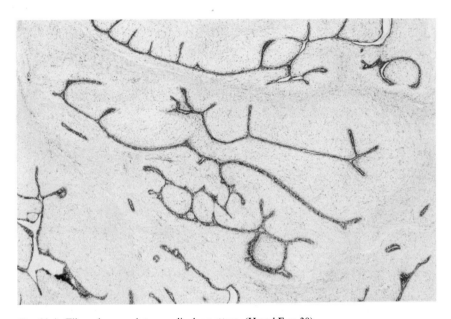

Fig. 11.4. Fibroadenoma: intracanalicular pattern. (H and E × 30)

Fibroadenomas may be complicated by infarction which may be partial or complete. This usually occurs during pregnancy as a result of a relative decrease in blood supply. Often there is a history of pain and a lump is palpable. The condition may then be confused with a carcinoma either clinically or on frozen section examination.

Variations of fibroadenoma

Giant fibroadenoma

This term can mean a very large but otherwise typical fibroadenoma, a benign cystosarcoma phyllodes or a juvenile fibroadenoma. The term therefore requires qualification before use.

Juvenile fibroadenoma

Although most fibroadenomas that arise in adolescent girls are of the typical adult variety described above, a distinct entity known as a juvenile fibroadenoma occurs in some cases. This is often large and may compress the skin causing thinning and even ulceration. Histologically, the epithelial component is exuberant and the stroma is cellular. It may sometimes resemble a cystosarcoma phyllodes. The prognosis is excellent after resection.

Papillary Lesions of the Breast

An intraduct papilloma is a benign lesion which usually occurs in a large breast duct. If the duct becomes blocked and grossly distended with fluid, the lesion is termed a papillary cystadenoma. A papillary carcinoma is a malignant tumour with a papillary pattern. When confined to the breast ducts it is one variant of intraduct carcinoma, and when invasive it is a variant of invasive carcinoma. Papillomatosis is used by some (mainly American) authorities to describe epitheliosis and by others to describe multiple intraduct papillomas. Therefore, the term should only be used if qualified. Juvenile papillomatosis is a specific lesion described below.

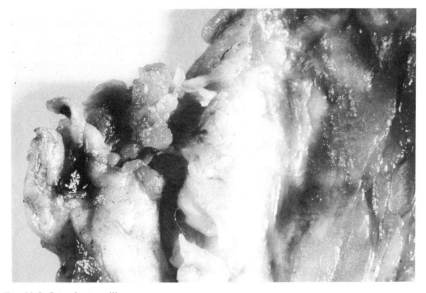

Fig. 11.5. Intraduct papilloma.

Intraduct papilloma

An intraduct papilloma usually occurs near the nipple in a large breast duct and presents with a nipple discharge which is often blood stained. Careful palpation of the surrounding tissue may or may not reveal a mass, but the position of the papilloma may be detected by inference if pressure expresses blood from one duct opening on the nipple. Opening the affected duct will reveal a papillary tumour which may be very small and rarely exceeds 3 mm in size (*see Fig.* 11.5). Microscopically, a papillary pattern is seen in which the fronds of connective tissue are covered by both an epithelial and a myoepithelial layer.

Occasionally, multiple papillomas occur in the large breast ducts and in these patients the risk of recurrence and carcinoma formation at the same site is much increased. The minimum recommendation for treatment is excision of all diseased tissue and very careful follow-up.

Papillary carcinoma

These also appear grossly as papillary tumours and distinction from intraduct papilloma is at the microscopic level. They probably arise *de novo* and not in pre-existing intraduct papillomas. Malignant tumours have less connective tissue stroma in their fronds and paradoxically the cells may have a more uniform appearance than the benign lesion. This is because two cell types are present in the benign lesion whereas only the epithelial cells are proliferating in malignant tumours. When intraduct papillary carcinomas become invasive, the invasive part usually loses its papillary pattern.

Juvenile papillomatosis

This occurs in young women and adolescent girls. It is a circumscribed lesion with many cysts and dilated ducts and has the appearance of Swiss cheese on gross inspection. Histologically, the presence of many cysts is confirmed and florid epithelial hyperplasia is seen. Although development of cancer has not been reported, careful follow-up is advised since many patients have a strong family history of breast cancer.

Adenoma of the Nipple

This rare condition consists of a proliferation of tubules in the nipple region. It may erode the nipple skin to give fissuring and ulceration and can therefore be confused with Paget's disease of the nipple. Clinically, a lump is palpable in the nipple. Histology confirms the presence of a proliferation of tubules containing the benign feature of two cell layers. Some foci of solid cells may occur which can cause confusion with invasive carcinoma, especially at frozen section. The condition may also be seen in men.

Very rarely, malignant change has been described and local recurrence may arise. Treatment should be excision of the complete nipple.

In-situ Breast Carcinoma

In-situ breast carcinoma is of two types, intraduct carcinoma and lobular carcinoma-in-situ. Although some authorities consider it to be an over-simplification, for practical purposes intraduct carcinoma arises from the epithelium of ducts whereas lobular carcinomas-in-situ arise from the epithelium of breast lobules. The two diseases have markedly different behaviour patterns and will be discussed separately.

Intraduct carcinoma

An intraduct carcinoma is confined to the breast ducts without invasion of the surrounding breast tissue. It may come to the surgeon's attention in one of several ways. A lump or breast thickening near the nipple is the most usual, occurring in up to 75% of cases, but a nipple discharge (present in about a third) and Paget's disease of the nipple (seen in up to a quarter—Westbrook and Gallager 1975) are also common. Occasionally, the tumour is discovered on screening mammography or as an incidental microscopic finding in a breast biopsy taken for other reasons.

Morphology

Intraduct carcinoma consists of a proliferation of malignant cells within the breast ducts. It may be difficult to distinguish from severe epitheliosis, causing frozen section examination sometimes to be equivocal. Microscopically, intraduct carcinoma is distinguished from epitheliosis by both the pattern of growth and the cell morphology.

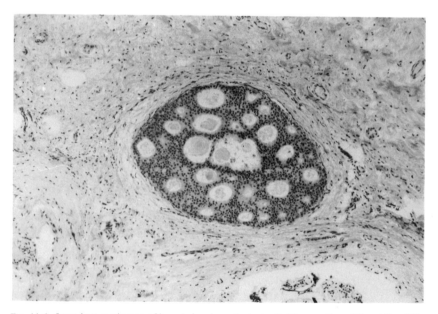

Fig. 11.6. Intraduct carcinoma of breast showing a typical cribriform pattern. (H and E × 75)

Several basic patterns of intraduct carcinoma are recognized. The comedo type is characterized by an area of central necrosis, contrasting with the solid type in which the duct is completely filled with malignant cells. The cribriform type is especially characteristic of intraduct carcinoma and here the malignant tissue is perforated by a series of neatly rounded holes caused by cell necrosis (*see Fig.* 11.6). Papillary intraduct carcinomas are discussed on p. 301. In all these patterns the individual cells bear no relationship to each other, being dissociated with loss of cell polarity. In epitheliosis, however, the cells do bear a relationship to each other, some polarity is retained and the spaces which are formed are irregular both in size and shape.

Examination of individual cell morphology shows that the cells in intraduct carcinoma are rounded and often have distinct cell membranes. In intraduct carcinoma, only epithelial cells are proliferating, whereas in epitheliosis, both epithelial and myoepithelial cells are proliferating. The former may therefore have a more monotonous cellular appearance, although there are abnormal mitotic figures and variations in nuclear shape.

Prognosis

Several important points about intraduct carcinoma influence the prognosis.

1. After simple biopsy, residual tumour tissue is found in a large proportion of patients due to the frequent multicentric origin of the lesion. In one study, residual tumour tissue was found in 32 out of 38 patients (Carter and Smith 1977).
2. Axillary lymph nodes are infiltrated by tumour in less than 5% of cases of pure intraduct carcinoma. The metastases may arise from a small area of invasion, not recognized at the time of histological examination.
3. Up to 67% of non-invasive carcinomas will progress to invasive carcinoma if left untreated over a 10–20 year period and 17% of patients will develop invasive carcinoma in the opposite breast (Editorial 1984).
4. If all tumour tissue is removed, patients with an intraduct carcinoma have an excellent long-term prognosis. One study reported 62 out of 64 patients disease-free after a minimum follow-up of four years (Westbrook and Gallager 1975).

Lobular carcinoma-in-situ

Lobular carcinoma-in-situ arises in the acini of breast lobules. While the lesion is still in-situ there is no invasion of surrounding stroma. When the surrounding stroma is invaded the condition becomes invasive lobular carcinoma.

Unlike ductal carcinoma, lobular carcinoma-in-situ is invariably an incidental finding in a breast biopsy carried out for other reasons.

Morphology

The condition is not recognized macroscopically. At microscopic examination all, or nearly all, the acini of one or more lobules are distended by cells and their lumina are obliterated (*see Fig.* 11.7). The cells which distend the acini have rounded nuclei and a characteristic monotonous appearance with few mitotic figures. The lesion may spread along the breast ducts in a Pagetoid fashion between the normal ductal epithelium and its basement membrane, but they do not reach the nipple surface and Paget's disease of the nipple is therefore not a feature.

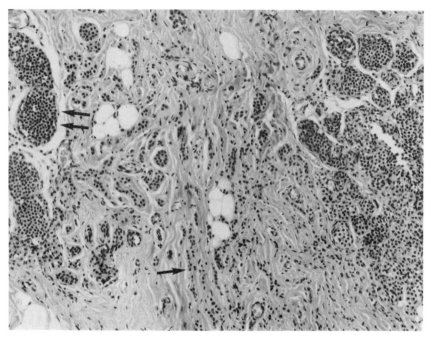

Fig. 11.7. Invasive lobular carcinoma showing an 'Indian file pattern' (single arrow) with areas of lobular carcinoma-in-situ (double arrow). (H and E × 350)

Prognosis

A diagnosis of lobular carcinoma-in-situ does not invariably mean that the patient will develop invasive lobular carcinoma. Andersen (1977) followed up patients with lobular carcinoma-in-situ for an average of 15·9 years and reported that 20% developed invasive carcinoma in the affected breast and almost 10% developed invasive carcinoma in the contralateral breast.

Invasive Breast Cancer

Epidemiology

Breast cancer accounts for 12 000 deaths annually in England and Wales. The disease is 100 times more common in women than in men and the incidence increases rapidly with age until 40 years, after which it levels out. Breast cancer is six times more common in the USA and UK than in Africa or Asia, although in recent years there has been a dramatic rise in Japan. Studies on second generation Japanese women living in the United States suggests that environmental factors are important in determining an increasing incidence.

Women who have a first degree relative with the disease have double the risk of developing breast cancer when compared with the general population. This may partly be explained by the sharing of similar environmental factors. A patient who develops breast cancer has a four to five times greater than average risk of developing malignancy in the contralateral breast.

There is some epidemiological evidence that women with excessive exposure to oestrogens, particularly when unopposed by progesterone, have a high incidence of breast cancer. Thus, an early menarche and a late menopause both increase the duration of exposure to oestrogen and both are associated with about double the average risk of developing breast cancer. Nulliparous women also have a greater risk, possibly because they have not had the protective effect of progesterone during pregnancy. Women who have their first child when over the age of 30 years also have a greater than average risk. Patients with oestrogen secreting ovarian tumours have an increased risk of developing breast cancer, while patients who have bilateral oophorectomy before the age of 35 years have a greatly reduced risk. Obese women are also at increased risk, probably as a result of hormonal factors (Doll and Peto 1983).

There is considerable controversy as to whether the oral contraceptive pill is associated with an increased risk of breast cancer. Recently, the weight of evidence seems to be against any link between breast cancer and 'the pill' (Diggory 1984). Women who take oestrogens for menopausal symptoms may have an increased risk approximately a decade later.

The risk for patients with fibrocystic disease developing cancer has been discussed on p. 298.

Aetiology

HORMONAL FACTORS: Oestrogen causes cellular proliferation in the breast whereas progesterone tends to stimulate differentiation. Relatively unopposed oestrogen activity has therefore been implicated as a promoting agent in breast cancer and as an explanation for several of the epidemiological factors described above. It might be expected that breast cancer patients have some deficiency in progesterone production, such as an inadequate luteal phase of the menstrual cycle. In fact, however, both 'high risk women' and women with breast cancer have normal luteal phase progesterone production. Follicle stimulating hormone, luteinizing hormone and prolactin levels are also normal.

In order to explain these apparent contradictions, Korenman (1980) proposed the 'oestrogen window hypothesis' of breast cancer. This hypothesis suggests that cancer induction by carcinogens occurs in a breast which is made susceptible by the unopposed action of oestrogen and that this unopposed action takes place at two distinct periods of a woman's life, during which time the oestrogen window is said to be open. The first oestrogen window opens at age 8 to 10 years, during which time oestrogen levels start to rise. After an average of 2·3 years the menses are established but the early menstrual periods may be anovulatory with resultant poor progesterone production. The ease of cancer induction by carcinogens declines with the establishment of normal cycles (i.e. the oestrogen window closes) and becomes very low during pregnancy, presumably due to the high levels of circulating progesterone at this time. This may explain why women who have a very early first pregnancy have a lower than average risk of developing breast cancer. The second oestrogen window opens at the time of the menopause when, again, anovulatory cycles occur and oestrogen is unopposed. Women with a late menopause have a longer period of luteal deficiency thus explaining why a late menopause is associated with an increased risk of breast cancer.

Support for the oestrogen window hypothesis comes from the study of the life span of atomic bomb survivors in Hiroshima and Nagasaki (Korenman 1980). These data showed a rise in breast cancer incidence only if exposure took place at a time when the oestrogen window was open (a statistically significant increase if exposure was during the time of the first oestrogen window, but a statistically non-significant increase if exposure took place at the time of the second oestrogen window).

During the post-menopausal phase, a large percentage of oestrogen comes from the peripheral conversion of androstenedione (which is produced by the adrenal) to oestrone. This conversion takes place in fat cells and the percentage conversion increases with body weight, possibly explaining the association between body weight and breast cancer.

Table 11.1. Clinical classification of breast cancer

TNM System	
Tis	Carcinoma-in-situ
T0	No evidence of primary tumour
T1	< 2 cm
T2	2–5 cm
T3	> 5 cm
T4	Extension to chest wall or skin—
	(a) chest wall
	(b) skin oedema, or infiltration, or ulceration
	(c) both chest wall and skin
N0	No nodes palpable
N1	Mobile axillary—
	(a) not considered involved by tumour
	(b) considered involved by tumour
N2	Fixed axillary nodes
N3	Palpable supraclavicular nodes
M0	No distant metastases
M1	Distant metastases
Manchester System	
Stage I	Tumour confined to breast. Not adherent to pectoral muscles or chest wall. If skin adherence, this must be smaller than size of tumour.
Stage II	Primary tumour as in Stage I, with the addition of mobile ipsilateral lymph nodes.
Stage III	Skin involvement larger than tumour; tumour fixed to pectoral muscles but not to chest wall. Fixed nodes in axilla.
Stage IV	Distant spread either blood- or lymph-borne. Invasion of skin wide of breast. Palpable supraclavicular nodes. Involvement of opposite breast. Bone, brain, lung, liver involvement.

VIRAL FACTORS: The Bittner factor is an oncogenic virus found in mice. It is transmissible through the mother's milk and causes breast cancer in the suckling young. Electron microscopy studies have found similar particles in human breast cancer cells. A high percentage of Parsee women in India, who have a very high incidence of breast cancer, have these viral particles in their milk. Reverse transcriptase, an enzyme which occurs only in oncogenic RNA viruses, has also been identified in human breast milk. Although there is substantial evidence that viruses occur in human breast cancer cells, it is unknown whether or not they play a primary role in cancer development.

Although the exact aetiology of breast cancer is unknown, a working hypothesis is that genetically predisposed individuals who have prolonged periods of unopposed oestrogen stimulation are susceptible to cancer induction by carcinogens which, in some cases, may be viral.

Classification

The two commonly used clinical staging systems of breast cancer are shown in *Table* 11.1. A simple pathological classification of breast carcinoma which is based mainly on microscopic features is given in *Table* 11.2. Only the more important histological types will be discussed.

Table 11.2. Classification of breast cancer*

1.	Lobular
	A. In-situ
	B. Invasive
2.	Ductal
	A. In-situ
	B. Invasive
	i. Not otherwise specified (the most common type)
	ii. Medullary carcinoma with lymphoid stroma
	iii. Pure mucoid
	iv. Tubular
	v. Squamous
	vi. Adenoid cystic
	vii. Apocrine
	viii. Lipid rich
	ix. Juvenile
	x. Carcinomas with noteworthy clinical manifestations
	(a) Inflammatory carcinoma
	(b) Paget's disease of nipple
3.	Uncertain—either ductal or lobular
4.	Mixture of ductal and lobular
5.	Carcinoma arising in a pre-existing benign tumour
6.	Carcinosarcoma
7.	Unclassified

* Adapted from Azzopardi (1979).

Lobular carcinoma

This accounts for about 12% of infiltrating carcinomas in the United Kingdom.

Macroscopically, a lobular carcinoma tends to be rubbery and often lacks the classical features of the more common ductal carcinoma described below. Microscopically, the most important feature of lobular carcinoma is infiltration of a fibroblastic stroma by single cells and lines of cells arranged in single file, the so-called Indian file pattern. The cells are small and monotonous. The single files are frequently disposed in concentric circles around a breast duct giving a 'targetoid lesion'. Areas of lobular carcinoma-in-situ are often seen in the same breast (*see Fig.* 11.7 on p. 304). Other less characteristic patterns with more solid areas of infiltrating tumour are seen but are less typical. A feature of lobular carcinomas of importance to the clinician is that they are almost invariably oestrogen receptor positive (*see* p. 313).

Ductal carcinoma

The majority of breast carcinomas are infiltrating ductal in type with no specific features (the 'not otherwise specified' category in *Table* 11.2). Macroscopically, two different types are seen, stellate and circumscribed. The stellate type (*see Fig.* 11.8) is the more common and has the classic macroscopic features of breast cancer. The edge is highly irregular with long strands of tumour infiltrating the breast tissue (the cancer crab). No capsule is seen. The tumour has a hard consistency due to the dense stroma and hence this type used to be termed 'scirrhous'. A gritty sensation is felt on cutting and the cut surface assumes a concave shape. Yellow streaks which used to be described as areas of necrosis but which are now considered to be elastosis are often visible. The circumscribed tumours are less common. Although the edge of the tumour is well defined, it is often multilobular

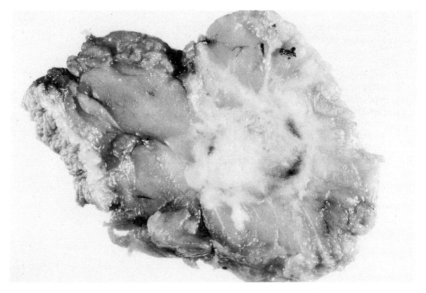

Fig. 11.8. Breast carcinoma (stellate type).

and appears to grow in a pushing fashion rather than by infiltration. There is evidence that circumscribed tumours have a better prognosis than the stellate variety.

Histologically, invasive ductal carcinoma has a great variation both in the type of epithelial component and in the amount and type of stroma. Bloom and Richardson (1957) suggested a histological grading depending on the amount of tubular differentiation, the degree of nuclear pleomorphism and the number of mitotic figures. Grade one tumours are well differentiated with well formed tubules, little pleomorphism and few mitoses. Grade two is the common pattern (about 50% of ductal carcinomas) and consists of a mixed pattern of clumps and trabeculae of malignant cells with some attempted tubule formation. Grade three tumours are anaplastic with considerable nuclear pleomorphism and a high mitotic count but no tubule formation (*see Fig.* 11.9). This grading system is related to prognosis (*see below*). Several patterns may be seen in one tumour and frequently areas of intraduct carcinoma are also seen.

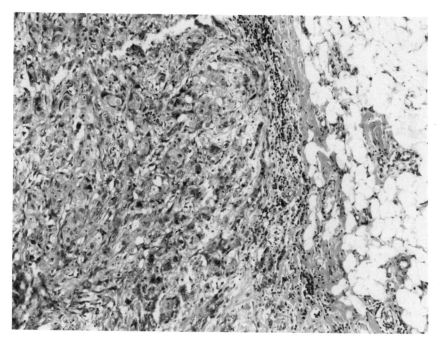

Fig. 11.9. Poorly differentiated ductal carcinoma of breast. (H and E × 80)

Variants of ductal carcinoma

MEDULLARY CARCINOMA WITH LYMPHOID STROMA: The term 'medullary' formerly implied a soft breast tumour (sometimes also termed 'encephaloid' tumour). The term is now more specific and has been incorporated into the phrase 'medullary carcinoma with lymphoid stroma' in order to describe a distinct variant of breast cancer. The tumour is characteristically well circumscribed and histologically consists of nests of syncytial malignant cells surrounded by a stroma which is heavily infiltrated by lymphocytes. It has a better prognosis than some other forms of invasive breast cancer.

MUCOID CARCINOMA: This variant also has a circumscribed outline and relatively good prognosis. The gross appearance is characteristically gelatinous and, on microscopic examination, groups of malignant cells are seen in a 'sea of mucin' (*see* Fig. 11.10).

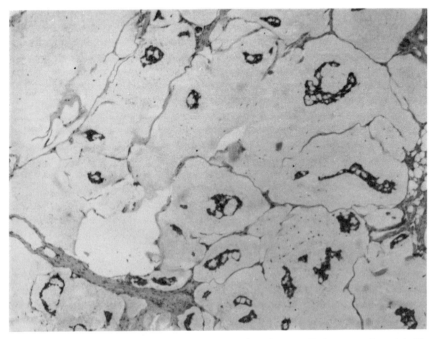

Fig. 11.10. Mucinous carcinoma of breast. Clumps of malignant cells in a 'sea of mucin'. (H and E × 30)

TUBULAR CARCINOMA: This is another distinct variant and also has a favourable prognosis. It is often detected in screening clinics as it is frequently calcified and can be observed by mammography before it is palpable. The tumour is small with an irregular outline and, on microscopy, consists of a proliferation of small irregular and angulated tubules in a fibrous stroma. The lesion may be difficult to distinguish from sclerosing adenosis.

SQUAMOUS CARCINOMA: This variant is rare and arises in the breast substance rather than the overlying skin. It is often cystic. Microscopically, it has the characteristic features of squamous carcinoma.

ADENOID CYSTIC CARCINOMA: This tumour is similar to the adenoid cystic carcinoma of the salivary gland but does not have such a good prognosis. Histologically, it shows the characteristic multiple cyst-like spaces which are lined by small dark uniform cells. (*See Fig.* 1.9, p. 24.)

JUVENILE: The juvenile or secretory variant of breast cancer is usually seen in children although it may also be found in adults. It is rare. Histologically, it consists of large pale staining cells which form irregular tubules. The tubules are filled with an eosinophilic secretory product. The prognosis is good compared with the other varieties.

INFLAMMATORY CARCINOMA: This condition is characterized by extensive dermal permeation of lymphatics. This causes gross oedema and redness of the overlying skin simulating an inflammatory condition. The prognosis is poor.

PAGET'S DISEASE OF THE NIPPLE: Sir James Paget (1814–1899) first described this condition in 1874. The clinical features include eczema, ulceration, discharge, bleeding, fissures and surrounding inflammation. The fact that it is unilateral helps to distinguish it from simple eczema of the nipple. Distinction from the rare conditions of Bowen's disease and superficial spreading melanoma may be more difficult. An underlying intraduct or infiltrating ductal carcinoma is invariably present and may be palpable in some cases. Of the 50 cases reviewed by Paone and Baker (1981), all had underlying tumour (palpable in 31, impalpable in 19).

Microscopically, the epidermis of the nipple is infiltrated by Paget's cells which are either single or in clusters (*see Fig.* 11.11). These are large cells with prominent nucleoli and abundant cytoplasm. The nuclei are often surrounded by a clear zone or halo. The underlying dermis is inflamed. Examination of the rest of the breast reveals either an intraduct or infiltrating ductal carcinoma.

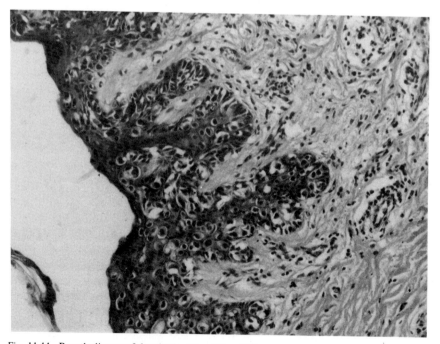

Fig. 11.11. Paget's disease of the nipple. (H and E × 150)

The origin of the Paget cell has given rise to controversy. The earlier work suggested that Paget's cells arose in the underlying ductal carcinoma and permeated along the duct onto the nipple skin. More recent work, however, has failed to show an anatomical connection between the carcinoma and the nipple, and it has therefore been proposed that Paget's cells arise in the epidermis, perhaps as part of a generalized field change. In support of this theory is the ultrastructural finding of epidermal features such as desmosomes between Paget's cells and adjacent epithelial cells. No firm conclusion has yet been reached.

The prognosis of Paget's disease of the nipple depends on whether or not the underlying tumour is palpable. When a tumour is palpable (and therefore more likely to be invasive), the prognosis and behaviour is similar to ordinary invasive breast cancer. When no tumour is palpable, lymph node metastases are rare and the prognosis is excellent. Betsill *et al.* (1978) showed that one-third of patients with intraduct carcinoma treated by biopsy alone developed recurrent disease after 10 years.

Prognosis of breast cancer

The single most important prognostic feature in breast cancer is the presence or absence of axillary lymph node metastases. Alderson *et al.* (1971) followed up 258 patients with breast cancer and carried out a computer assisted analysis to determine the relevant importance of 21 separate prognostic features. The most important factors influencing prognosis were (in decreasing order of importance): (1) lymph node status, (2) tumour size, (3) stromal reaction, (4) histological grade.

Haybittle *et al.* (1982) also found that lymph node status, histological grade and tumour size were statistically significant in determining prognosis.

It is important that lymph nodes should only be considered involved with tumour if this is confirmed histologically; a clinical impression can be misleading. In one large study 35% of clinically normal nodes were histologically positive while 13% of clinically enlarged nodes were histologically negative (Smart *et al.* 1978). The American College of Surgeons (1979) showed that the five year survival rate for patients with one, four and five nodes involved were 48%, 38% and 29% respectively. Lymph node metastases less than 2 mm in diameter may be missed on routine histological study but there is general agreement that these micrometastases do not influence survival (Millis 1984).

The size of the primary tumour is also a determinant of prognosis in that the larger the tumour the worse the five year survival (Fisher *et al.* 1969). This may be partly due to the fact that larger tumours are more often associated with lymph node metastases. Some authorities use the term 'minimal breast carcinoma' which has most recently been defined as in-situ carcinoma or invasive carcinoma of less than 1 cm in diameter. These tumours have a much better prognosis than more extensive tumours. There is also evidence that tumours with well defined contours have a better prognosis than stellate tumours.

Stromal reaction also influences prognosis and this is particularly noted in the good prognosis of those tumours classified as medullary carcinoma with lymphoid stroma. This may partly be due to an immunological host reaction to the malignant tissue.

Bloom and Field (1971) have given five year survival rates analysed by histological grade (described on p. 309). The figures were 81%, 54% and 34% for grades one, two and three respectively.

Hormone receptors and breast cancer

Two main types of hormone receptor are present in normal breast epithelial cells, oestrogen receptor (ER) and progesterone receptor (PgR). ER is a cytoplasmic protein which has a high affinity for binding to oestrogen.* When oestrogen enters the cell (either by diffusion or possibly by an active uptake mechanism) it binds to ER and the resultant complex enters the cell nucleus where it binds to specific areas of the chromatin known as acceptor sites. This results in the production of messenger RNA by transcription. The messenger RNA enters the cytoplasm and produces various enzymes and proteins, one of which is progesterone receptor. The oestrogen/ER complex also induces DNA synthesis and cell growth although the mechanism for this is not yet known (*see Fig. 11.12*).

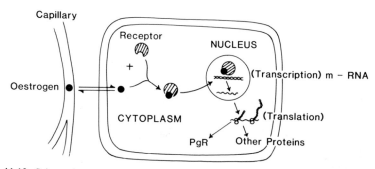

Fig. 11.12. Schematic representation of the oestrogen receptor mechanism showing that an intact mechanism is necessary for the production of progesterone receptor (PgR). (Adapted from Forrest 1982.)*

When breast epithelial cells undergo malignant transformation, the ER system may remain intact, become damaged at one or more stages of the process or be completely destroyed. In general, the system tends to remain intact in well differentiated tumours whereas it tends to be destroyed in poorly differentiated tumours.

Various methods are available for the assay of cytoplasmic oestrogen receptors in tumour tissue and it is known that 50–60% of women with ER positive tumours respond to endocrine therapy, whereas less than 10% of ER negative patients respond. When ER and PgR are both positive the response rate rises to 80%. This is because PgR, being an end product of the ER system, is a measure of whether or not a major part of the system is intact, whereas the presence of ER only indicates that the first stage is intact. In the 20% who do not respond, despite having both receptors, it appears that only that part of the ER mechanism which influences DNA synthesis and growth is defective.

ERs occur more commonly in the primary tumour than in metastatic deposits, although the demonstration of ERs in secondary deposits may help identify an occult primary site in the breast.

---

*The traditional view that ER is located in the cytoplasm has been challenged by some workers who believe that it is situated in the nucleus (Welshons *et al.* 1981).

Although conflicting reports have appeared, the weight of evidence suggests that women with ER positive tumours have an overall improved survival (Howell *et al.* 1984).

Cystosarcoma Phyllodes (Phyllodes Tumour)

Cystosarcoma phyllodes (also spelt phylloides) was so named at a time when the term sarcoma merely meant fleshy and did not necessarily imply malignancy. In fact, only about 20% of these tumours are malignant and therefore some authorities prefer the term 'phyllodes tumour'. The tumour presents as a breast mass. The age range is wide though patients with malignant phyllodes tumours tend to be slightly older than those with the benign type. Phyllodes tumours are composed of an epithelial component (benign) and a stromal component (either benign or malignant). Grossly, all phyllodes tumours are fleshy on cut section and are lobulated. Within the lobules, characteristic clefting is seen (*see Fig.* 11.13). They are frequently large and although well circumscribed they tend to have small surface protrusions which, if left behind at the time of surgery, will lead to recurrence.

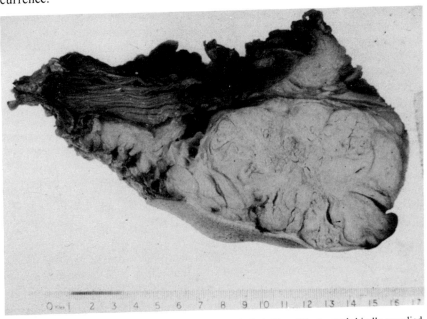

Fig. 11.13. Cystosarcoma phyllodes showing the typical clefting. (Photograph kindly supplied by Dr R. Millis and reproduced by permission of M.T.P. Press.)

Microscopically, the features are similar to those of a fibroadenoma with a prominent intracanalicular pattern (*see* p. 299). The lesion is distinguished from a fibroadenoma by its characteristic hypercellular stroma. Benign and malignant phyllodes tumours are distinguished from each other by the higher mitotic rate and stromal overgrowth seen in the malignant variety. The edges of malignant tumours are also likely to be infiltrative rather than pushing.

Spread of the malignant variety is via the blood stream to lung and bone and only rarely to regional nodes, although regional nodes may be clinically enlarged due to reactive change. The tumour can also be locally invasive. The benign tumours must be widely excised due to their surface projections while malignant tumours require mastectomy.

Breast Sarcomas

True sarcomas of the breast do occur but they must be distinguished from carcinomas with metaplasia and phyllodes tumours with stromal overgrowth.

Grossly, they tend to be rubbery with areas of necrosis and haemorrhage. Histologically, they are usually fibrosarcomas but areas of metaplasia to bone, cartilage, muscle or fat are sometimes seen.

Angiosarcomas arising in the breast are important as they can be confused with benign angiomas or even granulation tissue. The skin overlying these tumours may have a blue appearance and microscopically there is variation in pattern from well formed vascular channels to solid overgrowth of endothelium.

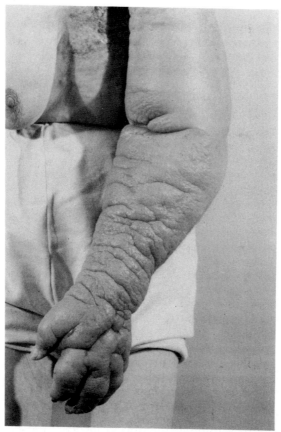

Fig. 11.14. Stewart–Treves syndrome.

Sarcomas spread via the blood stream and, therefore, axillary lymph node sampling or dissection is less important than with carcinoma.

Post-mastectomy lymphangiosarcoma (Stewart–Treves syndrome)

Lymphangiosarcomatous change may occur in some women who develop post-mastectomy chronic lymphoedema of the arm (*see Fig.* 11.14). The tumour presents as multiple subcutaneous haemorrhagic nodules in the arm. Microscopically, a lymphangiosarcomatous pattern is seen with endothelial lined vascular spaces. Some authorities have suggested that the tumour represents multiple carcinomatous secondary deposits arising in the arm as a result of retrograde spread. However, the weight of evidence including immunohistochemical and ultrastructural techniques indicates an endothelial origin. The prognosis is exceedingly poor.

The Male Breast

Gynaecomastia

Gynaecomastia is enlargement of the male breast. It may be discussed under several headings.

1. PUBERTAL: A transient breast enlargement, which is usually but not always bilateral, is common in adolescent boys. It usually subsides within two years and may be due to the rise in oestradiol which occurs before the rise in testosterone at puberty. Histologically, the enlargement is chiefly due to excess fibrous tissue, which may be associated with hyperplasia of duct epithelium.

2. SENESCENT: A mild degree of breast enlargement is not uncommon in men, often in the sixth decade. It presents as a firm mass, deep to the nipple, which may be unilateral or bilateral. There may be clinical confusion with a carcinoma. Histologically, there is excessive fibrous tissue enclosing scattered ducts. The swelling usually regresses within one year.

3. ENDOCRINE CAUSES: Patients with thyrotoxicosis, Cushing's syndrome, feminizing tumours of the adrenal cortex, testicular tumors and Klinefelter's syndrome may develop gynaecomastia. There is also an association with hepatic cirrhosis, possibly due to decreased oestrogen breakdown by the liver.

4. DRUG INDUCED: Oestrogen therapy for prostatic carcinoma may be complicated by gynaecomastia. It may also be caused by digoxin, phenothiazines, isoniazid, spironolactone, cimetidine and regular cannabis smoking.

Carcinoma of the male breast

This is a rare disease accounting for approximately 0·7% of all breast cancers (Ribeiro 1977), although the incidence is much higher in certain areas such as Egypt. This is perhaps due to the high incidence of gynaecomastia seen in that country as a result of schistosomal fibrosis of the liver. Carcinoma of the male breast is usually a disease of elderly men in the seventh and eighth decade.

Possible aetiological factors include exogenous oestrogen exposure, Klinefelter's syndrome, gynaecomastia, chest wall trauma and a positive family history (Crichlow 1972).

Most patients present with a hard breast lump beneath the areola. Histologically, the tumours are similar to carcinoma of the female breast and most have a marked desmoplastic reaction, thus accounting for the hardness on palpation. Axillary node metastases are common and most authors believe that breast cancer in the male has a worse prognosis than in the female due to early infiltration of the chest wall and late presentation. One series reported 5 and 10 year survivals of only 38% and 17% respectively (Spence *et al.* 1985).

References

Alderson M. R., Hamlin I., Staunton M. D. (1971) The relative significance of prognostic factors in breast carcinoma. *Br. J. Cancer* **25**, 646–56.

American College of Surgeons Commission on Cancer (1979) Final report on long-term follow-up patient care evaluation study for carcinoma of the female breast. 1–42.

Andersen J. A. (1977) Lobular carcinoma-in-situ of the breast. An approach to rational treatment. *Cancer* **39**, 2597–602.

Apps M. C. P., Harrison N. K., Blauth C. I. A. (1984) Tuberculosis of the breast. *Br. Med. J.* **288**, 1874–5.

Azzopardi J. G. (1979) *Problems in Breast Pathology*. London, W. B. Saunders.

Betsill W. L., Rosen P. P., Lieberman P. H., Robbins G. F. (1978) Intraductal carcinoma. Long-term follow up after treatment by biopsy alone. *J.A.M.A.* **239**, 1863–7.

Bloom H.J.G., Field J. R. (1971) Impact of tumour grade and host resistance on survival of women with breast cancer. *Cancer* **28**, 1580–9.

Bloom H. J. G., Richardson W. W. (1957) Histological grading and prognosis in breast cancer. *Br. J. Cancer.* **11**, 359–77.

Carter D., Smith R. R. (1977) Carcinoma-in-situ of the breast. *Cancer* **40**, 1189–93.

Crichlow R. W. (1972) Carcinoma of the male breast. *Surg. Gynecol. Obstet.* **134**, 1011–19.

De Hertogh D. A., Rossof A. H., Harris A. A., Economou S. G. (1980) Prednisone management of granulomatous mastitis. *N. Engl. J. Med.* **303**, 799–800.

Diggory P. (1984) Cancer and the pill. *Lancet* **2**, 166.

Doll R., Peto R. (1983) Epidemiology of cancer. In: Weatherall D. J., Le Dingham J. G. G., Warrell D. A. (eds.) *Oxford Textbook of Medicine*. Oxford, Oxford Medical.

Dupont W. D., Page D. L. (1985) Risk factors for breast cancer in women with proliferative breast disease. *N. Engl. J. Med.* **312**, 146–51.

Editorial (1984) Intraduct carcinoma of the breast. *Lancet* **2**, 24.

Fisher B. F., Slack N. H., Bross I. D. (1969) Cancer of the breast: size of neoplasm and prognosis. *Cancer* **24**, 1071–80.

Forrest A. P. M. (1982) Beatson: Hormones and management of breast cancer. *J. R. Coll. Surg. Edinb.* **27**, 253–63.

Gardecki T. I., Melcher D. H., Hogbin B. M., Smith R. S. (1980) Aspiration cytology in the preoperative management of breast cancer. *Lancet* **2**, 790–2.

Hadfield G. J. (1976) Benign diseases of the breast. In: Hadfield J., Hobsley M. (eds.) *Current Surgical Practice*, Vol. 1, pp. 250–61. London, Edward Arnold.

Haybittle J. L., Blamey R. W., Elston C. W. *et al.* (1982) A prognostic index in primary breast cancer. *Br. J. Cancer* **45**, 361–6.

Holaday W. J., Assor D. (1974) Ten thousand consecutive frozen sections. A retrospective study focusing on accuracy and quality control. *Am. J. Clin. Pathol.* **61**, 769–77.

Howell A., Harland R. W. L., Bramwell V. H. C. *et al.* (1984) Steroid-hormone receptors and survival after first relapse in breast cancer. *Lancet* **1**, 588–91.

Korenman S. G. (1980) The endocrinology of breast cancer. *Cancer* **46**, 874–8.

Millis R. R. (1984) *Atlas of Breast Pathology*. Lancaster, MTP Press.

Page D. L., Van der Zwaag R., Rogers L. W., Williams L. T., Walker W. E., Hartmann W. H. (1978) Relation between component parts of fibrocystic disease complex and breast cancer. *J. Natl. Cancer Inst.* **61**, 1055–63.

Paone J. F., Baker R. R. (1981) Pathogenesis and treatment of Paget's disease of the breast. *Cancer* **48**, 825–9.

Ribeiro G. G. (1977) Carcinoma of the male breast: a review of 200 cases. *Br. J. Surg.* **64**, 381–3.

Smart C. R., Myers M. H., Gloeckler L. A. (1978) Implications from SEER data on breast cancer management. *Cancer* **41**, 787–9.

Spence R. A. J., Mackenzie G., Anderson J. R., Lyons A. R., Bell M. (1985) Long-term survival following cancer of the male breast in Northern Ireland. *Cancer* **55**, 648–52.

Welshons W. V., Lieberman M. E., Gorski J. (1984) Nuclear localization of unoccupied oestrogen receptors. *Nature* **307**, 797–9.

Westbrook K. C., Gallager H. S. (1975) Intraductal carcinoma of the breast. A comparative study. *Am. J. Surg.* **130**, 667–70.

Chapter 12

The Heart

Normal Structure

The adult heart weighs about 300 g and is the shape of a cone. The base points posteriorly and is formed mainly of the left atrium. The apex points to the left and is composed of the tip of the left ventricle. The heart lies within the pericardial sac and is suspended by the great vessels. The atria and ventricles are separated by a fibrous atrioventricular ring to which the muscle fibres are attached.

The right atrium receives both the superior and inferior vena cavae and is prolonged as the atrial appendage which overlaps the base of the aorta. An external groove between the superior vena cava and the right atrial appendage (the sulcus terminalis) corresponds to the crista terminalis internally, which is a ridge of heart muscle in the wall of the right atrium. The smooth atrial wall between the great veins is derived embryologically from the sinus venosus while the remaining free wall and appendage are derived from the primitive atrium and are trabeculated. The opening of the coronary sinus lies near the septal cusp of the tricuspid valve and the lower interatrial septum has a depression (fossa ovalis) which represents the closed foramen ovale. This has a prominent margin, the limbus fossa ovalis, which represents the free edge of the septum secundum.

The right ventricle muscle is separated from the right atrium externally by the atrioventricular groove in which lies the right coronary artery. Internally, the muscle is in ridges (trabeculae carneae). The moderator band is a distinct band of muscle which connects the anterior wall of the ventricle to the interventricular septum. The ventricle funnels towards the pulmonary orifice and this part is the smooth walled infundibulum. The latter represents part of the bulbus cordis which has become incorporated into the right ventricle.

The tricuspid valve has three cusps attached by their bases to the fibrous atrioventricular ring. The cusps are septal, inferior (sometimes called posterior) and anterior; the edges of their ventricular surfaces receive the chordae tendineae which arise from the papillary muscles. The chordae are glistening white fibrous cords mainly composed of collagen.

The pulmonary valve consists of three semilunar cusps attached to a fibrous thickening in the wall of the pulmonary trunk. There are two anterior cusps (right and left) and one posterior cusp. Opposite the semilunar cusps, the wall of the pulmonary trunk has three dilatations—the sinuses of Valsalva.

The wall of the left atrium is thicker than that of the right. It originates chiefly from incorporated pulmonary veins and the internal surface is therefore smooth. There is a small atrial appendage and the four pulmonary veins enter the main cavity in a symmetrical fashion. Occasionally, the atrium may only receive three pulmonary veins but fewer than three is exceedingly rare.

The walls of the left ventricle are three times thicker than those of the right and the interventricular septum tends to bulge into the right ventricle. The trabeculae are well developed and two papillary muscles project into the cavity and give rise to the chordae tendineae of the mitral valve cusps. The papillary muscles are anterior and posterior. The outflow track of the ventricle is smooth compared with the marked trabeculation seen elsewhere in the ventricular wall.

The interventricular septum has a thick wall similar to that of the rest of the left ventricle and is trabeculated except at its attachment to the fibrous skeleton where it is thin and membranous.

The mitral valve consists of a large anterior (septal) and a small posterior cusp. Occasionally there is a small accessory leaflet between the two major cusps. The cusps are attached to the chordae of the papillary muscles.

The aortic valve consists of three semilunar cusps, one anterior and two posterior (right and left) and above each cusp is a dilatation (the aortic sinuses). The right coronary artery arises from the anterior sinus while the left coronary artery originates from the posterior sinus. The valve cusps may also be termed right coronary, left coronary and non-coronary.

Structurally, the heart has three layers: endocardium, myocardium and epicardium. The endocardium is an inner layer of endothelial cells which lies on a subendocardial layer of connective tissue. This allows movement of the endocardium, without damage, during contraction of the heart. The myocardial cells form a branching network. The cells have central nuclei, cross striations similar to those seen in skeletal muscle and are separated from each other by intercalated discs. The intercalated discs are areas of low electrical resistance which allow the rapid spread of electrical activity so that the heart muscle acts as a functional syncytium. The epicardium consists of a flattened layer of cells which lies on a layer of areolar connective tissue in which the major coronary arteries are embedded.

The conducting system of the heart comprises the sino-atrial (SA) node, the atrio-ventricular (AV) node, the atrio-ventricular (AV) bundle of His, the left and right branches of the AV bundle and the Purkinje fibres. The SA node is a pacemaker, situated at the upper end of the crista terminalis. From here, electrical impulses spread through the atrial walls to the AV node which lies in the septal wall of the right atrium, just above the opening of the coronary sinus. From here, impulses pass through the fibrous ring of the heart via the AV bundle. The left and right branches of the AV bundle are distributed to the ventricles and they terminate in the Purkinje fibres. Part of the right branch passes through the moderator band from the interventricular septum to the anterior wall of the right ventricle.

The blood supply of the heart is discussed with ischaemic heart disease (see p. 333). The venous drainage of the heart is mainly by the coronary sinus. Its main tributary is the great cardiac vein which ascends the anterior interventricular sulcus to turn around the left border of the heart where it becomes the coronary sinus. Several other veins drain to the coronary sinus before it enters the right atrium.

Congenital Heart Disease

A congenital heart lesion occurs in 6–8 per 1000 live births. Approximately 8% of cases of congenital heart disease have a definite genetic basis, 2% are due to environmental causes alone and 90% are due to a combination of genetic and environmental factors (Nora and Nora 1978). There is a three- to five-fold increase in the incidence of congenital heart disease in the first degree relatives of affected patients and certain inherited syndromes have an association with specific defects. Trisomy-21 (Down's syndrome) is associated with atrio-ventricular canal defects and patent ductus arteriosus; Turner's syndrome is associated with coarctation of the aorta, aortic stenosis and atrial septal defects; Ehlers–Danlos syndrome is associated with atrio-ventricular valve regurgitation and aortic dissection; Marfan's syndrome is associated with aortic dissection and mitral valve prolapse; osteogenesis imperfecta is associated with aortic regurgitation; and Friedreich's ataxia and Duchenne's muscular dystrophy are associated with cardiomyopathies.

There is strong evidence that certain drugs, infections and disease processes in the mother predispose to congenital heart disease. Alcohol consumption is implicated in the cause of ventricular and atrial septal defects and patent ductus arteriosus; anti-convulsants are associated with pulmonary and aortic stenosis, aortic coarctation and patent ductus arteriosus; maternal sex hormones predispose to transposition of the great arteries, tetralogy of Fallot and ventricular septal defects; thalidomide was associated with tetralogy of Fallot, persistent truncus arteriosus and septal defects; maternal rubella is associated with septal defects, patent ductus arteriosus and peripheral pulmonary artery stenosis; maternal diabetes is associated with a higher than normal risk of transposition of the great arteries, ventricular septal defects and aortic coarctation.

Embryology

The two endocardial tubes which appear in early embryological life fuse to form one tube. Constrictions in this single tube mark off chambers which form the truncus arteriosus, bulbus cordis, ventricle, atrium and sinus venosus. Dorsal and ventral endocardial partitions develop between the ventricle and atrium and eventually form the atrio-ventricular (AV) valves. The sinus venosus becomes absorbed into the atrium. The ridge between the bulbus cordis and ventricle disappears, thus incorporating the bulbus into the ventricle. Longitudinal spiral endocardial cushions form in the truncus arteriosus and finally fuse in order to separate the aorta from the pulmonary artery (see Fig. 12.1).

Congenital heart disease can be classified as acyanotic (with and without a left to right shunt) and cyanotic.

Acyanotic congenital heart disease with left to right shunt

Atrial septal defect (ASD)

Normally, the common atrium is at first separated by the septum primum which grows downwards towards the AV endocardial cushions. The gap between the septum primum and the AV cushions is termed the ostium primum. Further downgrowth obliterates the ostium primum, although communication between the left and right atrium is maintained by breakdown of the upper part of the septum primum to form the ostium secundum. The septum secundum grows down on the right side of the septum primum. It also has a defect (the foramen ovale) which is opposite an intact part of the septum primum. The flap valve so formed allows blood flow from right to left during fetal life, but prevents left to right flow when

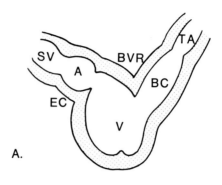

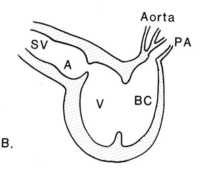

A.

B.

Fig. 12.1. Development of the heart: TA—truncus arteriosus; BC—bulbus cordis; V—ventricle; A—atrium; SV—sinus venosus; BVR—bulbo-ventricular ridge; EC—endocardial cushions; PA—pulmonary artery. (Adapted from Fleming and Braimbridge 1974.)

atrial pressures are reversed after birth (*see Fig.* 12.2). Abnormalities of the embryological separation of the atria lead to a variety of atrial septal defects.

1. SECUNDUM DEFECT (90%): The septum secundum is abnormal, leaving a defect which does not extend as far as the AV valves. The defect is usually at the site of the foramen ovale in the mid-portion of the septum.

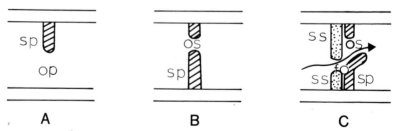

A   B   C

Fig. 12.2. Development of the atrial septum: SP—septum primum; OP—ostium primum; OS—ostium secundum; SS—septum secundum; FO—foramen ovale. (Adapted from Fleming and Braimbridge 1974.)

2. PRIMUM AND ENDOCARDIAL CUSHION DEFECTS (5%): There is a failure of the septum primum and the AV endocardial cushions to meet in the centre of the heart. Several abnormalities may arise. An ostium primum defect in isolation is a rare cause of an atrial septal defect which is low and adjacent to the AV valve. More commonly, the ostium primum defect is associated with a cleft mitral and/or tricuspid valve.

3. SINUS VENOSUS DEFECT (5%): Failure of the sinus venosus to become incorporated into the atrium leads to a high atrial septal defect near the orifice of the superior vena cava.

Patients with secundum defects usually present in adult life with atrial fibrillation or right ventricular failure. Alternatively, a murmur may be heard during routine medical examination. Patients with primum defects and AV valve abnormalities do less well and present at an early stage with heart failure and arrhythmias. Occasionally, in adults, late pulmonary hypertension and eventually, right to left shunting may occur. In patients without pulmonary hypertension, surgical repair using either direct suture or a patch has a mortality of less than 1%.

Ventricular septal defect (VSD)

The ventricular septum forms from three parts (*see Fig.* 12.3): (1) the membranous septum grows down from the AV endocardial cushions towards the muscular septum; (2) the bulbar septum is a downward continuation of the spiral septum (which separates the aorta from the pulmonary artery); and (3) the muscular septum. The three components meet at the crista supraventricularis. VSDs may occur in any of these three areas. Supracristal defects occur in the bulbar septum and are found just below the aortic valve. Membranous VSDs are the commonest (90%) and are seen just below the tricuspid valve. The bundle of His runs in the posterior edge of the defect. Defects of the muscular septum are less common and may be single or multiple.

Small VSDs (0·5 cm in diameter or less) may cause no symptoms, although a systolic murmur may be noticed on routine examination. Larger defects present in infancy or early adult life, depending on the size of the opening. They cause left ventricular failure, poor feeding, tiredness and recurrent pulmonary infections.

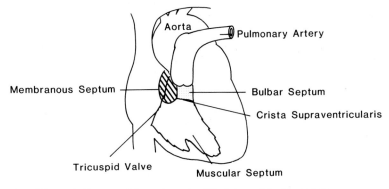

Fig. 12.3. Schematic diagram of the main parts of the interventricular septum.

Later, a right to left shunt may occur if pulmonary hypertension develops. Small defects may become smaller or close spontaneously. Larger defects are usually surgically closed at age 2–3 years, unless symptoms are severe, in which case earlier closure is undertaken. In the absence of pulmonary hypertension, operative mortality is less than 5%, but if the defect is near the AV node, heart block may follow the procedure.

Persistent ductus arteriosus (PDA)

The ductus arteriosus runs from the left pulmonary artery (near the pulmonary bifurcation) to the descending thoracic artery which it enters just distal to the left subclavian artery. It closes shortly after birth due, initially, to muscular contraction and then fibrous obliteration. Prostaglandins appear to play a role in closure. Persistence of a lumen of 2 mm or greater after the first week of life is considered abnormal.

Small defects may cause no symptoms whereas large defects cause cardiac decompensation and failure to thrive in infancy. The left to right shunt continues throughout both systole and diastole (as aortic pressure is always greater than pulmonary artery pressure) giving rise to a typical continuous 'machinery' type murmur. Later, pulmonary hypertension and eventual right to left shunting may occur with cyanosis more severe in the feet than in the hands (differential cyanosis).

Usually, division of the patent ductus is undertaken between ages 2–5 years and, in uncomplicated cases, mortality is less than 1%. Complications of the surgery include damage to the phrenic or recurrent laryngeal nerves and chylothorax. In view of the role of prostaglandins in the closure of the ductus, there is recent interest in using indomethacin to encourage medical closure, especially in premature infants.

Complications of left to right shunts

1. CARDIAC FAILURE: The heart has to cope with the normal cardiac output and also the shunt of blood which can cause overload and failure. An ASD causes right ventricular failure, a PDA causes left ventricular failure and a VSD causes failure of both ventricles.

2. INFECTIVE ENDOCARDITIS: This may be further complicated by metastatic abscesses elsewhere, especially in the brain.

3. INCREASED PULMONARY VASCULAR RESISTANCE: In some (but not all) patients with left to right shunts, the pulmonary arterioles become narrowed by intimal thickening and medial hypertrophy, thus producing an increase in pulmonary vascular resistance. Initially, as pulmonary arterial pressure rises, there is a reduction in the magnitude of the left to right shunt. A further rise in pulmonary resistance causes a balanced shunt (with approximately equal quantities of blood going in each direction). Finally, as pulmonary vascular resistance rises further, the shunt is reversed and the patient becomes cyanosed (the Eisenmenger syndrome).

4. PARADOXICAL EMBOLISM: An embolism originating in the venous system may pass into the systemic circulation via the defect and lodge in the arterial tree affecting organs such as the brain, spleen and gut.

Acyanotic congenital heart disease without left to right shunt: right heart lesions

Pulmonary valve stenosis

This is a relatively common lesion and most cases of pulmonary stenosis are congenital in origin. The pulmonary valve, which can be either bicuspid or tricuspid, is thickened and the cusps are fused. Right ventricular hypertrophy and post-stenotic dilatation of the pulmonary artery develop. The patient may have no symptoms or may have syncopal attacks and develop right heart failure in more serious cases. Usually there is no cyanosis unless there is severe outflow obstruction when a right to left shunt may develop via an atrial septal defect. Recently a balloon catheter technique has been described for dilatation of a stenotic pulmonary valve (Kan *et al.* 1982) and infants with severe symptoms of heart failure or high right ventricular pressures require valvotomy. The complication of pulmonary regurgitation after surgery is relatively well tolerated and mortality from valvotomy is less than 1% unless the infant is very ill.

Infundibular pulmonary stenosis

This is a condition in which the bulbo-ventricular ridge persists, causing narrowing of the lumen of the right ventricle below the pulmonary valve. The effect is similar to pulmonary stenosis.

Pulmonary artery stenosis

This exists in several varieties depending on whether the constrictions are in the main pulmonary trunk or its branches. The effects are similar to pulmonary stenosis.

Ebstein's anomaly

This is an abnormality of the tricuspid valve in which the medial and posterior leaflets are adherent to the ventricular wall. The origin of the free part of the valve cusp therefore comes off the ventricular wall low-down at some distance from its normal origin at the AV ring. That part of the ventricle above the valve attachment is thin walled, dilated and acts functionally as part of the atrium. The incompetent tricuspid valve and small right ventricle produce a reduction in pulmonary blood flow and a high pressure right atrium. If there is an atrial septal defect (a common association) the right atrium becomes decompressed by a right–left shunt which causes cyanosis. Paradoxical embolism and brain abscess are common complications.

These patients develop fatigue and dyspnoea due to the low cardiac output. The Wolff–Parkinson–White syndrome and arrhythmias are common. Symptomatic patients may require valvuloplasty or tricuspid replacement. Prognosis is poor in patients with severe forms of Ebstein's anomaly and one-third are dead by age 12 years.

Acyanotic congenital heart disease without left to right shunt: left heart lesions

Aortic stenosis

The cusps of the aortic valve are thickened and fused to varying degrees, often producing a bicuspid valve or sometimes a unicuspid valve. Usually there is fusion of the commissure between the right and left coronary cusps. Severe cases present in infancy with left ventricular outflow obstruction and less severe cases present in adult life when the abnormal valve becomes calcified (calcific aortic stenosis—*see* p. 345).

Infants with severe stenosis usually require surgery and even relatively asymptomatic older patients require operation if the gradient across the obstruction is more than 60 mmHg.

Supravalvular aortic stenosis

The aorta is stenosed just above the aortic valve and the constriction may produce an hour-glass type of deformity. In other cases there is a perforated diaphragm across the aortic lumen or a tubular narrowing over some distance. Supravalvular aortic stenosis is associated with abnormal facies (broad forehead and wideset eyes) and hypercalcaemia. The coronary arteries arise from a high pressure area below the narrowing and are therefore subject to premature atheroma. If the lesion is localized, excision with a patch on the wall gives good results.

Subvalvular aortic stenosis

Congenital subvalvular aortic stenosis may be due to a perforated diaphragm or a fibromuscular ring below the aortic valve. Presentation is similar to aortic stenosis. Excision of the membrane gives good results but care must be taken not to damage the mitral or aortic valves.

Mitral valve lesions

Several anomalies of the mitral valve may cause congenital stenosis. The valve may be of normal construction but small (miniaturization). The so-called parachute lesion is one in which all the chordae are inserted into a single papillary muscle so that the valve resembles a parachute; the interchordal spaces tend to become obliterated causing mitral stenosis. A double orifice mitral valve is also associated with stenosis.

These patients present with dyspnoea and other features of heart failure. The small mitral valve associated with the hypoplastic left heart syndrome is usually fatal. Conservative surgical treatment for congenital mitral valve lesions is difficult and valve replacement may be required.

Coarctation of the aorta

This is a congenital narrowing of the aorta, usually situated just distal to the left subclavian artery. The condition may be proximal or distal to the ductus arteriosus. Common co-existing congenital heart defects include bicuspid aortic valve, patent ductus arteriosus, ventricular septal defect and abnormality of the mitral valve. Aneurysms of the circle of Willis are also described.

POSTDUCTAL (ADULT TYPE): If the ductus remains open, the associated shunt is left to right and therefore no deoxygenated blood reaches the systemic circulation and cyanosis is not a feature. Unless very severe, the patients are asymptomatic until adult life, at which time proximal hypertension and distal hypotension are noted. The proximal hypertension may be complicated by left ventricular failure or aortic dissection. The dissection, however, characteristically stops at the point of coarctation.

The narrow segment (*see Fig.* 12.4) may extend over several centimetres or may be represented by a perforated membrane. The patients characteristically have left ventricular hypertrophy and collateral vessels are seen, especially in the region of the scapula. Collateral arteries include the internal mammary, intercostal, lateral thoracic and subscapular arteries.

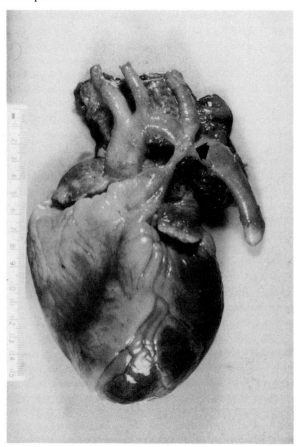

Fig. 12.4. Post-ductal coarctation of aorta (arrow) and persistent ductus arteriosus.

The mechanism of the hypertension above the coarctation is controversial. There are two theories: (1) the effect of the mechanical obstruction, and (2) increased renin and angiotensin levels secondary to decreased renal arterial pressure. Recent work suggests that the latter is the principal factor.

PREDUCTAL (INFANTILE TYPE): The pulmonary artery is at a higher pressure than the post-coarctation aorta and deoxygenated blood flows into the aorta distal to the left subclavian artery resulting in cyanosis of the lower limbs only (differential cyanosis). Other congenital defects such as an ASD and VSD are present in a large proportion of cases. These patients tend to present in infancy with heart failure.

Follow-up studies of patients reaching adulthood after successful childhood correction of coarctation have shown a high incidence of premature cardiovascular disease (Maron *et al.* 1973). This may be due to hypertension, coronary artery disease, cerebrovascular disease, aortic regurgitation and congestive heart failure.

Coronary artery anomalies

With the increasing use of coronary angiography, a wide range of coronary artery anomalies has been reported.

ANOMALOUS ORIGIN OF THE LEFT CORONARY ARTERY FROM THE PULMONARY ARTERY: This may present as myocardial infarction and death in the neonatal period. Those who survive the critical neonatal period (due to collateral circulation from the right coronary artery) develop symptoms of myocardial ischaemia and may suffer from sudden death in infancy or childhood. Aneurysmal dilatation of the ischaemic left ventricle may occur.

CORONARY ARTERY FISTULA AND ANEURYSM: Fistulas occur most commonly between the right coronary artery and the right ventricle or right atrium; a left to right shunt results and usually presentation is with cardiac failure or a murmur. Congenital aneurysm of the coronary artery has also been described. Complications include rupture and endocarditis.

Aortic arch abnormalities

Many aortic arch abnormalities have been reported but few require surgical correction. Three types of vascular rings which may require surgery for oesophageal or tracheal compression are described.

1. The double aortic arch occurs when neither of the two embryological aortic arches regresses. The ascending aorta bifurcates with a smaller arch to the left and anteriorly, while a larger arch lies posteriorly and to the right. The limbs rejoin behind the trachea and oesophagus to produce a ring.
2. Right aortic arch with left ligamentum arteriosum in which the aorta passes to the left behind the trachea and oesophagus to join the pulmonary artery anteriorly.
3. A retro-oesophageal right subclavian artery arises as a last branch of the arch and passes behind the oesophagus to the right and superiorly.

If symptoms occur in these anomalies they are usually due to tracheal and oesophageal obstruction with dysphagia and aspiration pneumonia. If symptoms are marked, surgical intervention is required.

Cyanotic congenital heart disease

Tetralogy of Fallot

An abnormality of the normal absorption of the bulbus into the ventricle leads to a series of defects: (1) persistence of the ventriculobulbar ridge which causes obstruction to the outflow of the right ventricle at the infundibulum; (2) failure of closure of the membranous part of the interventricular septum which produces a VSD; (3) abnormal rotation of the great arteries causing an over-riding aorta. These features, together with right ventricular hypertrophy, make up the classic tetralogy of Fallot, although variations exist. The presence of outflow obstruction of the right ventricle results in a right to left flow across the VSD and central cyanosis (*see Fig. 12.5*).

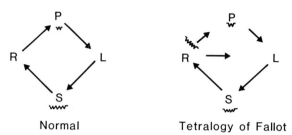

Normal   Tetralogy of Fallot

Fig. 12.5. Flow diagram of normal circulation and tetralogy of Fallot: R—right heart; L—left heart; P—pulmonary circulation: S—systemic circulation. The length of the resistance symbol is roughly proportional to the degree of resistance. (From Sherman 1974; reproduced with permission.)

In severe cases, cyanosis is present from birth or shortly after, but in less severe cases it may not be noticed for several months. The muscle of the infundibulum of the right ventricle increases in tone during crying and this may cause sudden deep cyanosis and syncope (the so-called cyanotic attack). These children characteristically squat so that pressure on the abdominal aorta increases systemic blood pressure thereby reducing the amount of the right to left shunt.

Complications include secondary polycythaemia, pulmonary infections and cerebral abscess. Palliative procedures aim to increase pulmonary blood flow and later total correction is carried out. Palliation is by systemic-pulmonary shunts such as pulmonary artery-subclavian artery anastomosis (Blalock–Taussig operation) and ascending aorta to right pulmonary artery anastomosis (Waterston operation). The other palliative approach is to decrease the right ventricular outflow obstruction by valvotomy or excision of part of the muscular infundibular stenosis (Brock operation). Total correction involves closure of the ventricular septal defect and relief of the outflow obstruction; the mortality is about 5%. Total correction may be carried out at the primary surgery or it may be preceded by a procedure aimed at increasing pulmonary blood flow.

Transposition of the great arteries (see Fig. 12.6)

The spiral septum of the truncus arteriosus develops abnormally so that the aorta arises from the right ventricle and the pulmonary artery arises from the left ventricle. Pulmonary and systemic circulations are therefore separate and flow in parallel rather than in series. Survival is only possible if there is a connection (PDA, ASD, or VSD) between the two circulations. An ASD is the most common association but it provides poor mixing so that presentation is with severe cyanosis in early infancy. A VSD provides better mixing but causes pulmonary hypertension unless there is an associated pulmonary stenosis. Anomalies of coronary artery anatomy are common associations.

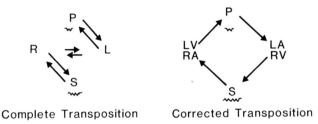

Complete Transposition   Corrected Transposition

Fig. 12.6. Flow diagram to represent complete and corrected transposition. (Adapted from Sherman 1974.)

Emergency procedures include the balloon atrial septostomy of Rashkind to create an ASD by passing a balloon catheter across the foramen ovale into the left atrium. The balloon is inflated and pulled back into the right atrium. More definitive treatment involves redirection of flow using a procedure such as the Mustard operation. More recently, total correction has been carried out to reconnect the aorta and pulmonary artery to the appropriate ventricles.

Corrected transposition (see Fig. 12.6)

In this lesion, the great arteries are transposed but inversion of the ventricles corrects the defect. Thus, the left ventricle flows into the pulmonary artery but receives its blood from the right atrium and vice-versa. Presentation may be with associated defects (VSD, ASD, etc.) or with arrhythmias due to the abnormal anatomy of the conducting system.

Total anomalous pulmonary venous connection (see Fig. 12.7)

There is no connection between the pulmonary veins and the left atrium. The pulmonary veins join the systemic veins (e.g. the superior vena cava, coronary sinus or hepatic veins) so that the venous return from the lungs enters the right atrium instead of the left. Survival is only possible if an ASD allows blood into the left side of the heart. There is therefore a right to left shunt with severe cyanosis from birth. Surgical reposition of the veins and enlargement of the left atrium is required.

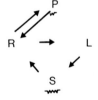

Fig. 12.7. Flow diagram to represent total anomalous pulmonary venous connection. (From Sherman 1974; reproduced with permission.)

Ischaemic Heart Disease

In the vast majority of cases, ischaemic heart disease is due to atheroma of the coronary arteries and its complications. Atheroma tends to be most severe in the proximal parts of the left coronary artery and its two main branches and in both the proximal and distal parts of the right coronary artery. Ischaemia may rarely be caused by atheroma in the ascending aorta which can block the coronary ostia. The aetiology and pathogenesis of atheroma are discussed on p. 354.

In the normal heart, the greatest resistance to flow lies in the arterioles. Obstruction in a proximal artery by atheroma generally does not provide greater resistance than the arterioles until about 75% of the lumen is obstructed.

Several mechanisms may make myocardial ischaemia worse. Firstly, hypotension due to shock (e.g. traumatic or surgical) reduces coronary perfusion, and, secondly, an increase in demand as occurs in exercise. Since the myocardium normally extracts up to 75% of the oxygen from blood, the increased demand must be accompanied by an increase in blood flow rather than by an increase in oxygen extraction. Finally, reduction in the oxygen carrying capacity of the blood, as in anaemia, will aggravate myocardial ischaemia.

Epidemiology

Approximately 156 000 deaths in England and Wales each year are due to ischaemic heart disease, this being 30% of all male deaths and 22% of all female deaths. The incidence of death from ischaemic heart disease increases with age. Death rates for women are less than for men up until the age of 75 years when they reach equality.

The death rate from ischaemic heart disease in Western countries has been rising steadily for most of this century, although in the United States a plateau was reached in the late 1960s and 1975 showed a statistically significant fall. This has been related to health education programmes which have reduced smoking and dietary fat.

Ischaemic heart disease is much less common in non-industrial countries and in Japan compared with the West. This has been related to environmental influences because migrants from low risk areas develop the risk of their adopted countries.

Certain risk factors for the development of ischaemic heart disease have been identified by prospective studies, particularly the Framingham Study (Kannel *et al.* 1976). The four most important risk factors found in this study were as follows:

1. HYPERLIPIDAEMIA: People with hypercholesterolaemia have a greatly increased risk of ischaemic heart disease. The hypercholesterolaemia may be due to one of the familial hyperlipidaemias or to diet, especially one which contains a high content of saturated fatty acids.

2. HYPERTENSION: High blood pressure, especially a high diastolic pressure, is associated with an increased risk of ischaemic heart disease. Patients with a diastolic pressure above 105 mmHg have a four times greater risk than those with a diastolic pressure below 85 mmHg.

3. CIGARETTE SMOKING: Men aged 45–54 years who smoke more than 40 cigarettes per day have a ten times greater incidence of death from ischaemic heart disease

than non-smokers of the same age. There appears to be a positive correlation between death rate and the number of cigarettes smoked.

4. DIABETES: Diabetics have about a two-fold increased risk of myocardial infarction compared with non-diabetics. Impaired glucose tolerance is positively correlated with increased mortality and morbidity from coronary artery disease. Diabetes mellitus is associated with hyperlipidaemia, increased platelet aggregability, a tendency towards hypertension and a diminished prostaglandin production. Control of diabetes may not affect the progression of atheroma.

Other less important risk factors include reduced physical activity, obesity, type A behaviour pattern (competitiveness and impatience), a positive family history and possibly long-term ingestion of the contraceptive pill. Unfortunately, the presence of two or more risk factors has a more than additive effect.

Ischaemic heart disease presents clinically as sudden death, angina pectoris or myocardial infarction. In addition, some patients present with a slow onset of left ventricular failure, without an acute event. Only angina pectoris and myocardial infarction will be considered further.

Angina pectoris

Angina pectoris describes the clinical situation of episodes of myocardial pain without evidence of actual myocardial infarction.

Stable angina is the common form in which episodes of pain are brought on by exertion and relieved by rest. These patients generally have severe stenosing atheroma of the main coronary trunks.

Prinzmetal or variant angina is characterized by episodes of pain which occur at rest. Prinzmetal et al. (1959) found that their patients had transient ST elevation on electrocardiogram and postulated that the syndrome was due to a sudden increase in smooth muscle tone at or adjacent to a severe stenosis. Maseri et al. (1978) subsequently showed that: (1) vasospastic myocardial ischaemia can occur in the presence of a very variable degree of coronary atheroma (from normal to severely diseased); (2) ST depression can also occur in these patients; and (3) transient vasospastic myocardial ischaemia can be accompanied by chest pain, or remain asymptomatic and can evolve into myocardial infarction and sudden death. The original syndrome as described by Prinzmetal et al. (1959) has therefore been broadened. The coronary artery spasm, which can be demonstrated at coronary angiography, causes a massive reduction in blood flow to one area of the myocardium and blood flow returns to normal when the spasm resolves. It has been shown that diseased coronary arteries retain the ability to contract since the atheroma tends to be patchy and does not involve the muscular media until the late stages of the disease. The reason for the coronary artery spasm is unknown.

Patients with unstable angina (also called acute coronary insufficiency or pre-infarction angina) have prolonged unrelieved pain often starting at rest, or else a rapid worsening of their usual stable angina. At post-mortem, these patients have extensive coronary atheroma.

Rarely, angina may be caused by an intramural position of one coronary artery (commonly the left anterior descending) which results in compression by the overlying myocardial muscle during systole. In some cases, the condition has been relieved by myotomy of the myocardial bridge.

Morphologically, patients with exertion related angina pectoris have severe atheroma of at least one and usually two or three of the main coronary arteries. They develop patchy necrosis of individual fibres of the myocardium which heal by fibrosis.

Myocardial infarction

Myocardial infarction occurs in two main morphological forms, transmural and diffuse subendocardial, although mixtures of these two morphological types may co-exist. The pathogenesis of transmural myocardial infarction is controversial, particularly as to whether coronary thrombosis is a primary or a secondary event.

The primary role of coronary thrombosis as the cause of myocardial infarction is supported by the following evidence: (1) when a thrombus is identified at post-mortem, it usually occurs on a damaged or 'cracked' atheromatous plaque, indicating that local trauma to the plaque has predisposed to thrombus; (2) some coronary angiography studies show a higher proportion of thrombus four hours after infarction than at 24 hours after infarction, possibly because of lysis of the thrombus.

The secondary role of thrombus is suggested by the following evidence: (1) a thrombus cannot be identified in all cases of myocardial infarction; (2) theoretically vasospasm could lead to damage of an atheromatous plaque with resultant myocardial infarction and secondary thrombosis in the region of the traumatized plaque.

The aetiological role of coronary thrombosis in causing myocardial infarction is therefore unclear, although current evidence suggests that coronary thrombosis is the primary event in most cases (DeWood et al. 1980).

Subendocardial myocardial infarctions are probably the result of an overall or global reduction in myocardial perfusion due to extensive coronary atheroma. These cases are only infrequently associated with an identifiable coronary thrombosis. Since the blood vessels of the heart run from the epicardial to the endocardial surfaces, subendothelial fibres tend to have the most tenuous blood supply and are therefore the first to be affected by a global hypoperfusion.

Haemorrhage into an atheromatous plaque has also been postulated as a cause of myocardial infarction. Recent studies suggest that the vasa vasorum of the coronary arteries are particularly prominent in regions of atheroma, while in areas of normal artery, vasa vasorum are rarely observed. This implies neovascularization in the area of atheroma, extending from the adventitia, through the media and into the thickened intima. These vessels are fragile and may precipitate medial haemorrhage. It is possible that this neovascularization may be a response to tissue injury and may be induced by macrophages, especially in areas of low oxygen tension (Barger et al. 1984).

Other possible causes of myocardial infarction include coronary artery spasm (see p. 332), embolization and a failure of flow in a stenosed artery to rise and meet an increased demand.

The myocardium is supplied by the right coronary artery (RCA) and the left coronary artery (LCA) which rapidly divides to form the left anterior descending (LAD) and the left circumflex arteries, thus providing a total of three main vascular channels.

Normally the area of distribution and therefore associated infarction for each vessel is: RCA—posterior wall of the left ventricle, posterior one-third of the interventricular septum and the adjoining part of the right ventricle; LAD—anterior wall of the left ventricle, anterior two-thirds of the interventricular septum and the adjoining part of the right ventricle; left circumflex—lateral wall of the left ventricle. Although generally only the left ventricle becomes infarcted, the infarct may extend into the right ventricular wall, especially the posterior right ventricular wall in cases of RCA occlusion.

Although the left and right coronary arteries were formerly considered to be end-arteries, it is now recognized that anastomoses occur between them. Thus occlusion of one artery may cause an infarct in the territory of another if that territory had been relying on collateral circulation due to stenosis of its own artery. Therefore, the correlation between the site of a coronary artery occlusion and its related myocardial infarction is not perfect.

In approximately 90% of cases, the RCA gives rise to the posterior descending artery and this situation is known as 'right dominance'. In about 10% of cases, the left circumflex gives rise to the posterior descending artery and this is termed 'left

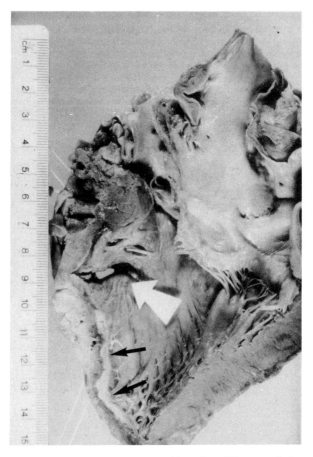

Fig. 12.8. Myocardial infarction (black arrows) with perforated interventricular septum (white arrow).

dominance'. This is important since the posterior descending artery supplies the AV node and therefore arrhythmias are more likely if the dominant artery is affected.

Grossly, an area of infarction of the myocardium is not apparent for 12–18 hours at which time it is seen as a pale-coloured area. Shortly afterwards, the infarct becomes encircled by a border of hyperaemia and by the end of the first week it appears as a yellow central area of necrosis with a dark hyperaemic rim (*see Fig.* 12.8). Eventually the infarct is replaced by scar tissue which appears as a thin grey area of the ventricular wall.

Histologically, the early changes occurring in the first few days are oedema (seen as separation of the myocardial fibres), neutrophil infiltration and coagulation necrosis which is characterized by eosinophilia of the myocardial fibres, the nuclei of which become pyknotic (*see Fig.* 12.9). Surrounding the area of coagulation necrosis, an area of so-called contraction band necrosis may be seen. This is characterized by thick cross bands of eosinophilic material in the myocardial fibres and it probably represents hypercontraction of cells in the 'border zone' of the infarct. There is some evidence that this change may be reversible and that the infarct border zone may benefit from rapid reperfusion.

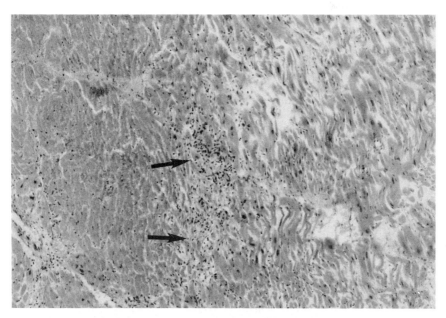

Fig. 12.9. Myocardial infarction: necrotic myocardial fibres to the left, some surrounding inflammatory cells (arrowed) and 'wavy' but viable myocardial fibres to the right. (H and E × 30)

The number of neutrophils peak in the first week and then they are replaced by lymphocytes, plasma cells and macrophages. Necrotic myocardial cells are removed and replaced by connective tissue. After three or four weeks, the inflammatory cells decrease in number and the connective tissue becomes hypocellular and sclerotic, thus forming a scar (*see Fig.* 12.10).

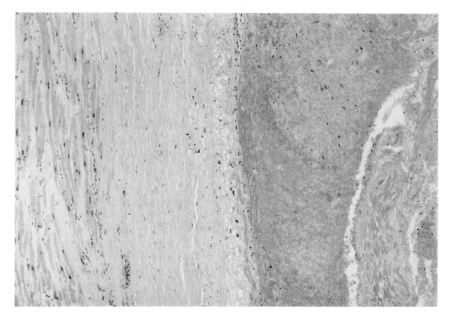

Fig. 12.10. Healed myocardial infarct (to the left) with a mural thrombus (to the right). (H and E × 30)

In the experimental situation, reperfusion of the ischaemic myocardium within 40 minutes reduces the infarct size by 60–70% and reperfusion within 3 hours salvages 20% of the area at risk. Beyond 6 hours, there is little or no salvage since severe swelling of the ischaemic endothelial and myocardial cells eventually blocks the capillaries and results in persistent ischaemia, even after the coronary artery occlusion has been released; this 'no reflow' phenomenon was first described in the brain.

These experiments provide a pathological basis for attempting early surgical reperfusion, although it is difficult to set up cardiopulmonary bypass within 6 hours of the onset of symptoms (Laffel and Braunwald 1984). Alternatively, attempts may be made to undertake thrombolysis using intravenous or intra-coronary artery streptokinase.

Complications of myocardial infarction

ARRHYTHMIAS: Bradyarrhythmias are more prominent in posterior and inferior infarcts as these are usually the result of right coronary artery occlusion. When the right coronary artery is dominant (as it usually is), it supplies the AV node (*see above*).

RUPTURE OF THE VENTRICULAR WALL: Rupture may be of the free wall which produces cardiac tamponade and death, or of the septum in which case survival is possible in some cases (*see Fig. 12.8*). About half of free wall ruptures occur within the first 24 hours after the onset of the infarction although they may be seen up to 12 weeks after the event.

RUPTURE OF A PAPILLARY MUSCLE: This complication usually occurs in the first week after infarction and involves one of the papillary muscles of the left ventricle. The patient suffers sudden haemodynamic deterioration and a loud systolic murmur of mitral regurgitation is heard. The posterior muscle of the mitral valve is more often affected than the anterior as it is situated in the watershed zone between the right coronary and the left circumflex areas of distribution. Papillary muscle dysfunction without actual rupture can occur in cases of severe ischaemia and in cases where the muscle origin is in an area of ventricular aneurysm.

MURAL THROMBUS: This occurs on the dyskinetic area of the ventricular wall and may give rise to emboli to other organs. (*See Fig.* 12.10.)

CARDIOGENIC SHOCK: Substantial loss of left ventricular muscle (over 40%) gives rise to cardiogenic shock characterized by hypotension, poor urinary output and poor peripheral perfusion.

VENTRICULAR ANEURYSM: This is an out-bulging of the left ventricular wall which can occur as an acute complication of infarction or as a dyskinetic fibrotic scar in the late stages. Aneurysms are more common in the anterior wall than in the posterior wall. Ventricular aneurysms cause inefficient ventricular contraction and can therefore be responsible for left ventricular failure or angina pectoris. They may also be a focus of arrhythmias or they can be the origin of thrombotic emboli. Surgical removal of the aneurysm may be necessary for these complications.

Occasionally, a rupture of the ventricular free wall may be locally contained, resulting in a false aneurysm which characteristically has a narrow neck.

Prognosis of ischaemic heart disease

Patients with stable angina who are receiving medical therapy probably have a mortality of between 3% and 5% per year (Hurst *et al.* 1982). Those with severe left main coronary disease have the worst prognosis. Survival for patients with left main coronary disease is improved by bypass surgery as shown by the Veterans' Administration trial (Takardo *et al.* 1976). The same is true for patients with triple vessel disease and also probably for those with double vessel disease.

Approximately 40–50% of patients who have a myocardial infarction die within twenty days. Half of these deaths occur within one to two hours of the onset of symptoms. Survival at three years after a first infarction ranges between about 30% and 60%, depending on such factors as the development of chronic angina pectoris, significant hypertension, residual electrocardiographic changes and cardiomegaly (Hurst *et al.* 1982).

Pathology of aorto-coronary bypass grafts

A reversed saphenous vein is the usual material for coronary artery bypass. Initial failure may be due to faulty technique such as (1) too short a graft causing tension and therefore narrowing; (2) too long a graft causing kinking; (3) suturing the distal end of the graft just proximal to an atheromatous plaque which may lead to thrombosis at the anastomotic site, poor distal run-off or dissection of the coronary artery.

Early failure within the first week may be due to thrombosis of the graft. The thrombus may be precipitated by endothelial damage which in turn may have been due to trauma to the graft at the time of surgery. Ischaemia, high pressure within the graft and poor flow caused by inadequate run-off, all also predispose to thrombosis.

Intimal fibrous proliferation occurs as a late complication and is usually not apparent until at least one month after surgery. The intima becomes thickened by deposition of fibrous tissue which, in some cases, eventually produces complete obliteration of the graft. The cause may again be trauma to the graft at the time of surgery. The condition tends to stabilize and is rarely progressive after one year.

In addition to complications in the graft itself, aorto-coronary bypass surgery may cause myocardial damage and infarction. Occasionally, return of blood flow to an ischaemic myocardium causes hypercontraction and the so-called 'stone heart syndrome' which is characterized histologically by the presence of contraction bands (*see* p. 335).

Rheumatic Heart Disease

Epidemiology and aetiology

Rheumatic fever is an acute illness mainly affecting children aged 4–14 years. Rheumatic heart disease is a chronic disease of the heart, principally affecting the valves, which follows attacks of rheumatic fever after a variable time. The epidemiology of rheumatic heart disease therefore parallels that of rheumatic fever. The annual incidence of rheumatic fever has reduced in Western countries over the past few decades due to: (1) a higher standard of hygiene and less over-crowding, both of which reduce the incidence of streptococcal sore throats; (2) prophylactic antibiotic treatment of children after one attack of rheumatic fever in order to prevent other attacks; and (3) possibly reduced virulence of the Strepto-coccus. This reduction in incidence has not taken place in the Third World, the annual incidence of rheumatic fever in India being over 200 per 100 000 compared with an incidence of 2·9 per 100 000 in the United States.

Rheumatic fever appears to be caused by antibodies to the M protein of the streptococcal wall cross-reacting with antigens in myocardial connective tissue and heart valves. They also cross-react with neuronal antigens in the basal ganglia and with antigens elsewhere in the body. Rheumatic fever follows infection of the throat (but not elsewhere) with group A beta-haemolytic streptococci. At the onset of the symptoms of rheumatic fever, the throat swab is usually negative although elevated titres of anti-streptolysin-O (ASO) and anti-DNA-ase indicate a previous streptococcal infection.

The subsequent inflammatory lesions in the joints, pericardium and myo-cardium heal without clinical consequence, although those in the heart valves heal by fibrosis with consequent distortion and malfunction.

Clinical features

Rheumatic fever is a febrile illness which may be diagnosed by the presence of either two major Jones criteria or of one major and two minor criteria. The major Jones criteria are (1) carditis, (2) polyarthritis, (3) chorea, (4) erythema marginatum and (5) subcutaneous nodules. The minor criteria include fever, arthralgia, previous rheumatic fever, a prolonged PR interval on ECG, a raised ESR, and evidence of a previous streptococcal infection.

Rheumatic heart disease most commonly affects both the mitral and aortic valves or the mitral valve in isolation. In severe cases, the tricuspid valve is also affected. The aortic and tricuspid valves are rarely affected in isolation and in those cases where they are so affected, causes other than rheumatic heart disease should be considered. The pulmonary valve is rarely affected by rheumatic heart disease.

Rheumatic valvular disease of the heart leads to stenosis or incompetence of the affected valve. The various clinical features of these conditions are well known and will not be discussed further.

Morphology

Rheumatic fever may affect the endocardium, myocardium and epicardium, and frequently all three are affected (pancarditis). The inflammatory reaction due to the presumed immunological process is most marked in the interstitial connective tissue of the myocardium, particularly in perivascular areas. Grossly, the valves are thickened and inflamed and verrucae (small vegetations composed of fibrin, etc.) appear at the free edges on the side exposed to the forward flow of blood. The myocardium shows little abnormality on gross inspection. The histological hallmark of acute rheumatic fever is the presence of Aschoff bodies which are areas of fibrinoid necrosis of ground substance surrounded by a proliferative cellular

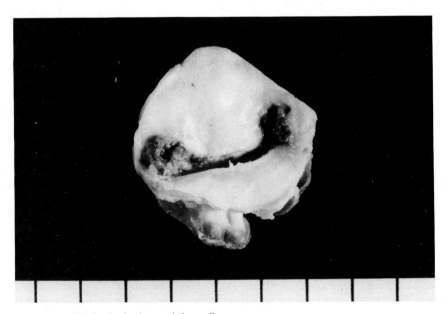

Fig. 12.11. Mitral valve in rheumatic heart disease.

reaction. This cellular reaction contains the Aschoff cells which may be multi-nucleated. Classical Aschoff bodies are found in the myocardium but rarely in the heart valve. Aschoff-like bodies are also seen in joint synovium.

In mitral stenosis, the cross-sectional area of the valve lumen is reduced from about five square centimetres down to about 1·6 square centimetres, at which point the symptoms of mitral stenosis occur (*see Fig.* 12.11). The valve cusps are thickened by fibrosis and calcification and they are vascularized. The anterior leaflet is less affected than the posterior leaflet and therefore mitral valve function may be maintained for some time. The valve leaflets are fused at the commissures for a variable distance thus causing a stenosing funnel-like or fish-mouth deformity and the chordae become fibrosed and shortened with consequent immobility of the valve leaflets. The left atrium becomes grossly dilated and occasionally contains a large ball thrombus. The left atrial appendage invariably contains thrombus which may give rise to thromboembolism. The immobile stenosed valve is invariably associated with some degree of mitral incompetence. In pure mitral incompetence, there is less commissure fusion and the main feature is fibrosis and retraction of the posterior valve which becomes fixed in the open position.

In aortic stenosis, the aortic valve undergoes thickening and shortening of its cusps which become adherent to each other along the commissures so that it may not be possible to distinguish whether the valve was originally bicuspid or tricuspid. The free edges of the cusps tend to roll and evert upwards and in the late stages the aortic valve becomes calcified. It may then be indistinguishable from the lesion of calcific aortic stenosis, although a concurrent diseased mitral valve suggests rheumatic heart disease. In pure aortic incompetence, there is fibrous retraction of the valve cusps without fusion at the commissures.

The tricuspid valve, when affected, resembles the diseased mitral valve.

Histologically, the valves in rheumatic heart disease show thickening, dense fibrosis, vascularization and calcification. These are non-specific features of a healed inflammatory valvulitis although in some cases of chronic rheumatic valve disease, occasional Aschoff bodies may be seen and these give a clue to the aetiology.

Prognosis

Patients with moderate aortic regurgitation have about 50% ten year survival and patients with mild aortic regurgitation have a good prognosis (over 90% alive at ten years). Patients with aortic stenosis have five and ten year survivals of 40% and 20% respectively and are prone to sudden death; therefore, patients who have aortic stenosis and symptoms of angina, syncope or congestive failure require valve replacement. The operative mortality is under 5%, provided ventricular decompensation is not severe. Five year survival following aortic valve replacement approaches 80%.

In mitral stenosis, once symptoms develop, five year survival ranges between 20% and 60%, depending on severity, and therefore patients with severe symptoms should be considered for surgery. Mitral regurgitation carries a five year survival of 75% overall, but if combined with stenosis, the prognosis drops to about a 60% five year survival. Operative mortality for mitral valve replacement is about 5%. Most types of mitral valve replacements carry a 70–80% five year survival.

Infective Endocarditis

In the UK, infective endocarditis tends to affect middle-aged and elderly patients. Thirty-three per cent were aged over 60 years in one UK study (Schnurr *et al.* 1977).

Aetiology and pathogenesis

About 90% of cases of infective endocarditis are due to either Streptococci or Staphylococci. *Strep. viridans* is especially important if the valves have been affected by rheumatic heart disease. Enterococci and group A beta haemolytic Streptococci may affect previously normal valves. Staphylococcal and Gram-negative infections may occur in main line drug addicts and diabetics. Fungal infections tend to be clinically indolent and occur in drug addicts or in patients with vascular catheters, or who are immunosuppressed. *Coxiella burnetii* (Q fever) is a further cause and some cases may be due to a mixed infection.

The source of the organisms in most cases is a transient bacteraemia. Transient bacteraemias occur in all people, but are normally dealt with by immune mechanisms. They often follow tooth extraction or urinary tract instrumentation and have been reported following gastrointestinal and bronchial endoscopy. Infection due to intravenous drug abuse affects the right heart valves.

In Schnurr *et al.'s* (1977) series there was no obvious pre-existing cardiac disease in about half the patients and rheumatic heart disease was the precipitating cause in about one-quarter of cases. Infective endocarditis more commonly affects incompetent valves than stenotic valves. Other valvular conditions which may be complicated by infective endocarditis include floppy mitral valve, bicuspid aortic valve and prosthetic heart valves. Small VSDs, PDAs, coarctations of the aorta and other congential heart diseases may also be affected.

Experimental studies show that if infected fluid is forced through a constriction at high pressure, the organisms settle out in low pressure 'sinks' immediately beyond the area of narrowing (Rodbard 1963). Thus, for example, vegetation occurs on the atrial aspect of an incompetent mitral valve and distal to a coarctation. A high pressure jet also damages the endothelium where it impinges and this predisposes to satellite lesions.

Clinical features

Patients may present with a slow ('sub-acute') onset characterized by pyrexia, weight loss, weakness and the classical findings which include Osler's nodes, splinter haemorrhages, etc. Some patients develop peripheral emboli. A heart murmur is not necessarily present and if it is present, the classical changing character is rarely encountered. Alternatively, patients may present acutely with rigors, heart failure and peripheral emboli.

Morphology

The most striking gross feature is the presence of large friable vegetations. They occur on the atrial aspects of the atrioventricular valves and on the ventricular aspects of the aortic and pulmonary valves. The mitral valve is the one most frequently affected, followed by the aortic and tricuspid. The pulmonary valve is rarely affected. Satellite lesions are found on the right ventricular wall opposite a VSD.

Histologically, the early vegetations consist of platelets and fibrin with polymorphs and colonies of bacteria. Later chronic inflammatory cells are seen and finally, organization occurs. The adjacent valve cusp may undergo necrosis.

Complications

The physical presence of the vegetation may interfere with the normal valve function, causing stenosis or incompetence with consequent cardiac failure. The infection weakens the valve cusp and produces aneurysmal dilatation or perforation of the leaflet with associated severe incompetence. Incompetence may also result from extension of infection to the chordae or the papillary muscles. Infection of the aortic valve may spread to the conducting system and cause complete heart block.

Systemic complications may be produced by embolization or by immune phenomena. Right heart vegetations embolize to the lungs and left heart vegetations embolize to the brain, spleen and kidney, etc. The bacteraemia may produce disseminated intravascular coagulation and the antigen/antibody reaction can cause glomerulonephritis, vasculitis and arthritis.

Prognosis

In Schnurr *et al.'s* study, overall mortality was 34%; the highest mortality was in those patients with *Staph. aureus* infections.

Heart Valve Prostheses

Prosthetic heart valves may either be tissue valves or non-tissue valves. The non-tissue valves are of two types: (1) those which have a central occluder and blood must swirl around it—these are termed lateral flow prostheses and an example is the Star–Edwards ball and cage valve; (2) those in which a tilting occluder permits a semicentral flow—an example is the Bjork–Shiley tilting disc prosthesis. Tissue valves allow a central flow, similar to that of normal heart valves. They also are of two types: (1) homografts which are from a cadaver—an example is fresh aortic valve, although these have a high incidence of infection and aortic regurgitation; (2) heterografts, the most popular of which is the porcine graft. These are treated with glutaraldehyde which destroys the antigenicity and increases the durability by stabilizing collagen cross-linkages.

The complications of prosthetic heart valves are as follows.

1. MECHANICAL: Mechanical problems tend to present as early complications. A dehiscence may occur along the suture line between the prosthesis and the valve ring. Calcification or myxomatous change in the valve ring and infection all predispose to dehiscence. There may be a disproportion, i.e. the valve is too large or too small, and this can lead to dysfunction of the valve or ulceration of the valve into the heart tissue. Ulceration, in turn, can cause perforation and arrhythmias. Angu-

lation of the valve is due to its being wrongly placed and it may cause dysfunction. Misplaced sutures may damage vital structures, such as the conducting system. Late mechanical failure depends on the durability and design of the valve.

2. THROMBUS FORMATION: This is more likely in non-tissue than in tissue valves. Thrombosis may occur acutely and cause obstruction to the valve and death. The thrombi tend to occur in areas of stasis in the valve and at component interfaces (e.g. where cloth and metal meet). Thrombus on a heart valve predisposes to embolization and to infection.

3. INFECTION: Early infection (usually *Staph. aureus*) is probably introduced at the time of surgery. Later, infection may be due to transient bacteraemia, such as occurs with genitourinary instrumentation. The infection causes dysfunction and tissue valves may perforate. Dehiscence may occur and the infection may spread to the valve ring with subsequent abscess formation and destruction of the conducting system.

4. TURBULENCE AND HAEMOLYSIS: Turbulence is a problem with non-tissue prostheses, especially those of the lateral flow type. The turbulence may eventually lead to fibromuscular thickening of the endocardium or aortic intima distal to the prosthesis, and in the latter case this can cause narrowing of the coronary artery ostia. The turbulence gives rise to red cell haemolysis and anaemia which is rarely severe. Lactate dehydrogenase is released from the red cells and its serum level gives a guide to the degree of haemolysis.

The Floppy Mitral Valve Syndrome
(Mitral valve prolapse; mid-systolic click syndrome)

There is some confusion regarding the significance of mitral valve prolapse. In one study in Framingham, evidence of mitral valve prolapse was found in 5% of the general population (especially young women) on echocardiography, although only a few of these had auscultatory findings of a systolic click and murmur (Savage *et al.* 1983). Symptoms were no more common in those people with echocardiographic mitral valve prolapse than in the general population. The relationship between the incidental finding of asymptomatic mitral valve prolapse and the clinical syndrome of mitral valve prolapse with valvular dysfunction and ruptured chordae will not be known until the Framingham cohort is followed up. In the meantime, three groups can be considered: (1) those with mitral valve prolapse on echocardiography but with no signs or symptoms, and who are regarded as a variant of normal by Oakley (1984); (2) those with mitral valve prolapse on echocardiography and auscultatory findings who are regarded as possible candidates for complications and who should be protected against endocarditis (Oakley 1984); and (3) those with actual mitral valve dysfunction. This discussion is confined to the last group.

The essential abnormality is laxity of the mitral valve leaflet and chordae associated with myxomatous change so that instead of closing at the normal position the valve prolapses into the left atrium during systole.

The aetiology of the condition is unknown. A similar valvular lesion occurs in

Marfan's syndrome and some authorities consider the floppy mitral valve syndrome to be a *forme fruste* of Marfan's syndrome. The pathogenesis of the weakness and laxity of the valve is also unknown with some authorities suggesting that myxomatous change is the important factor, while others claim that an abnormality of collagen is the primary defect with the myxomatous change occurring as a secondary phenomenon. Mitral regurgitation may occur in the otherwise uncomplicated case, although more commonly it is the result of rupture of the weakened chordae. The deformed valves may be affected by infective endocarditis or by thrombosis.

On gross examination, the posterior mitral valve leaflet is much more frequently affected than the anterior leaflet. The valve cusp has a larger than normal surface area and tends to be hooded (*see Fig.* 12.12). On sectioning the valve, the central myxomatous area can be seen. The chordae are attenuated and abnormally anchored to the valve cusp in such a way that parts of the cusp are completely devoid of chordal attachment, thus permitting interchordal hooding. This results in abnormal closure of the mitral valve. Later, the valve and chordae become thickened and fibrosed. Microscopically, the main feature is the presence of a layer of myxomatous tissue, composed of acid mucopolysaccharides sandwiched in the middle of the valve cusp; embedded in this myxomatous matrix are numerous stellate cells. Ultrastructural studies show defects in collagen fibres which may be the cause of the valve weakness.

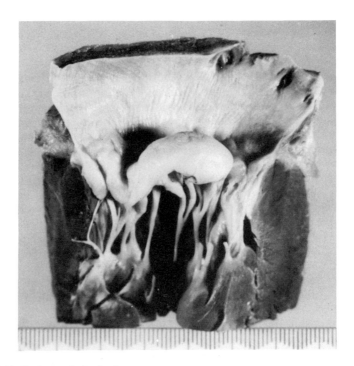

Fig. 12.12. Prolapse of mitral valve.

Calcific Aortic Stenosis

As discussed earlier, it is now realized that many cases of aortic stenosis are on a non-rheumatic basis. Congenital bicuspid valves are prone to wear and tear phenomena which eventually produce fibrous thickening and calcification, although otherwise normal tricuspid valves may also be affected. Patients may present clinically with aortic stenosis which on X-ray shows calcification in the aortic valve cusps. At surgery, the cusps of the valve are thickened, deformed and calcified.

Other Diseases of the Heart Valves

As well as rheumatic heart disease, the heart valves may be affected by rheumatoid arthritis (which gives a granulomatous response) and by systemic lupus erythematosis (characterized by the verrucae of Libman and Sacks which are attached to the affected valve). The latter rarely causes significant valvular dysfunction.

Marfan's syndrome, the Ehlers–Danlos syndrome and osteogenesis imperfecta are all associated with weakening of the valve leaflets and consequent valve dysfunction.

Whipple's disease may cause deformity, similar to that seen in rheumatic heart disease, and, histologically, macrophages packed with eosinophilic material are seen within the cusps. Similar macrophages are found in the small bowel in this condition.

Loeffler's endomyocardial fibrosis with eosinophilia affects middle-aged men and is characterized by eosinophilia, skin rash and endomyocardial fibrosis with eosinophilic infiltrates. It may cause valve dysfunction.

In the carcinoid syndrome, the right side of the heart becomes affected in up to 50% of cases. The full carcinoid syndrome of flushing, cramps, diarrhoea and wheezing, etc., usually only complicates carcinoids which have metastasized to the liver. Carcinoids located in the gut drain into the portal circulation with subsequent degradation of their secretory products. The cardiac lesions are probably due to the effects of 5-hydroxytryptophan, bradykinin or other products of the tumour which increase capillary permeability, cause oedema and, eventually, a fibroblastic reaction with thickening of the valve. Grossly, the lesions are characterized by fibrous plaques on the pulmonary and tricuspid valves and in the nearby endocardium. Histologically, the plaques consist of fibroblasts, smooth muscle cells and other cells embedded in a stroma of collagen and ground substance.

Cardiomyopathy and Specific Heart Muscle Disease

In the older terminology, cardiomyopathy was divided into primary (no known cause or association) and secondary (with a known cause or association). More recently, the term cardiomyopathy has been defined as heart muscle disease of unknown cause whereas those cases with a known cause or association have been termed 'specific heart muscle disease'.

Cardiomyopathy

This is classified into three pathological forms:

1. *Dilated cardiomyopathy*

These patients develop progressive heart failure and morphologically there is dilatation of either the left or both ventricles. There is an increase in heart weight, although dilatation prevents thickening of the ventricular wall. The histological features are non-specific with fibrosis and small foci of inflammatory cells. Surgical treatment, except for transplantation, is inappropriate.

2. *Hypertrophic cardiomyopathy*

This condition was formerly called hypertrophic obstructive cardiomyopathy (HOCM) or asymmetrical septal hypertrophy. Both these terms are now considered unsatisfactory as outflow obstruction is not always a feature. Cases have been described in which the whole of the left ventricular muscle, as opposed to just the septum, shows hypertrophy.

Morphologically, there is gross thickening of the wall of the left, right or both ventricles, with a predilection for the septum, and the ventricular cavities are grossly reduced in size. A characteristic feature is a white plaque on the septal wall of the left ventricle, just below the aortic valve where the anterior cusp of the mitral valve comes into contact during systole.

Histologically, the characteristic feature is disorganization of the normal orderly arrangement of myocardial fibres. The individual fibres tend to be short and broad with bizarre hyperchromatic nuclei. In hypertrophic cardiomyopathy, the change is very extensive, although small foci of similar changes can be seen in an otherwise normal heart. Thus, caution must be exercised in the interpretation of small myocardial biopsies.

Recently, it has been shown that the main physiological defects are failure of diastolic relaxation and an abnormally rapid systolic ejection rather than obstruction to the outflow tract by the hypertrophied interventricular septum. The high pressure gradient generated during systole is, therefore, due to rapid ejection rather than to obstruction. An additional characteristic abnormality is impact between the anterior leaflet of the mitral valve and the ventricular septum during each systole. This 'systolic anterior movement' is a helpful diagnostic feature in echocardiography.

The realization that the physical abnormality is not entirely due to obstruction has led to a reappraisal of the surgical procedures used to thin the ventricular septum.

3. *Restrictive/obliterative cardiomyopathy*

The ventricular wall is resistant to diastolic filling and therefore high diastolic filling pressures are required. This occurs in endocardial fibro-elastosis, a disease mainly of infants in which there is gross thickening of the endocardium. In adults, endomyocardial fibrosis is a condition in which there is fibrosis and thickening of the endocardium and the inner third of the myocardium. If there is an infiltrate of the eosinophils, it is termed Loeffler's syndrome. A mural thrombus is characteristic of this condition and organization of this obliterates the ventricular lumen.

Specific heart muscle disease

A very large number of conditions may cause disease of the myocardium and result in myocardial failure. These include toxins (e.g. alcohol and cobalt), metabolic diseases (e.g. haemochromatosis and thiamine deficiency), neuromuscular disease (e.g. Friedreich's ataxia) and neoplastic infiltration (e.g. leukaemia). These conditions tend not to be treated surgically and therefore are not considered further.

Cardiac Tumours

Most cardiac tumours are benign. Myxomas are the most common type and are further discussed below. Rhabdomyomas are much less common and occur as circumscribed tumour masses in the ventricular wall. Malignant cardiac tumours include angiosarcomas, rhabdomyosarcomas and mesotheliomas. They are exceedingly rare.

Cardiac myxomas

These are by far the most common cardiac tumours. Wold and Lie (1980) reported 59 patients with atrial myxomas seen at the Mayo Clinic. The mean age was 47 years and the lesion was three times more common in women than in men. Seventy per cent of the tumours were in the left atrium, the rest being present in the other chambers and occasionally on the heart valves.

Both organizing thrombus and a true benign tumour have been suggested to explain the pathogenesis of cardiac myxomas. Ultrastructural and tissue culture studies are strongly in favour of a true benign neoplastic nature.

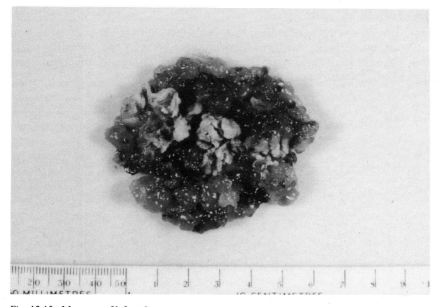

Fig. 12.13. Myxoma of left atrium.

Clinical symptoms may be due to obstruction of the AV valves (which can cause sudden death) or to emboli. Some patients develop constitutional symptoms such as fever and weight loss and the condition should be especially considered in young patients who develop recurrent emboli. It is imperative that any peripheral embolus removed surgically is sent for histological examination.

The typical macroscopic appearance is a pedunculated soft gelatinous tumour with a papillary surface (*see Fig.* 12.13). However, smooth, hard, non-pedunculated types are also seen.

Histologically, the tumour cells are embedded in a mucoid matrix. Stellate cells and 'lipidic' cells arranged singly or in clusters are seen together with smooth muscle cells, macrophages and other cell types.

The prognosis after removal is excellent (Rowlands 1983). However, tumour recurrence can occur and long-term follow-up is required.

The Pericardium

Congenital defects and cysts

Defects of the parietal pericardium are rare and usually found as incidental findings at autopsy. They are usually due to arrested development of the pleuropericardial membranes and are frequently associated with other developmental abnormalities of the heart and lungs. The defects are usually asymptomatic, although they can predispose to herniation of the ventricles and consequent coronary artery occlusion.

Pleuro-pericardial cysts (spring water cysts) are discussed on p. 416.

Acquired defects and cysts

Acquired defects of the pericardium may be due to injury to the heart or they may follow cardiac surgery. Acquired pericardial cysts may be parasitic (usually hydatid) or neoplastic (e.g. cystic lymphangioma). Pseudocysts are due to loculation of an inflammatory exudate.

Pericarditis

Acute non-specific pericarditis

This is an idiopathic condition occurring predominantly in males aged between 20 and 40 years. The likely cause is viral. The patient develops a pericardial serosanguinous effusion which very occasionally causes tamponade.

Infective pericarditis

VIRAL: Viral pericarditis is usually associated with a myocarditis and the common agents are Coxsackie A and B and ECHO viruses. A serosanguinous effusion develops with a fibrinous exudate and histologically the inflammatory infiltrate mostly consists of lymphocytes. Tamponade is unusual and constrictive pericarditis is a rare sequel.

BACTERIAL: This is a serious life-threatening condition. It is most common in Third World countries, although in the West there is a subgroup of cases which follow cardiac surgery. The most common organisms responsible are Gram-negative bacilli and *Staph. aureus*. In the majority of cases, there is a predisposing factor such as uraemia, diabetes mellitus, neoplasia or myocardial infarction.

The patient is toxic and has haemodynamic abnormalities. Tamponade is not uncommon.

Grossly, the visceral pericardium is covered with a thick shaggy fibrino-purulent exudate and, histologically, there is an intense polymorph infiltrate. The exudate may become loculated and drainage is frequently required. Mortality is about 40%.

Tuberculous pericarditis is usually secondary to a focus elsewhere in the body. The clinical onset is insidious. Initially, there is an effusion containing lymphocytes and later a granulomatous reaction is seen. The effusion becomes thick and opaque and later a fibroblastic proliferation causes thickening of the pericardium and obliteration of the pericardial space. Finally, constrictive pericarditis may ensue.

OTHER INFECTIONS: Fungal diseases may rarely cause pericarditis, especially in the immunosuppressed patient. Amoebic infection is usually secondary to a liver abscess which ruptures into the pericardial sac. Survivors may develop late constrictive pericarditis. Toxoplasmosis and filariasis are other rare causes.

Miscellaneous causes of pericarditis
Pericarditis may occur in association with a myocardial infarction, either early (during the first seven days) or late (after several weeks or months). The latter is termed Dressler's syndrome. Several generalized diseases such as renal failure, diabetes mellitus, rheumatoid arthritis and other collagen diseases may be associated with pericarditis. Tumour infiltration may cause a blood stained effusion and pericarditis has been described in association with certain drugs.

Constrictive pericarditis
Acute constrictive pericarditis develops within weeks of an acute pericarditis, while the chronic type (Pick's disease) develops over several years. About half the cases are idiopathic and some of these may be due to a previous unrecognized viral infection. Tuberculosis causes about one-third of cases and some follow pyogenic pericarditis.

Chronic constrictive pericarditis occurs in the fourth and fifth decades and is more common in males than females (male to female ratio 2:1). The heart is encased in an adherent fibrous pericardium up to 1 cm or more thick and the pericardial cavity is obliterated. Calcification is seen in 50% of cases. The fibrosis is usually diffuse, although a localized form has been described.

Tumours of the pericardium
Metastatic tumours of the pericardium are twenty times more common than primary tumours. Benign primary tumours include lipomas, which are often

misdiagnosed clinically as pericardial cysts. Malignant mesothelioma of the pericardium is a rare tumour which can give the symptoms of acute or chronic pericarditis. There appears to be no association with asbestos. Histologically, they are similar to pleural mesotheliomas. Sarcomas of the pericardium are exceedingly rare.

References

Barger A. C., Beeuwkes R., Lainey L. L., Silverman K. J. (1984) Hypothesis: Vasa vasorum and neovascularization of human coronary arteries. *N. Engl. J. Med.* **310**, 175–7.

DeWood M. A., Spores J., Notske R. *et al.* (1980) Prevalence of total coronary occlusion during the early hours of transmural myocardial infarction. *N. Engl. J. Med.* **303**, 897–902.

Fleming J. S., Braimbridge M. V. (1974) *Lecture Notes in Cardiology,* 2nd ed. Oxford, Blackwell Scientific Publications.

Hurst J. W., King S. B., Walter P. F., Friesinger G. C., Edwards J. E. (1982) Atherosclerotic coronary heart disease: angina pectoris, myocardial infarction and other manifestations of myocardial ischaemia. In: Hurst J. W. (ed.) *The Heart Arteries and Veins.* New York, McGraw-Hill.

Kan J. S., White R. I., Mitchell S. E., Gardner T. J. (1982) Percutaneous balloon valvuloplasty: a new method for treating congenital pulmonary-valve stenosis. *N. Engl. J. Med.* **307**, 540–2.

Kannel W. B., McGee D., Gordon T. (1976) A general cardiovascular risk profile: The Framington study. *Am. J. Cardiol.* **38**, 46–51.

Laffel G. L., Braunwald E. (1984) Thrombolytic therapy. A new strategy for the treatment of acute myocardial infarction (1). *N. Engl. J. Med.* **311**, 710–17.

Maron B. J., Humphries J. O., Rowe R. D., Mellits E. D. (1973) Prognosis of surgically corrected coarctation of the aorta. A 20 year post-operative appraisal. *Circulation* **47**, 119–26.

Maseri A., Severi S., Nes M. D. *et al.* (1978) 'Variant' angina: one aspect of a continuous spectrum of vasospastic myocardial ischemia. Pathogenetic mechanisms, estimated incidence and clinical and coronary arteriographic findings in 138 patients. *Am. J. Cardiol.* **42**, 1019–35.

Nora J. J., Nora A. H. (1978) The evolution of specific genetic and environmental counselling in congenital heart diseases. *Circulation* **57**, 205–13.

Oakley C. M. (1984) Mitral valve prolapse: harbinger of death or variant of normal? (editorial). *Br. Med. J.* **288**, 1853–4.

Prinzmetal M., Kennamer R., Merliss R., Wado T., Bor N. (1959) Angina pectoris: I. A variant of angina pectoris. Preliminary report. *Am. J. Med.* **27**, 375–88.

Rodbard S. (1963) Blood velocity and endocarditis. *Circulation* **27**, 18–28.

Rowlands D. J. (1983) Left atrial myxoma. *Br. J. Hosp. Med.* **30**, 415–20.

Savage D. D., Garrison R. J., Devereux R. B. *et al.* (1983) Mitral valve prolapse in the general population. 1. Epidemiological features: The Framingham Study. *Am. Heart J.* **106**, 571–6.

Schnurr L. P., Ball A. P., Geddis A. M., Gray J., McGhie D. (1977) Bacterial endocarditis in England in the 1970s. A review of 70 patients. *Quart. J. Med.* **46**, 499–512.

Sherman F. E. (1974) Congenital right to left shunts and bidirectional shunts. In: Edwards J. E., Lev M., Abell M. R. (eds.) *The Heart International Academy of Pathology Monograph.* Baltimore, Williams and Wilkins.

Takardo T., Hultgren H. N., Lipton M. J., Detre K. M. (1976) The VA co-operative randomized study of surgery for coronary arterial occlusive disease II. Subgroup with significant left main lesions. *Circulation* **54**, (Suppl. 3), 107–17.

Wold L. E., Lie J. T. (1980) Cardiac myxomas. A clinicopathologic profile. *Am. J. Pathol.* **101**, 219–40.

Chapter 13

The Blood Vessels

Normal Structure

The whole of the vascular system has a basic three layer structure consisting of an inner tunica intima, a tunica media and an outer connective tissue tunica adventitia. The structure of these three layers, especially the media, varies greatly in different types of vessels.

In the large elastic arteries (aorta, great vessels, pulmonary artery), the intima consists of an endothelium lying on a subendothelial layer of collagen, elastic fibres and scattered fibroblasts. In the deeper layers of the intima there are small bundles of smooth muscle. The media consists of numerous distinct elastic membranes, 40–70 in number, between which are scattered fibroblasts and smooth muscle cells. The adventitia is thin and blends with the surrounding connective tissue.

The muscular arteries (also termed the distributing arteries) include the radial, ulnar and anterior and posterior tibial arteries. The intima has three layers consisting of endothelium, subendothelial layers of elastic tissue and a prominent elastic membrane which separates the intima from the media (the internal elastic membrane). The media consists of up to forty layers of muscle cells with some collagen and a few elastic fibres. The adventitia contains a diffuse external elastic lamina and connective tissue.

Arterioles have lumina less than about 0·3 mm in diameter. The intima consists of endothelium and an internal elastic lamina with very little connective tissue in between. The media consists of 1–5 layers of muscle cells and the adventitia is a thin loose layer of connective tissue.

The capillaries are 3–4 μm in diameter and drain into the venules.

The smallest venules consist only of endothelium surrounded by collagenous fibres. At 50 μm diameter, they acquire smooth muscle fibres, and by 200 μm diameter, the venule has acquired a media of circular muscle fibres 1–3 cells thick. The adventitia is thick and consists of longitudinal collagen and elastic fibres and fibroblasts.

The small and medium sized veins include all the named veins, except the great veins of the trunk. The intima is thin with endothelial cells on an inconspicuous subendothelial layer. The media is also thin and consists of bundles of circular muscle fibres separated by collagen and elastic fibres. The adventitia is well developed and forms the greatest part of the wall. It is composed of loose connective tissue with collagen bundles and a few smooth muscle cells.

The large veins include the cavae and portal veins and their main tributaries. The intima is similar to that seen in smaller veins, but the media is poorly defined with few fibres. The adventitia is thick and has three zones—inner and outer layers of collagen and elastic connective tissue—between which is a layer of longitudinal muscle fibres.

The veins of the limbs and uterus have a rich smooth muscle wall, while the cerebral, meningeal, penile and bone veins have a minimal muscle coat.

Most veins have valves to prevent reflux of blood. Each valve is formed by reduplication of the intima, strengthened by connective tissue and elastic fibres. Both sides of the valves are covered by endothelium. On the surface of the valve next to the vein wall the endothelial cells are arranged transversely, while the cells facing the current of blood flow are arranged longitudinally. The wall of the vein on the proximal side of the valve is expanded into a sinus. Valves are numerous in the veins of the lower extremities and tend to be absent or few in number in very small and very large veins.

Limb Ischaemia

Peripheral vascular disease frequently presents as limb ischaemia which may be acute or chronic. The lower limbs are more often affected than the upper limbs. Similar disease processes are seen in both upper and lower limbs although their relative frequency is different.

Lower limb ischaemia

Acute lower limb ischaemia may be due to embolism, thrombosis (arterial or venous), trauma or aortic dissection. The classical clinical presentation is with a painful, cold, pale leg with varying degrees of numbness and paralysis.

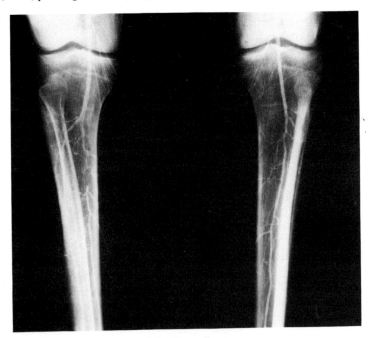

Fig. 13.1. Angiogram showing severe below knee atheroma.

The common cause of chronic lower limb ischaemia is atheroma (*see Fig.* 13.1). This may be aorto-iliac disease, femoro-popliteal disease or infra-patellar disease. Infra-patellar disease and small vessel disease, especially in a relatively young patient, suggests the possibility of diabetes. Less common causes of chronic lower limb ischaemia include thromboangiitis obliterans (Buerger's disease) and other vasculidities, entrapment syndromes, Raynaud's syndrome and other rare conditions. The classical symptom of chronic lower limb ischaemia is intermittent claudication.

Upper limb ischaemia

Acute upper limb ischaemia is due to the same conditions as cause acute lower limb ischaemia, although embolism is relatively less common in the arm compared with the leg.

Chronic ischaemia of the arm is much less common than in the leg. Ischaemia due to proximal arterial disease may be on the basis of atheroma of the innominate or subclavian artery, cervical rib or the thoracic inlet syndrome. Other diseases such as thromboangiitis obliterans, other forms of arteritis and Raynaud's syndrome tend to affect the more peripheral arteries. Recurrent microemboli may arise as complications of the thoracic inlet syndrome and cause a unilateral episodic ischaemia of the digits (similar to Raynaud's syndrome) and, finally, chronic ischaemia of the hand.

Arteriosclerosis

Arteriosclerosis is a non-specific term meaning 'hardening of the arteries'. There are three recognized causes: (1) Atheroma. (2) Mönckeberg's medial calcific sclerosis in which rings of calcification are seen in the media of large and medium sized arteries, especially the femoral. These give the affected artery a nodularity on palpation and they are seen on X-ray, although there is no obstruction and the condition is of little clinical importance. (3) Arteriolosclerosis affects arterioles, the walls of which are thickened by the deposition of a hyaline material with consequent luminal narrowing. Hypertensive and diabetic patients are particularly affected. The peripheral site of the lesions explains why some diabetic patients have severe ischaemia of the toes in the presence of normal limb pulses. Of these three conditions, atheroma is the one which most concerns the surgeon and it will be discussed in more detail.

Atheroma

The epidemiology of atheroma parallels that of ischaemic heart disease (*see* p. 331).

Atheroma typically causes slowly progressive ischaemia of the lower limbs and less commonly of the upper limbs. The patients complain of coldness of the feet, numbness and intermittent claudication. Claudication pain affects the buttocks and calf in aorto-iliac disease, calf muscles predominantly in femoral disease and the foot in tibial and peroneal disease. Later in the disease process, ischaemic ulcers occur in the skin and the patient develops rest pain. Eventually gangrene ensues.

This gradual process may be interrupted by sudden deterioration due to thrombosis occurring over an ulcerated atheromatous plaque.

Pathogenesis

The numerous complex theories of the pathogenesis of atheroma will not be considered in detail. An excellent review is given by Robbins *et al.* (1984). The most widely accepted concept is the 'reaction to injury' hypothesis which will be considered in outline only. This hypothesis suggests the following series of events: (1) the arterial endothelium becomes injured; (2) platelets adhere to, and plasma constituents enter, the injured wall; (3) factors released from the platelets and plasma cause smooth muscle proliferation; (4) lipid accumulates within smooth muscle cells, macrophages and in the intercellular space. Each of these steps will be discussed separately.

1. ENDOTHELIAL DAMAGE: Endothelial injury may be caused by haemodynamic shearing forces thus explaining the predilection for atheroma at arterial bifurcations (where stress is greatest) and its common occurrence in hypertensive patients. There is also evidence that the endothelium may be damaged by cigarette smoking and by hyperlipidaemia.

2. PLATELET ADHERENCE AND ENTRY OF PLASMA CONSTITUENTS: The platelets adhere to the points of injury and release various factors including platelet derived growth factor (PDGF) which stimulates proliferation of smooth muscle. Smooth muscle proliferation may also be stimulated by low density lipoproteins (*see* below) and by factors released by macrophages. Hyperlipidaemia tends to favour platelet aggregation.

3. SMOOTH MUSCLE PROLIFERATION: Under the influence of the above factors, smooth muscle cells migrate from the arterial media into the intima and undergo proliferation. In doing so they lay down extracellular ground substance such as collagen and proteoglycans which are important constituents of the atheromatous plaque.

4. ACCUMULATION OF LIPIDS: Lipid is carried in plasma in four forms: (i) chylomicrons, (ii) very low density lipoproteins (VLDL), (iii) low density lipoproteins (LDL), which have a very high cholesterol content, and (iv) high density lipoproteins (HDL). Exogenous (i.e. ingested) lipids are absorbed and transferred in the form of chylomicrons to the liver where they are metabolized. Endogenous lipoprotein is transported from the liver to other tissues in the form of VLDL which are metabolized to LDL prior to uptake by the extrahepatic cells where they are used to construct and repair cell membranes. The LDL enters the cell by one of two mechanisms. Firstly, absorption may take place by cell membrane LDL receptors which are under a negative feedback control (i.e. when LDL accumulate in the cell, the number of receptors on the cell wall is reduced). Secondly, absorptive endocytosis may occur. This is not receptor mediated and is therefore not under feedback control. When cell membranes break down, the resultant excess lipid is transported away as HDL. Any abnormality of these complex homeostatic mechanisms may lead to lipid accumulation in the cells and extracellular space. Possible

abnormalities include: (1) Hypercholesterolaemia, either inherited or as a result of diet. (2) Modification of the LDL which results in it being taken up by endocytosis rather than by the receptor mechanism. Since endocytosis has no feedback control, this causes lipid accumulation in smooth muscle cells and macrophages which eventually become foam cells. Factors released by platelets may cause modification of LDL. (3) Simple insudation of plasma lipoproteins across the damaged endothelium which produces accumulation of lipids in the extracellular spaces.

These mechanisms explain the positive correlation between serum LDL and atheroma and the negative correlation between serum HDL (which removes excess lipid) and atheroma.

Morphology

Atheroma occurs in discrete plaques (presumably at the points of former injury), although in advanced cases the plaques may coalesce to form an atheromatous mass. The vessels most affected are the abdominal aorta, the coronary, popliteal, femoral and internal carotid arteries and the circle of Willis. There is a special predilection for atheromatous plaques to occur at the point where the profunda

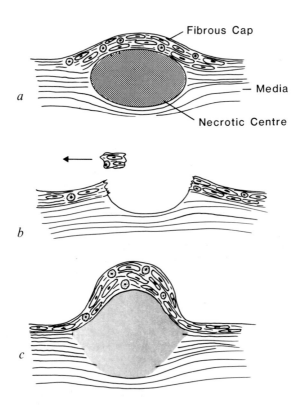

Fig. 13.2. *a*. Schematic diagram of a plaque of atheroma; *b*. Atheromatous embolus; *c*. Haemorrhage into an atheromatous plaque.

femoris artery branches from the common femoral artery and in the lower part of the femoral artery just below the site where it passes behind the adductor magnus tendon. Ischaemia of the arm may be caused by plaques in the innominate or proximal subclavian arteries.

Grossly, each plaque has a luminal covering of firm white tissue (the fibrous cap) overlying the centre of thick yellow viscous fluid which contains cell debris and lipid. Plaques are initially confined to the intima, although in the later stages the media is also affected (*see Fig.* 13.2*a*).

Histologically, the luminal covering or cap consists of smooth muscle cells with surrounding collagen, proteoglycans and lipid. Lipid accumulation in the smooth muscle cells and macrophages results in numerous foam cells. The necrotic centre is a mass of amorphous material with cell debris and cholesterol clefts (*see Fig.* 13.3). Calcification is frequently seen in long-standing plaques.

The basic atheromatous plaque may be complicated in several ways. Ulceration of the overlying cap allows debris to escape and form emboli (*see Fig.* 13.2*b*). Thrombosis may occur in ulcerated areas causing vessel occlusion, and haemorrhage into the plaque may also cause sudden occlusion (*see Fig.* 13.2*c*).

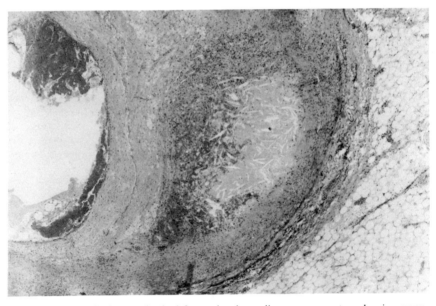

Fig. 13.3. Plaque of atheroma in the left anterior descending coronary artery showing many cholesterol clefts. (H and E × 30)

Arterial Thrombosis

Primary arterial thrombi occur in previously normal arteries and are rare. Aetiological factors include direct injury, generalized infections such as typhoid and meningococcal septicaemia, polycythaemia and prolonged bed rest. Thrombosis of the popliteal artery may be due to repeated minor injury as in the popliteal entrapment syndrome.

Secondary arterial thrombosis is usually due to an ulcerated atheromatous plaque. Other causes are Buerger's disease, giant cell arteritis and Takayasu's disease.

Arterial thrombi may remain *in situ* or they may embolize. In either event, the result is distal ischaemia. The sudden onset of the ischaemia may make clinical distinction between thrombosis and embolism difficult.

Arterial thrombi are structurally similar to other ante-mortem thrombi and the presence of lines of Zahn (*see below*) distinguishes them from post-mortem thrombi. If left undisturbed, they eventually organize and become recanalized.

Arterial Embolism

Embolism is defined as the transportation of undissolved material in the circulation and its subsequent impaction. Emboli are either solid or gaseous and either infected or sterile.

Thrombo-embolism is the main solid type of embolus. The most common site of origin is a diseased heart (mural thrombus secondary to a myocardial infarction or atrial thrombus secondary to atrial fibrillation and rheumatic mitral stenosis). Less than 5% arise from thrombus on an ulcerated atheromatous plaque in the aorta or its main branches; about 1% arise in arterial aneurysms. In 5–10% there is no obvious cause.

The common sites of lodgement of emboli are the distal extremities and the cerebral circulation (*see* p. 610). They have a predilection to lodge at arterial bifurcations.

Thrombi which arise in fast flowing blood (e.g. over a myocardial infarct) have a high proportion of white thrombus, which is composed mainly of platelets and fibrin. This forms prominent laminations between which is red thrombus (many red blood cells). These alternating layers of red and white thrombus are known as the lines of Zahn. Emboli arising on atheromatous plaques also tend to be composed of white thrombus together with atheromatous debris. Thrombi forming in slowly moving blood (e.g. the left atrium in atrial fibrillation) often have a high proportion of red thrombus and the lines of Zahn may not be distinct.

Occasionally, thrombi arising in the deep veins of the leg reach the right atrium and pass through an atrial septal defect into the systemic circulation (paradoxical embolism).

Emboli arising from atheromatous plaques may consist either of thrombus (as discussed above) or of atheromatous material. The atheromatous material contains cholesterol and lodges in arterioles 100–200 µm in diameter. They may cause transient ischaemic attacks (*see* p. 608).

Other causes of systemic arterial embolism are rare. Cardiac myxomas may embolize to the lower limbs and therefore all material removed at embolectomy should be sent for histology. Infected emboli may arise in infective endocarditis (*see* p. 341). Amniotic fluid and Wharton's jelly are well recognized types of emboli.

Iatrogenic emboli may arise from prosthetic heart valves, and from various parts of intravenous catheters. Various synthetic substances used for therapeutic embolization such as gelfoam may become misdirected. Caval filters used to prevent pulmonary thrombo-embolism may rarely migrate to the heart and pass through septal defects into the systemic circulation.

Air embolism may follow thoracic procedures and operations in the posterior cranial fossa. Fat embolism is discussed on p. 590.

Entrapment Syndromes

Of the many entrapment syndromes, only four will be described.

Popliteal artery entrapment

The tendon of the medial head of gastrocnemius passes laterally to the popliteal artery and compresses it against the lateral aspect of the medial femoral condyle. The anomaly is due either to an abnormal insertion of the gastrocnemius or to an abnormal course of the popliteal artery.

Most patients who present with symptoms are males between 20 and 40 years old, who complain of claudication which may be precipitated by thrombosis of the artery. Claudication is frequently unilateral although the anomaly is usually bilateral.

Post-stenotic dilatation of the artery occurs and this may go on to aneurysm formation.

Coeliac artery compression

A high origin of the coeliac axis from the aorta may cause its compression by the median arcuate ligament of the diaphragm. Lateral aortograms show extrinsic compression of the anterior wall of the artery. Correlation with abdominal pain is poor and the effect of surgery is unpredictable.

Subclavian artery compression

A cervical rib may compress the subclavian artery against the scalenus anterior muscle with resultant symptoms in the arm. Local thrombosis may occur and post-stenotic dilatation is common. This may go on to aneurysm formation. Emboli arising from the area of thrombosis tend to enter the radial artery or, if small, the digital arteries.

Other causes of subclavian artery compression include abnormal scalene muscles and an abnormal first rib (due to congenital anomaly, fracture callus or tumour).

If the subclavian artery is occluded proximally and the ipsilateral vertebral artery is patent, the subclavian steal syndrome may develop.

Persistent ischiadic artery

The iliac artery appears to run an anomalous course from the aorta to the groin and it becomes trapped behind the psoas muscle. The anomaly probably represents failure of the external iliac artery to develop so that the proximal embryonic ischiadic artery persists and anastomoses with the femoral artery.

Arteriovenous Fistulas

An arteriovenous fistula is an abnormal communication between an artery and a vein. It may be congenital or acquired.

The embryonic vascular plexus differentiates into both arteries and veins and failure of the process leads to a congenital arteriovenous fistula which usually has multiple connections between veins and arteries. They usually affect either the limbs or the viscera. Congenital arteriovenous fistulas of the limbs may be localized or diffuse and cardiac overload is rare in both types. The localized variety presents as a warm pulsatile mass with surrounding varicose veins. The diffuse type affects part or all of a limb and is accompanied by an increase in the length and circumference of the limb. The increased limb length is due to bone overgrowth which in turn may be due to increased bone temperature. The patients often develop severe venous insufficiency with varicose veins and ulceration. Visceral arteriovenous fistulas may be small or large and single or multiple. Large visceral arteriovenous fistulas may lead to high output cardiac failure.

Acquired arteriovenous fistulas may be traumatic, infective, spontaneous, or due to rupture of an aneurysm. They most commonly arise where an artery or vein run close together. Traumatic causes include stabbing and crushing injuries. Iatrogenic arteriovenous fistulas may follow mass ligation of the renal, splenic or superior thyroid pedicles. Operation on the lumbar discs may lead to an aortocaval fistula or to a fistula between the right common iliac artery and the left common iliac vein. Renal biopsy may occasionally cause a renal arteriovenous fistula. Arteriovenous fistulas on the forearm are constructed to allow vascular access for haemodialysis.

Spontaneous arteriovenous fistulas may arise in the Ehlers–Danlos syndrome due to defective connective tissue.

Rupture of an aortic aneurysm into the inferior vena cava causes an aortocaval fistula which is associated with hypotension, heart failure and bilateral leg oedema. Thrombus from the aneurysmal sac may pass through the fistula into the venous system and cause massive pulmonary embolism.

In general, the arteriovenous connection in an acquired fistula tends to be single and it may be direct or via a false aneurysmal sac. Collateral vascular channels form between those branches of the artery above the fistula and those below the fistula. Increased numbers of venous collaterals also occur.

The effects of arteriovenous fistulas are systemic and local.

If the fistula is large enough to cause a fall in peripheral resistance, this leads to a rise in heart rate in order to maintain blood pressure. The heart hypertrophies and if decompensation occurs there is a rise in central venous presssure and a fall in arterial pressure. The arteriovenous oxygen difference is diminished.

Locally there is an increased blood flow in the artery proximal to the fistula. The proximal artery becomes widened, lengthened and tortuous. Atheroma and aneurysmal dilatation eventually occur in the region of the fistula. The proximal and distal veins become lengthened, thickened and dilated. The haemodynamics of blood flow through the fistula and the distal artery and vein are complex and depend on the size of the fistula, the development of venous and arterial collaterals and the competency of the venous valves. The subject is reviewed by Sumner (1977). There is a threat to the blood supply of the peripheral tissues which can lead to absent pulses, pallor, ischaemic ulceration and gangrene.

Vasculitis

Vasculitis is characterized by a primary inflammatory process of a vessel wall, usually affecting arteries but occasionally also veins. Vasculitis is divided into several subgroups: (1) polyarteritis nodosa which is a disease of small and medium sized muscular arteries; (2) hypersensitivity vasculitis which affects small vessels and includes causes such as Henoch–Schoenlein purpura and connective tissue diseases; (3) temporal arteritis; (4) Takayasu's arteritis; (5) thromboangiitis obliterans (Buerger's disease). The last three will be considered briefly as the surgeon may be involved in their management.

Temporal arteritis (giant cell arteritis)

This condition affects elderly patients who present with headache and tenderness over the temporal artery. Involvement of the ophthalmic artery may cause blindness. About half of the patients have polymyalgia rheumatica with its associated systemic symptoms including muscle aching.

The aetiology is unknown although an autoimmune reaction to the vessel wall has been postulated. Grossly, nodular thickening can be palpated along the length of the temporal artery. Some patients may have involvement of other vessels such as the coronary and mesenteric arteries and the aortic arch.

The classical histological lesion is giant cell granulomas associated with fragmentation of the internal elastic lamina of the artery (*see Fig.* 13.4). However, some cases may only have a non-specific inflammatory infiltrate of the vessel wall or intimal fibrosis.

When taking a temporal artery biopsy it is desirable to palpate and remove a nodular segment of the artery. Up to 40% of biopsies are negative as the condition is patchy; therefore, a negative biopsy does not rule out the diagnosis.

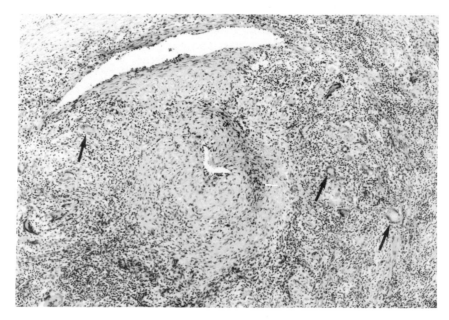

Fig. 13.4. Giant cell arteritis. Inflammatory reaction in the wall of the temporal artery with numerous giant cells (some of which are arrowed). (H and E × 30)

Takayasu's arteritis

Takayasu's arteritis is an inflammatory and stenosing condition mainly affecting the aortic arch and the origins of the great vessels. It is also known as the aortic arch syndrome or pulseless disease. Up to 90% of cases affect females who are usually under 30 years old. The disease was first described in Japan and subsequently cases have been seen in Western countries. The aetiology is unknown but an autoimmune basis has been suggested.

Clinically, the common presentation is with neurological symptoms such as visual disturbances and weakness due to cerebral ischaemia. There is associated weakening of the pulses and low blood pressure in the upper limbs. There may be associated fever, malaise and arthritis.

Grossly, there is substantial thickening of the aortic wall in the region of the arch with consequent narrowing of the lumen. The origins of the great vessels are narrowed and this is responsible for the pulseless limbs and neurological disturbance. There may be associated aneurysm formation.

Histologically, there is an infiltrate of mononuclear cells in the wall of the artery, sometimes with granulomas formation. Later, there is dense fibrosis.

Thromboangiitis obliterans (Buerger's disease)

This condition almost invariably affects young males (usually less than 35 years old) who are heavy cigarette smokers. The pathogenesis is unknown although the vessel wall may be subject to a genetic susceptibility to damage by cigarette smoke. However, the disease is extremely rare in female smokers.

Grossly, the small arteries in both upper and lower limbs, generally distal to the popliteal and brachial, are affected, resulting in distal ischaemia and eventually gangrene. There may also be a migratory phlebitis. Histologically, there is first an acute inflammatory reaction in the arterial wall with an associated overlying thrombus which characteristically contains small micro-abscesses. Later there is fibrosis of the arterial wall with spread to involve and encase nerves and veins so that the entire neurovascular bundle is affected. Organization of the thrombus and recanalization of the lumen may occur.

Raynaud's Syndrome

Primary Raynaud's syndrome (also called Raynaud's disease) is an exaggerated vasoconstrictor response in otherwise normal digital arteries.

Secondary Raynaud's syndrome (also called Raynaud's phenomenon) is due to a normal vasoconstrictor response acting on arteries which are abnormally narrowed by disease.

Patients with primary Raynaud's syndrome are usually women who complain of a series of colour changes (white then blue then red) in their fingers, or less commonly toes, stimulated by cold or emotion. This is due to reversible vasoconstriction and therefore ischaemic ulceration or gangrene of the finger tips very rarely occurs. Investigation of many of these patients reveals an underlying connective tissue disease which puts them into the category of secondary Raynaud's syndrome.

Patients with secondary Raynaud's syndrome complain of similar colour changes. However, since the affected vessels are already abnormal, ischaemia, ulceration and gangrene of the fingers may occur. The associated diseases include connective tissue diseases (especially scleroderma), atheroma, those brought about by drugs (ergot and the contraceptive pill), increased blood viscosity (e.g. polycythaemia rubra vera) and thromboangiitis obliterans.

Cystic Degeneration of the Popliteal Artery

This mainly affects young men and is probably traumatic in origin. Patients complain of claudication, coldness of the feet, pallor of the toes and the distal pulses may disappear on flexion of the knee joint. An asymmetrical filling defect is seen on arteriography and this is due to a ganglion-like, multiloculated cyst in the arterial media. There may be an overlying secondary thrombosis.

Idiopathic Popliteal Arterial Thrombosis and Dissection

This syndrome may or may not be preceded by trauma to the popliteal fossa. The patient develops sudden unilateral claudication due to a localized dissection of the popliteal artery with intramural haematoma. In many cases there is an associated thrombosis.

Aneurysms

An aneurysm is an abnormal dilatation of an artery or a vein. They can be classified according to site, shape, aetiology and whether they are true or false.

1. SITE: About 75% of aneurysms are situated in the aorta and iliac vessels. The next commonest site is the popliteal artery. The less frequent sites include femoral, subclavian, splenic, carotid and intracranial arteries.

2. SHAPE: A berry aneurysm is a small spherical dilatation on the wall of an artery. Larger spherical aneurysms are termed saccular. These two types have lumina which are not in direct continuity with the blood flow and therefore they tend to be filled with thrombus. The fusiform type is one in which there is gradual dilatation of the vessel to form a spindle shaped aneurysm, the lumen of which is in direct contact with the blood flow. Dissecting aneurysms are described under a separate heading.

3. AETIOLOGY: Most aneurysms are thought to be on the basis of atheroma although this has been challenged (see below). Other causes are infection (mycotic aneurysm), post-stenotic aneurysms, connective tissue disorders and trauma. The causes of berry aneurysms, dissecting aneurysms and inflammatory aneurysms are discussed elsewhere.

4. TRUE OR FALSE: A true aneurysm is formed from the distended layers of the vessel wall itself. A false aneurysm (commonly due to trauma or arterial catheterization) is one in which the wall is formed by surrounding connective tissue and not by the actual vessel wall.

Abdominal aortic aneurysms (*see Fig.* 13.5)

The incidence of intact abdominal aneurysms in the general population in England is said to be about 2% in people over 50 years of age. The majority of the patients are elderly males, the male to female ratio being about 4 : 1.

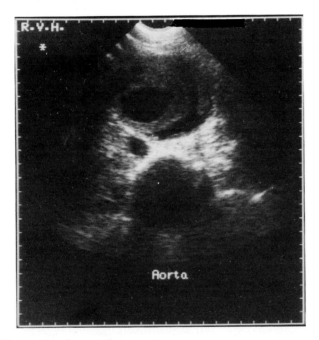

Fig. 13.5. Ultrasound to show aortic aneurysm.

Clinically, unruptured aneurysms present as abdominal or back pain. Alternatively, a pulsating mass may be found incidentally by the physician or by the patient.

Aetiology and pathogenesis

Classically, abdominal aneurysms are said to be due to atheroma. Although atheroma is basically an intimal disease, large plaques cause attenuation and weakening of the aortic media with consequent dilatation. The lower abdominal aorta is especially at risk due to reflection of the pressure wave from the aortic bifurcation. Once dilatation starts a vicious cycle is set up due to the fact that the tension in the aneurysm wall is proportional to the radius of the vessel; therefore, as the lesion enlarges, tension increases and causes further enlargement and finally rupture (Law of Laplace).

Bloor and Humphreys (1979) have challenged this classical view on the basis that: (1) the topography of aneurysms is not the same as the topography of atheroma, and (2) affected patients have a lower incidence of peripheral vascular disease and a better long-term survival than would be expected if they suffered from widespread atheroma. These authors suggest that abdominal aortic aneurysms are due to an unexplained weakness of the aortic wall with transudation of blood constituents across the wall. If an autoimmune reaction is set up to this transudate an inflammatory aneurysm (*see* below) results.

In support of the theory that there is intrinsic weakness of the aortic wall is the evidence that there is an increased elastase and collagenase activity in the walls of aneurysms and that the proportion of elastin and collagen in the walls of aneurysms appears to be significantly less than normal. Tilson (1982) has shown that patients with abdominal aortic aneurysms have a tissue copper deficiency and he has proposed that a sex-linked inherited copper deficiency decreases collagen cross-linking and predisposes to aneurysm formation.

An inflammatory aneurysm is a recently described sub-group and accounts for about 10% of abdominal aortic aneurysms. These patients may have a systemic illness with weight loss and raised ESR. Surgery relieves these symptoms even though the aneurysm wall is not removed, probably because further transudation of blood constituents is prevented so that the autoimmune reaction (mentioned above) ceases.

Morphology

The majority of abdominal aortic aneurysms start 2–3 cm below the renal arteries and frequently they involve the common iliac arteries. In only about 2% of cases they extend above the renal arteries. The origin of the inferior mesenteric artery is usually blocked and in those cases of upward extension, to and beyond the renal arteries, the superior mesenteric and coeliac arteries may also be involved.

In some patients the aneurysm extends up to the thoracic aorta, thus forming a thoraco-abdominal aneurysm which presents major surgical difficulties, although recently successful complete aortic replacement has been reported.

The aneurysm almost invariably contains clot which in most cases is anteriorly situated. This tends to prevent anterior rupture which would result in intraperitoneal haemorrhage and sudden death. Posterior rupture with containment by the retroperitoneal tissues is more common.

The gross appearance of the inflammatory variant is characteristic. The aneurysm wall is thick due to shiny white fibrous tissue which is continuous into the retroperitoneal area and may involve retroperitoneal structures such as the duodenum and ureters (the ureters may be pulled medially on a pre-operative IVU). The resected specimen shows a chronic inflammatory infiltrate in the aortic media and adventitia on histological examination. Surgery is more difficult than for ordinary aneurysms, particularly due to adherence of the duodenum to the aortic wall.

As well as rupture, abdominal aortic aneurysms may be complicated by embolism to the lower limbs (from the contained thrombus); occlusion of vessels (e.g. the vertebral branches of the spinal cord) due to thrombus; direct pressure and compression of adjacent structures such as the ureter; and aorto-caval or aorto-enteric fistulas may occasionally develop. The latter is usually to the duodenum and may present with small repeated haematemeses or with catastrophic haemorrhage.

Prognosis
Currently, most authorities believe that all aortic aneurysms below the renal arteries should be resected, provided the patient is fit for surgery. The operative mortality for an elective resection is 5–8% while mortality for a ruptured aneurysm was over 40% in one large British series (Fielding *et al.* 1981). Five year survival after resection is about 65%.

Thoracic aortic aneurysm

The classical cause of aneurysms of the thoracic aorta is tertiary syphilis, although currently atheroma may be a more common cause.

The aneurysm of tertiary syphilis is saccular or fusiform and may be very large so as to cause erosion of vertebrae, ribs or sternum. Characteristically, on gross examination, grey plaques of fibrous tissue are seen subintimally.

Histologically, the typical feature is an obliterative endarteritis of the vasa vasorum and the vessels are surrounded by a chronic inflammatory infiltrate. This causes ischaemia of the media with loss of elastic fibres and smooth muscle cells. Areas of fibrous scarring eventually appear.

Popliteal artery aneurysms

These usually arise on the basis of atheroma. There is predilection for aneurysm formation at the popliteal site due to continuous bending and to the post-stenotic effect of the adductor magnus hiatus. These patients frequently have associated aortic aneurysms and in 60% of cases they are bilateral. The aneurysm usually involves the upper two-thirds of the artery, sparing the lower segment proximal to its division.

The common presentation is an incidental finding of a pulsatile mass. Lower limb ischaemia may result from embolism or occlusion of the artery by thrombosis.

Femoral aneurysms

True femoral aneurysms are thought to be due to atheroma and are associated with aneurysms at other sites in about two-thirds of cases. They may be asymptomatic or they may present with thrombosis or rupture.

False femoral aneurysms are now more common than the true type, the majority being the result of disruption of an anastomosis between a synthetic graft and the artery. False aneurysms of the femoral artery may also be due to the Seldinger technique of catheterization or to stabbing or gunshot wounds.

Subclavian artery aneurysms

These classically occur as a post-stenotic dilatation associated with a cervical rib. Presentation is with embolism to the digital arteries, a pulsatile mass or as chest pain. Half of these aneurysms are intrathoracic and half are extrathoracic.

Splenic artery aneurysms

The common type of splenic artery aneurysm is found at the bifurcation of the splenic artery at the splenic hilum and is due to a congenital defect of the arterial wall. Atheroma associated aneurysms are found more proximally.

Splenic artery aneurysms are more common in females than males and they have a predilection to rupture during pregnancy.

Mycotic aneurysms

Peripheral arteries may become infected by septic emboli from a proximal site such as the heart, or by bacteria from a distant extravascular focus, or by contiguous spread of infection. Recently, cryptogenic mycotic aneurysms have been described with no obvious source of infection. The arterial wall shows an acute inflammatory reaction and it later becomes weakened producing a mycotic aneurysm. They tend to occur at bifurcations where emboli lodge and they frequently rupture while still small (1–2 cm in diameter). The commonest sites for mycotic aneurysms are aorta, superior mesenteric, splenic and coronary arteries; they are multiple in up to 25% of cases.

Dissecting Aneurysm of the Aorta

Dissecting aneurysm is characterized by splitting of the aortic media and dissection of blood within the aortic wall for a variable distance. Since there is little dilatation of the aortic wall, some authors suggest that the term 'aortic dissection' be used rather than dissecting aneurysm. The condition is about two times more common in men than women and the peak age incidence is 40–60 years. The incidence is thought to be relatively slightly increased during pregnancy. Aortic dissection may be more common than is generally considered as it may be responsible for some cases of sudden death in which no autopsy is carried out.

Aetiology and pathogenesis

The aetiology and pathogenesis of this condition are unknown. However, two major aetiological factors are often quoted, hypertension and abnormality of the aortic wall.

Left ventricular hypertrophy indicates previous hypertension in 90% of patients with aortic dissection who have an autopsy. Patients with coarctation have a high incidence of aortic dissection and it invariably occurs in the pre-stenotic high pressure area.

A high proportion of patients with aortic dissection have an abnormality of the aortic wall, in particular Erdheim's cystic medial necrosis. This is typified by fragmentation of the elastic laminae of the media and the development of mucoid filled cystic spaces. This type of change can be seen to some extent as an ageing process in otherwise normal patients without dissection. However, patients with Marfan's syndrome (who have a high incidence of dissection) have a high incidence of cystic change of the media. Klima *et al.* (1983) found a high incidence of elastic fragmentation and cystic change in non-Marfan's aortic dissection patients, especially the young, thus indicating that these patients have a 'tissue insufficiency', possibly on the basis of a *forme fruste* of Marfan's syndrome. The cause of the tissue abnormality in Marfan's syndrome is defective collagen cross-linking and a similar problem may be present in the non-Marfan's aortic dissection patients. Experimental evidence for this comes from the fact that animals fed with compounds which inhibit the enzymes necessary for the cross-linking of collagen develop a syndrome called lathyrism which is characterized by connective tissue weakness. Many of these animals die of aortic dissection.

The dissection is precipitated by a tear in the aortic intima. It is possible that cystic change in the media allows the inner part of the aorta (intima and inner media) to slip backwards and forwards on the outer media and adventitia during systole and diastole. The aorta, therefore, functions as two units, thus allowing shearing forces (which are greater in hypertensive patients) to buckle and eventually tear the inner layer.

Morphology

Grossly, specimens of aortic dissection show separation of the media by haematoma. In at least 90% of cases an intimal tear can be found. In 70% of these the tear is in the ascending aorta, in 20% it is in the descending thoracic aorta and in the remainder it is in the aortic arch or rarely in the abdominal aorta. The intimal tear and subsequent dissection usually affect about half the circumference of the aorta rather than the entire circumference. At the region of the aortic arch the 'greater curve' is more commonly affected than the 'lesser curve' and therefore the great vessels are frequently involved. A re-entry tear is found only in about 10% of cases.

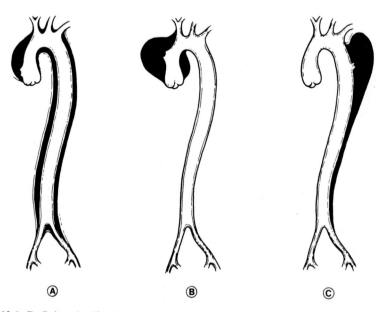

Fig. 13.6. De Bakey classification of aortic dissecting aneurysm.

The dissection takes place in the outer part of the media and therefore the outer wall of the dissection tract is thin and predisposed to rupture.

Once started, the blood dissects in a distal direction and less commonly in a proximal direction. The subsequent dissection is extensive unless it is stopped by a coarctation or by an atheromatous plaque. Dissection, therefore, tends to be more extensive in younger patients who do not have advanced atheroma.

Dissecting aneurysms have been classified by De Bakey into types A, B and C, as shown in *Fig.* 13.6.

Histologically, there is obvious splitting of the media (*see Fig.* 13.7) and fragmentation of the elastic fibres is seen in over 90% of cases. If Erdheim's cystic medial necrosis is present this is seen as fragmentation of the elastic fibres of the media together with small cystic spaces filled with ground substance.

Complications

The most serious complication is rupture of the aorta if the outer wall of the dissection track gives way. Since the pericardium is inserted into the aorta just proximal to the innominate artery, rupture of the ascending aorta causes haemopericardium, cardiac tamponade and death. The aortic arch ruptures into the mediastinum and the descending aorta ruptures into the left pleural cavity. The abdominal aorta ruptures into the retroperitoneal tissues.

Dissection of a branch of the aorta may cause ischaemia of the organ supplied and thus myocardial infarction, stroke, renal infarcts and lower or upper limb ischaemia may occur.

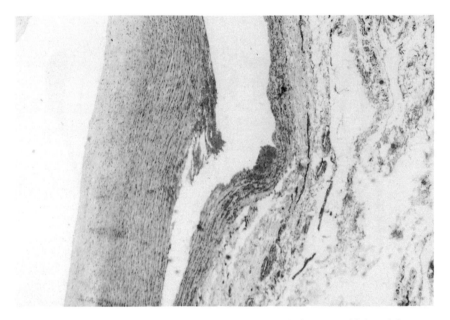

Fig. 13.7. Dissecting aneurysm of aorta. The split is between the inner two-thirds and the outer one-third of the aortic wall. (H and E × 30)

Retrograde dissection in the ascending aorta involves the aortic root with loss of support for one or more of the aortic valve cusps which causes aortic regurgitation.

Circumferential haematoma of the aorta in some cases causes narrowing of the lumen and 'true aortic stenosis' (as opposed to stenosis of the aortic valve).

Rarely, when the dissection ruptures back into the aortic lumen (causing a re-entry tear), the patient survives and the dissection becomes endothelial lined to form a double-barrelled aorta.

Prognosis

In specialized centres, with early recognition and treatment, up to 75% of patients who reach hospital alive survive. There is evidence that patients with proximal dissection do better with surgery while patients with distal dissection do better with medical therapy (Vecht *et al.* 1980).

Veins

Primary varicose veins

These are varicose veins without an obvious predisposing cause. They are more common in women than men (male to female ratio 1 : 3) and increase in frequency with age. About 20% of the population eventually develop some degree of varicose veins. Obese people are more commonly affected than the non-obese. More than half of all patients having surgery for varicose veins have a positive family history of the disorder.

The venous return to the lower limb is by two systems, termed deep and superficial, depending on the relationship to the deep fascia. The superficial system consists of the long saphenous and the short saphenous veins. The deep veins run with the named arteries. The two systems are connected by perforating veins which pass through the deep fascia. The most important perforating veins are in the medial part of the lower third of the leg.

Throughout the deep, perforating and superficial veins are the venous valves. They are not usually present in the venous sinuses of the soleus and gastrocnemius muscles. The valves are usually bicuspid and are frequently situated just distal to entering tributaries so that they prevent reflux. The valves of the perforating veins allow blood to flow only from the superficial to the deep veins.

The venous return of the lower limb depends on: (1) the muscular pump/venous valve system, (2) the negative intrathoracic pressure, and (3) the capillary blood pressure. A defect in these mechanisms leads to venous hypertension and dilatation.

The initiating cause of primary varicose veins is unknown, although the defect seems to be in the vein wall. The valves, whose cusps are essentially normal, become incompetent as they cannot meet in the dilated vein. One theory suggests that affected patients have a generalized abnormality of connective tissue, so that the vein tends to dilate abnormally in response to prolonged hydrostatic pressure. Another theory suggests that there is an inherited absence of a functioning valve in the femoral vein just above the sapheno-femoral junction.

Factors which aggravate varicose veins include pregnancy and occupations which require prolonged standing. Straining at stool associated with a Western diet has also been implicated.

Clinically, the patients may complain of aches in the legs, mild swelling and a cosmetic defect.

On gross examination, the venous dilatation is irregular, causing outpouchings, rather than cylindrical. The vein increases in both length and diameter. Histologically in the early stage, there may be a minor degree of smooth muscle proliferation but this soon becomes replaced by fibrous tissue.

Several complications of varicose veins may arise. Minor trauma tends to cause severe venous haemorrhage and superficial thrombophlebitis is common (*see* below). Dermatitis, skin pigmentation and skin irritation are associated with chronic venous stasis. The pigmentation is due to rupture of the cutaneous capillaries and deposition of haemosiderin from extravasated red blood cells. Finally, the skin may break down to form gravitational ulcers (*see* below).

Secondary varicose veins

Patients with secondary varicose veins have an identifiable cause.

Deep venous thrombosis may be followed by the post-phlebitic syndrome (*see* p. 373). The venous thrombosis damages the valves of the perforating veins and causes obstruction to the deep veins. Blood, therefore, tends to flow in a retrograde direction through the perforating veins into the superficial veins which become varicose. This condition is important to recognize clinically, as removal or ligation of the superficial veins will further impede venous return from the leg. A venogram may assist in the diagnosis.

Tumour masses in the pelvis may press on the ileofemoral veins and cause secondary varicose veins. Tricuspid incompetence is a rare cause of secondary varicose veins.

Gross varicose veins in patients below the age of 18 years may be due to congenital anomalies such as multiple congenital arteriovenous fistulas or the absence of venous valves. Varicose veins associated with congenital or acquired arteriovenous fistulas may show arterial pulsation.

Venous Thrombosis

Venous thrombo-embolism is more common in Northern Europe and the USA than in Asia and Africa. The difference has been attributed to differences in diet, fibrinolytic activity, ethnic origin and climate. Race alone does not appear to have a major influence on the varying incidence.

Risk factors in venous thrombo-embolism

AGE AND SEX: The incidence of venous thrombosis at autopsy increases with advancing age but age itself may not be an independent variable as diseases such as cardiovascular and neoplastic conditions also become more common with increasing age. Venous thrombo-embolism is more common in women than men.

VENOUS DISEASE: If a patient has had a previous deep vein thrombosis, there is a significantly higher risk of a further thrombotic episode. Monitoring with ^{125}I-fibrinogen has shown a postoperative incidence of 60% in these patients. Patients with varicose veins probably have about a two-fold increased incidence of postoperative deep vein thrombosis.

HEART DISEASE: Using labelled fibrinogen, deep vein thrombosis has been detected in 30–40% of non-anticoagulated patients with acute myocardial infarction. This high incidence is related to venous stasis and altered circulatory dynamics.

CANCER: The risk of deep vein thrombosis detected by scanning is increased to up to three times in patients with cancer. Pulmonary emboli are found at autopsy in 35% of patients with pancreatic carcinoma and in 20% of patients with lung cancer.

TRAUMA: Trauma to the lower limbs and pelvis significantly increases the risk of thrombo-embolism. Pulmonary emboli are found at autopsy in 45–60% of patients with lower limb fractures and in 27% of patients with pelvic fractures. Death has been attributed to pulmonary embolism in up to half of patients dying following fracture of the hip.

OPERATION: ^{125}I-fibrinogen leg scanning in patients over 40 years of age undergoing major surgery has shown a frequency of deep vein thrombosis of 15–50% (Kakkar et al. 1970). Although traditionally calf venous thrombosis has been considered of less importance than popliteal or femoral thrombosis, it has been shown that 25% of 'serious' pulmonary emboli arise from thrombi located inferior to the popliteal vein (Havig 1977). Thrombi usually start to form on the day of the operation but patients undergoing extensive preoperative work-up may develop thrombi prior to surgery. Surgery to the back, pelvis and legs (especially amputations and hip procedures) have the highest rates of thrombo-embolism (Williams et al. 1975).

PREGNANCY AND PUERPERIUM: The risk of deep venous thrombosis is increased by about five-fold during pregnancy and the post-partum period although fatal pulmonary emboli are rare. The risk of thrombosis is doubled if the patient is delivered by caesarean section compared with a vaginal delivery. Post-partum thrombosis is 3–6 times more frequent than ante-partum thrombosis.

ORAL CONTRACEPTIVES—OESTROGEN THERAPY: Oral contraceptives produce a 4–7-fold increase in the risk of venous thrombo-embolism (Vessey and Doll 1968) and the risk persists for at least one month after the pill is stopped. When oestrogens are administered for suppression of lactation or prostatic cancer, the risk is similarly increased and the higher the dose of oestrogen, the greater the risk. The risk of postoperative thrombo-embolism is increased 4–6-fold in women taking an oral contraceptive in the month prior to surgery.

PARALYSIS: Prolonged immobilization with no calf muscle activity increases the risk of thrombo-embolism. In acute stroke, 60% of the paralysed legs develop thrombosis compared with 7% of the non-paralysed legs (Warlow et al. 1976).

A high incidence of thrombo-embolism has been found in patients with acute paraplegia and in the Guillain–Barré syndrome.

OBESITY: Patients who are 20% or more overweight have a 1·5–2·0 increased risk of thrombo-embolism.

BLOOD GROUP: Some studies have shown that patients with blood group A have an increased risk compared with those who are group O.

FAMILY HISTORY: Patients with a deficiency of antithrombin III may have a family history of thrombo-embolism.

GRAM-NEGATIVE SEPSIS: Patients with endotoxaemia tend to develop intravascular coagulation and have a high risk of thrombo-embolism (Coon 1984).

OTHER ASSOCIATIONS: Statistically, patients with chronic ulcerative colitis have a three-fold increase in risk but the significance of this is unclear. Finally, patients with Cushing's disease appear to have an increased risk.

Pathogenesis
The pathogenesis of thrombosis is classically considered under the three headings of Virchow's triad:

1. CHANGES IN THE VEIN WALL: Although injury to the arterial endothelium is a well known cause of arterial thrombosis, the role of intimal injury in deep venous thrombosis of the leg veins is less well established. It is possible that localized hypoxia, especially in the valve pockets, may cause endothelial damage. When the flow of blood is pulsatile (due to the muscle pump) the Po_2 in the valve pockets is the same as in the luminal blood. However, when the flow is streamline and non-pulsatile, the valve pockets are undisturbed and the contained blood becomes hypoxic. Damage to the endothelium exposes subendothelial collagen with the result that tissue thromboplastin is released and thrombosis occurs.

2. CHANGES IN BLOOD FLOW: Stasis of blood in the deep veins is considered to be an important factor in the pathogenesis of deep venous thrombosis. Sevitt (1974) showed that valve pockets frequently contain tiny aggregates of red cells, white cells and fibrin. Whereas normally these would be washed away in the stream of blood, stasis may allow an accumulation and subsequent thrombus formation.

3. CHANGES IN THE COAGULABILITY OF BLOOD: It seems likely that blood may be in a hypercoagulable state in many conditions which predispose to deep venous thrombosis including malignancy, pregnancy and surgery, although in many of these conditions the exact mechanism of the hypercoagulability is unknown.

Clinical features
Thrombosis in a vein causes an inflammatory reaction in the wall of the vein and this gives rise to the clinical features of pain, tenderness and pyrexia. Venous

obstruction causes oedema. The relationship between deep venous thrombosis and pulmonary embolism is discussed on p. 392

Morphology

A venous thrombus is said classically to evolve through five phases (Walter and Isreal 1979). (1) A primary platelet thrombus is deposited due to minor endothelial injury. If stasis is present, clotting factors accumulate and promote fibrin deposition. (2) Further platelet accumulation takes the form of upstanding laminae growing across the blood stream. Between the laminae there is complete stasis and fibrin accumulates. The fibrin traps red and white blood cells and the result is alternate pale and dark layers known as coralline thrombus. The platelet laminae remain elevated above the surface and are known as the lines of Zahn. (3) The coralline thrombus eventually occludes the vein and blood flow ceases. (4) The stationary column of blood beyond the occlusion coagulates up to the next venous tributary. (5) Propagated thrombus develops beyond the next venous tributary (*see Fig. 13.8*).

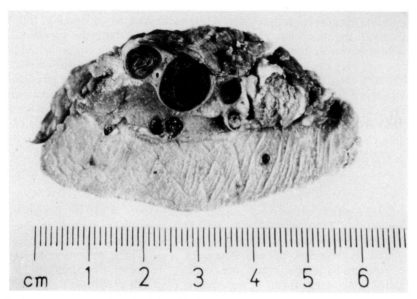

Fig. 13.8. Deep venous thrombosis in calf veins.

The initial occluding thrombus is firmly attached to the vein wall and is pale in colour. The propagated thrombus is red, loosely attached and may break off to form an embolus.

If the thrombus remains *in situ* it becomes organized by an ingrowth of capillaries and fibroblasts. Recanalization occurs and eventually the lumen is restored.

Complications of deep venous thrombosis

1. PULMONARY EMBOLISM: This is discussed on p. 392

2. POSTPHLEBITIC SYNDROME: This syndrome consists of pain on standing, dependent oedema and the later development of brawny, tender induration of the

subcutaneous tissues of the medial lower leg (lipodermatosclerosis). Subcutaneous fibrosis may progress to produce a 'champagne bottle leg'. Pruritus and eczematous skin changes occur and many patients develop secondary superficial varicose veins. Chronic indolent venous ulcers are frequently found and occasionally a squamous carcinoma may arise at the edge of an ulcer (Marjolin's ulcer). Most patients with the syndrome have a history of antecedent deep venous thrombosis and usually symptoms develop within three years of the thrombotic event although they may come much later. The usual sequence is deep vein thrombosis, followed by recanalization with destruction of the venous valves and the development of venous hypertension in the deep venous system during exercise.

3. VENOUS ULCERATION: This is discussed below.

4. OTHER SEQUELAE: Direct sequelae include oedema and cyanosis of the affected area.

Following deep venous thrombosis and organization of the thrombus, the valves are irreparably damaged and some degree of venous insufficiency often remains.

Phlegmasia alba dolens is the painful white swollen leg which develops following thrombosis of the iliac veins and causes obstruction of both the superficial and deep venous flow from the limb. It occurs most often in the puerperium and pelvic infection may play a role, producing also an element of lymphatic obstruction.

Phlegmasia caerulea dolens is rare and occurs with near total venous occlusion. It may progress to venous gangrene with a mortality of about 25% and an amputation rate approaching 50%. Presentation is with massive oedema, severe pain, shock and absent peripheral pulses. Treatment with streptokinase may be of benefit (Elliot *et al.* 1979).

Venous (Gravitational) Ulcers

These ulcers typically occur on the lower medial aspect of the leg just above the medial malleolus. The ulceration is associated with venous hypertension and most patients have varicose veins and/or a history of deep venous thrombosis. The exact pathogenesis is, however, unclear. The high venous pressure causes leakage of plasma from capillaries with consequent oedema. However, this cannot be the sole explanation, since other forms of leg oedema (e.g. due to cardiac failure) do not predispose to venous ulceration. Burnand *et al.* (1982), using biopsy specimens from venous ulcer bearing skin, have shown that the tissue contains an abnormally high number of capillaries and that the capillaries have surrounding layers of fibrin. These authors postulate that chronic venous hypertension increases the leakage of large molecules from capillaries into tissue spaces. This results in fibrinogen escaping from the capillaries into the tissues where it is converted into fibrin which is not broken down since these patients have a locally deficient fibrinolytic system. A peri-capillary cuff of fibrin forms and acts as a diffusion barrier for oxygen with resultant lipodermatosclerosis and ulceration, both of which appear to be a response to local ischaemia.

Grossly, venous ulcers are covered with grey slough which if removed reveals granulation tissue. The margin of the ulcer is pink and the surrounding skin is pigmented. The surrounding tissues are brawny and indurated (lipodermato-sclerosis). The site of predilection on the lower medial leg is probably due to incompetence of the perforators in this region.

Superfical Thrombophlebitis

This is a common condition appearing as tender red areas on superficial veins. The vein becomes occluded by thrombus which usually remains firmly adherent to the vein due to the inflammatory reaction. Local extension may occur and cause a cellulitis but significant embolism is rare.

Predisposing causes include pre-existing varicose veins, intravenous cannulae (especially if hypertonic solutions are used) and injection sclerotherapy. Thrombophlebitis migrans is a superficial thrombophlebitis associated with visceral malignancy (usually pancreatic carcinoma). Mondor's disease is discussed on p. 295.

Lymph Vessels

Primary lymphoedema

Primary lymphoedema occurs without an obvious acquired cause.

Congenital lymphoedema occurs at or soon after birth and in some of these cases the condition is hereditary (Milroy's disease). Lymphoedema praecox presents at age 10–25 and is more common in women than in men. It presents with spontaneous swelling of one foot or ankle which becomes progressive over a period of months. Lymphoedema tarda presents after the age of 35 years. It is likely that these three forms of primary lymphoedema represent different parts of the same spectrum of disease in which there are various developmental anomalies of the lymphatics. These anomalies include varicose dilatation, aplasia and hypoplasia which result in lymphatic obstruction. The obstruction causes distal dilatation and incompetent lymphatic valves which further aggravate the situation.

In primary lymphoedema the abnormality is generally confined to the superficial tissues which become grossly swollen and eventually hard in consistency.

Secondary lymphoedema

Secondary lymphoedema is caused by an acquired obstruction of the lymphatic channels. The obstruction causes distal dilatation and secondary incompetence of the lymphatic valves.

The commonest cause of secondary lymphoedema world-wide is filariasis (due to infestation with *Wuchereria bancrofti*). Surgical excision of lymphatics, as in a radical mastectomy or in radical groin dissection, may be followed by lymphoedema. Other causes include infiltration with malignant disease, radiotherapy, burns, tuberculosis, lymphogranuloma venereum and fungal infections.

The commonest complication of lymphoedema is cellulitis, usually caused by Streptococci. A late complication is the development of lymphangiosarcoma originating in the lymphatic endothelium.

Tumours of lymphatic vessels

These are discussed in Chapter 18. The Stewart–Treves syndrome is discussed in Chapter 11.

References

Bloor K., Humphreys W. V. (1979) Aneurysms of the abdominal aorta. *Br. J. Hosp. Med.* **21**, 568–83.

Burnand K. G., Whimster I., Naidoo A., Browse N. L. (1982) Pericapillary fibrin in the ulcer-bearing skin of the leg: the cause of lipodermatosclerosis and venous ulceration. *Br. Med. J.* **285**, 1071–2.

Coon W. W. (1984) Venous thromboembolism. Prevalence, risk factors and prevention. *Clin. Chest Med.* **5**, 391–401.

Elliot M. S., Immelman E. J., Jeffery P. *et al.* (1979) The role of thrombolytic therapy in the management of phlegmasia caerulea dolens. *Br. J. Surg.* **66**, 422–4.

Fielding J. W., Black J., Ashton F., Slaney G., Campbell D. J. (1981) Diagnosis and management of 528 abdominal aortic aneurysms. *Br. Med. J.* **283**, 355–9.

Havig O. (1977) Deep vein thrombosis and pulmonary embolism. An autopsy study with multiple regression analysis of possible risk factors. *Acta Chir. Scand.* (Suppl) **478**, 1–120.

Kakkar V. V., Howe C. T., Nicolaides A. N., Renney J. T. G., Clark M. B. (1970) Deep vein thrombosis of the leg. Is there a 'high risk' group? *Am. J. Surg.* **120**, 527–30.

Klima T., Spjut H. J., Coelho A. *et al.* (1983) The morphology of ascending aortic aneurysms. *Human Pathol.* **14**, 810–17.

Robbins S. L., Cotran R. S., Kumar V. (1984) *Pathologic Basis of Disease,* 3rd ed. Philadelphia, W. B. Saunders.

Sevitt S. (1974) The structure and growth of valve-pocket thrombi in femoral veins *J. Clin. Pathol.* **27**, 517–28.

Sumner D. S. (1977) Hemodynamics and pathophysiology of arterial disease. In: Rutherford R. B. (ed.) *Vascular Surgery*, pp. 25–46. Philadelphia, W.B. Saunders.

Tilson M. D. (1982) Decreased hepatic copper levels. A possible chemical marker for the pathogenesis of aortic aneurysms in man. *Arch. Surg.* **117**, 1212–13.

Vecht R. J., Besterman E. M., Bromley L. L., Eastcott H. H., Kenyon J. R. (1980) Acute dissection of the aorta: long-term review and management. *Lancet* **1**, 109–11.

Vessey M. P., Doll R. (1968) Investigation of relation between use of oral contraceptives and thromboembolic disease. *Br. Med. J.* **2**, 199–205.

Walter J. B., Isreal M. S. (1979) *General Pathology.* 5th ed. Edinburgh, Churchill Livingstone.

Warlow C., Ogston D., Douglas A. S. (1976) Deep venous thrombosis of the legs after strokes. Part I. Incidence and predisposing factors. *Br. Med. J.* **1**, 1178–81.

Williams J. W., Britt L. G., Eades T., Sherman R. T. (1975) Pulmonary embolism after amputations of the lower extremity. *Surg. Gynaecol. Obstet.* **140**, 246–8.

Chapter 14

The Lung, Pleura and Mediastinum

LUNG

Normal Development and Structure

At the fourth week of fetal life, a median laryngotracheal groove forms in the ventral wall of the pharynx and this eventually forms a laryngotracheal tube. The tube is lined by endoderm and from this the respiratory epithelium forms. The cranial end of the tube forms the larynx and the caudal end becomes the trachea. From the caudal end two lateral outgrowths arise to form the stem bronchi and right and left lung buds. These grow into the pleural coelom and become covered in splanchnic mesenchyme, from which the cartilage, smooth muscle and vasculature of the bronchi and lungs develop. The lung buds divide into lobules representing future lobes, three on the right and two on the left. Multiple further subdivisions produce the air sacs.

The adult left lung is divided into upper and lower lobes by an oblique fissure. The right lung is divided into upper, middle and lower lobes by oblique and horizontal fissures. The horizontal fissure is complete in only 30% of individuals and is absent in 10%.

Each lobe is supplied by lobar bronchi and vessels. The lobes are composed of a number of bronchopulmonary segments, which are pyramidal in shape with their apices pointing towards the hilum. The bronchopulmonary segments are supplied by segmental arteries and bronchi.

The tracheal wall consists of C-shaped cartilage plates which are joined together by fibroelastic membranes. The gaps in the cartilage lie posteriorly and smooth muscle (trachealis) lies in the gap. The trachea is lined with respiratory mucous membrane containing many mucous and serous glands. The epithelium is ciliated pseudostratified columnar with goblet cells.

The bifurcation or carina lies at T4. Widening of the carina at bronchoscopy for a bronchial carcinoma may indicate neoplastic involvement of the sub-carinal glands and implies inoperability.

The right main bronchus is wider, shorter and more vertical than the left and therefore foreign bodies tend to lodge in the right. The structure and mucous membrane of the major bronchi is similar to that of the trachea. The tertiary bronchi supply the broncho-pulmonary segments and repeated branching occurs within the segments. Eventually the cartilage and submucosal glands disappear from the wall and at this level the airways are known as bronchioles. Further division forms the terminal bronchioles which are less than 2 mm in diameter. Each terminal bronchiole divides into 1–3 respiratory bronchioles which are characterized by having alveoli opening directly from their walls. The respiratory bronchioles are lined by ciliated cuboidal cells and by non-ciliated cells known as Clara cells. The respiratory bronchioles run into the alveolar ducts which immediately precede the alveolar sacs. The walls of the alveolar sacs are composed completely of alveoli. The acinus is that part of the lung distal to a terminal bronchiole and is the functional unit of the lung (*see Fig.* 14.1).

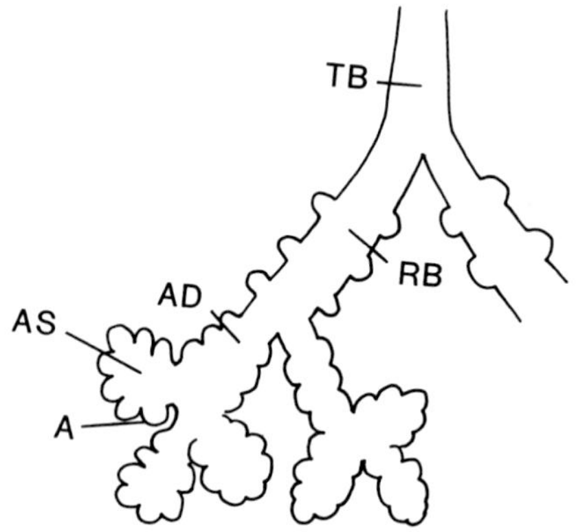

Fig. 14.1. Schematic diagram of the microstructure of the lung: TB—terminal bronchiole; RB—respiratory bronchiole; AD—alveolar duct; AS—alveolar sac; A—alveolus.

The alveoli are separated from each other by interalveolar septa in which lie the connective tissue elements of the respiratory tissue and the capillary beds of the pulmonary blood supply.

The epithelial lining of the alveoli consists of two cell types. The type I pneumocyte is a flattened attenuated cell which forms most of the alveolar surface. The remainder of the alveolar surface is composed of type II pneumocytes which are rounded cells projecting into the alveolar lumina. Their free surfaces are covered with microvilli. The type II cells produce surfactant, a phospholipid which forms a thin film on the alveolar surface. Type I cells cannot proliferate after damage. However, the type II cells proliferate rapidly after alveolar damage and quickly reform the epithelial lining. They appear to have the ability to then differentiate into type I cells.

Within the alveoli are the alveolar macrophages which phagocytose inhaled dust particles and extravasated red blood cells.

The bronchial tree is supplied by the bronchial arteries which are direct branches from the aorta. They supply the bronchi from the carina to the respiratory bronchioles. The bronchial veins drain into the azygos vein on the right and the hemiazygos vein on the left. The alveoli have a rich capillary plexus fed with deoxygenated blood by the pulmonary artery. The pulmonary artery branches tend to run with the segmental bronchi and the pulmonary veins tend to run in the intersegmental septa. There is both a submucous and a peribronchial lymphatic plexus. The lymph drainage is towards the hilum, along with the bronchi and pulmonary artery branches, to the bronchopulmonary nodes. It then goes to the tracheobronchial nodes at the bifurcation of the trachea and thereafter to paratracheal nodes and the mediastinal lymph trunks.

Bronchial and Pulmonary Biopsy

Tissue may be obtained at bronchoscopy by bronchial biopsy, transbronchial lung biopsy, brush biopsy, or bronchoalveolar lavage. Percutaneous biopsy techniques include cutting needle biopsy, high speed trephine biopsy and fine needle aspiration. Tissue can also be obtained at thoracoscopy or by open biopsy.

Pleural biopsy using an Abrams' needle has a limited place in the presence of pleural effusions. In the absence of fluid, the Menghini needle may be used to biopsy solid pleural lesions.

Other sources of tissue in pulmonary disease include supraclavicular lymph nodes, either by aspiration or by open biopsy. Such nodal tissue may aid the diagnosis of neoplasm, sarcoidosis, tuberculosis or lymphoma. Mediastinoscopy of the superior mediastinum with biopsy of the paratracheal nodes may be helpful in the diagnosis of the same conditions. Mediastinoscopy has also been used to stage carcinoma of the lung but there is significant morbidity, including bleeding and left recurrent laryngeal nerve palsy.

Transbronchial biopsy is frequently used to investigate diffuse lung infiltrates. The diagnostic rate is only 40–65% for some conditions, although in conditions with specific histology, such as sarcoidosis and diffuse malignancy, the diagnostic rate is much higher (up to 80% positive).

Major complications of fibre-optic bronchoscopy and biopsy occur in 2% of patients overall and mortality is 0·2%. Pneumothorax, not always requiring treatment, occurs in 5·5%. Haemorrhage of over 50 ml occurs in 1–4% of otherwise normal individuals but is more frequent in immunosuppressed patients (25%) and in uraemic patients (45%) (Fulkerson 1984).

Percutaneous biopsy of peripheral lung lesions which cannot be seen at bronchoscopy is useful. Percutaneous needle aspiration provides tissue for cytology and microbiological examination. A positive diagnosis of malignancy can be made in over 80% of cases (MacFarlane 1985). False positives are rare but the cytological tumour cell typing is inaccurate in about 30% of cases. The technique is less useful for diffuse infiltrative lung disease. A radiological pneumothorax occurs in about one-third of patients (Johnson et al. 1983) although less than 10% require drainage. Bleeding, air embolism and tumour seeding are very rare and overall mortality is 0·1%.

Percutaneous cutting needle biopsy of lung nodules gives accurate histology in 90% of cases although tumour seeding may occur occasionally (Harrison et al. 1984).

Open biopsy permits a representative sample of tissue to be obtained and the diagnostic rate in diffuse lung disease is 90% with a mortality of 0·3–1%.

One study compared the value of percutaneous needle aspiration, percutaneous cutting needle biopsy, transbronchial biopsy and open biopsy in patients with diffuse lung shadowing. The diagnostic yields were 29%, 53%, 59% and 94% respectively (Burt et al. 1981).

Congenital and Developmental Abnormalities

Failure of development of one primary bronchus causes agenesis of one lung. Variation in the arrangement of segmental bronchi is common and usually of little importance, although minor malformations of segmental bronchi can cause air trapping and congenital lobar emphysema.

Hypoplasia of one or both lungs may be associated with other congenital anomalies, such as diaphragmatic hernia. Very rarely, there is total lack of mucous glands in the respiratory tract.

Bronchogenic cysts

Bronchogenic cysts are congenital cysts of bronchial origin. They are usually closely related to the trachea, the lung hilum or the oesophagus and often present as an asymptomatic mediastinal cyst seen on chest X-ray.

The lining is of respiratory type. The lumen, which usually does not connect with the bronchial tree, is filled with mucoid material and the wall is composed of connective tissue which may contain cartilage.

Bronchogenic cysts may cause external pressure on a bronchus with consequent obstruction. Other complications include haemorrhage and infection.

Pulmonary cysts

Pulmonary cysts differ from bronchogenic cysts in that: (1) they are embedded in the pulmonary parenchyma, (2) they are connected to the airways and therefore contain air, and (3) their walls do not contain cartilage.

They may cause respiratory problems some time after birth due to compression of surrounding lung tissue, as air is trapped in the cysts. Other complications include haemorrhage, infection and pneumothorax.

Sequestration

This refers to an abnormal mass of lung tissue which is supplied by the systemic circulation (often from a branch of the aorta) and has either no, or else an abnormal, communication with the tracheobronchial tree.

They are probably derived from accessory lung buds growing out from the foregut. This theory is supported by the frequent finding of connections via fibrous cords with foregut structures (the oesophagus or stomach).

An extralobar sequestration lies outside the lung. It may be in the thorax or below the diaphragm near the kidney.

An intralobar sequestration is within the lung parenchyma and because of its abnormal drainage, it often gives rise to infection. The most frequent site is the posterior basal segments of the left or right lower lobe. Clinically the condition may mimic bronchiectasis.

Histologically, dilated inflamed airways with intervening alveolar structures are often seen. The vessels characteristically are of systemic rather than pulmonary type.

Congenital cystic adenomatoid malformation

In this condition a cystic mass replaces all or part of a lung or lobe of lung. It causes respiratory distress soon after birth and is seen on chest X-ray as an intrapulmonary mass.

The mass is composed of intercommunicating cysts which are lined by tall columnar cells and this gives them the appearance of large glands (thus the name adenomatoid). Solid areas may also be seen.

Surgical removal of the mass may be curative.

Accessory pulmonary lobes

An azygos lobe is occasionally found on the medial aspect of the right upper lobe, separated from it by a fold of pleura and the azygos vein.

The cardiac lobe (medial basal lobe) is sometimes separated from the right lower lobe.

A tracheal lobe is occasionally found arising from the right side of the trachea just above the bifurcation.

Congenital vascular anomalies

Aplasia

Aplasia of a pulmonary artery occurs with equal frequency on the right and left sides. In half of the cases an anomalous systemic artery arises from the aorta to supply the lung on the affected side. In the remaining cases, collateral circulation from the bronchial arteries supplies the affected side. Hypoplasia of the pulmonary artery also occurs and although the anomaly may be symptomless, recurrent pulmonary infection is a common complication.

Stenosis

This may take the form of single or multiple strictures affecting either the main pulmonary arteries or their segmental branches. There is post-stenotic dilatation and there may be accompanying cardiac anomalies.

Pulmonary arteriovenous fistula

This is a shunt between the pulmonary artery and pulmonary vein; the condition may be single or multiple. Polycythaemia, finger clubbing, cerebral complications and cyanosis occur. Hereditary haemorrhagic telangiectasis is seen in half of the cases.

Pulmonary Infection

Bacterial pneumonia

The filtering function of the nasopharynx and the cough reflex prevent bacteria from entering the lungs. Normally organisms which do enter the lung are cleared by ciliary action in the bronchial tree and by alveolar macrophages. Anything that damages these mechanisms may lead to bacterial pneumonia. In the postoperative patient, the cough reflex is suppressed. Surgical patients are especially compromised if they smoke, since cigarette smoke damages the ciliary action and reduces alveolar macrophage activity. Accumulation of secretions and pulmonary oedema also predispose to infection, as do general debility and immunosuppression. Bacterial pneumonia is usually divided morphologically into bronchopneumonia and lobar pneumonia.

Bronchopneumonia

This may be due to a wide range of organisms, including Staphylococcus, Streptococcus, Pneumococcus, *Haemophilus influenzae* and Coliforms. Bronchopneumonia is the common morphological type of pneumonia in postoperative patients and in elderly and debilitated subjects.

Grossly, the lungs on cut section show patchy areas of consolidation. These are seen as poorly demarcated pale areas which feel firmer than the surrounding lung parenchyma.

Histologically, the areas of inflammation are centred on bronchioles and affect the surrounding alveoli. The infiltrate is mainly of acute inflammatory cells (*see* Fig. 14.2).

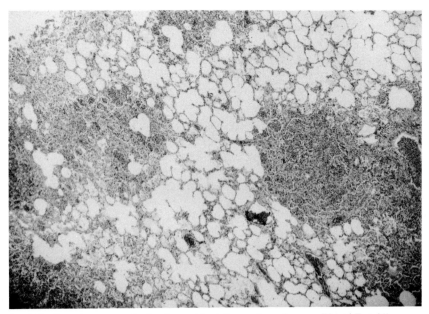

Fig. 14.2. Bronchopneumonia showing patchy inflammatory changes. (H and E × 30)

Lobar pneumonia

In these cases, an entire lobe is consolidated. The commonest organism to cause this is the Pneumococcus which is particularly virulent. Its capsule hinders phagocytosis and the organism can thus spread rapidly between alveoli through the pores of Kohn. Other organisms which can cause this morphological pattern include Klebsiella (in which case the cut section of the involved lobe has a mucoid appearance), Staphylococcus and Streptococcus. Males tend to be more commonly affected than females.

Pathologically the condition classically has four phases, although nowadays, these are rarely seen due to early antibiotic treatment.

1. *Congestion*: The lung is heavy. Histologically, vascular engorgement and intra-alveolar fluid are seen.
2. *Red hepatization*: The lung is solid, red and liver-like. Histologically, the alveoli are stuffed with neutrophils and fibrin.
3. *Grey hepatization*: The lung is still solid but paler in colour. Histologically, more fibrin is seen together with degenerating white cells and red cells.
4. *Resolution*: The exudate is digested to produce a granular debris and finally the lung returns to normal, except in rare cases when organization and subsequent fibrosis occur.

Atypical pneumonia

These patients have a variable clinical presentation. Infection is caused by a variety of non-bacterial organisms, the commonest of which is *Mycoplasma pneumoniae*. Other organisms include influenza virus, respiratory syncytial virus, Coxsackie virus and ECHO virus.

The main morphological feature is that the inflammation is in the inter-alveolar walls which are widened by an exudate of mononuclear inflammatory cells (interstitial pneumonitis).

Pulmonary tuberculosis

Pulmonary tuberculosis is caused by the organism *Mycobacterium tuberculosis*.

Two species of *M. tuberculosis* affect humans. *M. tuberculosis hominis* is spread by inhalation of infected droplets and the initial infection is usually in the lungs. *M. tuberculosis bovis* is transmitted by the ingestion of milk and the initial infection is in the tonsils or intestine. Infection by *M. tuberculosis bovis* is rare in Western countries because of strict regulations for dairy herds. Several mycobacteria which are related to *M. tuberculosis* may cause pulmonary infection. These are termed 'atypical mycobacteria' and the common types to cause pulmonary infection are *M. kansasii* and *M. avium-intracellulare*. This account is restricted to infection caused by *M. tuberculosis hominis*.

When the tubercle bacilli enter the lung in a non-sensitized individual, they initially evoke a non-specific inflammatory response and the organisms are phagocytosed by macrophages. After some time, a hypersensitivity reaction appears and the inflammatory reaction becomes granulomatous. The hypersensitivity reaction is cell-mediated by T-lymphocytes, which liberate lymphokines. Lymphokines are chemotactic to macrophages, stimulate them to aggregate and activate them, so that their ability to phagocytose and destroy tubercle bacilli is enhanced. The hypersensitivity reaction is associated with caseous destruction of lung tissue which lowers oxygen tension and pH, both of which hinder the growth of the tubercle bacilli. At the same time, the host's resistance, or immunity, toward the tubercle bacilli is increasing. It is unclear whether the host's resistance is part of the hypersensitivity reaction or whether it is mediated by a different T-cell sub-set.

Primary infection

In a patient who has not previously been infected by tubercle bacilli and has no immune responsiveness to tubercle bacilli, the initial infection takes the form of a single lesion, usually in a subpleural location in either the lower part of the upper lobe or the upper part of the lower lobe of one lung. This is known as a Ghon focus. Grossly, at first, it is an area of consolidation which then develops a soft caseous (cheese-like) centre. Histologically, the caseous necrosis is seen as an eosinophilic granular area. At the edge of the Ghon focus, granulomas are seen. These are typically composed of a centre of caseous necrosis, surrounded by epithelial cells and Langhans giant cells, which are surrounded, in turn, by a mantle of lymphocytes. The regional lymph nodes are usually involved and the combination of the Ghon focus and the involved lymph nodes is known as the primary or Ghon complex.

Usually primary tuberculosis heals by fibrosis and calcification, although viable organisms may be present within the fibrous tissue. Less commonly, there is spread within the lung to form progressive primary tuberculosis or invasion into a pulmonary vessel causing blood-borne spread and miliary tuberculosis.

Secondary infection

Reinfection by organisms, or reactivation of latent organisms, stimulates a prompt hypersensitivity reaction in the already sensitized patient. The lesion is usually in the apex of one or both lungs, since the intra-alveolar oxygen tension is greatest here. Reinfection starts as a small focus of consolidation which may progress in several ways. In many cases there is progressive fibrosis and walling off to leave finally a fibrous and calcified scar. In fibrocaseous tuberculosis, many granulomas coalesce to form a caseous cavity. This may erode into a bronchiole and subsequent expectoration of the caseous material leaves an open tuberculous cavity. Entry of air into this cavity increases the oxygen tension, which stimulates the organisms to grow with consequent progression of the disease. Blood vessels may be seen crossing these cavities and, although usually thrombosed, some may remain patent and rupture causing massive haemoptysis. The cavity may become superinfected with *Aspergillus fumigatus* to form an aspergilloma. Obstruction of bronchi or destruction of lung tissue leads to bronchiectasis. Spread of organisms along the mucosal lining of the bronchi and trachea causes ulceration and inflammation (endobronchial and endotracheal tuberculosis). Aspiration of infected material causes diffuse tuberculous bronchopneumonia. Entry of organisms into lymphatics may cause spread of tuberculosis within the lung or to distant organs. Erosion of infected material into a pulmonary artery causes miliary spread to the part of the lung supplied by that artery. Erosion into a pulmonary vein may result in widespread miliary tuberculosis throughout the body.

The mainstay of treatment is antituberculous chemotherapy. Surgical resection may be used in cases of progressive disease with resistant organisms or in cases of persistent tuberculous cavities, especially if complicated by massive or repeated haemoptysis or by the development of an aspergilloma. Surgery may also be considered for bronchiectasis localized to a segment or lobe.

Fungal infections

Pulmonary fungal infections are likely to occur in patients who have some generalized systemic abnormality such as severe malnutrition or diabetes mellitus, or in those patients receiving steroids, broad spectrum antibiotics or immunosuppressive drugs. Fungal infection may also complicate an underlying pulmonary disease such as tuberculosis, cancer or bronchiectasis.

Candidiasis (moniliasis)

This is usually due to infection with *C. albicans* which can appear as rounded yeast forms or as branching mycelia. It may give rise to a bronchopneumonia or to a miliary candidiasis of the lung.

Aspergillosis

The most common species to infect man is *A. fumigatus*, although *A. nigra* and others also are found. The organism can cause an asthmatic-like condition (allergic aspergillosis), or invasive lung infections which can take the form of a granulomatous reaction, a lobar pneumonia or an abscess. The manifestation most frequently encountered by the surgeon is an aspergilloma. This is not an invasive infection, but rather a saprophytic fungus ball (mycetoma) which is found complicating bronchiectasis or cavities resulting from tuberculosis, a lung abscess or a necrotic lung tumour.

Grossly, the cavity is filled with a brown or grey material. On X-ray the typical finding is an opacity capped by a bubble of air.

Histologically, the mycetoma is composed of a tangled mass of mycelia together with cell debris (*see Fig.* 14.3).

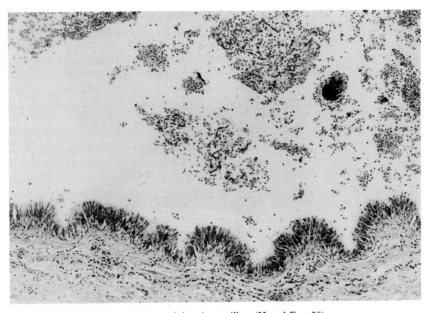

Fig. 14.3. Bronchiectatic cavity containing Aspergillus. (H and E × 30)

Cryptococcosis

This is caused by *C. neoformans*, a rounded yeast-like organism. It causes primary and secondary infections, similar to tuberculosis. Clinically, it may present as a diffuse pulmonary infiltrate or as an isolated pulmonary nodule which can be confused with a peripheral carcinoma. Histology, however, shows a granulomatous mass. A disseminated infection may occur. There is a good response to amphotericin.

Histoplasmosis

H. capsulatum in North America and *H. duboisii* in Africa are the organisms concerned. The disease is rare in the UK but does occur. The organism is oval and yeast-like and there is a close clinical resemblance to tuberculosis, with a primary infection and a secondary cavitating infection. The latter is very similar grossly and radiologically to tuberculosis. Histologically, however, fungi are seen.

Lung abscess

This is a localized suppurative lesion within the lung substance. It is usually secondary to some predisposing condition, the commonest of which is aspiration pneumonia. Certain specific organisms tend to produce abscesses and these include Staphylococcus, Actinomyces, Klebsiella and Amoebae. Bronchial occlusion due to benign or malignant tumours, foreign bodies or sputum plugs (as in postoperative atelectasis), predispose to distal infection and subsequent abscess formation. A pulmonary infarct may become secondarily infected and form an abscess; septic emboli are rare except among drug addicts. Pulmonary haematomas secondary to blunt or penetrating trauma may be complicated by an abscess. General predisposing causes include immunosuppression by disease or by drugs.

Abscesses secondary to aspiration tend to be colonized by a mixture of organisms, such as *Haemophilus influenzae,* Pneumococci, anaerobic Streptococci, Spirochaetes and fusiform bacilli. The right lung is affected more often than the left, probably due to the more direct course of the right main bronchus. Abscesses may be single or multiple and appear as spherical lesions on chest X-ray. At thoracotomy there may be pleurisy overlying the affected area of the lung. The wall of the abscess is formed by fibrous tissue with surrounding compressed lung substance. An abscess can rupture into a bronchus and the contents may then be expectorated, although a state of chronic infection may be produced. Rupture into the pleural cavity produces an empyema. Metastatic abscess formation in the brain is a well documented complication. Occasionally, considerable haemorrhage with severe haemoptysis occurs from the abscess cavity and long-standing abscess cavities may be complicated by superinfection with fungi.

Bronchiectasis

Bronchiectasis is an irreversible dilatation of the bronchi associated with infection. The prevalence of bronchiectasis in children and young adults has declined markedly since the 1950s due to the more effective treatment of childhood pulmonary infections with antibiotics. Obstructive-type bronchiectasis is, however, still commonly seen in patients with bronchial carcinoma.

Aetiology and pathogenesis

Although the term bronchiectasis covers a wide range of disorders of different aetiology, there are generally considered to be two major factors in the pathogenesis: (1) tension in the bronchial wall, and (2) weakening of the bronchial wall.

TENSION IN THE BRONCHIAL WALL: The negative intrapleural pressure constantly attempts to expand the lung to fill the pleural cavity. If there is loss of volume in one part of the lung, the rest of the lung expands to fill the space. Thus, if the parenchyma around a bronchus is destroyed or collapsed, the resulting tension in the bronchial wall causes it to dilate. This can happen in several ways: (1) Obstruction of distal airways occurs during acute respiratory infections in childhood, such as measles and whooping cough. The parenchyma distal to the obstruction collapses and the bronchi proximal to the obstruction dilate. This is less likely to occur in adults since the bronchioles are wider and less likely to obstruct and the inter-alveolar pores are better developed thus allowing collateral ventilation. (2) Chronic lung infections may cause progressive destruction of lung parenchyma with resultant loss of lung volume. (3) Obstruction of a major bronchus by tumour or foreign body causes collapse of the parenchyma with bronchial dilatation which is made worse by accumulation of secretions.

WEAKENING OF THE BRONCHIAL WALL: The most important cause of bronchial wall weakness is infection. Once the initial dilatation of the bronchi takes place, there is predisposition to infection. Infection by organisms such as Staphylococcus and particularly *H. influenzae* weakens the bronchial wall and perpetuates the condition, thus setting up a vicious cycle.

Tuberculosis not only weakens the bronchial wall but also can damage the lung parenchyma with subsequent loss of lung volume. In addition, bronchial obstruction may occur due to hilar lymphadenopathy. Viral infection appears to be important in the cause of follicular bronchiectasis (*see below*) and one study found evidence of adenovirus infection in 11 out of 18 children with this form of the disease (MacFarlane and Sommerville 1957).

Several conditions are associated with bronchiectasis on the basis of predisposition to infection:

1. Kartagener's syndrome is an autosomal recessive condition characterized by bronchiectasis, sinusitis and situs invertus. It is now known that these patients have a defect in ciliary motility due to a morphological defect of the cilia which can be demonstrated on electron microscopy. The immobile cilia cannot carry out the usual bacterial clearance in the sinuses or bronchi and, therefore, infection occurs. Males are infertile due to immotile sperm.
2. Cystic fibrosis patients have severe saccular bronchiectasis due to a defect in exocrine function which is associated with viscous secretions, bronchial obstruction and superimposed infection.

3. Immune deficiency states are also associated with bronchiectasis on the basis of predisposition to infection.

Weakening of the bronchial wall may also be due to a congenital defect of cartilage formation.

Once established, the bronchiectasis becomes self-perpetuating since the bronchial dilatation itself predisposes to further infection. Ulceration and squamous metaplasia of the mucous membrane causes a defect in ciliary clearance and the normal bronchomotor tone, which moves secretions in an upwards direction, is lost.

Clinical features

Some cases of bronchiectasis are asymptomatic and are found as an incidental finding on chest X-ray. The symptomatic patients often have a history dating back to respiratory infections in childhood. They complain of large quantities of foul sputum and associated haemoptysis. In some cases the sputum volume is low (dry bronchiectasis) and these patients often have severe haemoptysis. Affected children may fail to thrive.

Morphology

A classification of bronchiectasis based on aetiology will be described. There is some overlap between these groups; for example, some cases of post-obstructive bronchiectasis may be associated with infection (*see Fig.* 14.4).

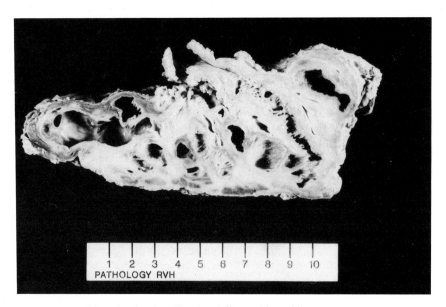

Fig. 14.4. Bronchiectasis, showing dilated and distorted bronchi.

Post-infective bronchiectasis

1. FOLLICULAR BRONCHIECTASIS: This occurs in children, usually under the age of seven years. These cases are frequently associated with adenovirus infection (*see* above). Sectioning of the lung shows bronchial dilatation in a cylindrical or fusiform fashion. The bronchi are visible right up to the pleural surface whereas normally bronchi are no longer visible several centimetres proximal to the pleural surface.

Histologically, the characteristic feature is the presence of many lymphoid follicles in the walls of the dilated bronchi. Areas of ulceration lined by granulation tissue are seen in place of the mucosal surface.

2. SACCULAR BRONCHIECTASIS: This presents at a later stage than follicular bronchiectasis, although there is often a history of pulmonary infection in childhood. The medium-sized bronchi are severely damaged.

Grossly, pus-filled sacs are seen in the lung parenchyma, most commonly in the lower lobes (especially the left).

Histologically, the sacs have thin walls which contain no muscle or cartilage. They are lined by granulation tissue or by epithelium which has undergone squamous metaplasia. Large dilated blood vessels are seen in the walls of the dilated bronchi. These are due to bronchopulmonary arterial anastomoses which develop in this condition and rupture of these may cause severe haemoptysis.

Post-collapse bronchiectasis

1. PROXIMAL OBSTRUCTION: Proximal obstruction of large bronchi leads to atelectasis of the parenchyma distal to the obstruction, due to absorption of air from the alveolar spaces. There is consequent dilatation of the bronchi in order to compensate for the loss of lung volume. Causes of obstruction include bronchial carcinoma, foreign body, mucous plugging and enlarged lymph nodes (e.g. due to tuberculosis). The bronchus to the right middle lobe is especially prone to this form of bronchiectasis as it is longer, of smaller diameter and has less cartilage than other bronchi. In addition, the lymph nodes surrounding it drain both the middle and lower lobes and therefore an inflammatory lesion in either area may cause obstruction due to lymphadenopathy. Bronchiectasis of this distribution is termed the 'right middle lobe syndrome'.

Grossly, there is uniform dilatation (as opposed to saccular dilatation) of all bronchi distal to the obstruction.

Histology confirms the dilatation of bronchi which show various degrees of inflammatory change in their walls. The surrounding lung tissue is collapsed.

2. DISTAL OBSTRUCTION: In cases of widespread obstruction of small bronchioles due to mucus or inflammation, collapse of alveoli is associated with compensatory dilatation of proximal bronchi in an attempt to retain lung volume. This may be seen in adults with asthma and viral pneumonia. Widespread distal obstruction is also important in the pathogenesis of post-infective bronchiectasis of childhood.

Congenital bronchiectasis

1. ARRESTED DEVELOPMENT OF SMALL BRONCHI: This causes the proximal bronchi to undergo gross dilatation. The condition presents in early childhood.

2. KARTAGENER'S SYNDROME AND CILIAL DYSFUNCTION: This has been discussed above. Ciliary dysfunction leads to infection and severe generalized bronchiectasis arising at an early age.

Respiratory Complications of Surgery
Predisposing factors

1. *Pre-existing pulmonary disease*
The two most important lung diseases which may be exacerbated by surgery are chronic bronchitis and emphysema. Often the two conditions co-exist and they can be considered as a spectrum from pure emphysema, through a mixture of the two, to pure chronic bronchitis.

Chronic bronchitis is defined as a persistent cough with sputum production for at least three months in at least two consecutive years. Two factors are important in the aetiology and pathogenesis. (i) Chronic irritation, especially by cigarette smoke, causes an increase in the number of submucosal mucus secreting glands with consequent excessive mucus secretion. Mucous plugging of bronchioles and inflammation with fibrosis of bronchiolar walls lead to airways obstruction. (ii) Infection appears to be of secondary importance and is probably the cause of exacerbations.

Emphysema is defined as 'an abnormal permanent increase in the size of the air spaces distal to the terminal bronchiole with destruction of their walls'. It, therefore, has a morphological definition as opposed to chronic bronchitis which has a clinical definition. Although in some cases, air trapping due to chronic bronchitis obstructing the bronchioles (*see* above) may be the cause, in other cases, a deficiency of alpha-1-antitrypsin (α-1-AT) has been implicated. Deficiency of α-1-AT is inherited and patients may be homozygous (very low levels) or heterozygous (intermediate levels). Homozygotes have a greatly increased risk and heterozygotes probably have an increased risk of developing emphysema. The α-1-AT normally inhibits proteases such as elastase which would otherwise cause destruction of the lung parenchyma. Smoking exacerbates any α-1-AT deficiency since it causes aggregation of neutrophils (which produce proteases) within the lung and decreases the activity of α-1-AT.

Morphologically, emphysema can be detected by examining sections of lung with a hand lens. Several patterns are recognized: (i) centriacinar, in which part of the acinus around the respiratory bronchiole is affected, (ii) panacinar, in which the whole acinus is affected, and (iii) paraseptal, in which the peripheral part of the acinus is affected so that the emphysema is worse in areas adjacent to the pleura and along the connective tissue septa.

Other pre-existing diseases which may require special attention include bronchial asthma, bronchiectasis (*see* p. 386) and the various diffuse interstitial lung diseases (e.g. occupational lung disease, sarcoidosis, extrinsic allergic alveolitis and cryptogenic fibrosing alveolitis.)

2. *Cigarette smoking*
Cigarette smoking causes a significant increase in postoperative lung complications (Wightman 1968). As well as exacerbating pre-existing lung disease it reduces the activity of alveolar macrophages and paralyses cilia.

3. *Obesity*

Wightman (1968) did not find that obesity contributed significantly to postoperative respiratory infection although these patients do tend to be less mobile, and less willing to breath deeply, than average.

4. *Age*

The arterial oxygen tension declines with age and therefore elderly patients are more easily tipped into respiratory failure.

5. *Heart disease*

Congestive cardiac failure with pulmonary oedema exacerbates pulmonary disease.

6. *Inadequate analgesia*

Craig (1981) showed that poor pain relief was associated with respiratory complications and that epidural analgesia was more effective than systemic narcotic administration.

7. *Type of incision*

Craig (1981) found that separate abdominal and thoracic incisions are preferable to a thoraco-abdominal incision and that for cholecystectomy, a subcostal incision is preferable to a vertical incision.

8. *Reflex inhibition of diaphragm*

Ford and Guenter (1984) have shown that surgical patients may develop reflex neurological inhibition of the diaphragm, independent of the site of incision or the degree of pain. Reversal to normal takes place in 24–48 hours.

Lung changes after surgery

1. *Exacerbation of pre-existing pulmonary disease*

The various predisposing factors listed above may combine to tip a patient with pre-existing chronic bronchitis, emphysema or other lung disease into respiratory failure. Thus a simple chronic bronchitis may become infected to give a mucopurulent bronchitis. Bronchopneumonia or atelectasis may further worsen lung function.

2. *Atelectasis*

Atelectasis is collapse of part of the lung. Small plugs of mucus which are not adequately cleared cause obstruction of small airways with absorption of air from the airways beyond. This causes an upset in the ventilation/perfusion ratio and predisposes to infection.

3. *Adult respiratory distress syndrome*

This results from severe alveolar damage which might occur before or at operation. The condition is discussed on p. 397.

4. *Pulmonary embolus, bronchopneumonia, pneumothorax*

These may all occur as postoperative complications. They are discussed elsewhere.

Prevention of postoperative pulmonary complications

Laszlo *et al.* (1973) showed that preoperative physiotherapy or antibiotic treatment did not influence the postoperative respiratory complications in patients with bronchitis. Adequate analgesia and careful selection of incision do reduce respiratory complications.

Celli *et al.* (1984) found that intermittent positive pressure breathing, incentive spirometry (by which the patient can assess his progress) and deep breathing exercises all have good effects on lung function.

Bullous Disease of the Lungs

A bulla is defined as an emphysematous space of more than one centimetre diameter in the distended state. It is clinically important as a cause of recurrent pneumothorax, especially in elderly patients.

The pathogenesis is unclear. Some may represent a localized area of advanced paraseptal emphysema (*see* p. 390) whereas in other cases the surrounding lung is normal, suggesting that emphysema is not the cause. These latter types may represent an inherited defect.

Grossly, they are seen as air filled sacs in the subpleural region, commonly at the lung apices, along the anterior margins of the upper lobes or on the undersurface of the lower lobes. Radiologically, they may be distinguished from pneumothorax by the presence of fibrous bands which can be seen as radio-opaque lines crossing the otherwise lucent space.

If complicated by recurrent pneumothorax, they may be surgically excised.

Pulmonary Embolism

Pulmonary emboli are found at autopsy in up to 50% of patients dying in hospital. They are particularly common in surgical patients. The condition is fatal in approximately one-third of those who have symptoms and up to 90% of fatal pulmonary emboli occur in patients aged over 50 years. The sexes are affected approximately equally, although women on the contraceptive pill have a higher than average incidence for their age group.

The vast majority of pulmonary emboli arise from deep venous thrombosis in the veins of the legs and pelvis, the aetiology and pathogenesis of which are described on p. 370). Other sources of emboli include right atrial thrombi, tricuspid endocarditis (often related to drug abuse), tumours, amniotic fluid, fat and air.

Non-embolic thrombosis may occur in the pulmonary artery in cases of chest trauma.

The relationship between deep venous thrombosis of the legs and pelvis and pulmonary embolism is controversial. Bell and Simon (1982) have reviewed the literature and their conclusions were; (1) about 15–20% of thrombi in the legs embolize; (2) major emboli are more likely to arise from thrombi in the large veins proximal to the knee, but occasionally they arise from calf veins; and (3) thrombi usually originate in calf veins and propagate proximally to the larger veins above the knee, although occasionally they originate in the iliac or femoral veins.

Pathophysiology

A severe upset in blood gases results from several factors. The ventilation of under-perfused alveoli causes an abnormal ventilation/perfusion ratio. Dissolution of the clot with subsequent re-perfusion may not aid the situation as the affected lung tissue often undergoes atelectasis. The atelectasis is probably due to a combination of loss of pulmonary surfactant which occurs when arterial flow is occluded, and to bronchiolar constriction which results from humoral mediators derived from platelets in the embolus. The bronchospasm also causes a generalized increase in airways resistance which aggravates the hypoxia.

Intrapulmonary shunting, due to opening up of pre-existing pulmonary arterio-venous anastomoses, contributes to the blood gas abnormalities. In some patients the increase in right atrial pressure produces intracardial shunting through a patent foramen ovale (15% of individuals have a potentially patent foramen ovale).

Pulmonary infarction usually does not develop although episodes of infarction due to minor emboli may antedate the symptoms of massive embolus.

Classification and clinical features

Several clinical syndromes of pulmonary embolism are recognized depending on the size of the embolus and the rapidity of onset of symptoms (Miller 1983).

1. ACUTE MASSIVE PULMONARY EMBOLISM: Haemodynamic changes occur if 50% of the pulmonary arterial tree is obstructed in an otherwise healthy individual, although less obstruction is required in patients with cardiopulmonary disease. There is a significant rise in pulmonary arterial pressure (to > 25 mmHg). If 75% of the pulmonary arterial circulation is occluded, a pressure of over 50 mmHg is necessary to maintain pulmonary perfusion, and as the right ventricle cannot generate more than 50 mmHg acute, right ventricular failure occurs. Patients with acute massive pulmonary embolism develop severe cardio-respiratory symptoms and the condition may be fatal.

2. ACUTE MINOR PULMONARY EMBOLISM: If less than 50% of the pulmonary arterial tree is obstructed in an otherwise healthy individual, no haemodynamic changes occur and thus there are no haemodynamic symptoms. This syndrome is, therefore, only symptomatic if there is associated pulmonary infarction. Infarction of normal lung does not occur with obstruction of the pulmonary artery because

the bronchial arteries provide adequate circulation. However, when there is pre-existing cardiopulmonary disease, such as pulmonary oedema due to left ventricular failure, infarction with necrosis of the alveolar walls does result. This situation is common in the older age groups. Younger patients with pulmonary embolism but no underlying cardiopulmonary disease who develop pleuritic pain haemoptysis and a wedge-shaped shadow on chest X-ray are thought to have incomplete infarction (see below) which is characterized by intra-alveolar haemorrhage and oedema without actual alveolar wall necrosis.

3. SUBMASSIVE PULMONARY EMBOLISM: These are patients with massive pulmonary embolism in which the symptoms are of gradual onset. They develop increasing dyspnoea and haemoptysis over a period of several weeks.

4. CHRONIC PULMONARY EMBOLISM: This is thought to be due to recurrent small emboli which lead to a gradual onset of pulmonary hypertension.

A further classification is that of Greenfield and Langham (1984) which is based on treatment.

GROUP I: No signs or symptoms and pulmonary arterial occlusion less than 20%; no treatment.

GROUP II: Tachypnoea, 20–30% pulmonary arterial occlusion and mean pulmonary artery wedge pressure < 20 mmHg; anticoagulation only.

GROUP III: Hypoxia and collapse, 30–50% pulmonary arterial occlusion and mean pulmonary artery wedge pressure > 20 mmHg; anticoagulation and caval filter.

GROUP IV: Shock, more than 50% pulmonary arterial occlusion and mean pulmonary artery wedge pressure > 30 mmHg; embolectomy with a suction catheter and caval filter and, if the patient has arrested, open embolectomy is required.

GROUP V: Cor pulmonale (chronic pulmonary hypertension), pulmonary arterial occlusion > 50% and mean pulmonary artery wedge pressure > 40 mmHg; anticoagulation and caval filter.

Groups I and II are roughly equivalent to the clinical group of acute minor pulmonary embolism and groups III and IV are roughly equivalent to acute massive pulmonary embolism and acute submassive pulmonary embolism. Group V is roughly equivalent to chronic pulmonary thrombo-embolism.

Morphology (see Fig. 14.5)
In cases of fatal pulmonary embolism, the clot is usually found in the pulmonary trunk or as a saddle embolism occluding both pulmonary arteries. The embolus is coiled and the valvular markings of the vein of origin may be seen. Smaller emboli are found more peripherally, often astride the bifurcation of a vessel. Within a few hours the embolus characteristically retracts in size and allows the blood flow to pass. This allows fibrinolysis to occur due to contact between fibrinolysins and the

embolus. However, it may also cause fragments to be washed off and become impacted further along the pulmonary tree.

Histologically, the clot has the characteristic laminated appearance of ante-mortem thrombus. Its contours do not correspond to the vessel wall in which it is lodged, thus indicating an embolic episode rather than a local thrombosis. Within 24 hours, the embolus has an endothelial surface. Fibroblasts invade the clot from its points of contact with the vessel wall as organization begins. Endo-thelial lined clefts appear as recanalization occurs. Eventually the only remnant of the embolus is a series of fibrous bands stretching across the vessel lumen.

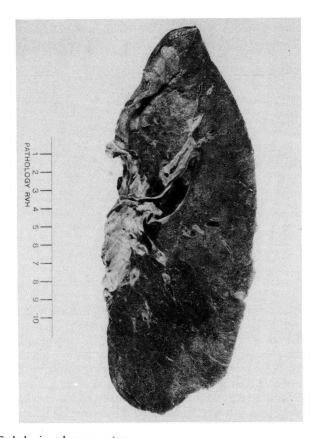

Fig. 14.5. Embolus in pulmonary artery.

Pulmonary infarcts are seen grossly as fairly sharply demarcated wedge-shaped areas of red solid tissue. The base lies on the pleural surface which has a fibrinous exudate and the apex points towards the hilum. An embolus may be seen in a pulmonary artery near the apex.

Histologically, a complete infarct shows intra-alveolar haemorrhage with necrosis of the inter-alveolar septa, bronchioles, etc. (*see Fig.* 14.6). This heals by fibrosis and leaves a scar. Incomplete infarction shows intra-alveolar haemorrhage without necrosis of lung substance. This completely resolves.

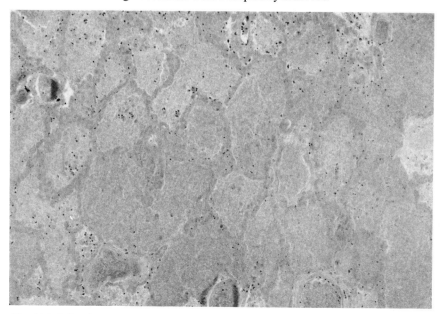

Fig. 14.6. Infarction of lung. The ghost outlines of the alveolar walls are visible. (H and E × 75)

Prognosis

Death occurs in 8–12% of cases of pulmonary embolism and pulmonary infarction occurs in 10–15% (Giudice *et al.* 1980). The impacted tissue may become infected with subsequent abscess formation. In 70–80% of cases there is resolution of the embolus. This occurs by two mechanisms: (1) Fragmentation may occur on impact of the thrombus in the pulmonary artery and/or by reshaping of the clot. This accounts for the spontaneous reduction in pulmonary vascular resistance which produces the early improvement in cardiac output within minutes or hours of the acute episode. (2) Resolution of the embolus also takes place by endogenous fibrinolytic mechanisms during the days and weeks after the event. This probably occurs completely or almost completely in most patients. The improvement in pulmonary perfusion may be as high as 80% at the end of the first week and over 90% by four weeks (Murphy and Bulloch 1968). The most likely cause of apparent delay in resolution is recurrent embolism rather than failure of lysis of a large clot. Patients who have a high risk of recurrent embolism include those with a large total initial perfusion defect (> 35%), associated heart disease and overt co-existing deep vein thrombosis.

Chronic pulmonary hypertension is a late sequela in about 5% of all cases of pulmonary embolism, although it is unusual after acute pulmonary embolism (Paraskos *et al.* 1973).

Adult Respiratory Distress Syndrome

The adult respiratory distress syndrome is acute respiratory failure due initially to pulmonary oedema of non-cardiogenic origin and later to diffuse pulmonary fibrosis. Synonyms include shock lung, traumatic wet lung, Da Nang lung, blast lung, pump lung, adult hyaline membrane disease, respirator lung and stiff lung syndrome.

Aetiology and pathogenesis

The adult respiratory distress syndrome (ARDS) is associated with numerous conditions, some of which are listed in *Table* 14.1. All these conditions appear to cause diffuse alveolar damage which leads to increased capillary permeability with subsequent interstitial and intra-alveolar oedema, fibrin exudation and hyaline membrane formation. A reparative response to this damage produces diffuse interstitial and alveolar fibrosis in the later stages of the syndrome (*see Fig.* 14.7). There is good evidence that the various causes of ARDS act through a final common pathway of complement activation, which is a common consequence of trauma, sepsis, etc. Complement activation releases the peptide fragment C5a which in turn causes neutrophil aggregation in the lungs. Neutrophils cause endothelial and epithelial damage in two main ways: (1) by releasing superoxide radicals as a by-product of phagocytosis, and (2) by releasing proteases which destroy structural protein such as collagen and elastin. These proteases also cleave and activate fibrinogen, complement and the Hageman factor thus causing intravascular coagulation and further neutrophil aggregation. In normal circumstances, proteases are inactivated by protease inhibitors such as alpha-1-antitrypsin. In ARDS, the protease inhibitors are inactivated by the superoxides which are released from neutrophils.

Table 14.1. Some conditions associated with ARDS

Trauma
Burns
Haemorrhagic shock
Septic shock
Oxygen therapy
Extra-corporeal circulation
Radiation
Paraquat poisoning

Animal experiments in which activated complement was infused into sheep caused an ARDS-like syndrome, thus adding support to the activated complement hypothesis of pathogenesis.

Although activated complement is of primary importance, other studies have shown that disseminated intravascular coagulation (DIC) may also be of importance in the pathogenesis of ARDS. Fibrin degradation products which result from DIC are found in patients with ARDS and when infused into dogs cause increased alveolar capillary permeability.

As discussed above, neutrophil aggregation can result in intravascular coagulation; also, the by-products of intravascular coagulation can cause neutrophil aggregation. Therefore, the two mechanisms can amplify each other by positive feedback systems.

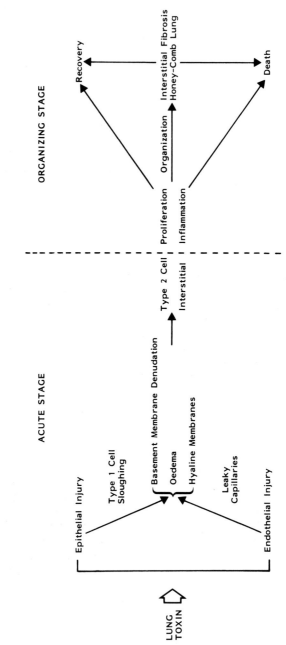
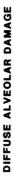

Fig. 14.7. Pathogenesis of diffuse alveolar damage. (Reproduced with permission from Katzenstein and Askin 1982.)

Arachidonic acid metabolites may also cause pulmonary damage. Neutrophils, platelets and pulmonary endothelium can manufacture arachidonic acids and their metabolites may cause bronchoconstriction, pulmonary vasoconstriction and increased pulmonary vascular permeability. These metabolites include prostaglandins E2, F2, H2 and thromboxane A2. A further metabolite, leukotriene B4, is known to stimulate enzyme release and superoxide generation by human neutrophils.

The combined results of these factors are epithelial and endothelial damage. Capillary permeability is increased and this causes interstitial and intra-alveolar oedema. The type I pneumocytes undergo necrosis and form part of the hyaline membrane (see below). Functional damage to type II pneumocytes causes loss of surfactant with resultant atelectasis.

Those patients who survive enter a reparative phase. Type II pneumocytes proliferate and line the alveolar walls. The interstitial tissue which has been damaged by proteases, etc., is invaded by fibroblasts. The fibrosis characteristically develops exceedingly rapidly and appears to be detectable in all patients who survive 12 or more days. It eventually results in a condition similar to idiopathic interstitial fibrosis.

Clinical features

The criteria for the diagnosis of ARDS include: (1) a clinical history of a pulmonary or non-pulmonary catastrophic event (aspiration, trauma, sepsis, etc.); (2) exclusion of cardiogenic pulmonary oedema or chronic pulmonary disease as the main cause of respiratory failure; (3) clinical respiratory failure with hypoxaemia, tachypnoea and dyspnoea; (4) diffuse pulmonary infiltrates on chest X-ray. Respiratory function tests reveal hypoxia, reduced pulmonary compliance, increased shunting and increased dead-space ventilation. A biopsy is rarely required (Stevens and Raffin 1984).

Morphology

In those patients who die in the early course of the disease, the lungs are exceptionally heavy and solid. On cut section they are congested and blood stained and oedema fluid is seen.

The initial histological changes are intra-alveolar and interstitial oedema and fibrin deposition in small vessels. These are rapidly followed by the formation of hyaline membranes which are seen as amorphous eosinophilic masses of fibrin and necrotic epithelial cells lying in the alveolar spaces. The type I alveolar epithelial cell is more sensitive to injury than the more resistant cuboidal type II cell.

After about five days, the surviving type II pneumocytes regenerate and line the alveolar spaces. These are thicker than normal type I pneumocytes and therefore appear as low cuboidal cells. In those patients who survive for more than a few weeks, the interstitial spaces are thickened by fibrosis (chiefly in the alveolar ducts) (see Fig. 14.8).

Prognosis

Recovery from ARDS depends on the age of the patient, the severity of lung injury and the presence of other organ complications. The overall mortality is 50% and

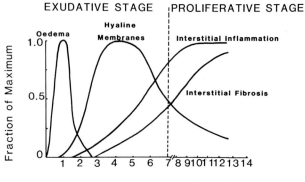

Fig. 14.8. Sequence of events in 'shock lung'. (Reproduced with permission from Katzenstein and Askin 1982.)

abnormal pulmonary function is found in about 40% of survivors after six months. Lung volumes, carbon dioxide diffusing capacity and Po_2 with exercise are all reduced (Boggis and Greene 1983; Fein et al. 1982).

Pulmonary Hamartoma

This is a peripheral lung mass which is usually found as an incidental finding on chest X-ray. Although considered to be a hamartoma by some, others consider it to be a true neoplasm and term it a fibrochondrolipoma.

They are well circumscribed and encapsulated and measure up to a few centimetres in diameter. Some grow into a bronchus. On sectioning, they are usually cartilaginous.

Histologically, the usual appearance is of lobules of cartilage which are separated from each other by fat or fibrous tissue. The fibrous tissue typically contains slit like spaces which are lined by alveolar or respiratory epithelium. These latter elements are thought to have been entrapped in the growing lesion.

Malignant change is exceedingly rare.

Benign Lung Tumours

Multiple papillomatosis is a condition of young people and occurs in association with juvenile papillomatosis of the larynx. The condition may be viral in origin. Grossly, the papillomas are seen in the main bronchi or more distally. Histologically, they consist of a connective tissue stalk with an overlying squamous epithelium. They can cause obstructive problems but tend to regress completely after puberty.

Solitary papillomas occur in older patients in segmental or larger bronchi. Grossly, they appear as warty growths. Histologically, the connective tissue core is covered with squamous epithelium. There is a tendency for them to undergo malignant change which may be indicated by dysplasia of the epithelium.

Adenomas, similar to the pleomorphic adenoma and the monomorphic adenomas of the salivary glands, occasionally occur. They are usually situated in the wall of a main bronchus and are therefore visible at bronchoscopy.

The clear cell tumour is a benign lesion which often presents as a peripheral opacity on chest X-ray. Histologically it consists of sheets of clear cells with little pleomorphism. The cell cytoplasm contains much glycogen, and thus the alternative name is 'sugar tumour'.

Other benign tumours such as neurofibroma, chondroma, lipoma, leiomyoma and fibroma are rare.

Malignant Lung Tumours

Malignant tumours of the trachea, bronchi and lungs accounted for over 26 000 male deaths and over 8000 female deaths in England and Wales in 1981. They were the commonest single cause of death from malignant disease in males and second to breast cancer in females. The peak incidence is between 65 and 75 years of age. The incidence of lung cancer has risen in the United Kingdom during this century due to cigarette smoking and the male to female ratio has fallen in recent years due to a relative increase in female smokers. Females have a relatively higher incidence of adenocarcinomas when compared with males. While the mortality is still increasing in the elderly, death rates in young people are now falling (Coggon and Acheson 1983).

Aetiology

SMOKING: In 1950, Doll and Hill (1964) started their prospective study on the smoking habits of British doctors. This has shown (1) that there is a virtual linear relationship between the number of cigarettes smoked per day and the mortality from lung cancer (*see Fig.* 14.9*a*), and (2) that the reduction in smoking amongst doctors has been associated with a reduction in mortality from lung cancer but not from other cancers (*see Fig.* 14.9*b*). In animal experiments it has been shown that cigarette smoke fractions can cause skin cancer when painted onto the skin of mice. It is also likely that the cumulative effects of passive smoking increases an individual's risk of developing lung cancer. This risk increases with each member of a household who smokes over the individual's life-time (Sandler *et al.* 1985).

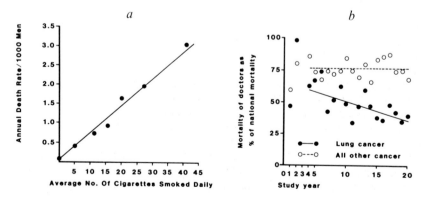

Fig. 14.9 *a.* The relationship between cigarettes smoked daily and the annual death rate from lung cancer. (Reproduced with permission from Doll and Hill 1964.) *b.* Fall in mortality from lung cancer amongst British doctors. (Reproduced with permission from Doll and Peto 1976.)

It is unclear which component of the cigarette smoke is responsible. It is likely that more than one carcinogen is responsible since cigarette smoke is a complex mixture of carcinogens, both in the gaseous phase (e.g. nitrosamine) and in the particulate phase (e.g. polycyclic hydrocarbons).

AIR POLLUTION: People living in rural areas have a lower incidence of lung cancer than those living in urban areas. The differences may be partly due to smoking and occupational differences as well as to differences in air pollution (Coggon and Acheson 1983).

ASBESTOS EXPOSURE: Asbestos is a mineral containing silicate and other compounds. Several varieties exist and all have the property of separating into small fibres. All the major forms of asbestos are associated with the development of lung cancer and mesotheliomas. About 20% of people occupationally exposed to asbestos die from lung cancer (Selikoff et al. 1968). In those tumours arising in the lung (as opposed to the pleura), the distribution of histological types is the same as occurs in non-exposed individuals. Studies have shown that it is the size of the fibre rather than the chemical composition which is important in the causation of cancer (the fibre size hypothesis).

OTHER INDUSTRIES: An increased incidence of lung cancer has been noted in people who have worked with chromium, nickel, beryllium, arsenic and coal gas. A high mortality from lung cancer has been noted in Central Europe among miners who have worked with ore of high uranium content. Small cell carcinomas predominate in radiation associated cancers.

PRE-EXISTING SCARS: Between 20% and 30% of adenocarcinomas and a small proportion of squamous and large cell carcinomas arise in scars. The scars may be due to healed infarcts, healed tuberculosis or trauma. The tumours may arise in the proliferating cells which occur at the interface between the scar and the normal lung parenchyma. Some authorities have suggested that the fibrous scar arises as a result of the tumour rather than before it.

Pathogenesis

Although the stages of the early development of lung cancer are unknown, it is possible that at least some cases arise in areas of abnormal respiratory mucosa. Two abnormalities are recognized. (1) Squamous metaplasia occurs when the normal ciliated epithelium becomes squamous in type. In animal experiments, damage to the normal ciliated epithelium, followed by chronic irritation, leads to squamous metaplasia. Smokers have a higher incidence of squamous metaplasia than non-smokers and it is seen commonly in the bronchial mucosa surrounding squamous carcinomas. Dysplasia of the squamous epithelium is seen when atypical cells are present, and when they replace the full thickness of the epithelium, the condition is termed carcinoma-in-situ. These dysplastic changes are considered to be pre-malignant. (2) Basal cell hyperplasia occurs when the normal 2–3 layers of basal cells which lie under the ciliated epithelium become increased in number. This is also more common in smokers than in non-smokers and atypical cells may be seen. The condition is probably pre-malignant and may give rise to poorly differentiated squamous carcinomas or possibly to oat cell tumours.

Clinical features

The presenting symptoms may be due to the following. (1) The tumour itself —cough and haemoptysis are the classical symptoms and when the tumour has spread locally, presentation may be with superior vena cava obstruction, the Pancoast syndrome or pleural effusion. (2) A metastasis, for example a pathological fracture or a suspected primary brain tumour. (3) A non-metastatic effect of malignancy. Endocrine symptoms are common in lung cancer, especially in the oat cell type. Cushing's syndrome may occur although it is often atypical and not fully developed. There is associated adrenal cortical hyperplasia and Crooke cells appear in the pituitary (*see* p. 480). Inappropriate ADH secretion causes water retention and hyponatraemia which results in lethargy and disorientation. The carcinoid syndrome, hypercalcaemia, hypoglycaemia, gynaecomastia, acromegaly and hyperthyroidism have all been described. Hypercalcaemia is commoner in squamous and adenocarcinomas than it is in oat cell carcinoma. (4) The general debility of malignant disease.

Morphology

The WHO classification of the common lung tumour is given in *Table* 14.2.

Table 14.2 Malignant tumours of the lung (WHO classification)

Squamous cell carcinoma
Small cell carcinoma:
   1. Oat cell
   2. Intermediate cell type
   3. Combined oat cell carcinoma

Adenocarcinoma:
   1. Acinar
   2. Papillary
   3. Bronchiolo-alveolar
   4. Solid with mucus formation

Large cell carcinoma:
   1. Undifferentiated
   2. Giant cell
   3. Clear cell

Adenosquamous

Carcinoid

Bronchial gland carcinomas:
   1. Adenoid cystic
   2. Mucoepidermoid

SQUAMOUS CARCINOMA: This is the commonest histological type and it is strongly associated with cigarette smoking. Grossly, approximately 90% arise in sub-segmental or larger bronchi (*see Fig.* 14.10). They tend to grow into the bronchial lumen and form a fungating mass which can be seen at bronchoscopy. The tumour tends to spread upwards towards the main bronchus. On sectioning a lobectomy or pneumonectomy specimen, the point of origin from the bronchus can usually be identified and this rules out the possibility of secondary tumour. The tumour infiltrates the surrounding lung parenchyma, bronchi and lymph nodes and spread to the mediastinum may cause superior vena cava obstruction. Changes seen in the

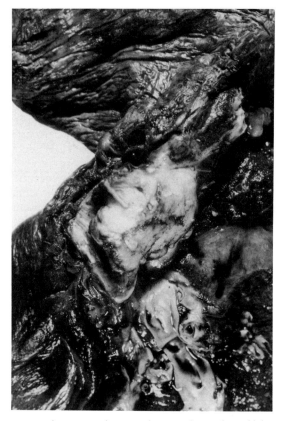

Fig. 14.10. Squamous carcinoma growing as an intra- and extra-bronchial mass.

lung parenchyma distal to the lesion include bronchopneumonia, bronchiectasis and lung abscess, all of which may give rise to systemic symptoms (*see Fig.* 14.11).

Pre-malignant conditions (including carcinoma-in-situ) can be detected at bronchoscopy as red or white plaques on the bronchial epithelium. If these changes are seen extending proximally away from a carcinoma, more extensive surgery than would otherwise be done may be necessary.

Histologically (*see Fig.* 14.12), well differentiated squamous tumours show the features of squamous epithelium which are stratification, intercellular bridges and keratin formation. Keratin may be in individual cells or at the centre of a whorl of squamous cells (keratin pearls). Well differentiated tumours showing all these features are relatively uncommon in the lung and the finding of a well differentiated squamous tumour in a cervical lymph node should suggest the possibility of a primary tumour in the oropharynx, oesophagus or larynx, rather than in the lung. Moderately or poorly differentiated tumours are more common. The former show some areas of easily recognized squamous cells whereas the latter show only poorly differentiated cells which are seen to be of squamous origin on the basis of intercellular bridges and occasional keratinization.

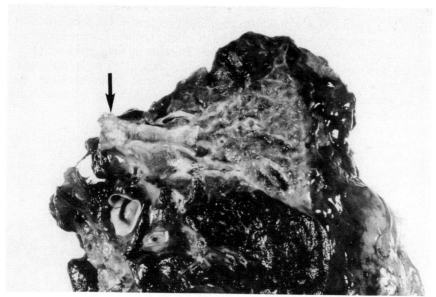

Fig. 14.11. Carcinoma of lung. A small squamous carcinoma (arrow) has blocked a segmental bronchus and caused a distal segmental shaped area of bronchiectasis and consolidation.

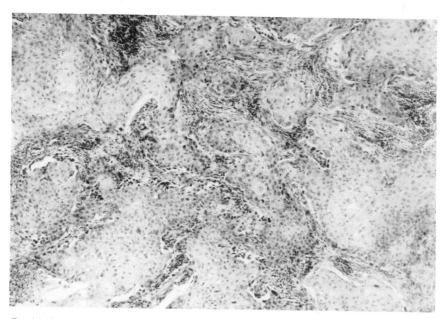

Fig. 14.12. Squamous carcinoma of lung. (H and E × 75)

SMALL CELL CARCINOMA: The various histological subdivisions of this cell type all behave in a similar highly malignant fashion. Frequently, the terms oat cell and small cell are used synonymously, although strictly speaking, oat cell carcinomas form a subdivision of small cell carcinomas. They are all associated with cigarette smoking and they are most commonly centrally located. Grossly, although they arise from the bronchial epithelium, an origin is not commonly seen. As the tumour enlarges, it invades the surrounding lung parenchyma, bronchi and hilar nodes to form an expanding mass. Unlike squamous tumours, they rarely form fungating intrabronchial masses.

Histologically, oat cell tumours consist of small darkly-staining round to oval shaped cells with little visible cytoplasm (see Fig. 14.13). They are arranged into sheets, ribbons and trabeculae; streaming of cells or rosette formation may be seen. A characteristic feature is the presence of basophilic material in the associated blood vessels which has been shown to be DNA.

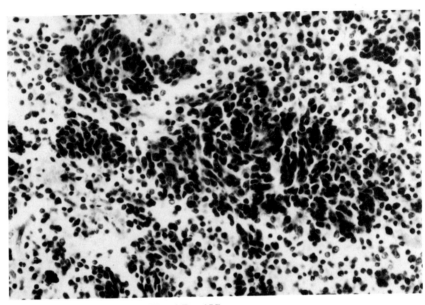

Fig. 14.13. Oat cell carcinoma. (H and E × 175)

The intermediate cell type consists of slightly larger cells, often polygonal in shape and with some visible cytoplasm.

Combined oat cell tumours consist of areas which are oat cell in type, together with squamous or adenocarcinomatous areas.

The cell of origin of small cell tumours is not known, although it is suspected that bronchial carcinoids and oat cell tumours are the benign and malignant tumours of bronchial argyrophil cells which are similar to the endocrine cells of the gut. Supporting evidence for this is the finding of neurosecretory granules in some small cell tumours on electron microscopy.

ADENOCARCINOMAS: These tumours tend to arise in the peripheral bronchi and appear on chest X-ray as a mass in the lung parenchyma. Grossly, they tend to be peripherally situated spherical masses which pucker the overlying pleura. They are hard and fibrotic on cutting. Histologically, several patterns are seen. When gland formation is prominent they are termed 'acinar' (*see Fig.* 14.14). This type causes a desmoplastic reaction so that the irregularly shaped glands are embedded in dense fibrous tissue. Papillary adenocarcinomas are recognized as a sub-group but have a similar prognosis to the acinar type. Solid tumours are similar in appearance to large cell tumours (*see* below) except that the former produce mucin.

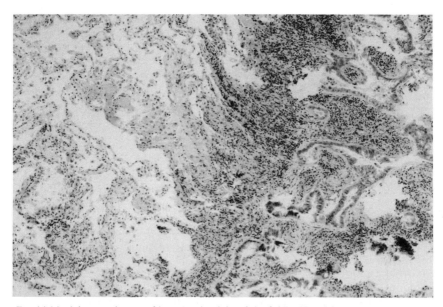

Fig. 14.14. Adenocarcinoma of lung (to the right of the field). (H and E × 30)

It is of clinical importance to realize that it is usually histologically impossible to distinguish between a primary adenocarcinoma of the lung and a secondary adenocarcinoma from the gut or elsewhere. It is therefore essential to rule out the possibility of a secondary tumour before the diagnosis of primary lung adenocarcinoma can be made.

The bronchiolo-alveolar carcinoma (alveolar cell carcinoma) is a distinct subdivision of adenocarcinoma. They probably arise from type II pneumocytes or Clara cells. Grossly, they appear as single or multiple peripheral nodules and some are discovered incidentally on chest X-ray.

Histologically, the characteristic feature is that the malignant cells spread along the alveolar walls without destroying the architecture of the lung. The alveoli are, therefore, lined by tall, columnar mucus-secreting cells or by less well differentiated cells showing nuclear atypia (*see Fig.* 14.15). This characteristic growth pattern may be mimicked by secondary tumour, for example from breast or pancreas, and, therefore, as with all adenocarcinomas, a primary tumour from another site must be ruled out in all cases.

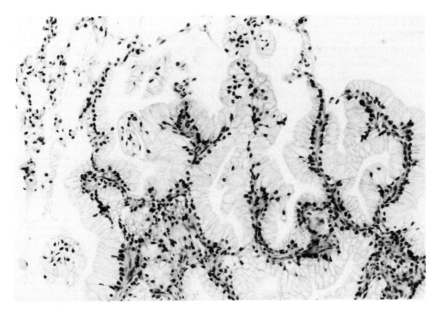

Fig. 14.15. Bronchiolo-alveolar carcinoma. (H and E × 75)

LARGE CELL TUMOURS: These tumours appear as large soft masses with haemorrhage and necrosis; half are central and half are peripheral. Histologically, the tumours are composed of sheets of large pleomorphic cells showing no particular pattern. Two histological variations are recognized: (1) the giant cell type which tends to be peripherally situated and characteristically shows bizarre giant cells—they are highly malignant; (2) the clear cell type which must be distinguished from secondary renal cell carcinoma.

ADENOSQUAMOUS TUMOURS: The WHO recognizes a tumour consisting of adenocarcinoma and squamous carcinoma components. Behaviour is similar to that of adenocarcinoma.

Spread of lung cancer

Direct spread within the lung causes disruption of the parenchyma and bronchi. Spread within the inter-alveolar septa causes lymphangitis carcinomatosa in which prominent Kerley B lines are seen on chest X-ray. Direct spread into the mediastinum may cause superior vena cava obstruction and spread to the brachial plexus will cause a Pancoast syndrome.

Lymphatic spread causes hilar lymphadenopathy or cervical lymphadenopathy. Blood-borne metastases occur most frequently to the liver, adrenal and brain and are found most commonly in cases of adenocarcinoma and oat cell carcinoma. Vascular invasion may be demonstrated histologically, especially in the latter.

Staging of lung cancer

The TNM system of staging is summarized in *Table* 14.3. Preoperative staging is carried out by clinical findings and by various investigations. Clinically, mediastinal disease may be identified by superior vena cava obstruction and dysphagia. Cervical lymph nodes may be palpable and chest X-ray may show enlarged mediastinal glands. Mediastinoscopy with biopsy gives a more accurate assessment of mediastinal glands and up to 25% of patients with lung cancer who have a normal mediastinal appearance on chest X-ray have positive findings on mediastinoscopy. The upper limit of normal diameter for mediastinal nodes is 1·5 cm and enlarged nodes may be detected by CT scanning. In many cases, however, the enlargement is due to non-specific hyperplasia or previous inflammatory changes such as tuberculosis and therefore the specificity of CT scanning is less than mediastinoscopy.

Table 14.3. Summary of TNM classification of lung cancer (T = tumour)

Tis	Preinvasive (carcinoma-in-situ)
T0	No evidence of primary T.
T1	T <3 cm in greatest dimension, surrounded by lung or visceral pleura. No evidence of invasion proximal to lobar bronchus on bronchoscopy.
T2	T >3 cm, or any size of T invading visceral pleura, or any size of T associated with obstructive pneumonitis extending to the hilar region. At bronchoscopy, proximal extent must be 2 cm distal to carina.
T3	T any size with direct extension to adjacent structures, e.g. chest wall, diaphragm, mediastinal contents, or T at bronchoscopy <2 cm from carina, or any T associated with obstructive pneumonitis of entire lung or pleural effusion.
Tx	Not assessable.
N0	No regional nodes.
N1	Peribronchial and/or homolateral hilar nodes involved.
N2	Mediastinal nodes involved.
Nx	Not assessed.
M0	No distant metastases.
M1	Evidence of distant metastases.
Mx	Not assessed.

With accurate preoperative staging, the resectability rate in those patients who come to operation should be around 95%. At surgery, mediastinal glands, including those in the sub-carinal area should be sampled, to provide further information for staging and prognosis.

Prognosis of lung cancer

The various TNM combinations may be divided into three groups:

Stage I   T1, N0, M0; T1, N1, M0; T2, N0, M0
Stage II   T2, N1, M0
Stage III   T3, any N or M; N2, any T or M; M1, any T or N

The overall five year survival for lung cancer patients is less than 10%.

For Stage I and Stage II surgically treated non-small cell tumours, five year survival rates of 54% and 35% respectively have been reported. The five year survival rate for inoperable non-small cell tumours approaches zero. The natural history of squamous cell cancers appears to be more favourable than the natural history of adenocarcinomas, and adenocarcinomas are more favourable than large cell tumours.

Very occasionally, early small cell lesions (T1 N0) have been resected with some success (60% five year survival). However, for most small cell tumours, the stage has little influence on survival and the prognosis is bad. With chemotherapy, median survival times of 18 months and 9 months have been reported for limited and extensive disease respectively. Small cell tumours respond better to chemotherapy than do the other cell types, probably because they have a shorter doubling time.

Rare malignant tumours

Carcinosarcoma

This rare tumour occurs most commonly in elderly men as a fungating bronchial mass. Histologically, malignant epithelial cells, usually squamous in type, are seen in a malignant sarcomatous stroma. They tend to be slow growing.

Pulmonary blastoma

This can occur at any age and has no predilection for infancy. Grossly, a lung mass is seen. Histologically, epithelial elements forming tubules and acini are embedded in a primitive mesenchyme similar to that seen in a Wilms' tumour of the kidney. Since it does not occur at the early age of other blastomas (e.g. Wilms' tumour) it is considered more likely to be a type of mixed epithelial and mesenchymal tumour than a true blastoma. They have a relatively good prognosis when compared with other lung cancers.

Lung tumours of low-grade malignancy

Carcinoid tumours

These are tumours of the endocrine Kulchitsky cells of the bronchus which are of foregut origin. They account for 5% of all lung tumours and are not associated with cigarette smoking. Together with adenoid cystic carcinoma and mucoepidermoid carcinoma, they are sometimes referred to as bronchial adenomas. This term is now considered inappropriate since all are of low-grade malignancy.

The majority of lung carcinoids are centrally situated in a segmental or larger bronchus. Grossly, they grow partly into the bronchial lumen and partly into the surrounding parenchyma so that they may form a dumb-bell shape with growth on both sides of the bronchial wall. They are usually 2–4 cm in diameter and on cut section are tan or red in colour. The overlying mucosa is usually not ulcerated and therefore sputum cytology is frequently negative.

Histologically, they are composed of characteristically uniform cells arranged in nests, ribbons and trabeculae; mitoses are rare (see Fig. 14.16). About 10% of bronchial carcinoids are peripherally situated and these tend to be spindle cell in type.

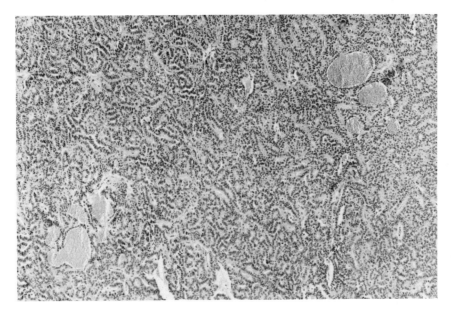

Fig. 14.16. Carcinoid tumour of lung showing a ribbon pattern. (H and E × 30)

Overall, only about 5% of lung carcinoids metastasize and in these cases the patients may develop the carcinoid syndrome. Although all histological types of carcinoid can metastasize, a sub-category termed 'atypical carcinoid' is recognized. They are characterized histologically by pleomorphic cells and up to 70% of this sub-type develop metastatic lesions.

Bronchial gland tumours

Bronchial glands contain both serous and mucinous elements similar to salivary glands and these give origin to several tumours similar histologically to salivary tumours. The adenoid cystic tumour has a similar gross appearance to a carcinoid and histology shows the characteristic pattern of adenoid cystic tumours of the salivary gland (*see* p. 23). These tumours used to be termed cylindromas and are sometimes inappropriately included with carcinoid and mucoepidermoid tumours as bronchial adenomas. They are of low-grade malignancy and, although they are locally invasive, they rarely metastasize.

Mucoepidermoid tumours are also of low-grade malignancy and are similar to the tumours of the same name which arise in the salivary glands.

Lymphoproliferative Disorders

The lung is subject to primary malignant lymphomas and to a series of other lymphoproliferative disorders, some of which are pre-malignant.

Primary malignant lymphoma

This accounts for a very small proportion of all lymphomas. The presentation may be with pulmonary symptoms, systemic symptoms or as an incidental shadow on chest X-ray. They probably arise in bronchial lymphoid tissue. Grossly, there may be one single lesion or multiple lesions. Histologically, they may be classified according to the Kiel classification (*see* p. 431)

Pseudolymphoma

This is a localized lymphoid proliferation in the lung. Histologically, there are lymphoid follicles with germinal centres and a mixture of cell types is seen. The prognosis is very good.

Lymphoid interstitial pneumonia

This term is used to describe a proliferation of mixed lymphoid cells within the interstitial spaces of the lung. It may develop into a lymphoma.

Lymphomatoid granulomatosis

This unusual condition occurs in all age groups and is more common in males than females. Patients present with cough and systemic symptoms. Chest X-ray shows multiple nodules which may be mistaken for secondary carcinoma. On cut section the nodules tend to have necrotic centres.

Histologically, there are two cardinal features: a necrotizing vasculitis and an infiltrate containing atypical lymphoid cells.

The relationship between lymphomatoid granulomatosis and lymphoma is unclear although many authorities consider the condition to be a lymphoma of T-cell origin.

PLEURA AND PLEURAL CAVITY

Pneumothorax

Air in the pleural space is often due to rupture of small subpleural blebs on the lung surface. These are thought to form when air tracks through congenital defects in alveolar walls. They occur at the lung apices, often bilaterally and usually in young persons. Bullae may complicate chronic bronchitis, emphysema or asthma, probably as a result of rupture of alveolar walls and rupture of a bulla is a common cause of pneumothorax in elderly patients. Hyperinflation of alveoli during intermittent positive pressure ventilation, dilatation and rupture of congenital pulmonary cysts, trauma, Staphylococcal pneumonia (which causes intrapulmonary cysts), tuberculosis and carcinoma are other causes.

A tension pneumothorax occurs when there is a valvular mechanism by which air enters the pleural cavity on inspiration but becomes trapped on expiration. This produces displacement of the mediastinum and kinking of the great vessels. It requires urgent treatment.

Rarely, a subpleural bleb ruptures while the visceral pleura remains intact. Air then tracks between the lung and visceral pleura to the hilum, mediastinum and into the neck thus producing surgical emphysema.

Empyema

The incidence of empyema is decreasing with improved antibiotic therapy. It can develop as a sequela to lung infections such as pneumonia, lung abscess, bronchiectasis or tuberculosis. Empyema can complicate penetrating wounds, haemothorax, thoracotomy and rupture of the oesophagus. Occasionally, a subphrenic abscess (pyogenic or amoebic) can spread above the diaphragm. Rarely, empyema follows osteomyelitis of the ribs or vertebrae.

Clinically the patients have rigors, malaise and weight loss in addition to the local signs of pleural effusion. If a bronchopleural fistula is present, the patient complains of a productive cough. With chronic empyema, anaemia and malaise are noted.

Initially an effusion containing protein and inflammatory cells forms and this becomes frank pus. Later, fibrin is deposited which becomes organized into fibrous tissue and this restricts chest wall and diaphragmatic movement. The underlying lung tissue is collapsed. Brain abscess and amyloidosis are late complications.

If a bronchopleural fistula is present, air as well as pus is present in the pleural space and the condition is termed a pyopneumothorax. The bronchopleural fistula may result from rupture of a lung abscess into the pleural space or from rupture of the bronchial stump after pneumonectomy. Pyopneumothorax may also occur as a complication of pleural aspiration and rarely gas forming organisms, such as Clostridia (associated with foreign bodies), are the cause.

In the acute form, appropriate antibiotic therapy with repeated aspiration or drainage may control the infection. For chronic empyema thoracotomy and decortication will frequently be required.

Chylothorax

Lymphatic fluid within the pleural cavity follows trauma to the thoracic duct or to the right bronchomediastinal lymph trunk. Trauma may be surgical (block dissection of neck, scalene node biopsy or oesophageal dissection) or due to sudden hyperextension of the spine. The latter produces rupture just above the diaphragm. Stab and gunshot wounds and injury at birth are rare causes. Obstruction of the thoracic duct by enlarged nodes (malignancy, tuberculosis or filariasis) may also produce a chylothorax.

Presentation is with pyrexia and dyspnoea and the clinical and radiological features of a pleural effusion are present. Presentation may be delayed for several days after the trauma.

The aspirate is white and oily with a high fat content. The patient may develop depletion of electrolytes, water, fat-soluble vitamins, proteins and lymphocytes.

About half close spontaneously. Some cases require ligation of the thoracic duct.

Malignant mesothelioma

About 500 new cases of mesothelioma are reported each year in the UK. The disease is more common in men than women. The association between asbestos exposure and both pleural and peritoneal mesothelioma is well established, although there is a long latent period between exposure and onset of the disease and there is little dose-response relationship. The asbestos fibres penetrate deeply into the airways as their long axes become orientated parallel to the air stream.

Chrysotile fibres do not penetrate as deeply into the lung as do Amphibole fibres because of their curved shape. Asbestos is not the only factor in the aetiology of mesothelioma as half of the patients have no history of exposure.

Clinically, patients with pleural mesothelioma present with chest pain and progressive shortness of breath. There may be a pleural effusion. Occasionally, the diagnosis may be made on a routine chest X-ray.

Peritoneal mesothelioma presents with abdominal cramps, ascites and intestinal obstruction. The ratio of pleural to peritoneal disease is 3 : 1. Pericardial mesothelioma has been reported but is rare.

Grossly, the lung is encased in a white or grey-yellow tumour which involves both visceral and parietal pleura. This obliterates the pleural space although a few loculi of fluid may be found. The tumour typically extends into the interlobar fissures, and the adjacent lung shows features of collapse (*see Fig.* 14.17). The tumour may also appear as a solid mass or as multiple nodules. Pleural mesotheliomas tend to be diffuse while peritoneal tumours are mainly nodular.

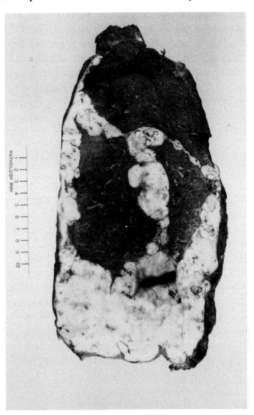

Fig. 14.17. Mesothelioma.

Several histological types are described. (1) The epithelial type which mimics a carcinoma with tubules, clefts and papillary areas. The cells are cuboidal or columnar. (2) The connective tissue type which mimics a sarcoma with spindle shaped cells and frequent mitoses. However, there are also areas of fibrosis and acellular hyaline material which may produce an erroneous benign diagnosis on a small biopsy. (3) The mixed type which is a combination of epithelial and connective tissue types. (4) Occasionally, undifferentiated tumours are found composed of large polygonal cells.

Diagnosis on a small biopsy is very difficult as is cytology of pleural fluid. Special techniques, including immunohistochemistry and electron microscopy, may help.

Hilar glands are involved in about 20% of cases. Distant blood spread is unusual but liver, bone and adrenals may rarely be involved.

A staging system for malignant mesothelioma is given in *Table* 14.4. Radical pleuropneumonectomy gives a few survivors at five years. Chemotherapy and radiotherapy have little to offer. Median survival times of 16, 9 and 5 months have been reported for Stage I, II and III disease respectively (Antman 1980).

Table 14.4. Staging of pleural malignant mesothelioma

Stage I	Tumour confined to ipsilateral pleura and lung
Stage II	Tumour involving chest wall, mediastinum, pericardium or contralateral pleura
Stage III	Tumour involving both thorax and abdomen or lymph nodes outside the chest
Stage IV	Distant blood-borne metastases

MEDIASTINUM

The mediastinum is divided into four compartments.

1. Superior:	Bounded by the manubrium and first four thoracic vertebrae anteriorly and posteriorly and by the thoracic inlet and a line through the manubriosternal joint above and below.
2. Anterior:	Between the sternum and pericardium.
3. Middle:	The pericardium, its contents and closely related structures.
4. Posterior:	Between the pericardium and the posterior chest wall.

Table 14.5. Location of mediastinal masses

Superior	Anterior	Middle	Posterior
Thyroid masses	Thymic lesions	Lymph node enlargement	Neural tumours
Lymph node enlargement	Lymphoma	Bronchogenic cysts	Thoracic meningocoele
Oesophageal tumours	Germ cell tumours	Enterogenic cysts	Oesophageal tumours
Aortic aneurysms	Pleuropericardial cyst		Aortic aneurysms
Parathyroid lesions	Paraganglioma		Paraganglioma
	Lymph node enlargement		

The various lesions of the mediastinum show predilections for the various compartments as indicated in *Table* 14.5. Clinically, many mediastinal masses are asymptomatic (95 out of 155 cases in one study; Ringertz and Lidholm 1956). Symptoms are often due to pressure on nearby structures causing dyspnoea, dysphagia, the superior vena cava syndrome, etc.

Developmental abnormalities

Thyroid masses

Most thyroid masses in the mediastinum represent retrosternal extension of an enlarged cervical thyroid. True mediastinal thyroids, due to an abnormality of thyroid descent (*see* p. 452) do occur and are subject to the spectrum of thyroid disease.

Parathyroid masses

One or both of the inferior parathyroids may descend into the mediastinum, where an adenoma may develop.

Pleuropericardial cysts

These probably represent a persistence of the central recess of the embryological pericardial sac. They are characteristically located anteriorly in the cardiophrenic angle.

Grossly, they are unilocular, up to 10 cm in diameter, and contain clear fluid (thus the term 'springwater cyst'). Histologically, a layer of mesothelial cells lines a connective tissue wall.

They are often asymptomatic and they do not undergo malignant change.

Bronchogenic and enterogenous cysts

These two types of cyst are closely related, since the respiratory system initially forms as a budding of the foregut. They are discussed elsewhere (*see* pp. 380 and 381).

Lymph node enlargement

Inflammatory and granulomatous conditions frequently cause mediastinal lymph node enlargement and may cause confusion with secondary carcinoma or lymphoma. The assessment of mediastinal lymph nodes in cases of lung cancer is discussed on p. 409.

Lymphomas of both Hodgkin's and non-Hodgkin's types may affect the mediastinal nodes. These conditions are discussed in Chapter 15.

Thymic masses

These are discussed in Chapter 15.

Germ cell tumours

Benign

The benign teratoma is found in the anterior mediastinum, often as an asymptomatic mass on routine chest X-ray. It is usually cystic, although it may have solid areas or be completely solid. Histologically, a mixture of tissues from all three germ layers is seen. These show various degrees of maturity, but no malignant tissue is present.

Benign teratoma may be complicated by infection. Malignant change occurs in up to a third of cystic teratomas and up to two-thirds of solid teratomas. They should, therefore, be surgically removed.

Malignant

Most malignant germ cell tumours occur in men of 20–40 years old. Extra testicular seminomas were mentioned on p. 271. Various types of malignant teratomas and yolk sac tumours may also rarely be found.

Neural tumours

These are the most common primary mediastinal tumours and they account for 75% of posterior mediastinal tumours. Symptoms may be due to pressure on thoracic structures, although root pain is sometimes a symptom. Extension through an intervertebral foramen may cause pressure on the spinal cord.

Neurilemmoma, neurofibroma, neurofibrosarcoma

The pathology of these tumours is discussed in Chapter 20. Most present in adults. About 10% of mediastinal nerve sheath tumours are malignant.

Ganglioneuroma, ganglioneuroblastoma, neuroblastoma

These appear to arise in the thoracic sympathetic chain. They represent a spectrum from mature and benign (ganglioneuroma) to immature and malignant (neuroblastoma). The morphology is identical to the tumours of the same names in the adrenal medulla (*see* p. 489).

Paragangliomas

These arise in extra-adrenal paraganglia tissue. In the mediastinum this is found in association with the sympathetic trunk and great vessels. The tumours are histologically similar to chemodectomas (*see* p. 26). Some authors classify functional paragangliomas (producing catecholamines) as extra-adrenal phaeochromocytes and non-functional tumours as chemodectomas. Some of these tumours show locally aggressive and metastatic behaviour.

Thoracic meningocoele

This is a cystic herniation of the spinal meninges which protrudes through a defect in the vertebral column. On chest X-ray it is similar to a neural tumour, although associated vertebral abnormalities give a clue as to the correct diagnosis. Myelography is diagnostic.

Rare mediastinal tumours

The various benign and malignant soft tissue tumours have been described in the mediastinum. They are often larger at the time of diagnosis than those at other sites. (*See* Chapter 18.)

Mediastinitis

Acute inflammation of the mediastinum occurs as a complication of oesophageal perforation (the most common cause), trauma, thoracic surgery, etc. A rapidly spreading cellulitis occurs and localized abscess formation may be seen. Tuberculosis and some rare fungal infections may cause a granulomatous mediastinitis.

Idiopathic mediastinal fibrosis

This is a diffuse replacement of the normal mediastinal connective tissue by a dense and white collagenous fibrous tissue.

The cause is unknown; some cases are associated with retroperitoneal fibrosis, Riedel's thyroiditis, and sclerosing cholangitis, and an autoimmune aetiology has been suggested. Other cases are associated with histoplasmosis and with the drug methylsergide.

Symptoms may be caused by compression of the superior vena cava, respiratory tree or great vessels. Treatment may be by removal of localized plaques of fibrosis or by a bypass procedure for superior vena cava obstruction. Steroids have been successful in a few patients.

References

Antman K. H. (1980) Current concepts: malignant mesothelioma. *N. Engl. J. Med.* **303**, 200–2.

Bell W. R., Simon T. L. (1982) Current status of pulmonary thromboembolic disease: pathophysiology, diagnosis, prevention, and treatment. *Am. Heart. J.* **103**, 239–62.

Boggis C. R., Greene R. (1983) Adult respiratory distress syndrome. *Br. J. Hosp. Med.* **29**, 167–74.

Burt M. E., Flye M. W., Webber B. L., Wesley R. A. (1981) Prospective evaluation of aspiration needle, cutting needle, transbronchial and open lung biopsy in patients with pulmonary infiltrates. *Ann. Thorac. Surg.* **32**, 146–53.

Celli B. R., Rodriguez K. S., Snider G. L. (1984) A controlled trial of intermittent positive pressure breathing, incentive spirometry, and deep breathing exercises in preventing pulmonary complications after abdominal surgery. *Am. Rev. Respir. Dis.* **130**, 12–15.

Coggon D., Acheson E. D. (1983) Trends in lung cancer mortality (editorial). *Thorax* **38**, 721–3.

Craig D. B. (1981) Postoperative recovery of pulmonary function. *Anesth. Analg.* **60**, 46–52.

Doll R., Hill A. B. (1964) Mortality in relation to smoking: ten years' observations of British doctors. *Br. Med. J.* **1**, 1399–410.

Doll R., Peto R. (1976) Mortality in relation to smoking: 20 years' observations on male British doctors. *Br. Med. J.* **2**, 1525–36.

Fein A. M., Goldberg S. K., Lippmann M. L., Fischer R., Morgan L. (1982) Adult respiratory distress syndrome. *Br. J. Anaesth.* **54**, 723–36.

Ford G. T., Guenter C. A. (1984) Toward prevention of postoperative pulmonary complications. *Am. Rev. Respir. Dis.* **130**, 4–5.

Fulkerson W. J. (1984) Current concepts. Fiberoptic bronchoscopy. *N. Engl. J. Med.* **311**, 511–15.

Giudice J. C., Komansky H. J., Gordon R. (1980) Pulmonary thromboembolism. 1. Current concepts in pathogenisis and diagnosis. *Postgrad. Med.* **67**, 64–77.

Greenfield L. J., Langham M. R. (1984) Surgical approaches to thromboembolism. *Br. J. Surg.* **71**, 968–70.

Harrison B. D., Thorpe R. S., Kitchener P. G., McCann B. G., Pilling J. R. (1984) Percutaneous trucut lung biopsy in the diagnosis of localised pulmonary lesions. *Thorax* **39**, 493–9.

Johnson R. D., Gobien R. P., Valicenti J. F. (1983) Current status of radiologically directed pulmonary thin needle aspiration biopsy. An analysis of consecutive biopsies and review of the literature. *Ann. Clin. Lab. Sci.* **13**, 225–39.

Katzenstein A.-L. A., Askin F. B. (1982) *Surgical Pathology of Non-Neoplastic Lung Disease*. Philadelphia, W.B. Saunders.

Laszlo G., Archer G. G., Darrell J. H., Dawson J. M., Fletcher C. M. (1973) The diagnosis and prophylaxis of pulmonary complications of surgical operation. *Br. J. Surg.* **60**, 129–34.

MacFarlane J. (1985) Lung biopsy. *Br. Med. J.* **290**, 97–8.

MacFarlane P. S., Sommerville R. G. (1957) Non-tuberculous juvenile bronchiectasis: a virus disease? *Lancet* **1**, 770–1.

Miller G. A. H. (1983) Pulmonary embolism. In: Ledingham J. G. G., Warrel D. A. (eds.) *Oxford Textbook of Medicine*. Oxford, Oxford Medical Publications.

Murphy M. L., Bulloch R. T. (1968) Factors influencing the restoration of blood flow following pulmonary embolization as determined by angiography and scanning. *Circulation* **38**, 1116–26.

Paraskos J. A., Adelstein S. J., Smith R. E. *et al.* (1973) Late prognosis of acute pulmonary embolism. *N. Engl. J. Med.* **289**, 55–8.

Ringertz N., Lidholm S. O. (1956) Mediastinal tumours and cysts. *J. Thorac. Surg.* **31**, 458–87.

Sandler D. P., Wilcox A. J., Everson R. B. (1985) Cumulative effects of lifetime passive smoking on cancer risk. *Lancet* **1**, 312–15.

Selikoff I. J., Hammond E. C., Churg J. (1968) Asbestos exposure, smoking and neoplasia. *J.A.M.A.* **204**, 106–12.

Stevens J. H., Raffin T. A. (1984) Adult respiratory distress syndrome I. Aetiology and mechanisms. *Postgrad. Med. J.* **60**, 505–13.

Stevens J. H., Raffin T. A. (1984) Adult respiratory distress syndrome II. Management. *Postgrad. Med. J.* **60**, 573–6.

Wightman J. A. (1968) A prospective survey of the incidence of postoperative pulmonary complications. *Br. J. Surg.* **55**, 85–91.

Chapter 15

The Lymphoreticular System

The immune defence of the body is mediated by two main cell types. Firstly, lymphocytes which are responsible for both humoral and cell mediated immunity, and secondly, monocytes/macrophages (known as monocytes when circulating in the blood and as macrophages or histiocytes when in tissue) which have a number of roles, including processing of antigen, presentation of antigen to immune-competent cells and phagocytosis.

Both these main cell types may be found circulating in the blood or in discrete aggregates known collectively as the lymphoreticular system. The main components of the lymphoreticular system are the lymph nodes, spleen, thymus, tonsils and adenoids. Less well formed aggregates are also present in the gut and in other tissues. Lymphomas, which arise in lymph nodes, are called nodal lymphomas whereas those arising in other parts of the lymphoreticular system are called extranodal lymphomas.

THE LYMPH NODES

Normal Structure and Function

The structure of a lymph node is shown diagrammatically in *Fig.* 15.1. Each lymph node is roughly kidney-shaped. Lymph enters the node via peripherally situated afferent lymphatics which drain into the subcapsular sinus. From here it flows to

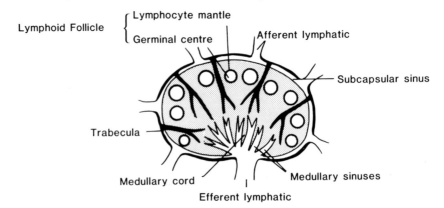

Fig. 15.1. Lymph node, schematic drawing.

the hilum of the node through medullary sinuses and finally exits through one or more efferent lymphatic channels. The outer part of the node around the periphery is termed the cortex and the inner part around the hilum is termed the medulla.

Within the cortex are spherical aggregates of densely packed lymphoid cells known as lymphoid follicles. Some of these have less densely packed and slightly paler staining centres known as germinal centres and these are composed of 'follicle centre cells'. The lymphocytes of the lymphoid follicles are mainly of B-cell origin (*see* below). Surrounding these lymphoid follicles, i.e. in the parafollicular zone of the cortex, the lymphocytes are of T-cell origin (*see* below). Extensions of the cortex into the medulla are termed medullary cords and these are composed of various lymphoid cells.

Lymphocytes

Lymphocytes are divided into B and T types and both types originate from the bone marrow. T-lymphocytes are so-called because they are modified by the thymus. B-lymphocytes are so-called because they are modified by the bursa of Fabricius in birds; the site of this modification in mammals is uncertain, although it may be the gut associated lymphoid tissue.

B-LYMPHOCYTES: These are found mainly in the lymphoid follicles of lymph nodes and spleen; they form only a minority of circulating lymphocytes. When stimulated by an antigen, they undergo a series of transformations (more fully discussed later) to form plasma cells which produce immunoglobulins. They are therefore responsible for humoral immunity.

T-LYMPHOCYTES: These constitute the majority of circulating lymphocytes and within lymph nodes they are found mainly in the parafollicular areas. They may also be transformed by antigen stimulation and are responsible for cell mediated immunity. Various sub-types of T-cells are also responsible for regulation of the immune system. T-helper cells 'help' both T- and B- cells to respond optimally to antigen. T-suppressor cells suppress the immune system.

Histochemical methods are available which differentiate between T- and B-cells and between various types of T-cells. These are useful in the differential diagnosis of non-Hodgkin's lymphomas but are limited by the fact that T-cell identification requires fresh rather than fixed tissue.

Monocytes/macrophages

These are present in the blood as circulating monocytes and in the tissues as monocytes and macrophages. In lymph nodes they form (together with endothelial cells) the lining of the lymphatic channels and they are also present in the cortex of the node. As well as their role in phagocytosis of unwanted material, such as antigen-antibody complexes, obsolete cells, etc., they also cooperate with T- and B-lymphocytes in the immune response. They process antigen and present it to the immune competent cells and they are attracted to the site of immunological activity by various products of T-cells (lymphokines).

Lymph Node Biopsy

The microscopic interpretation of abnormal lymph nodes is difficult. Of 226 cases initially diagnosed as reticular 'cell sarcoma', an error was made in 27% in one series (Symmers 1968) and in a more recent study discord was found in the classification of Hodgkin's disease between pathologists in one-third of cases (Neiman 1978). Biopsy of inguinal nodes frequently only shows chronic inflammatory changes and fibrosis which obscure the presence of other pathological processes. Therefore, if there is generalized lymphadenopathy, the surgeon should biopsy deep cervical or axillary nodes.

During laparotomy, if lymph node pathology is suspected, several nodes should be removed for biopsy and at any site the largest few nodes should be removed. The surgeon should be careful not to crush the node in forceps as the overall architecture is of diagnostic importance to the pathologist. The node should be sent intact to the pathologist, preferably fresh, so that part may be used for immunohistochemical techniques and/or electron microscopy. Frozen section is useful to confirm that the tissue removed is indeed lymph node as it may be difficult to ascertain this surgically in the case of a diffuse neck mass. If indicated, part of the node may be sent for bacteriological examination and for culture and identification of acid fast bacilli or fungi. Such material should be handled carefully and appropriate measures taken to avoid spread of infection.

A useful technique is touch imprinting of the cut surface of a fresh node onto a glass slide and staining with Giemsa solution (Velez-Garcia et al 1971). This is useful in the evaluation of lymphoma and leukaemia and is especially useful in the diagnosis of Burkitt's lymphoma. Needle biopsy of a lymph node is less useful except to confirm a diagnosis of metastatic carcinoma. Aspiration cytology requires the availability of an experienced cytologist.

Infective and Granulomatous Conditions of Lymph Nodes

Non-specific lymphadenitis

Acute lymphadenitis commonly occurs in the lymph nodes draining acutely infected lesions such as a dental abscess, etc. The nodes are swollen and tender to touch when pyogenic organisms are involved. They may undergo necrosis with abscess formation and this may rupture onto the skin surface leaving a sinus.

Viral infections may also give acute lymphadenitis and these are discussed below.

Chronic non-specific lymphadenitis due to persistent antigenic stimulation causes lymphadenopathy which may require lymph node biopsy. Histologically, the picture is one of follicular hyperplasia, i.e. the lymphoid follicles become enlarged and prominent. This may occasionally be confused with a follicular pattern of lymphoma (see p.432).

Viral lymphadenitis

Most viral diseases are diagnosed clinically and do not require lymph node biopsy. Occasionally, lymphadenopathy in an undiagnosed case of infectious mononucleosis leads to biopsy and this often causes concern as the histological features are bizarre. The parafollicular area of the lymph node is replaced by a sea of cells resembling centroblasts or immunoblasts (see later). This can replace the normal follicles, a feature which can lead to a mistaken diagnosis of malignant lymphoma.

Serological tests for infectious mononucleosis should therefore be carried out if bizarre lymph node histology is reported in a young patient.

Granulomatous lymphadenopathy

Several types of granulomatous reaction occur in lymph nodes. Classical epithelioid granulomas are seen in tuberculosis, sarcoidosis and Crohn's disease. Granulomas may also be seen in lymph nodes draining the site of a malignant tumour, such as the hilar nodes in bronchial carcinoma. Failure to realize this may lead to diagnostic confusion.

Sarcoidosis is a disease of unknown aetiology characterized by non-caseating granulomas. Clinical presentation is often with bilateral hilar lymphadenopathy and pulmonary disease, although granulomas may be widespread in other lymph nodes, spleen, liver, bone marrow and skin. Histologically, the granulomas are discrete and non-caseating (*see Fig.* 15.2). Identical granulomas may be seen in the lymph nodes in cases of Crohn's disease.

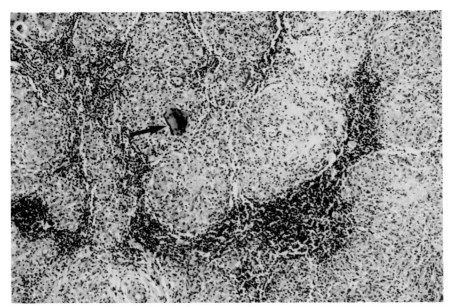

Fig. 15.2. Sarcoidosis of lymph node. Many granulomas are seen, one of which contains a giant cell (arrow). (H and E × 75)

The characteristic feature of tuberculous lymph nodes is the presence of central caseation in the granulomas although this feature is not always present. Tuberculosis should therefore be considered in the differential diagnosis of any granulomatous lymphadenopathy.

Large granulomas with central abscesses and pus formation are characteristic of cat-scratch disease, lymphogranuloma venereum and Yersinia infections.

Cat-scratch disease most commonly occurs in children. The cat-scratch is followed by a febrile illness and lymphadenopathy. It is a self-limiting disease and the causative organism has not been identified although a Gram-positive bacterium has recently been implicated (Gerber *et al.* 1985). Skin tests using an exudate from a known case may be used to confirm the diagnosis.

Lymphogranuloma venereum is a sexually transmitted disease caused by a chlamydial organism and most frequently affects the inguinal nodes.

Yersinia infections cause inflammation of the caecum and appendix and the characteristic lymph node changes are seen in the mesenteric nodes.

A further type of granulomatous lymphadenitis is characterized by scattered clusters of epithelioid cells rather than the classical discrete granulomas. This appearance is typical of toxoplasmosis which is caused by the parasite *Toxoplasma gondii*. Typically, young adults are infected and they develop lymphadenopathy, especially in the posterior triangle of the neck. The parasite is rarely seen histologically in lymph node sections, although the diagnosis can be confirmed by measuring antibody titres.

Acquired immune deficiency syndrome (AIDS) and progressive generalized lymphadenopathy (PGL) (*see also* page 531)

AIDS was originally defined as a 'disease, at least moderately predictive of a defect in cell mediated immunity, occurring in a person with no known cause for diminished resistance to that disease'. Such diseases include serious opportunistic infections (e.g. *Pneumocystis carinii* pneumonia) and Kaposi's sarcoma. This definition is now modified to take account of the Human T-Cell Lymphotrophic Virus Type III (HTLV-III), which is the presumed cause of the disease.

HTLV-III is a retrovirus which is cytopathic for T-helper cell (T4 cells) and it may also infect monocytes. The effects of infection include T-helper cell death with lymphopenia, a reduction in T-helper–B-cell co-operation, a reduction in T-helper–T-cell co-operation, and a failure of macrophages to respond to stimuli. Patients at risk from HTLV-III infection include male homosexuals, intravenous drug abusers and haemophiliacs. In the USA and Europe 90% of the cases occur in male homosexuals.

It is not known how many patients who carry the HTLV-III virus will develop disease. It appears that in many cases a steady state develops in which there is a balance between viral expression and cell production. If, however, a potent antigenetic stimulus occurs, such as a bacterial or viral infection, this switches on virus production to a degree which results in cell death exceeding production with resultant clinical effects.

Infection with HTLV-III may remain asymptomatic. Alternatively, the patient may develop PGL (characterized by the presence of lymph nodes of 1 cm or more in diameter in two or more groups, excluding the inguinal group in male homosexuals), which may revert to an asymptomatic phase, or develop into AIDS either directly or via a prodromal AIDS phase. Asymptomatic patients may develop AIDS without passing through the PGL phase either directly or through a prodromal AIDS phase.

In PGL the lymph node histology is characterized by marked follicular hyperplasia. The germinal centres become enlarged and irregular in shape. With the onset of full blown AIDS, there is a reduction in the number of lymphoid follicles, lymphocyte depletion and vascular proliferation. Finally, there is nodal atrophy with fibrosis.

Hodgkin's Disease

It is now generally accepted that Hodgkin's disease is a neoplastic rather than an infective condition of the lymphoreticular system. It has a bimodal age incidence with peaks in the adolescence/early twenties age group and again after the age of 50 years. The annual incidences in males and females are 2 and 3 per 100 000 respectively in the UK.

The aetiology of Hodgkin's disease is unknown. There is some evidence for an infective aetiology: (1) Antibodies to Epstein–Barr virus are found more often in the serum of patients with Hodgkin's disease than in controls, although this may merely represent a particular susceptibility of patients with Hodgkin's disease to infection due to impairment of the immune system. (2) There is an epidemiological link between Hodgkin's disease and good housing, small family and higher education, all factors known to be associated with the late exposure to childhood infections. Thus, Hodgkin's disease may be due to late infection with some agent and in this respect it could be similar to poliomyelitis. (3) Several incidences of clustering of the disease have been described although these may merely have been due to chance.

Despite this evidence, no convincing organism has been demonstrated.

Clinically the common presentation is with enlarged lymph nodes, most frequently in the neck or axilla and less often in the groin or in the mediastinum. About one-quarter of patients have constitutional symptoms such as fever, malaise, weight loss and skin itching. The classical Pel–Ebstein fever (recurring fevers at intervals of a few weeks) is rarely seen.

Grossly, the enlarged lymph nodes tend to be pale, discrete and indistinguishable from non-Hodgkin's lymphoma, although the nodes in the nodular sclerosing variety of Hodgkin's disease may be firm and fibrous on sectioning.

On histological examination four variants are recognized (*see* below). All four types contain Reed–Sternberg cells which are essential for the diagnosis of Hodgkin's disease. Reed–Sternberg-like cells can be found in other conditions and therefore, although their presence is essential for the diagnosis of Hodgkin's disease, they are not pathognomonic of the condition.

The classical Reed–Sternberg cells are large and binucleate (*see* Fig. 15.3). The nuclei appear as mirror images of each other and each contains a prominent eosinophilic nucleolus, surrounded by a clear halo (owl-eye nucleoli).

It is generally believed that the Reed–Sternberg cells and their variants are the neoplastic cells of Hodgkin's disease. The other constituents seen histologically, such as lymphocytes and eosinophils, are probably reactive to the neoplastic condition. It is unclear which cell the Reed–Sternberg cell is derived from. The four main histological types of Hodgkin's disease are as follows.

1. LYMPHOCYTE PREDOMINANT (8·2%)*: In this variety the lymph node is replaced by large numbers of lymphocytes in a nodular or diffuse pattern and dispersed between these are occasional Reed–Sternberg cells. The classical Reed–Sternberg cell (as described above) is rarely seen but variants with polylobated nuclei are more easily identified.

2. MIXED CELLULARITY (17·5%)*: This has fewer lymphocytes than the last category and classical Reed–Sternberg cells are easily seen. Eosinophils, neutrophils and plasma cells are also commonly seen.

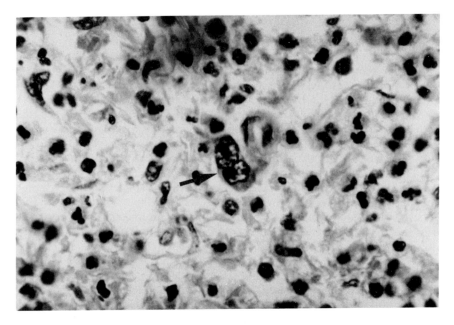

Fig. 15.3. Hodgkin's disease with a Reed–Sternberg cell (arrow). (H and E × 750)

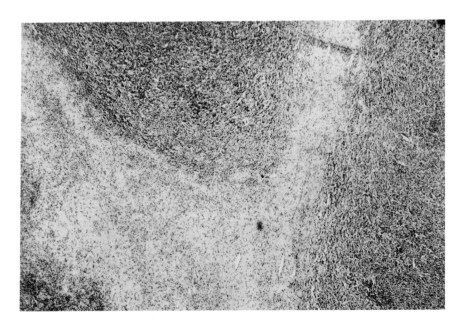

Fig. 15.4. Hodgkin's disease, nodular sclerosing type. The nodules of tumour are divided by bands of connective tissue. (H and E × 30)

3. NODULAR SCLEROSING (70·7%)*: This type is characterized by bands of fibrous tissue which divide the tumour into nodules (*see Fig.* 15.4). Within the nodules the tumour may resemble any of the other three variants of Hodgkin's disease, although the Reed–Sternberg cells tend to be a particular type characterized by contraction of the cell cytoplasm so as to give the impression that the cells are lying within lacunae; they are therefore termed lacunar cells.

4. LYMPHOCYTE DEPLETED (3·6%)*: In this variety the predominant cell is the Reed–Sternberg cell and its variants which may show considerable pleomorphism. Lymphocytes are not entirely absent and eosinophils, neutrophils and plasma cells may also be seen.

Spread, staging and prognosis
Unlike non-Hodgkin's lymphoma, Hodgkin's disease spreads from one area to an adjacent one in a contiguous fashion. The spread is therefore predictable and this gives a rational basis for staging. The Ann Arbor staging classification is widely used and is given in *Table* 15.1.

Table 15.1. Stages of Hodgkin's and non-Hodgkin's lymphomas (Ann Arbor classification)

I	Involvement of a single lymph node region or involvement of a single extralymphatic organ or site.
II	Involvement of two or more lymph node regions on the same side of the diaphragm alone, or with involvement of limited contiguous extralymphatic organ or tissue.
III	Involvement of lymph node regions on both sides of the diaphragm which may include the spleen and/or limited contiguous extralymphatic organ or site.
IV	Multiple or disseminated foci, or involvement of one or more extralymphatic organs or tissues, with or without lymphatic involvement.
A	Asymptomatic
B	Symptomatic.

The role of staging laparotomy in Hodgkin's disease is controversial. Although staging laparotomy does not appear to alter overall survival rates, its basis is that it assigns the patient to the most appropriate treatment category and hence it minimizes morbidity from unnecessary treatment modalities. The laparotomy protocol usually involves splenectomy, biopsy of splenic nodes, wedge biopsy of liver (usually left lobe), Menghini or Trucut needle biopsies from both liver lobes and biopsy of coeliac and porta hepatis nodes. Biopsies of para-aortic and mesenteric nodes and any additional masses are usually included. Most patients have had a marrow trephine prior to laparotomy and the place of oophoropexy is currently disputed. It has been established that the presence of intra-abdominal lymphoma, particularly in the spleen cannot be determined accurately with non-invasive imaging such as CT scanning. Spleen size is not an indication of involvement (Gill *et al.* 1980) and 30–45% of patients have their clinical staging altered by staging laparotomy.

*Percentage found in 1190 patients (Haybittle *et al.* 1985).

In one large series, one-third of the patients with clinical Stage I or II were upstaged to Stage III or IV (Glees *et al.* 1982).

However, with the increasing use of improved chemotherapeutic regimes, the place of staging laparotomy in Hodgkin's disease is becoming more limited. Excellent results have been reported from Toronto where the management does not involve staging laparotomy (Bergsagel *et al.* 1982). There is also a significant morbidity from splenectomy and laparotomy (major complications in 4%, minor complications in 31%). Laparotomy is still probably useful in those patients for whom treatment is to be radiotherapy alone, although if combination chemotherapy is to be used, there is probably currently no role for staging laparotomy.

The most important factor in determining prognosis is the stage of the disease when treatment is initiated. Five year survival rates for Stages I and II are in the region of 90% whereas for Stages III and IV this drops to about 75% and 60% respectively.

Traditionally, lymphocyte predominant and nodular sclerosing Hodgkin's disease tend to do better than mixed cellularity or lymphocyte depleted Hodgkin's diseases, although these differences have been narrowed by the newer more aggressive methods of treatment. More recently, Haybittle *et al.* (1985) have suggested that Hodgkin's disease should be divided into two histological grades. Grade I includes lymphocyte predominant and those cases of nodular sclerosis which do not have areas of lymphocyte depletion. Grade II includes mixed cellularity and those cases of nodular sclerosis with areas of lymphocyte depletion and pleomorphic cells. These authors found that for Stages I and IIA, a good prognosis was indicated by pathological Grade I, female sex, lack of mediastinal involvement and young age.

The Non-Hodgkin's Lymphomas

Non-Hodgkin's lymphomas occur most commonly in adults with a peak incidence during the seventh decade. The annual incidence in England and Wales is between 4 and 5 per 100 000. In about two-thirds of patients the primary lesion is in the lymph nodes and in the remaining one-third the primary lesion is extranodal (e.g. in the gut, skin, etc.). In children, a higher proportion is extranodal.

In most cases the aetiology of lymphomas is unknown. Several situations are, however, associated with a higher than normal incidence of lymphoma. (1) Graft recipients following therapeutic immunosuppression after organ transplantation can be infected with the Epstein–Barr (EB) virus, or the virus may be reactivated, as indicated by rising titres of antibodies to EB antigen and shedding of the virus in oral secretions. The loss of ability to control latent EB virus infections may be especially likely if cyclosporin A is used. This drug, by its action on suppressor T-cells, may specifically impair the normal immunological control of latent EB virus infection which may result in intense B-cell proliferation (Nagington and Gray 1980) and a lymphoproliferative response resulting in lymphoma-like lesions which appear to be clinically extranodal (Editorial 1984). The increase in the incidence of lymphomas has been well documented following transplantations of many organs including the heart (Austen and Cosimi 1984). (2) Patients with autoimmune diseases such as Sjögren's syndrome and rheumatoid arthritis. (3) Patients with primary immunodeficiency syndromes.

Clinically, patients with nodal lymphomas present with painless lymphadenopathy. The nodes are non-tender and initially feel rubbery and discrete. Later they may become a matted mass. Common sites such as the neck and the axilla may be affected or there may be generalized lymphadenopathy and hepatosplenomegaly.

Grossly, the individual nodes show generalized enlargement and the cut surface is grey or white; little necrosis or haemorrhage is seen.

Histologically, there is great variation in appearance and this has resulted in numerous classifications of non-Hodgkin's lymphomas. The Rappaport classification, which is shown in *Table* 15.2, divides lymphomas on the basis of histology only. It is still used in some centres although in others it has been replaced by either the Kiel or the Lukes–Collins' classification.

Table 15.2. Rappaport classification of non-Hodgkin's lymphomas

Well differentiated lymphocytic*
Poorly differentiated lymphocytic
Histiocytic
Mixed lymphocytic histiocytic
Undifferentiated (Burkitt's and non-Burkitt's)*

* These are only seen in a diffuse form; all others may be in a diffuse or nodular form.

Rappaport classification
The main contributions of the Rappaport classification were the division of lymphomas histologically into diffuse and nodular patterns and the realization that the nodular pattern has the better prognosis (*see Table* 15.2).

Well differentiated lymphocytic lymphoma
This occurs in diffuse form only and is composed of small darkly staining cells which are very similar to lymphocytes. In the later stages, spillage into the blood gives a picture similar to chronic lymphatic leukaemia. It may not be possible in these cases to distinguish between well differentiated lymphocytic lymphoma which has spread to the blood and chronic lymphatic leukaemia which has spread to the lymph nodes. Some patients may have plasma cells or plasma cell-like cells (plasmacytoid cells) within the lymphoma and these patients often have a monoclonal IgM in their serum (Waldenström's macroglobulinaemia).

Poorly differentiated lymphocytic lymphoma
A diffuse or nodular pattern may be seen in this type. The cells are larger than lymphocytes and characteristically have irregular nuclear indentations.

Histiocytic lymphoma
These also occur in a diffuse or nodular pattern. The cells are much larger than normal lymphocytes and their nuclei are pale staining with several prominent nucleoli.

Mixed lymphocytic histiocytic lymphoma

These contain a mixture of cells similar to those seen in both the poorly differentiated lymphocytic lymphoma and in the histiocytic lymphoma.

Undifferentiated lymphomas

These are composed mainly of small undifferentiated cells which have numerous nucleoli and a high mitotic rate. They are divided into the Burkitt's type and the non-Burkitt's type.

The Burkitt's lymphoma is again subdivided into an endemic type which is common in Central Africa, New Guinea and other tropical areas and a sporadic type which is seen occasionally in the rest of the world.

The endemic or African Burkitt's lymphoma is of interest because of its strongly suspected, though as yet not proven, aetiological link with the E–B virus. It is postulated that infection with the E–B virus causes a polyclonal proliferation of B-cells which in normal individuals would be self-limited due to T-immunoregulatory cells. If, however, there is an immunological abnormality (as might occur due to malarial infection which has a similar geographical distribution to Burkitt's lymphoma) this limitation does not occur and there is a resultant chronic and rapid proliferation of B-cells. The rapidly proliferating B-cells are liable to undergo chromosomal translocations and one of these translocations may cause a truly neoplastic clone of B-cells. The tumour cells of Burkitt's lymphoma often do in fact show chromosomal translocation.

The non-endemic or sporadic Burkitt's lymphoma has been reported in other parts of the world and is histologically identical to the African Burkitt's lymphoma, although the cells of the former do not contain the E–B virus DNA.

The African Burkitt's lymphoma occurs mainly in children with a peak age incidence of 6–7 years. Its commonest presentation is with swelling of the maxilla or mandible due to tumour involvement. The non-endemic variety presents most commonly with abdominal swelling.

Histologically, Burkitt's lymphoma is composed of monotonous cells, with rounded nuclei and inconspicuous nucleoli. The cells have a very high mitotic rate indicating the rapid growth of the tumour. Interspersed with these malignant cells are benign macrophages which are pale staining. On low powered microscopic examination, therefore, a dark sheet of cells with pale spots is seen giving the classical 'starry sky' appearance.

The non-Burkitt's undifferentiated lymphoma occurs in elderly patients. It has no association with the E–B virus and histologically shows great variation in cell size and shape.

Basis of the newer non-Hodgkin's lymphoma classifications

The newer classifications of lymphoma (e.g. Kiel and Lukes–Collins) are based on the fact that both T- and B-lymphocytes undergo a series of transformations when stimulated by antigens. Each stage of these transformations is represented by a particular cell type and each cell type may undergo malignant change to give a particular histological type of lymphoma.

B-cell transformation

It is now realized that the majority of lymphomas are of B-cell origin. B-lymphocytes which reside in the mantles of the lymphoid follicles of the lymph node cortex enter the follicle centre and undergo cell division when stimulated by an antigen. As they do so, they pass through a series of stages as shown in *Fig.* 15.5. The majority of B-cell lymphomas arise from these cells (as is expected since they are rapidly dividing) and are thus known as 'follicle centre cell lymphomas'. The various stages of transformation are given different names by the Lukes–Collins classification and the Kiel classification. In the Lukes–Collins classification the B-lymphocytes first become small cleaved cells, then large cleaved cells, then small uncleaved cells, followed by large uncleaved cells and finally immunoblasts which mature into either plasma cells or revert back to lymphocytes. The terms cleaved and non-cleaved refer to the presence or absence of a deep cleft in the cell nucleus. The Kiel classification terms both small and large cleaved cells as centrocytes and the small and large uncleaved cells as centroblasts. Immunoblasts have the same terminology in both classifications. The uncleaved cells (centroblasts and immunoblasts) resemble histiocytes and although they are now known to be of lymphocytic origin, lymphomas of these cells are termed 'histiocytic' in the Rappaport classification.

FOLLICULAR CENTRE CELL TRANSFORMATION

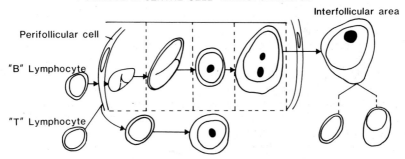

Fig. 15.5. Schematic diagram to show T-cell and B-cell transformation in the follicle centre. (*See text.*) (Reproduced with permission from Lukes and Collins 1975.)

T-cell transformation

T-cells in the parafollicular area of the node show a similar transformation without the stages of nuclear cleavage (*see Fig.* 15.5).

The Kiel classification of non-Hodgkin's lymphoma

Of the newer classifications, only the Kiel will be discussed briefly.

B-cell lymphomas

LYMPHOCYTIC LYMPHOMA: This is a lymphoma of elderly patients characterized by a proliferation of cells which resemble lymphocytes. The cells are identical to those seen in chronic lymphatic leukaemia and lymphocytic lymphomas can be regarded as the tissue phase of that disease. The equivalent Rappaport lesion is well differentiated lymphocytic lymphoma. Variants may have some cells which resemble plasma cells (lymphoplasmacytoid lymphoma) and some may have a scattering of mature plasma cells (lymphoplasmacytic lymphoma). In these cases, the lymphoma may secrete a paraprotein. Those composed entirely of plasma cells are termed plasmacytomas and in these cases a lymph node biopsy will not distinguish between an extramedullary plasmacytoma and lymph node involvement in generalized multiple myeloma.

FOLLICLE CENTRE CELL LYMPHOMA: These are the commonest forms of malignant lymphoma and are composed of cells similar to those seen in the normal follicle centre. The lymphomas, therefore, may be centrocytic, centroblastic or centrocytic/centroblastic. Centrocytes are larger than lymphocytes and have darkly staining, deeply indented irregular nuclei (the cleaved cells of Lukes–Collins) and centroblasts have large nuclei which are pale staining with a few prominent, peripherally situated nucleoli (the non-cleaved cells of Lukes–Collins). These tumours may show a follicular (*see Fig.* 15.6) or a diffuse pattern. The equivalent Rappaport terms are poorly differentiated lymphocytic for centrocytic and histiocytic for centroblastic.

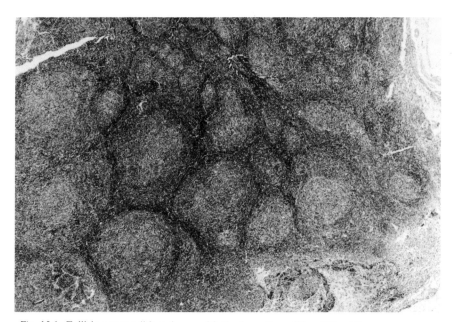

Fig. 15.6. Follicle centre cell lymphoma of follicular pattern. (H and E × 30)

B IMMUNOBLASTIC LYMPHOMA: These are lymphomas composed of immunoblasts which are large cells with abundant cytoplasm. The nuclei are also large, pale staining and each has a central prominent nucleolus.

BURKITT'S LYMPHOMA: This is discussed above. It may be derived from small centroblasts (small non-cleaved cells), although this is controversial.

T-cell lymphomas

Tumours of T-cells are much less common than B-cell lymphomas. The T-cell lymphomas tend at first to affect the parafollicular zone of the lymph node and they tend to stimulate endothelial cells so that venules become very prominent. The cell nuclei in T-cell lymphomas tend to be indented and folded (the so-called 'cerebriform nucleus'). T-cell lymphomas have a predilection for invading skin and some actually arise in the T-cells of the skin. The best described forms of T-cell lymphoma are the T-cell lymphocytic lymphoma (similar morphologically to B-cell lymphocytic lymphoma), cutaneous T-cell lymphoma (mycosis fungoides, Sézary's syndrome) and T-lymphoblastic lymphomas (lymphomas of precursor T-cells).

True histiocytic lymphomas

These are tumours of the monocyte/macrophage system. They were not included in the Kiel classification, but are mentioned here for completeness. Although many lymphomas are classified as histiocytic by Rappaport, most of these are now considered to be of follicle centre origin, leaving true histiocytic lymphomas as exceedingly rare tumours. Malignant histiocytosis of the gut is discussed on p. 111.

Spread, staging and prognosis of non-Hodgkin's lymphomas

Non-Hodgkin's lymphomas, unlike Hodgkin's disease, do not necessarily spread from one area to an adjacent area but instead spread in an unpredictable way. Spill-over into the blood may occur and nodal lymphomas may spread to other organs such as liver, bone marrow, gastrointestinal tract, etc. The same staging categories as in Hodgkin's disease can be used, although staging is less clinically relevant than in Hodgkin's disease due to the random nature of the spread. The prognosis of non-Hodgkin's lymphomas depends on the histological type and for this purpose they have been classified into high-grade or low-grade (*see Table* 15.3).

Table 15.3. High- and low-grade malignant lymphoma of non-Hodgkin's type (using Kiel terminology)

Low-grade lymphomas	High-grade lymphomas
Lymphocytic (T- or B-cell)	Centroblastic
Centrocytic	Lymphoblastic
Centrocytic/centroblastic	Immunoblastic
Mycosis fungoides	Burkitt's lymphoma
Sézary syndrome	

Patients with low-grade lymphoma of Stages I and II, treated by radiotherapy alone, have a five year survival of 70–75%. This drops to 50% for Stages III and IV treated by chemotherapy. Patients with high-grade lymphomas (excepting Burkitt's) with Stages I and II have five year survivals of 70% and 50% respectively and this drops to 10–30% for Stages III and IV.

The role of staging laparotomy in non-Hodgkin's lymphomas is even less clear than in Hodgkin's disease. The patients are often elderly and 60–80% have advanced disease at the time of presentation. Only 20% of clinical Stage I and II patients will be advanced to Stage III by laparotomy (Come and Chabner 1979).

Staging laparotomy in non-Hodgkin's lymphoma may have a place if radiotherapy is likely to be the treatment of choice, as the anatomical extent of the disease can be assessed.

Miscellaneous Causes of Lymphadenopathy

Histiocytosis X

Langerhans cells normally reside in the epidermis and are thought to have a role in antigen trapping. Histiocytosis X is a proliferation of Langerhans cells of unknown aetiology, although the condition is probably not neoplastic. It occurs in three different clinical forms. (1) Letterer–Siwe disease which affects infants and is generalized with a poor prognosis. (2) Unifocal eosinophilic granuloma which commonly affects bones and presents as a pathological fracture in children and young adults. (3) Multifocal eosinophilic granuloma (Hand–Schüller–Christian disease) in which multiple eosinophilic granulomas are found in different parts of the body, such as the lungs and particularly the posterior pituitary.

When lymph nodes are involved by histiocytosis X, lymphadenopathy may be massive. Young patients develop generalized lymphadenopathy whereas older patients often develop cervical lymphadenopathy.

Histologically, there is a proliferation of Langerhans cells, especially in the lymphatic sinuses of the lymph nodes. These Langerhans cells have abundant eosinophilic cytoplasm and a characteristic large folded nucleus. Mixed with these is a variable number of eosinophils and other inflammatory cells.

Angioimmunoblastic lymphadenopathy (AIL)

This condition presents as a systemic illness (fever, weight loss, etc.) with generalized lymphadenopathy. Elderly patients tend to be affected and there is frequently a history of drug ingestion, skin rash and arthralgia. The pathogenesis is unknown and, although it is considered to be a hyperplastic rather than a neoplastic reaction, malignant transformation does occur in some cases.

Histologically, the lymph node architecture is destroyed by an infiltrate of large cells with pale staining nuclei (immunoblasts). Very characteristically, there is an arborizing vascular proliferation of blood vessels within the infiltrate. Diagnosis is difficult and it is thought that some cases diagnosed as AIL are in fact examples of T-cell lymphomas.

The importance of angioimmunoblastic lymphadenopathy is because: (1) it is a rare cause of generalized lymphadenopathy, (2) the destruction of the lymph node architecture often leads to a mistaken diagnosis of lymphoma, and (3) patients frequently succumb to infection, probably due to an associated immunodeficiency.

Angiofollicular hyperplasia

Angiofollicular hyperplasia may occur at any age and presents with lymphadenopathy at single or multiple sites. Routine chest X-ray may show a mediastinal mass due to hilar node involvement. The degree of lymphadenopathy may be massive.

Histologically, the characteristic feature is replacement of the normal lymph node architecture by abnormal follicles. These abnormal follicles consist of concentric rings of lymphocytes around a central area of hyaline material in which a blood vessel is embedded. The condition is benign but is of importance in that it may be mistaken for malignant lymphoma.

Dermatopathic lymphadenopathy

Patients with any of the chronic dermatoses may develop lymphadenopathy which may be generalized or specific to the lymph drainage of the involved region.

Histologically, the lymph node sinuses are packed with histiocytic cells which compress the normal nodal architecture. When lymph node biopsy is carried out it is important that the surgeon informs the pathologist of any skin rash the patient may have so that the condition is not mistaken for malignancy.

Silicone lymphadenopathy

Silicone is used in mammoplasty procedures and in joint prostheses and it may cause local lymphadenopathy. Lymph node biopsy may be required to exclude recurrent carcinoma after implantation of a breast prosthesis. The lymph node shows reactive change with numerous giant cells containing refractile fragmented silicone.

Drug induced lymphadenopathy

Diphenylhydantoin (phenytonin) occasionally causes lymphadenopathy, which histologically shows bizarre cells, and thus the condition may be mistaken for lymphoma if the pathologist is unaware of the drug history.

SPLEEN

Normal Structure and Function

The spleen has diaphragmatic and visceral surfaces. The latter have gastric, renal, pancreatic and colic impressions. The lienorenal ligament contains the splenic vessels and the gastrosplenic ligament contains the short gastric vessels and the left gastroepiploic branches of the splenic artery. The adult spleen is usually 12 cm in length, 7 cm in width and 4 cm thick but decreases in size and weight with increasing age. The average adult weight is 150 g. Frequently, near the spleen, especially in the gastrosplenic ligament and greater omentum, small encapsulated nodules of splenic tissue may be found. These accessory spleens (splenunculi) may be isolated or connected to the spleen by bands of splenic tissue.

The spleen is encased in an external serous layer of investing peritoneum which is adherent to an underlying fibroelastic capsule. From the capsule, trabeculae pass into the spleen and carry with them the splenic vessels from the hilum. Arteriolar branches leave the trabeculae and their adventitial coats become replaced by a periarteriolar sheath of lymphatic tissue which accompanies the vessels until the capillaries are reached. These lymphatic sheaths form the white pulp of the spleen and are enlarged at intervals to form lymphoid follicles (Malpighian bodies) which are 0·25–1·0 mm in diameter and visible to the naked eye as grey flecks on the cut surface. The terminal arterioles divide and enter the red pulp.

The red pulp consists of sinusoids between which are many macrophages. The macrophages are supported by a reticulum network and are connected to each other by fine processes, thus forming an effective filter. These areas of macrophages are termed the splenic cords (of Billroth). Blood leaving the capillaries may pass directly through the sinusoids to the splenic veins (the 'closed circuit'). Alternatively, it may filter out through the discontinuous endothelium of the sinusoids into the splenic cords and penetrate through the labyrinth of macrophages before re-entering the circulation (the 'open circuit').

The spleen has several major functions. It removes ageing red cells from the circulation together with micro-organisms and cell debris. It phagocytoses antigen and brings it into contact with both T- and B-lymphocytes, thus initiating both cellular and humoral immunity. The spleen may be a source of extramedullary haemopoiesis in certain types of anaemia occurring in adult life and it may serve as a storage area for red blood cells, platelets and iron.

Splenomegaly and hypersplenism (*see Fig.* 15.7)

A list of some of the causes of splenomegaly is given in *Table* 15.4. Enlargement of the spleen may lead to hypersplenism which is usually defined as follows: a condition in which there is (1) splenomegaly, (2) a reduction in one or more of the cellular elements in the blood leading to anaemia, leucopenia or thrombocytopenia, or any combination of the three, associated with hyperplasia of the bone marrow, and (3) correction of the cytopenia(s) by splenectomy.

The cause of the cytopenia appears to be mainly due to excessive pooling of the cellular elements of the blood in the spleen. There is also evidence that red cells entrapped within the spleen have a reduced survival time due to a lack of glucose and a fall in pH.

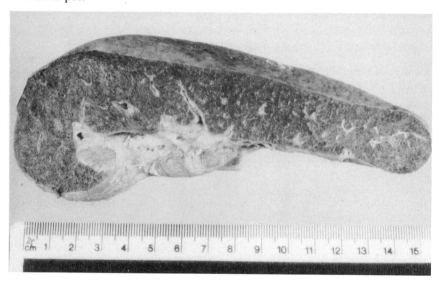

Fig. 15.7. Splenomegaly in portal hypertension.

Table 15.4. Some causes of splenomegaly

Infections	*Portal hypertension*
Infectious mononucleosis	Liver cirrhosis
Infective endocarditis	Portal vein thrombosis
Typhoid	Right heart failure
Brucellosis	
Tuberculosis	*Storage diseases*
Malaria	Gaucher's disease
Toxoplasmosis	Niemann-Pick disease
Kala-azar	Mucopolysaccharidoses
Schistosomiasis	
	Miscellaneous
Haematological	Felty's syndrome
Hodgkin's lymphoma	Connective tissue disorders
Non-Hodgkin's lymphoma	Cysts
Leukaemia	Primary tumours
Multiple myeloma	Secondary tumours
Myelofibrosis	
Polycythaemia rubra vera	
Haemolytic anaemias	
Thrombocytopenic purpura	

Congenital Anomalies of the Spleen

Congenital absence (asplenia, splenic aplasia, splenic agenesis) is rare and is usually associated with major cardiovascular abnormalities especially of the endocardial cushions. Visceral transposition and multiorgan defects are frequently found. Howell–Jolly bodies (*see* p. 435) are seen in the peripheral red blood cells and affected children have a predisposition to infection.

Hereditary splenic hypoplasia is exceedingly rare and predisposes to infection, especially during infancy.

Lobulation of the spleen is seen occasionally and is sometimes associated with cardiovascular anomalies.

Accessory splenic tissue (splenunculi) is present in 10% of the population and is most often found in the splenic hilum. They are usually less than 2 cm in diameter, dark in colour and spherical in shape. Larger splenunculi may project into the peritoneal cavity and have a serosal covering. If splenectomy is done for haematological reasons, such as hereditary spherocytosis, they may predispose to recurrence of the problem.

Splenic Trauma

The spleen is the commonest internal organ to be injured in blunt abdominal trauma, the cause usually being a blow or crush injury to the upper abdomen or lower left thorax (*see Fig.* 15.8). Penetrating injuries due to gunshot or stab wounds are common in some centres. A spleen which is pathologically enlarged is more prone to rupture than one which is not. Iatrogenic trauma occurs during fundoplication for hiatus hernia, gastrectomy and vagotomy, the risk being greater during revisional surgery (Cochrane 1980). These operative injuries are usually capsular tears due to pulling off adhesions. Spontaneous rupture is rare if the

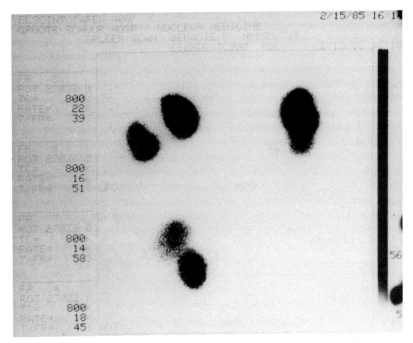

Fig. 15.8. Splenic scan showing post-traumatic splenic rupture. Two of the views show the spleen in two halves.

spleen is normal but is more common in enlarged spleens and has been reported in malaria, portal hypertension, polycythaemia rubra vera, glandular fever and other conditions.

The incidence of delayed splenic rupture secondary to a subcapsular or intrasplenic haematoma is uncertain.

Because of the risk of post-splenectomy sepsis (*see* p. 440) there is a current interest in preserving the spleen. This is especially applicable in children in whom the risk of post-splenectomy infection is significant and most paediatric centres now have a policy of non-operative management of trauma to the spleen unless there is life-threatening bleeding. If operation is required, many approaches to splenic conservation have been suggested, including topical agents such as microfibrillar collagen, thrombin and gelatin foam. Methods of splenorrhaphy include suture, omental wrap or polyglycolic mesh. Partial splenectomy based on a segmental arterial supply has also been advocated (Cooper and Williamson 1984).

If splenic conservation is not possible, transplantation of splenic fragments into an omental pouch has been used although a graft of 20–30 cm^3 is probably required (Corazza *et al.* 1984). However, there have been several reports of post-splenectomy sepsis in patients with splenosis (*see* p. 441) and it seems likely that an intact arterial supply is required for adequate Pneumococcal clearance.

Patients who require splenectomy should receive polyvalent Pneumococcal vaccine and some authorities give prophylactic antibiotics to post-splenectomy children.

While the conservative approach to splenic rupture in children is established, there is some controversy regarding the same approach in adults because of the much smaller risk of post-splenectomy sepsis.

Effects of splenectomy

Qualitative changes in circulating red cells include the presence of Howell–Jolly bodies and an increased proportion of target cells, siderocytes and red cells containing Heinz bodies. Howell–Jolly bodies are fragments of DNA of nuclear origin which normally occur in less than 2% of circulating red cells. Their presence may be due to a failure of the spleen to remove the nucleus from circulating normoblasts. Howell–Jolly bodies are found in congenital absence of the spleen and in cases of splenic atrophy as well as after splenectomy. Their absence from the blood of a patient who has had a splenectomy suggests that there is accessory splenic tissue present. Siderocytes are red cells containing granules of free iron. Heinz bodies consist of degraded haemoglobin and are found in ageing red cells.

A leucocytosis follows within hours of splenectomy. Neutrophils in particular increase in numbers in the postoperative period and this increase may persist for several weeks. Later there may be an absolute lymphocytosis or monocytosis. Eosinophils and basophils also increase in number.

A transient thrombocytopenia occurs during the first 24 hours after splenectomy, followed by a marked thrombocytosis which is maximal at 14 days postoperatively. The platelet count may reach $1 \times 10^{12}/l$. Platelet adhesiveness is increased after splenectomy and platelet function may be abnormal. The risk of spontaneous thrombosis may be increased after splenectomy although the data are unclear at present. Some authors, however, recommend anti-coagulation measures such as low dose heparin or the administration of aspirin.

The immunological effect of splenectomy is greatest with younger patients, especially those under one year old. Reported immune defects have included diminished phagocytic activity, loss of mechanical filtration of blood, decreased opsonin concentration, decreased serum IgM, depressed properdin titres, decreased tuftsin concentrations, altered T-helper and T-suppressor cell activity and impaired antibody production after intravenously administered antigens. Defective synthesis of specific antibodies in splenectomized patients is detectable many years after surgery and appears to be due to B-cell dysfunction. In addition, there appears to be a generalized inability of peripheral blood B-lymphocytes to differentiate into immunoglobulin secreting plasma cells. IgM levels are low for at least one year following splenectomy and gradually return to normal about four years postoperatively. Complement activity via the properdin pathway is defective initially but returns to normal several months later. All these factors predispose to a reduced ability to opsonize and phagocytose encapsulated organisms.

These immunological changes predispose to infection following splenectomy, especially in children, and there is a risk of developing 'overwhelming post-splenectomy infection' (OPSI) (see below). Splenectomy for trauma results in fewer changes in immune functions than splenectomy for other indications, possibly because implantation of splenic cells into the peritoneum at the time of capsular rupture (splenosis) may restore some splenic function (Pearson et al. 1978).

An increase in late deaths from ischaemic heart disease following splenectomy has been reported (Robinette and Fraumeni 1977). The increase was two-fold compared with age-matched controls. An increase in whole blood viscosity and a decrease in red cell deformability after splenectomy may contribute to this.

Other local sequelae of splenectomy which may occur in the postoperative period include pyrexia, atelectasis, left-sided pleural effusion, subphrenic abscess and damage to the stomach or pancreatic tail. Any splenunculi which are present tend to hypertrophy.

The mortality following splenectomy depends on the age of the patient and the indication for splenectomy. The operative mortality is less than 2% for cases of idiopathic thrombocytopenic purpura but may be up to 15–20% for myelosclerosis.

Post-splenectomy sepsis

It is now well recognized that the risk of infection is increased after splenectomy and the condition of 'overwhelming post-splenectomy infection' (OPSI) is well documented. King and Shumacker (1952) indicated that children after splenectomy were especially prone to infection, and Singer (1973)—and later Francke and Neu (1981)—attempted to quantify the risk. The overall incidence of sepsis after splenectomy is 5% and the overall risk of developing fatal post-splenectomy sepsis is about 2·5%. The risk is greater in children than in adults.

The risk of developing OPSI is greatest during the first year of life and it usually occurs within 24 months of splenectomy, although it may occur much later. Removal of the spleen for trauma carries a 1% risk of developing OPSI (60-fold increase over the normal population). The risk is higher after splenectomy for pathological conditions such as spherocytosis (200-fold increase), immune thrombocytopenic purpura (100-fold increase), thalassaemia, hypersplenism, and acquired haemolytic anaemia.

The risk of developing post-splenectomy sepsis in the adult is much less than in children but is still greater than in the general population, who have not undergone splenectomy.

OPSI is unlike septicaemia in patients who have an intact spleen in that the course is extraordinarily rapid and death may ensue within 18 hours. The onset is sudden with nausea, vomiting, confusion and later coma. The infecting organism is Pneumococcus in 50% of cases and the remaining cases are caused by Meningococcus, E. coli, Haemophilus influenzae, Staphylococcus and Streptococcus in decreasing frequency. Disseminated intravascular coagulation is frequent and hypoglycaemia, hypotension and electrolyte imbalance are common. Bacteria are seen on peripheral blood smears and at autopsy, multi-organ haemorrhage including the Waterhouse–Friderichsen syndrome (see p. 485) is often seen.

Frequently antibiotics fail to control the infection and while overall mortality is 50%, pneumococcal infections carry the highest mortality (50–80%).

Miscellaneous Conditions

Atrophy

This accompanies ageing and is also seen in intestinal malabsorption, thrombocythaemia and sickle cell anaemia (due to repeated infarcts). Splenic atrophy is one of the causes of hyposplenism (the others being splenectomy and splenic agenesis) which is characterized by the presence of Howell–Jolly bodies, target cells and siderocytes, together with thrombocytosis and leucocytosis in the peripheral blood.

Splenosis

This is multiple foci of splenic tissue on the serosa of the peritoneal cavity due to the seeding of splenic cells after splenic rupture. They are distinguished from splenunculi by their large number, irregular shape and wide distribution. There is usually a history of trauma. They occasionally cause complications such as intestinal obstruction.

Amyloidosis

The spleen is frequently involved in secondary amyloidosis and sometimes in primary amyloidosis. Spontaneous rupture may occur.

Splenic infarction (*see Fig.* 15.9)

Splenic artery embolism may be secondary to myocardial thrombus or to infective endocarditis. Other causes of infarction include thrombus superimposed on splenic artery atheroma, polyarteritis and sickle cell anaemia. Splenomegaly from any cause, especially chronic myeloid leukaemia, may be associated with splenic infarcts. The area of the infarct is wedge-shaped with the apex pointing to the hilum; there is an associated perisplenitis.

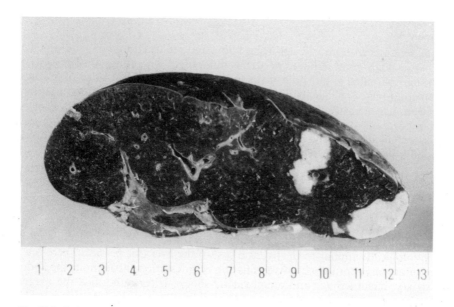

Fig. 15.9. Spleen with infarcts.

Torsion

This is rare and is due to congenital anomalies of the peritoneal folds. Haemorrhagic infarction ensues and rupture may occur.

Perisplenitis

This is associated with many pathological conditions of the spleen. A fibrinous exudate forms on the serosal surface and is associated with localized pain. The fibrinous exudate may later form fibrous adhesions. Chronic perisplenitis is a white thickening of the splenic capsule and it accompanies any cause of chronic splenomegaly. Histologically the capsule is covered in dense, hyaline collagenous tissue.

Splenic abscess

A splenic abscess may be the result of a septic embolus or a septicaemia as might happen in bacterial endocarditis, typhoid, paratyphoid, osteomyelitis and otitis media. Splenic abscess may also complicate a traumatic intrasplenic haematoma or portography.

The clinical presentation is with left hypochondrial pain, weight loss, rigors and splenomegaly. Rupture of the abscess may lead to a subdiaphragmatic abscess which may spread through the diaphragm and cause empyema. Rupture into the peritoneal cavity results in peritonitis.

If possible, the spleen should be removed, but dense adhesions may make drainage the only possibility.

Splenic Cysts

Pseudocysts

These are cysts with no true epithelial lining and are usually single, multiloculated and large. They contain blood or serous fluid, often with cholesterol crystals, and are usually situated at one pole of the spleen. The cyst wall is formed of fibrous tissue or compressed splenic tissue and it may calcify. The possible causes are trauma, infection, degeneration of an infarcted area, malaria and tuberculosis. They have been reported in otherwise normal spleens, in which case they probably represent degeneration of an old haematoma or infarct. They may rupture and produce considerable haemorrhage.

True cysts

Parasitic

Hydatid disease is the most common parasitic cyst of the spleen and it is morphologically similar to the hydatid cyst of the liver (*see* p. 162). There is a risk of spontaneous rupture with dissemination of infestation throughout the abdominal cavity, haemorrhage and anaphylactic shock. Ultrasound aids the diagnosis and splenectomy is required with care to avoid spillage of the cyst contents (Macpherson 1980).

Simple cysts (congenital cysts, serous cysts)

These are rare and have a cellular lining of flattened or cuboidal cells. Their origin is unclear and they may arise from infoldings of splenic peritoneum during embryological development. They are often multiple and are located near the splenic capsule. Others have suggested that they arise from dilated lymphatics.

Epidermoid cysts

These are rare and their origin is uncertain. They may be due to squamous metaplasia of a simple cyst, although some are considered to be true cystic neoplasms. They are unilocular, single, oval in shape and filled with straw-coloured fluid. They may be very large. The cyst wall is composed of dense fibrous tissue with a lining of stratified squamous epithelium without skin appendages. Most occur in females and tend to present in patients under 20 years of age. When large, the cysts cause pressure symptoms and occasionally they rupture or become infected. Treatment is by splenectomy.

Dermoid cysts

True dermoid cysts of the spleen are exceedingly rare. The wall contains keratinizing squamous epithelium with attached dermal appendages, such as sebaceous glands and hair follicles.

Splenic Tumours

Benign tumours

These are rare but splenic haemangiomas, lymphangiomas and hamartomas occur.

Haemangiomas

These may occur as an isolated finding or may be part of a more widespread vascular malformation. They are usually a small (less than 2 cm) solitary incidental finding at laparotomy. Occasionally they are large and cause pressure symptoms. Complications are thrombosis, infarction with fibrosis and rupture. They have no capsule and histologically large blood filled spaces are lined by endothelial cells and separated by fibrous septa. Splenectomy is curative.

Lymphangiomas

These are rare and may be hamartomas. They are seen as nodules consisting of cystic spaces filled with clear, yellow fluid. They slowly enlarge and splenomegaly may occur.

Hamartomas

These are uncommon and are formed of either lymphoid tissue (white pulp hamartomas) or a complex of sinuses equivalent to normal splenic pulp cords (red pulp hamartomas). They are well defined, occasionally multiple, non-encapsulated round nodules in the spleen substance, usually 2–4 cm in diameter. Most are discovered incidentally at autopsy or laparotomy.

Malignant tumours

Primary lymphoma

Lymphoma involving only the spleen is exceedingly rare and accounts for less than 0·5% of all malignant lymphomas. Involvement of the spleen in generalized lymphoma or leukaemia is much more common. A primary lymphoma may be of the Hodgkin's or non-Hodgkin's type. Macroscopically the cut surface may show diffuse involvement, nodular involvement (*see Fig*.15.10) or a single large tumour mass.

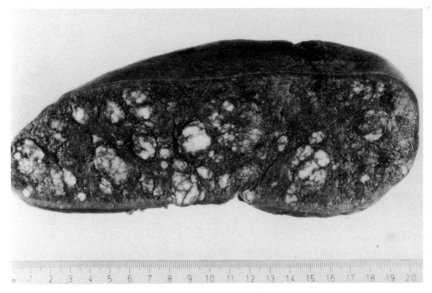

Fig. 15.10. Hodgkin's disease of the spleen showing nodules of tumour tissue.

Primary splenic lymphoma tends to occur in middle-aged and older subjects. Vague malaise and pyrexia associated with splenomegaly are the usual findings. If splenectomy is undertaken, the splenic nodes and the liver must be biopsied to stage the disease.

Haemangiosarcoma (angiosarcoma)

Although rare, this is the second most common malignant splenic tumour after lymphoma. It is uncertain whether the tumour arises from endothelial cells or pluripotential mesenchymal cells. There is a marked splenomegaly and the capsule is thickened with surrounding adhesions. Large grey tumour nodules, some of which are haemorrhagic, are seen on the cut surface. Histologically, the appearance is similar to that seen in haemangiosarcomas elsewhere (*see* p. 539). They grow rapidly and disseminate widely to liver, lymph nodes, bone and lungs. If the diagnosis is made during life, the prognosis is poor with a median survival of 4 months, even with splenectomy and chemotherapy.

Secondary (metastatic) splenic tumours

Although traditionally the spleen is said to be rarely the site of secondary tumours, about 10% of patients dying of carcinomatosis have obvious macroscopic deposits at autopsy. If careful microscopic examination of the spleen is undertaken, 20–30% of these patients have secondary deposits. Most probably arise from blood spread, although occasionally lymphatic spread occurs. The primary tumours which most commonly metastasize to the spleen are melanoma, cancer of lung, breast and ovary and choriocarcinoma. It has been considered that a splenic immunological factor may inhibit the growth of secondary deposits. The capsule of the spleen appears to be able to resist direct invasion from adjacent organs such as the stomach, colon and pancreas. Rarely a secondary tumour in the spleen may rupture spontaneously.

THYMUS

Normal Structure and Development

The thymus arises as a paired structure from the endoderm of the third branchial pouches during the sixth week *in utero*. By migration of the right and left lobes, the thymus finally lies in the anterior mediastinum, in front of the great vessels. The upper pole may remain in the neck applied to the trachea. In adult life it becomes yellow due to replacement by fat, whereas in early life it is pink, soft and lobulated. Small accessory nodules of thymic tissue may occur in the neck. The thymus varies in size with age, weighing 10–15 g at birth, 40 g at puberty, and, with atrophy in adulthood, its weight falls to 10 g by middle age. Its blood supply comes from multiple small tributaries of the inferior thyroid and internal thoracic arteries. The main veins drain into the left brachiocephalic, internal thoracic and inferior thyroid veins. The thymus is surrounded by a fibrous capsule and is divided into lobules by connective tissue. Histologically, each lobule, which is 3–5 mm in diameter, has a peripheral, darkly staining cortex and an inner pale medulla. The lobules consist of lymphocytic cells, epithelial cells and macrophages. The lymphocytes are numerous in the cortex and tend to obscure the epithelial cells in this region. In contrast, lymphocytes are fewer in the medulla, where they are scattered among numerous thymic epithelial cells. Macrophages are scattered throughout.

Thymic lymphocytes arise mainly by division of stem cells in the outer cortex. These stem cells have migrated to the thymus from bone marrow. Some thymic lymphocytes undergo degeneration while the remainder leave the thymus to form part of the circulating pool of lymphocytes.

Hassall's corpuscles are laminated keratinous bodies found only in the thymic medulla. They are complex tubular structures derived from aggregates of thymic epithelial cells. They increase in size and number during involution of the thymus.

There appears to be a barrier between the thymus and the circulation and injected particulate matter tends not to penetrate the extravascular spaces of the thymic cortex. This may indicate that this is an immunologically sequestrated site.

It is now accepted that the thymus is a primary lymphoid organ which is responsible for the production, differentiation and direction of small lymphocytes which are involved in cell mediated immunity and with 'memory' of a previous antigen stimulus. Thymus-dependent lymphocytes (T-lymphocytes) circulate in lymph and blood and are also found in the white pulp of the spleen and in the deep (paracortical) thymus-dependent zones of the lymph nodes. The T-cells require 'priming' by macrophages and the presence of the latter in the thymus is therefore of importance.

Thymic Aplasia and Hypoplasia

Aplasia and hypoplasia of the thymus are associated with various immunodeficiency states. They are all rare conditions, some of which are familial, and include Swiss-type hypogammaglobulinaemia and DiGeorge's syndrome.

Myasthenia Gravis and the Thymus

About 10–20% of patients with myasthenia gravis have an associated thymoma and this is discussed below. In the 80% of patients without a thymoma, changes are usually found in the thymus, especially in younger patients. The medulla contains many lymphoid follicles with active germinal centres and the gland may be enlarged, although its weight is frequently constant as the cortex undergoes involution. The lymphoid follicles in the medulla are similar to those found in lymph nodes but there is no connection between the number of follicles and severity of the myasthenia gravis. Other changes in the thymus include an increase in the numbers of lymphocytes and plasma cells and an increased number of Hassall's corpuscles. Classically these changes have been termed 'thymic hyperplasia'.

It is established that myasthenia gravis results from a reduction of available acetylcholine receptors at neuromuscular junctions, probably due to an autoimmune attack on the receptors. Antibodies to acetylcholine receptors are elevated in over 80% of patients and the incidence of elevated antibodies is particularly high in patients with thymomas, although the titres correspond only loosely to the severity of the disease. Following thymectomy the antibody titres to acetylcholine receptors tend to decrease but other autoantibodies persist. However, the fall in antibody correlates rather poorly with the good results obtained after thymectomy. The thymus itself does not produce the anti-receptor antibodies and the exact relationship between the thymus and myasthenia gravis is unclear. However, a thymic hormone (thymopoietin) has been identified in serum and this is decreased in most patients after thymectomy but remains elevated in those not improved after operation (Robinson 1983). This may act synergistically with receptor antibody to cause myasthenia gravis. Another theory suggests that Hassall's corpuscles, which resemble embryonic muscle cells (myoid cells), act as antigens and trigger an immune response which becomes directed at the acetylcholine receptors on the surfaces of the muscle cells. Finally, thymus-directed cell-mediated immunity against the neuromuscular junction may play a role.

Classically, it was considered that patients who benefited most from thymectomy were young females with a short history of myasthenia gravis. More recently, the indications for thymectomy in this disease have widened to include males and older patients.

In one series, thymectomy resulted in a 91% improvement with complete remission in about 10%. A short duration of disease, thymic hyperplasia with abundant germinal centres and acetylcholine receptor antibodies present before but absent after thymectomy were the best predictors of a good response. Thymic atrophy, incomplete excision, persistent antibodies and a very long duration of disease were predictive of a poor response. Response was independent of age and sex (Rubin *et al.* 1981).

Myasthenia gravis associated with a thymoma occurs at a later age and tends to be more severe and more refractory to treatment than cases with no thymoma. Usually the thymoma is of the mixed lymphocytic and epithelial type. Following thymectomy, the myasthenia may improve but the results are unpredictable (Shamji *et al.* 1984).

Tumours of the Thymus

Thymomas

Thymomas are tumours of the epithelial component of the thymus. Although many cases are heavily infiltrated by T-lymphocytes, it is generally considered that only the epithelial component is neoplastic. Thymomas which show no cytological atypia and no local invasion are slow growing and are termed benign. Those with little or no cellular atypia but which show local invasion are termed malignant thymomas. Rarely the tumour shows considerable atypia and this is called a thymic carcinoma.

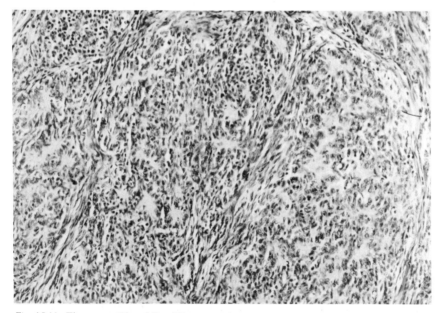

Fig. 15.11. Thymoma. (H and E × 75)

Thymomas may be an incidental finding on chest X-ray or may present as local pressure symptoms. Some are found during the investigation of one of the thymoma associated diseases which include myasthenia gravis, systemic lupus erythematosis, other collagen diseases, cytopenias and various non-thymic cancers. The usual age of presentation is in the 40–50 year age group.

Grossly, the cut section shows a lobular pattern and there may be cystic change.

Histologically (see Fig. 15.11), there is an epithelial component together with a lymphocytic component which may be heavy or scant. The epithelial cells may resemble normal thymic cells or they may be spindle shaped (spindle cell thymoma). Some cases may show squamous type epithelial cells.

About 90% of thymomas are benign and the prognosis after resection is good. Prognosis is not influenced by the presence or absence of myasthenia gravis (Shamji et al. 1984).

Teratomatous tumours of the thymus

Most teratomas in the anterior mediastinum are benign dermoid cysts. Usually thymic tissue can be found in the wall but whether the tumour arises in the thymus de novo or whether the tissue is merely compressed thymus is unclear.

Other thymic tumours

Non-Hodgkin's and Hodgkin's lymphomas may be found in the thymus and must be distinguished from thymoma. The latter was formerly termed 'granulomatous thymoma'.

Thymolipoma is a rare hamartoma consisting of adipose and thymic tissue. Some are very large.

Secondary involvement of the thymus in malignant tumours

Any form of lymphoma or leukaemia may involve the thymus at any stage of the disease process and distinction from a thymoma with a heavy lymphocytic infiltrate may be very difficult. Secondary invasion from bronchial carcinoma or mediastinal lymph node neoplasm may occur. It is rare for the thymus to be the seat of secondary deposits from a distant primary tumour.

Thymic Cysts

Small cysts are common due to degeneration of Hassall's corpuscles in the involuting thymus. Large cysts also occur and have a capsule of compressed thymic tissue. They are lined by epithelial tissue of either columnar, squamous or ciliated type. Some may be derived from remnants of the branchial endoderm or ectoderm of the cervical sinus. Most probably originate from degenerating Hassall's corpuscles and are acquired. Cystic degeneration may be seen in a thymoma.

References

Austen W. G., Cosimi A. B. (1984) Heart transplantation after 16 years. N. Engl. J. Med. 311, 1436–8.

Bergsagel D. E., Alison R. E., Bean H. A. et al. (1982) Results of treating Hodgkin's disease without a policy of laparotomy staging. Cancer Treat. Rep. 66, 717–31.

Cochrane J. P. (1980) Ruptured spleen. *Br. J. Hosp. Med.* **398**, 398–404.

Come S. E., Chabner B. A. (1979) Staging in non-Hodgkin's lymphoma: approach, results and relationship to histopathology. *Clin. Haematol.* **8**, 645–56.

Cooper M. J., Williamson R. C. N. (1984) Splenectomy: indications, hazards and alternatives. *Br. J. Surg.* **71**, 173–80.

Corazza G. R., Tarozzi C., Vaira D., Frisoni M., Gasbarrini G. (1984) Return of splenic function after splenectomy: how much tissue is needed? *Br. Med. J.* **289**, 861–4.

Editorial (1984) Lymphoma in organ transplant recipients. *Lancet* **1**, 601–3.

Francke E. L., Neu H. C. (1981) Postsplenectomy infection. In : Cooperman A. M. (ed.) *Surgical Clinics of North America: Liver, Spleen, and Pancreas*, Vol. 61, No. 1, pp. 135–55. Philadelphia, W. B. Saunders.

Gerber M. A., Sedgwick A. K., MacAlister T. J., Gustafson K. B., Ballow M., Tilton R. C. (1985) The aetiological agent of cat scratch disease. *Lancet* **1**, 1236–9.

Gill P. G., Souter R. G., Morris P. G. (1980) Results of surgical staging in Hodgkin's disease. *Br. J. Surg.* **67**, 478–81.

Glees J. P., Barr L. C., McElwain T. J., Peckham M. J., Gazet J. C. (1982) The changing role of staging laparotomy in Hodgkin's disease: a personal series of 310 patients. *Br. J. Surg.* **69**, 181–7.

Haybittle J. L., Hayhoe F. G. J., Easterling M. J. et al. (1985) Review of British national lymphoma investigation studies of Hodgkin's disease and development of prognostic index. *Lancet* **1**, 967–72.

King H., Shumacker H. B. (1952) Splenic studies I. Susceptibility to infection after splenectomy performed in infancy. *Ann. Surg.* **136**, 239–42.

Lukes R. J., Collins R. D. (1975) New approaches to the classification of the lymphomata. *Br. J. Cancer* **31** (Suppl. 2), 1–28.

Macpherson A. I. S. (1980) The spleen. Cysts and tumours. *Br. J. Hosp. Med.* **24**, 413–15.

Nagington J., Gray J. (1980) Cyclosporin A immunosuppression, Epstein–Barr antibody and lymphoma. *Lancet* **1**, 536–7.

Neiman R. S. (1978) Current problems in the histopathologic diagnosis and classification of Hodgkin's disease. *Pathol. Ann.* **13** (Pt. 2), 289–328.

Pearson H. A., Johnston D., Smith K. A., Touloukian R. J. (1978) The born-again spleen. Return of splenic function after splenectomy for trauma. *N. Engl. J. Med.* **298**, 1389–92.

Robinette C. D., Fraumeni J. F. (1977) Splenectomy and subsequent mortality in veterans of the 1939–45 war. *Lancet* **2**, 127–9.

Robinson C. L. (1983) The role of surgery of the thymus for myasthenia gravis. *Ann. R. Coll. Surg. Engl.* **65**, 145–51.

Rubin J. W., Ellison R. G., Moore H. V., Pai G. P. (1981) Factors affecting response to thymectomy for myasthenia gravis. *J. Thorac. Cardiovasc. Surg.* **82**, 720–8.

Shamji F., Pearson F. G., Todd T. R., Ginsberg R. J., Ilves R., Cooper J. D. (1984) Results of surgical treatment for thymoma. *J. Thorac. Cardiovasc. Surg.* **87**, 43–7.

Singer D. B. (1973) Postsplenectomy sepsis. *Perspect. Pediatr. Pathol.* **1**, 285–311.

Symmers W. S. C. (1968) Survey of the eventual diagnosis in 226 cases referred for a second histological opinion after an intitial biopsy diagnosis of reticulum cell sarcoma. *J. Clin. Pathol.* **21**, 654–5.

Velez-Garcia E., Fradera J., Grillo A. J., Velazquez J., Maldonado N. (1971) A study of lymph node and tumour imprints and aspirations. *Bol. Assoc. Med. P.R.* **63**, 188–203.

Chapter 16

The Endocrine Glands

THYROID

Normal Development, Structure and Function

The thyroid develops as a tubular endodermal structure arising from the posterior aspect of the tongue at 21 days of fetal life. It descends anterior to the hyoid bone and larynx, bifurcates and fuses with elements from the fourth branchial pouches. The downgrowth forms the thyroglossal duct, the proximal end of which forms the foramen caecum of the tongue. The distal end proliferates to form the thyroid. The duct itself usually atrophies although remnants can remain. Abnormalities of descent result in an ectopic thyroid. The ultimobranchial pouches (parts of the fourth branchial pouches) form the parafollicular calcitonin secreting C-cells which are part of the APUD system (see p. 108).

The thyroid consists of two lobes united by an isthmus. It is situated anterior to the larynx, cricoid cartilage and upper tracheal rings. The pyramidal lobe is present in 50% of cases; it extends towards the hyoid bone from the isthmus. Accessory thyroid glands are small detached portions of thyroid tissue sometimes found in the vicinity of the lobes or above the isthmus.

The vascularity of the thyroid may cause a problem with haemostasis during surgery. Each lateral lobe receives a superior thyroid artery (a branch of the external carotid) and an inferior thyroid artery (a branch of the thyrocervical trunk). The inferior artery has a close but variable relationship with the recurrent laryngeal nerve. The superior and middle thyroid veins enter the internal jugular vein and the inferior thyroid veins drain to the innominate vein. There is a rich supply of lymphatics which run in the interlobular connective tissue and frequently surround the arteries. They communicate in a network situated in the capsule of the gland and drain to nodes along the internal jugular and innominate veins. They are of great importance in the spread of thyroid carcinoma.

The gland consists of follicles (just visible to the naked eye) containing yellow viscous colloid. The follicles are separated by vascular connective tissue. Each follicle is lined with a single layer of cuboidal epithelium and the shape of the follicle depends on the activity of the gland. The lining cells are flattened in the inactive colloid-filled follicles and columnar when the gland is active in which case the follicles contain little colloid.

The function of the thyroid follicles is to secrete thyroxine (T4) and tri-iodothyronine (T3). The cells trap iodide by an active process, oxidize it and transport it into the follicle centre. The follicular cells also manufacture the glycoprotein, thyroglobulin, and secrete it into the follicles where it forms colloid, seen as deeply eosinophilic material on H and E sections. At the interface between the colloid and the follicular cells, iodination of the amino acid tyrosine takes place to form mono- and di-iodotyrosine (MIT and DIT). Coupling of MIT and DIT or of DIT and DIT form T3 and T4 respectively and these are stored in the colloid. In the secretion process, colloid is ingested by the thyroid cells where T3 and T4 are released by proteolysis and then secreted into the circulation. A major source of T3 is peripheral conversion of T4 to T3. T3 and T4 have the effect of increasing the metabolic rate of most tissues.

Thyroid secretion is under the control of thyrotrophin (also called thyroid stimulating hormone or TSH) which is produced in the pituitary. Thyrotrophin in turn is under the control of hypothalamic thyrotrophin-releasing hormone (TRH). Thyroid hormones suppress the release of both thyrotrophin and TRH, thus providing a feedback mechanism. The parafollicular C-cells produce calcitonin which is involved in calcium metabolism.

Biopsy of the Thyroid

Prior to surgery, thyroid tissue may be examined by fine needle aspiration cytology or by large needle biopsy. At surgery, tissue may be taken for immediate frozen section examination or for routine postoperative histological examination. In addition, the contents of a thyroid cyst can be examined by cytology.

Fine needle aspiration cytology is carried out in a similar way to that described for breast (see p. 292). The technique is useful for the diagnosis of a solitary thyroid nodule. If the nodule is a papillary carcinoma or part of a multinodular goitre or a medullary carcinoma, diagnosis is usually possible and further treatment can be planned if necessary. The technique is also useful for the diagnosis of Hashimoto's disease, thyroiditis and lymphoma. Distinction between a follicular adenoma and a follicular carcinoma depends in many cases on the presence or absence of capsular invasion which cannot be assessed by this technique.

Fine needle aspiration cytology gives a positive diagnosis in almost two-thirds of cases and this is useful in planning treatment. In the remainder there is a failure to establish a diagnosis and further biopsy is usually required.

Complications of fine needle aspiration cytology are exceedingly rare. Seeding of the tract by tumour does not appear to be a risk. Although false negative results are common, most studies have not had a false positive diagnosis of malignancy (e.g. Löwhagen et al. 1979).

Large needle biopsy (e.g. by a Tru-cut needle) provides a core of tissue which can be examined in the normal histological way. This has a slightly greater tendency to cause a haematoma but false negative results are less frequent than with fine needle aspiration cytology.

Frozen section examination of a solitary thyroid nodule, at the time of surgery, gives the diagnosis in most conditions. The distinction between a follicular adenoma and carcinoma is, however, still difficult. The minimal biopsy for a solitary thyroid nodule recommended by Wade (1983) is a lobectomy.

In the case of an extensive non-resectable thyroid malignancy, a biopsy can be taken from the isthmus. This has the dual purpose of releasing the trachea and providing tissue for diagnosis.

The examination of the fluid aspirated from a cyst or of fine needle aspirates is dependent on the availability of an experienced cytologist.

Presentation of Thyroid Disease

Thyroid disease most commonly presents as hyperfunction, hypofunction, a swelling of the gland or pain.

The symptoms of hyperthyroidism include weight loss in the presence of a good appetite, heat intolerance with excessive sweating, palpitations, muscular weakness, diarrhoea and an anxiety state. The signs of hyperthyroidism include a goitre (sometimes with a murmur heard over it), exophthalmos, lid lag, warm moist skin, tachycardia (sometimes with atrial fibrillation), muscle wasting, tremor and brisk tendon jerks. In some middle-aged or elderly patients, atrial fibrillation or cardiac failure are the predominant features.

The common causes are Graves' disease, toxic multinodular goitre and a solitary toxic adenoma, all of which are discussed later. Less common causes include thyroid carcinoma, inappropriate TSH secretion, subacute thyroiditis, ingestion of thyroid hormones and occasionally thyroid carcinoma. Very rare causes include struma ovarii (thyroid tissue in an ovarian teratoma), choriocarcinoma and hydatidiform mole. The last two can secrete TSH-like material.

Hypothyroidism is seldom treated by the surgeon. Common causes are primary idiopathic myxoedema and Hashimoto's thyroiditis. Less common causes are hypopituitarism, hypothalamic defects, developmental abnormalities (including dyshormonogenesis), severe iodine deficiency, ingestion of goitrogens (e.g. phenylbutazone and lithium) and peripheral resistance to thyroid hormones. Hypothyroidism may also result from therapy (e.g. surgical or radioactive iodine) for hyperthyroidism.

In children, thyroid deficiency causes cretinism and in the adult it causes myxoedema.

A swelling of the thyroid gland is termed a goitre. Although this can be a discrete mass (solitary thyroid nodule), most physicians mean a generalized enlargement when using the term goitre. The common causes of a solitary thyroid nodule are cysts, adenomas, dominant nodules in a multinodular goitre, and malignant tumours. Patients with a diffuse thyroid swelling may be hyperthyroid (e.g. Graves' disease and toxic multinodular goitre), hypothyroid (e.g. Hashimoto's disease and dyshormonogenesis), or euthyroid (e.g. diffuse non-toxic goitre, non-toxic multinodular goitre and malignant tumours). Midline swellings adjacent to the thyroid may be due to thyroglossal duct remnants.

Pain may be the presenting complaint in some forms of thyroiditis, especially infective thyroiditis and subacute thyroiditis. Pain may also be due to haemorrhage into an adenoma.

Developmental Abnormalities

Ectopia (*see Fig.* 16.1)
Occasionally the thyroid gland is not in its normal cervical position but lies beneath the epithelium of the tongue at the site of the foramen caecum. This is termed a lingual thyroid. It is usually small and is often the only thyroid tissue present. Radioactive iodine scanning aids diagnosis. An interesting feature of lingual thyroids is that they do not develop medullary carcinomas as they do not

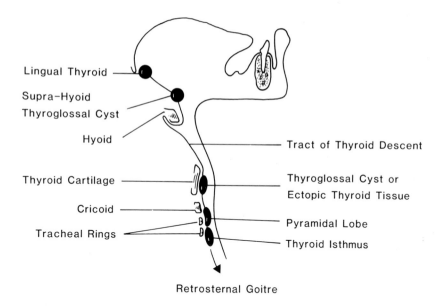

Lingual Thyroid

Supra-Hyoid
Thyroglossal Cyst

Hyoid

Thyroid Cartilage

Cricoid

Tracheal Rings

Tract of Thyroid Descent

Thyroglossal Cyst or
Ectopic Thyroid Tissue

Pyramidal Lobe

Thyroid Isthmus

Retrosternal Goitre

Fig. 16.1. Schematic diagram to show the descent of the thyroid and the abnormalities which are found at the different levels.

fuse with the ultimobranchial pouches and therefore do not contain parafollicular C-cells.

Partially descended glands which lie along the line from the foramen caecum to the normal site are rare.

The excision of a lingual thyroid requires great care because the gland is well vascularized by the lingual arteries. Malignancy appears to be more common than in normal thyroids. Some authors have suggested that lingual thyroids should be treated with thyroxine in an attempt to reduce their size.

Absence or hypoplasia

Although this is rare, it is important that it is recognized early in life as treatment with thyroxine leads to normal growth and development. In most Western countries screening of the newborn is now routine.

Dyshormonogenesis

These are biochemical disorders affecting the different enzyme pathways necessary for the production of T3 and T4. They are usually inherited in an autosomal recessive pattern. A goitre may develop under the influence of TSH stimulation. These enzyme defects are responsible for many cases of cretinism. Dyshormonogenesis may be associated with congenital nerve deafness and this combination is termed Pendred's syndrome.

Lateral aberrant thyroid

Although occasionally benign thyroid follicles may be found in cervical lymph nodes, it is now considered by most authorities that masses of thyroid tissue situated lateral to the main gland usually represent metastases from a papillary thyroid carcinoma.

Abnormalities of the thyroglossal tract (*see Fig.* 16.1)

The foramen caecum of the tongue and the pyramidal lobe of the thyroid gland are normal remnants of the thyroglossal duct. Between these structures is a very small epithelial tube usually broken in several places. Occasionally these fragments hypertrophy, secrete fluid and form cysts. The cysts can occur anywhere between the foramen caecum above and the manubrial notch below and they are the commonest midline neck cyst. Occasionally the thyroglossal duct persists and communicates with the skin forming a thyroglossal sinus. By pressure necrosis or surgical interference, a thyroglossal cyst can also form a fistula to the overlying skin. Thyroglossal cysts usually present in childhood (mean age of presentation 5 years), although an age range for presentation from birth to old age has been reported. Ninety per cent are midline and in the minority which deviate most are on the left. The majority occur at the level of the hyoid bone (75%); 15% occur at the thyroid cartilage level. Thyroglossal cysts are lined by columnar, ciliated or squamous epithelium and contain mucoid material secreted by the lining cells. Frequently, especially if a fistula is present, there are inflammatory changes in the wall.

At the time of surgery it is necessary to remove the entire sinus or cyst to avoid recurrence. In some cases this may necessitate removing a portion of the hyoid bone as the thyroglossal tract is often in close association with it.

Very rarely, carcinoma may arise within the thyroglossal duct. The tumour is nearly always a papillary thyroid carcinoma and may be suspected because of the firmness of a midline neck mass. The lesion may be difficult to distinguish from a metastatic deposit of primary thyroid carcinoma. However, the presence of nearby normal thyroid follicles indicates that the tumour has arisen in ectopic thyroid tissue.

Thyroiditis

Infective thyroiditis

This term, by tradition, includes those forms of thyroiditis caused by an infective agent other than a virus. One type of thyroiditis is presumed to be caused by a virus and this is discussed below under 'subacute thyroiditis'. Most cases of infective thyroiditis are due to bacteria although occasionally fungi and parasites are the pathogens. Presentation is usually as an acute septic thyroiditis and the resulting abscess may point and rupture onto the skin or into the trachea or oesophagus. On microscopic examination, a typical abscess cavity is seen. Tuberculosis rarely involves the thyroid. It may be a primary or secondary infection and typical caseating granulomas are seen. In the later stages of tuberculosis, profound fibrosis may cause confusion with Riedel's thyroiditis.

Subacute thyroiditis (de Quervain's thyroiditis)

This term is restricted to a distinctive clinical condition, probably of viral aetiology, in which there are generalized symptoms, thyroid inflammation and characteristic thyroid histology. Adult females are most commonly affected. The patient has a rapid onset of a febrile type illness, usually with thyroid pain and tenderness, although painless varieties have been described. The gland is enlarged and transient thyrotoxicosis may occur. The disease is usually a self-limiting condition lasting a few weeks or months. Many patients have antibodies to Coxsackie virus and in view of this a viral aetiology is considered likely. However, no viral particles have been found by electron microscopy.

Although a needle biopsy may be carried out to exclude tumour, most cases do not come to surgery. In those that do, however, the gland is loosely adherent to surrounding structures and on section white foci of involved tissue are seen in areas of normal thyroid parenchyma. Microscopically, initially there is destruction of the thyroid parenchyma followed by an infiltration of neutrophils. Macrophages enter the damaged follicles and later multinucleate giant cells appear. The follicles then take on the appearance of granulomas each of which surrounds a pool of colloid. Fibrosis is found in the late stages.

Hashimoto's disease

Hashimoto's disease is a common cause of hypothyroidism and commonly affects middle-aged women who present with clinical hypothyroidism in the presence of a smooth firm goitre and circulating thyroid antibodies.

Autoimmunity is strongly implicated in the aetiology and pathogenesis of Hashimoto's disease. Antibodies to thyroid microsomal antigen, thyroglobulin, and TSH receptors are found in a majority of patients. TSH receptor antibodies mimic the action of TSH on the thyroid and can be divided into thyroid stimulating immunoglobulins (which increase hormone production) and thyroid growth immunoglobulins (which increase thyroid growth). In Hashimoto's disease there are elevated levels of the thyroid growth immunoglobulin which cause the goitre. However, thyroid stimulating immunoglobulin is either not produced or else an antibody which blocks it is formed; thus there is no hyperfunction. Graves' disease (see p. 461) is different in that both types of TSH receptor antibody are often present. There may be an underlying defect in antigen specific suppressor T-cell function in both Hashimoto's disease and in Graves' disease and this may permit the immunological attack on the thyroid.

It is unclear how the destruction of thyroid parenchyma takes place. Experimental evidence suggests that killer lymphocytes are activated by immune complexes (the so-called 'antibody dependent cellular cytotoxicity').

Grossly, the gland is firm and symmetrically enlarged with a bosselated surface. The cut surface frequently shows white or yellow lobules surrounded by fibrous tissue. There is a homogeneous appearance without necrosis, cysts or haemorrhage (see Fig. 16.2).

The most characteristic histological feature is a heavy infiltrate of lymphocytes and plasma cells. This occurs initially in the interstitium and is accompanied by fibrosis. Later, large areas of parenchyma are replaced by lymphoid tissue which often contains germinal centres. Any thyroid follicles which remain are small and frequently show Hürthle cell change, i.e. the lining epithelial cells become large

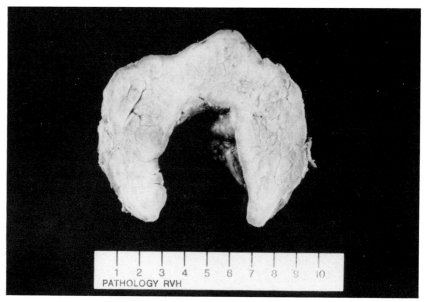

Fig. 16.2. Thyroid in Hashimoto's disease.

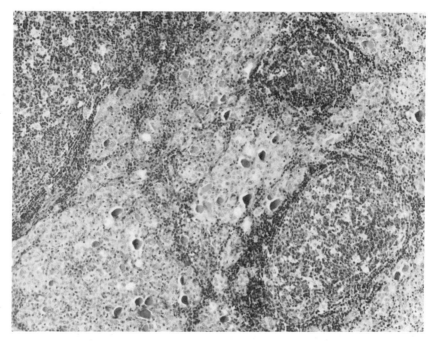

Fig. 16.3. Hashimoto's disease. Part of the thyroid has been replaced by a lymphocytic infiltrate with lymphoid follicles. The remaining thyroid shows Hürthle cell change. (H and E × 30)

with abundant eosinophilic cytoplasm. Some follicles become disrupted with the result that nests of epithelial and Hürthle cells are seen in the lymphoid background (*see Fig.* 16.3).

Children may develop a form of Hashimoto's disease, sometimes termed lymphocytic thyroiditis of childhood. In these cases, Hürthle cells and lymphoid follicles are rarely seen histologically.

The fibrous variant of Hashimoto's disease is well recognized and is characterized by profound fibrosis to the extent that the condition may be confused with Riedel's thyroiditis. However, the former does not show the fibrosis of surrounding tissues which is seen in Riedel's thyroiditis.

There is controversy as to whether Hashimoto's disease predisposes to an increased incidence of thyroid malignancy. Most authorities consider that there is insufficient evidence to prove an increased incidence of carcinoma in Hashimoto's disease although there is strong evidence for an increased incidence of lymphoma. One study estimated that the relative risk for developing thyroid lymphoma in Hashimoto's disease is 67 (Holm *et al.* 1985).

Riedel's thyroiditis

In this condition part of the thyroid is replaced by fibrous tissue which characteristically extends outside the thyroid capsule to involve other neck structures such as the trachea and carotid sheath. The patient presents with a stony hard neck lump and in some cases obstructive symptoms such as stridor occur.

The aetiology is unknown and it appears to be unrelated to other forms of thyroiditis. Thyroid antibodies are rarely present. Some patients develop mediastinal or retroperitoneal fibrosis or sclerosing cholangitis, thus suggesting a generalized abnormality.

Grossly, the involved tissue is grey or white and is gritty on cutting. There is almost complete obliteration of the involved thyroid parenchyma and any remaining follicles are shrunken. Usually only one lobe or even part of a lobe is affected with a sharp demarcation between abnormal and diseased tissue.

Non-toxic Goitre

Non-toxic goitre is a non-inflammatory non-neoplastic diffuse or nodular enlargement of the thyroid. The condition may be endemic in iodine deficient areas or it may be sporadic. In most sporadic cases the cause is unknown. The majority of patients of both varieties are euthyroid and present with a goitre which may give local symptoms only.

Aetiology and pathogenesis

ENDEMIC GOITRE: Lack of iodine is the major cause of goitre in the world. A daily intake of 100–300 µg of iodine is desirable for adults and levels may be inadequate in mountainous regions such as the Andes and Himalayas. Endemic goitre, in some areas, may be due to intake of goitrogens which occur, for example, in cabbage and similar vegetables. Calcium chloride in the water supply may also induce goitre.

In all these cases there is a reduced ability of the thyroid gland to produce T3 and T4. Therefore it is stimulated by TSH in an attempt to maintain the patient in an euthyroid state. This causes the initial enlargement which is characterized histologically by hyperplastic follicles. If iodine subsequently becomes more plentiful, or if demand for T3 and T4 reduces, part of the gland then undergoes involution and the follicles in this area become enlarged and filled with colloid. This is the so-called 'diffuse non-toxic' or 'colloid' goitre. At a later stage, some of the larger follicles may rupture with resultant haemorrhage, cyst formation and fibrosis. The fibrous tissue tends to enclose islands of follicles giving a nodular appearance and the condition then becomes a 'multinodular non-toxic goitre'. Fluctuating levels of TSH stimulation therefore probably account for the varied morphology (*see Fig.* 16.4).

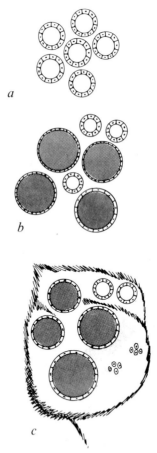

Fig. 16.4. Schematic diagram to show the development of a multinodular goitre. *a.* Initially TSH stimulation causes hyperplasia of the glands and the follicles have a high epithelial lining and scant colloid. *b.* Some of the follicles become inactive; they enlarge, have a flattened epithelial lining and are filled with colloid (colloid goitre). *c.* Some of the enlarged follicles rupture, releasing free colloid and epithelial cells; this stimulates fibrosis and, consequently, nodularity (multinodular goitre).

SPORADIC GOITRE: Although the cause of sporadic goitre is usually unknown, in some cases a relative iodine deficiency is at least a contributory factor. Known cases of enzyme defects are classified as dyshormonogenic goitre. It is possible that many cases of sporadic goitre are due to defects in iodine metabolism which are not detectable either because the patient is heterozygous for a particular enzyme defect or because the defect is very minor. Autoimmunity has been implicated in some cases. As with endemic goitre, fluctuating levels of stimulation by TSH are probably responsible for the morphology.

Morphology

The morphology of endemic and sporadic goitre is the same. In the early stages, under TSH stimulation, the gland is diffusely and smoothly enlarged. Later, when some of the follicles undergo involution, the gland has a glistening appearance on cut section due to colloid accumulation. Later still when the haemorrhage and degeneration with fibrosis occurs, irregular scarring develops giving a nodular appearance. This encapsulation of islands of thyroid tissue is similar to that found in adenomas and therefore the other term for multinodular goitre is 'adenomatous goitre'. Follicles within a nodule may break down resulting in haemorrhage and cyst formation. Calcification is also a common feature. One nodule may become dominant and present clinically as a solitary thyroid nodule.

Histologically, in the initial hyperplastic phase the follicles appear very active due to TSH stimulation. They are small with a tall epithelial lining and contain little colloid. The condition is rarely seen histologically at this early stage. When involution occurs, groups of follicles become much enlarged and distended with

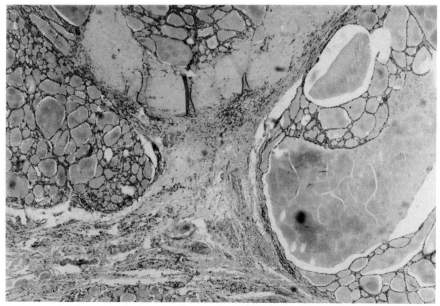

Fig. 16.5. Multinodular goitre. Nodules of thyroid tissue separated by fibrous tissue. (H and E × 30)

colloid. The epithelium then becomes flat and the appearances are those of inactivity. Some groups of follicles, however, retain their hyperplastic appearance and therefore the overall appearance of this stage (diffuse non-toxic or colloid goitre) is one of islands of hyperplastic follicles among large involuted follicles. The hyperplastic areas are responsible for maintaining hormone output.

When the stage of multinodular goitre is reached the pattern becomes variable with nodules of colloid filled follicles compressing the surrounding tissue and becoming encapsulated by fibrous tissue (see Fig. 16.5). Areas of haemorrhage are seen. The follicular walls within these nodules may break down to form a 'colloid cyst' and remnants of the follicular walls form projections into the cyst. Nodules composed of hyperplastic follicles may occur and if these are encapsulated they may be very difficult to distinguish from a follicular adenoma. In those cases which present as a solitary thyroid nodule, any of the histological patterns just described may be seen within it.

Complications

1. ONSET OF THYROTOXICOSIS (TOXIC NODULAR GOITRE): The onset of thyrotoxicosis may occur in two ways. Firstly, the thyrotoxicosis may have the clinical features of Graves' disease including (rarely) ophthalmopathy. In these cases the hyperfunctioning tissue is found in the internodular areas and the condition appears to be Graves' disease superimposed on a simple multinodular goitre. Secondly, one or more nodules may become hyperfunctional for reasons which are unclear. Histologically, the tissue within these toxic nodules is hyperplastic in appearance while the internodular tissue is inactive. This complication occurs after 15–25 years and is termed 'Plummer's disease' or 'multiple toxic adenomas'.

The introduction of iodine into an area of endemic multinodular goitre may precipitate an epidemic of thyrotoxicosis (Jod–Basedow effect).

2. PRESSURE SYMPTOMS: A large goitre may cause stridor or dysphagia. This is especially the case in retrosternal goitres when enlargement occurs downward into the mediastinum. In addition to stridor and dysphagia, superior vena cava obstruction may result. Fortunately the retrosternal goitre keeps its normal blood supply and therefore it can usually be delivered in the neck at the time of surgery, thus avoiding sternotomy.

3. MALIGNANT CHANGE: Careful examination of operative specimens of nodular goitre will reveal a carcinoma in up to 17% of cases (Cole et al. 1949) and this suggests a strong association between the two. However, these patients had had surgery and therefore represented a highly selected, unrepresentative group. There is, in addition, discrepancy between the actual annual death rate from thyroid cancer in endemic goitre areas and the expected death rate if the figure suggested above is correct. Furthermore, the introduction of iodine prophylaxis into endemic areas has not led to a reduction of thyroid cancer comparable to the reduction in the number of goitres. In view of this, Sokal (1960) has calculated that only 1% of patients with nodular goitre develop thyroid cancer (usually the follicular type) and most authorities currently do not recommend excision of a goitre for the purpose of cancer prophylaxis.

Graves' Disease

The cardinal features of Graves' disease are: (1) diffuse enlargement of the thyroid gland; (2) hyperthyroidism; (3) ophthalmopathy. Females are affected up to eight times more frequently than males. It is most common in young adults.

Aetiology and pathogenesis

There is strong evidence that Graves' disease is autoimmune in origin. It has long been known that these patients have circulating IgG antibodies (e.g. long acting thyroid stimulator and long acting thyroid stimulator protector) which stimulate the activity of the thyroid gland. These autoantibodies act on TSH receptors on the thyroid epithelial cell membranes and mimic the actions of TSH. The 'TSH receptor antibodies' are of two functional types; thyroid stimulating immunoglobulins (which increase thyroid hormone production), and thyroid-growth immunoglobulins (which increase thyroid growth). In Graves' disease, both types are often present, thus producing both a goitre and hyperfunction of the gland.

Okita *et al.* (1981) have proposed that there is a (probably genetic) defect in antigen-specific T-lymphocyte function in both Hashimoto's disease and Graves' disease. This defect allows the escape of a forbidden clone of thyroid directed T-helper lymphocytes, which interact with their complementary antigen on thyroid cell membranes and set up a local cell mediated immune response. The helper T-cells co-operate with B-lymphocytes which then produce the TSH receptor antibodies.

The ophthalmopathy of Graves' disease may be due to a specific IgG which binds with a retro-orbital antigen (Kendall-Taylor *et al.* 1984).

Morphology

The thyroid is diffusely and symmetrically enlarged. However, this enlargement is not as great as occurs in many other types of goitre. On cut section, the thyroid is soft and has a red appearance similar to muscle.

Histologically, the gland consists of hyperplastic follicles which are small and lined by a high columnar epithelium. Colloid is very scarce and what remains is scalloped at the edges and stains poorly (*see Fig.* 16.6). Within the follicles papillary projections form and in some cases this appearance may be confused with a papillary carcinoma. An important feature is the presence of a lymphocytic infiltrate, sometimes with lymphoid follicles, in the stroma. This classical description is modified by preoperative treatment and is therefore only rarely seen histologically. Iodine, in particular, causes involution of some of the follicles and devascularization.

Prognosis

The mortality from thyroidectomy in experienced hands approaches zero. Morbidity from tetany (0·3%) and recurrent laryngeal nerve damage (0·6%) is also low. The incidence of permanent hypothyroidism (which reaches 20%) is dependent on remnant size, amount of lymphocytic infiltrate in the gland and the preoperative concentration of antithyroglobulin and antimicrosomal antibodies. Hypothyroidism can become apparent up to twenty years after surgery.

Recurrent hyperthyroidism occurs in about 5% of patients after surgery.

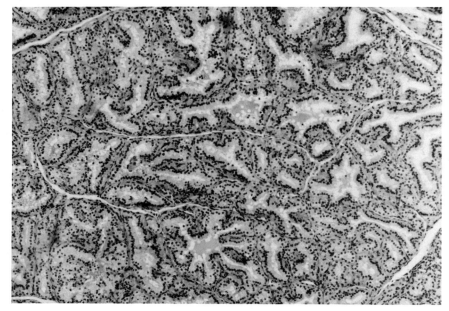

Fig. 16.6. Thyrotoxicosis. The follicles show high epithelial cells and papillary infoldings. They are depleted of colloid. (H and E × 30)

Thyroid Adenomas

A classification of thyroid neoplasms (based on the WHO Classification) is given in *Table* 16.1.

Table 16.1. Classification of thyroid tumours

EPITHELIAL
   Benign:
      Follicular adenoma
      Atypical adenoma

   Malignant:
      Papillary carcinoma
      Follicular carcinoma
        Invasive
        Encapsulated angio-invasive
      Anaplastic carcinoma
        Spindle cell
        Giant cell
        Mixed
      Medullary carcinoma
      Squamous carcinoma
      Metastatic

NON-EPITHELIAL
      Lymphomas
      Sarcomas

Thyroid adenomas are true benign neoplasms of the thyroid as opposed to nodules within a multinodular goitre which are non-neoplastic. They occur most commonly between the ages of 20 and 60 years and are up to seven times more common in females than males.

Morphology

They present clinically as a solitary thyroid nodule. When the thyroid lobe is removed and transected the adenoma stands out as a solitary encapsulated nodule, perhaps 3–4 cm in diameter, composed of firm tissue which may be pale and fleshy or reddish brown in appearance (*see Fig.* 16.7). Hürthle cell adenomas (*see* below) tend to be tan-coloured. The remaining thyroid tissue is typically normal. Within the adenoma, haemorrhage, cystic change and calcification are common.

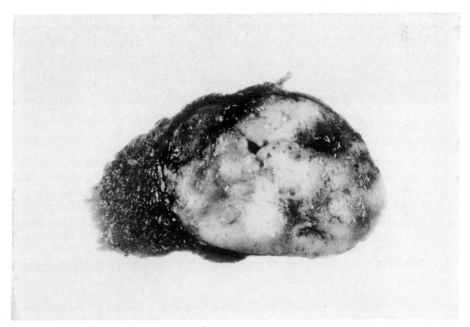

Fig. 16.7. Follicular adenoma of thyroid.

FOLLICULAR ADENOMA: Microscopic examination confirms that the lesion is completely encapsulated. The adenoma is made up of thyroid follicles but the architecture is distinctly different from the area of normal thyroid outside the capsule (*see Fig.* 16.8). There is much variation in follicle size both within individual adenomas and between different adenomas. Since the tumour expands centrifugally, there is characteristically an area of compressed follicles surrounding the capsule. Areas of haemorrhage and cystic degeneration are frequently encountered. Several variants are recognized although they have no prognostic significance. An embryonal or trabecular adenoma has cords of cells resembling those seen before follicles appear in embryological life. In fetal adenomas, the pattern consists of very small follicles which contain very little colloid.

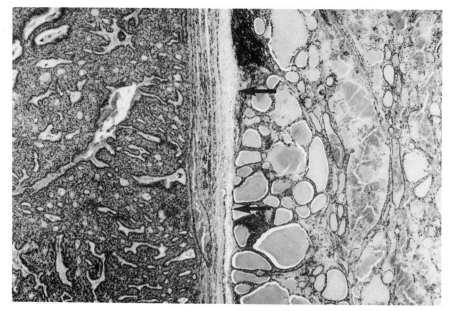

Fig. 16.8. Follicular adenoma (to the left of picture). Note the well defined capsule (arrowed) with the different architecture on either side. (H and E × 30)

Rarely the Hürthle cell variant is seen. It is composed of large cells with abundant eosinophilic granular cytoplasm. Hürthle cells characteristically have pleomorphic nuclei and therefore malignancy may be suspected in these cases.

A follicular adenoma may easily be confused histologically with a nodule arising in a multinodular goitre. The latter, however, may not be completely encapsulated, is more subject to haemorrhage and, if the entire lobe has been removed at operation, other smaller nodules will be seen.

The distinction between a follicular adenoma and a follicular carcinoma is much more important and is dealt with later.

PAPILLARY ADENOMAS: Since the behaviour of papillary lesions of the thyroid is unpredictable most pathologists consider all papillary lesions to be varying grades of carcinoma.

ATYPICAL ADENOMAS: This term is applied to those adenomas which have increased cellularity and cellular atypia. Although easily confused with a malignant lesion they are, however, encapsulated and no invasion of the capsule or vascular channels is seen. It has been shown that they run a benign course (Hazard and Kenyon 1954).

Complications

AUTONOMOUSLY FUNCTIONING ADENOMA: Occasionally a thyroid adenoma will produce thyroid hormones independent of TSH control. If the amount produced is too great the patient becomes thyrotoxic and the lesion is termed a 'toxic adenoma'.

More frequently, however, the nodule produces hormones approximately equal to requirement and it is then termed a non-toxic 'autonomous adenoma'. Thyroid scanning after TSH suppression shows the presence of a nodule which is persistently hot compared with the surrounding areas. In many cases an apparent toxic adenoma turns out to be one nodule in a toxic nodular goitre.

A non-toxic autonomous adenoma may safely be followed up with tests aimed at detecting impending toxicity, such as a rising T3 level. Toxic adenomas require treatment. Since an autonomous toxic nodule in the thyroid is almost invariably benign, limited surgery (lobectomy or even nodulectomy) or ablation with radioactive iodine is considered safe (Hamburger 1983).

SPONTANEOUS HAEMORRHAGE: Haemorrhagic infarction is relatively common in thyroid adenomas and is usually occult. Occasionally, however, haemorrhage may cause a sudden painful increase in size possibly with transient thyrotoxicosis as thyroid hormones are released from the gland. Blood is found on needle aspiration and this procedure may also be therapeutic.

THYROID CYST: Haemorrhagic infarction of an adenoma with resultant cyst formation accounts for many thyroid cysts (others may arise in nodular goitres). The cyst presents as a solitary thyroid nodule and the cystic nature is revealed by ultrasound. Subsequent aspiration may be curative provided cytological examination of the fluid shows no evidence of atypical cells.

Thyroid Cancer

The aetiology of thyroid cancer will be discussed in general, followed by an account of each individual type.

In some areas where goitre is non-endemic, for example the north-west of Norway, papillary thyroid cancer is exceedingly common, probably on a genetic basis. Some cases of medullary carcinoma are part of an inherited autosomal dominant syndrome (*see* later). Prolonged stimulation of the thyroid by TSH is thought to be responsible for the slightly increased incidence of thyroid cancer, especially of the follicular variety, in areas of endemic goitre. The growth of many follicular and papillary cancers is highly dependent on TSH production adding further evidence for the role of TSH in the aetiology of thyroid tumours. Irradiation received in childhood is associated with an increased risk of developing (usually) papillary thyroid cancer. This has been noted in atomic bomb survivors in Hiroshima and in children who have had thymic irradiation. Irradiation of the neck in young adults, for example for Hodgkin's disease, is also associated with a slightly increased risk.

Papillary thyroid cancer

This is the commonest form of thyroid cancer and accounts for at least 50% of all thyroid malignancy. This figure is even higher in children and in post-irradiation cases. The peak incidence is between 20 and 40 years and it is three times more common in women than in men.

Morphology

Typically, papillary tumours grow in an unencapsulated infiltrative fashion and tend not to have the well defined margins which are found in adenomas and follicular carcinomas. There is often marked fibrosis and small lesions may appear as a tiny scar (occult sclerosing carcinoma). On cutting there is a gritty sensation particularly if psammoma bodies are present. Cystic change is commonly seen and macroscopic papillary structures may be seen within the cyst. Actual necrosis is, however, rare compared with follicular and anaplastic tumours. Surrounding lymph nodes are commonly involved. When the main tumour is confined within the thyroid capsule it is termed intrathyroid, even if lymph node metastases are present. When the main tumour has invaded through the capsule it is termed extrathyroid.

The microscopic architecture of papillary cancer is very variable. Although papillary fronds with fibrovascular cores are seen, many tumours are composed partly or even mostly of follicular structures. It is important to note, however, that if papillary structures are present, even when the dominant pattern is follicular, the tumour behaves as papillary carcinoma and not as a follicular carcinoma. Solid and trabecular areas are also commonly seen. The individual cells are large and the chromatin is dispersed around the periphery of the nucleus making the centre pale staining. This is the characteristic clear or 'Orphan Annie eye' nucleus (*see Fig.* 16.9). This helpful diagnostic feature is unfortunately not seen in all cases and is also occasionally seen in benign conditions. The nuclei tend to be irregularly placed in the cells giving a disorganized appearance often with nuclear crowding and overlap. These nuclear features are seen both in papillary and follicular areas.

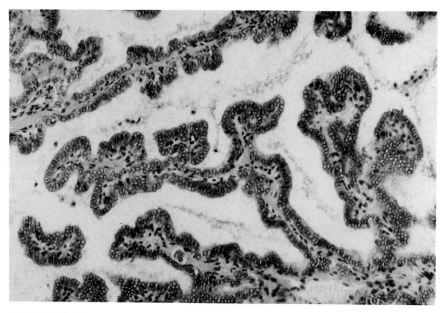

Fig. 16.9. Papillary carcinoma. Note the typical nuclei (*see* text). (H and E × 150)

Psammoma bodies (laminated calcific spherules) are present in 40–50% of cases and may be in the surrounding thyroid tissue as well as in the tumour. Microscopic examination of the rest of the thyroid may show other primary tumours. Papillary tumours are multifocal in 20–80% of cases but multifocal primaries are difficult to distinguish from multiple intraglandular metastases which are also common.

Spread and prognosis

Papillary tumours classically spread via lymphatics both within the gland and outside the gland to involve cervical lymph nodes. Distant metastases are present in less than 1% of patients at the time of diagnosis (Mazzaferri and Oertel 1983). Lung metastases may occur as discrete nodules or as lymphatic permeation which gives a snow-storm appearance on chest X-ray.

The prognosis is relatively good. In one series of 576 patients followed up over 30 years, total mortality from cancer was only 1·2% (Mazzaferri and Young 1981). In general, the tumour tends to be more aggressive in patients over 40 years old.

The size of the primary tumour at the time of diagnosis is an important determinant of prognosis. Occult (not detectable clinically) and minimal (1 cm or less as detected on scanning) tumours have an especially good prognosis even in the presence of lymph node metastases. Intrathyroid tumours have a better prognosis than the extrathyroid tumours. Recurrence rates are doubled when lymph node metastases are found at the time of diagnosis. Distant metastases, especially if they do not take up radioactive iodine, substantially worsen the prognosis.

Follicular carcinoma

Follicular carcinoma accounts for 15–25% of thyroid cancers (slightly more in endemic goitre regions). The peak incidence occurs in an older age group (35–45 years) than papillary carcinomas. It is three times more common in females than in males.

Morphology

Most tumours are solitary, encapsulated and well defined in contrast to the infiltrating character of papillary tumours. Occasionally follicular tumours can appear as aggressive infiltrating growths with nodules of tumour outside the gland which can be easily confused with lymph nodes. Invasion of the capsule and plugs of tumour in vascular channels may be seen on gross inspection. Necrosis is commonly seen but cystic change is not.

Histologically, typical follicular carcinomas are composed of follicles of varying sizes, although there may be solid and trabecular areas present. Unlike papillary tumours the cell nuclei are uniform in shape, small and darkly staining. They are also more regularly arranged and do not appear to be crowded. In some cases the tumour is made up entirely of Hürthle cells—the so-called 'Hürthle cell carcinoma'.

The most important aspect of the histological diagnosis is to distinguish between a well differentiated encapsulated follicular carcinoma and a follicular adenoma. The presence of mitotic figures in the carcinoma may help but it is generally accepted that there are two features which indicate malignancy: (1) capsular invasion, (2) vascular invasion. When capsular invasion occurs the inner rim of the capsule appears irregularly eroded. Isolated follicles may be seen within the capsule but they are not proof of invasion as they may merely represent entrapped benign follicles. When vascular invasion occurs, the malignant follicles form a tongue of tissue pushing into the vessel, separated from the lumen only by endothelial cells. Free follicles within a vessel lumen may be artefacts.

Spread and prognosis

Follicular carcinoma metastases are blood-borne to the lungs, skeleton, brain, etc.; only about 5% metastasize to regional lymph nodes.

In general, the prognosis for follicular carcinoma is worse than for papillary carcinoma and 10 year survival rates range from 20–50%. However, if follicular carcinomas are divided into those with minimal capsular invasion (encapsulated angioinvasive) and those with obvious or extreme invasion (invasive), the latter have a distinctively worse prognosis. In the minimally invasive group only 3% die as a result of their disease, while 50% of the invasive group are dead within six years. Prognosis is better in younger patients and obviously worse in those with distant metastases, especially if these do not take up radioactive iodine. Hürthle cell carcinomas are said to have a worse prognosis than the ordinary follicular carcinomas.

Anaplastic carcinoma

These are thought to arise within well differentiated thyroid carcinomas. They comprise 10–20% of all thyroid malignancy and are commonest in elderly patients with a peak incidence in patients aged 60–70 years. The lesion is more common in

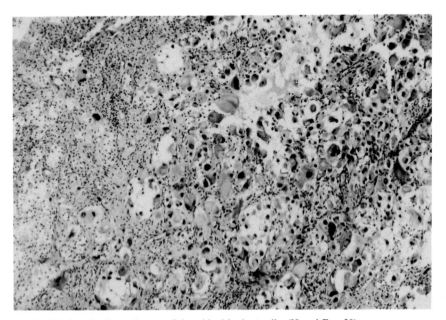

Fig. 16.10. Anaplastic carcinoma of thyroid with giant cells. (H and E × 30)

women than in men and in endemic goitre areas compared with non-endemic areas. Thomas and Buckwalter (1973) found that 80% of cases had a history of a long-standing goitre. The tumour is rapidly growing and causes hoarseness, stridor and dysphagia at an early stage.

Grossly the tumour is obviously malignant. It is firm or hard and infiltrates the surrounding structures. The cut surface often shows necrosis and haemorrhage.

Histologically, the tumour frequently consists of masses of spindle and giant cells. Some cases are predominantly spindle cells, some predominantly giant cells, whereas others are mixed (see Fig. 16.10). The cells show frequent mitoses and bizarre nuclear forms, and distinction from sarcoma may be difficult. Foci of papillary or follicular patterns may be seen. Other histological features include metaplasia to bone or cartilage.

Prognosis is exceedingly poor with very few cases surviving more than one year. It is rarely possible to carry out a total thyroidectomy because of local invasion. Usually only a biopsy and radiotherapy is possible and the benefit of the latter is questionable.

Squamous carcinoma

Squamous carcinoma is seen alone or in association with other thyroid tumours. It may arise in a squamous lined thyroglossal duct epithelium or in areas of squamous metaplasia. It usually occurs in middle-aged or elderly patients who have a history of goitre or chronic thyroiditis. They are rare and account for only 1% of thyroid tumours. The lesion is radio-resistant and highly malignant.

Medullary carcinoma

This is a tumour of the parafollicular or C-cells of the thyroid. These cells, which have a different embryological origin from the rest of the thyroid, normally secrete calcitonin. They are difficult to detect in H and E sections but contain cytoplasmic neurosecretory granules which can be demonstrated by silver stains and by electron microscopy.

Medullary carcinoma arises either sporadically or familially and accounts for about 7% of thyroid tumours. In the latter, medullary carcinoma is part of the multiple endocrine adenomatosis type 2 syndrome (MEA 2) which is discussed on p. 475. There is some evidence to suggest that medullary carcinomas rising in multiple endocrine adenomatosis syndromes are preceded by hyperplasia of the thyroid C-cells.

The commonest clinical presentation is with a painless lump or with local pressure symptoms such as dysphagia and hoarseness. Some are found as silent lesions when examining relatives of patients with familial medullary carcinomas. Some patients complain of diarrhoea. Many of the patients have elevated basal serum calcitonin which can be detected by radioimmunoassay. Others have elevated levels only in response to stimulation with pentagastrin or calcium. These tests are useful in screening relatives of patients with MEA 2. The tumour, in some cases, secretes other peptides such as ACTH or serotonin, which can cause Cushing's syndrome or carcinoid syndrome respectively.

Morphology

No macroscopic feature is diagnostic of medullary carcinoma. The tumour is firm and grey on cut section and is usually sharply demarcated from the surrounding thyroid tissue. The tumour is bilateral in about one-fifth of sporadic cases and in up to 80% of familial cases.

The most common microscopic pattern of medullary carcinoma of the thyroid described by Hazard *et al.* (1959) is one of solid sheets and islands of fairly regular polygonal cells interspaced with a stroma containing amyloid. Some nuclear variation is seen and binucleate cells are common. In some areas a nesting pattern is seen, similar to that seen in carcinoid tumours, and in others the cells are spindle in type. Occasionally tubules filled with amyloid may give a pseudo-follicular pattern. Several patterns may be seen in one tumour. A congo red stain is useful for the demonstration of amyloid which is seen in at least 95% of cases (*see Fig. 16.11*).

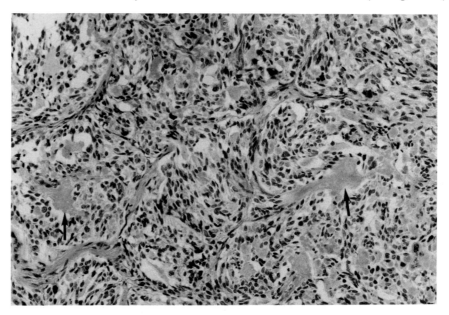

Fig. 16.11. Medullary carcinoma. The stroma (arrowed) stained strongly positive for amyloid. (H and E × 75)

Spread and prognosis

The tumour is more aggressive than papillary carcinoma and spreads directly via lymphatics and via the blood stream to give distant metastases.

In a study of 139 patients seen at the Mayo Clinic with medullary carcinoma of the thyroid, the overall five year survival was 67%. The figure was 86% for those without and 40% for those with lymph node metastases (Chong *et al.* 1975).

Malignant lymphomas of the thyroid

These may arise as primary tumours of the thyroid or as secondary involvement of the thyroid by a generalized lymphoma.

Primary thyroid lymphomas most commonly occur in middle-aged and elderly females. Many arise in a pre-existing Hashimoto's disease.

Preoperative diagnosis may be made by fine needle aspiration cytology or by surgical biopsy. It is usual to remove the thyroid isthmus for biopsy as this also frees the trachea.

Generally, the gland is enlarged and firm. Histologically, most lymphomas are of follicle centre cell type (see p. 432). It may be difficult to distinguish Hashimoto's disease from lymphoma. The latter tends to show invasion of blood vessels, the thyroid capsule and individual thyroid acini; this last feature is highly characteristic. It is now realized that many small cell tumours of the thyroid, formerly diagnosed as carcinomas, are in fact lymphomas.

After tissue diagnosis, treatment is by radiotherapy. One study reported a five year survival of 54% (Burke et al. 1977).

PARATHYROIDS

Normal Structure and Function

The parathyroid glands are yellow-brown ovoid bodies which vary in size. The dimensions average 6 mm × 4 mm × 2 mm and each weighs about 50 mg. The number can vary but there are usually two superior and two inferior glands.

They develop from the endoderm of the pharyngeal pouches—the inferior glands from the third pouch (parathyroids III) and the superior glands from the fourth pouch (parathyroids IV). The other part of the third pouch forms the thymus which migrates into the thorax. The inferior parathyroids may be found at any point along the course of migration. The usual site is at the lower pole of the thyroid, although they can be found as far up as the bifurcation of the common carotid artery and as low down as the mediastinum. The superior glands have a more constant position at the middle of the posterior border of each thyroid lobe.

The glands have a rich blood supply from the inferior thyroid arteries or the anastomoses between the superior and inferior thyroid vessels.

Histologically, a thin capsule is seen around the gland. The parathyroid hormone secreting cells are the chief cells which have pale staining cytoplasm. Oxyphil cells have a granular eosinophilic cytoplasm and their function is unknown. 'Transitional' cells are those with features of both types.

Human parathyroid hormone (PTH) is a linear polypeptide of 84 amino acids. It is synthesized as part of a larger molecule of 115 amino acids (prepro-PTH). The endoplasmic reticulum of the chief cells removes 25 amino acids to form pro-PTH and then the Golgi apparatus removes a further 6 amino acids to form PTH. The half-life of PTH in the circulation is less than 20 minutes. It acts directly on bone to increase reabsorption of calcium. It also increases phosphate excretion in the urine by decreasing phosphate reabsorption in the proximal tubules. The formation of 1,25-dihydroxycholecalciferol, the active metabolite of vitamin D, is also increased. The action of PTH on bone and kidney is via cyclic AMP.

Secretion of PTH is controlled by the negative feedback effect of ionized calcium on the parathyroid glands.

Primary Hyperparathyroidism (*see* also p. 584)

This syndrome results from excessive parathormone production in the absence of any known stimulus to the parathyroid glands.

Clinically, symptomatic patients present with the effects or complications of hypercalcaemia (especially renal disease, 60%; bone disease, 24%) or with associated conditions (peptic ulcer, 8%; pancreatitis, 2%). In many patients the symptoms are vague. Biochemical studies show that in primary hyperparathyroidism the serum calcium and PTH are raised and the serum phosphate is lowered.

The realization that hyperparathyroidism is frequently asymptomatic has led to a number of screening studies of normal populations for hypercalcaemia. Boonstra and Jackson (1971) found 50 cases of hypercalcaemia per 50 000 apparently healthy individuals. Other studies have given similar data. These studies raise the problem of the treatment of mild cases; no controlled trial has as yet found operation to be beneficial in this situation.

The causes of hyperparathyroidism in 914 cases seen in the Massachusetts General Hospital between 1930 and 1979 is given in *Table* 16.2. As in most series, a single adenoma is by far the most common cause.

Table 16.2. Causes of primary hyperparathyroidism seen in the Massachusetts General Hospital (1930–1979) (Silverberg 1983)

Cause of hyperparathyroidism	Patients	
Adenoma	758	82·9%
(Single)	(750)	(82·1%)
(Double)	(8)	(0·9%)
Hyperplasia	133	14·6%
(Chief cell)	(114)	(12·5%)
(Clear cell)	(19)	(2·1%)
Carcinoma	23	2·5%
Total	914	100·0%

Parathyroid adenoma

In the vast majority of cases the aetiology of parathyroid adenomas is unknown although prior exposure to head and neck irradiation is considered to be a cause in a few cases. Some studies have suggested that parathyroid adenomas are of multicellular origin and are therefore biologically similar to hyperplasia. This conclusion comes from work on women who were heterozygous for glucose-6-phosphate dehydrogenase and in whose adenomas two different isoenzymes were found, suggesting a multicellular rather than a unicellular origin. Other studies have, however, produced contradictory data.

Parathyroid adenomas most frequently involve only one gland, although occasionally two or more may be involved in which case differentiation from parathyroid hyperplasia is exceedingly difficult.

Grossly, usually the entire gland is involved and enlarged. Very small adenomas may, however, be no larger than the upper limit of normal parathyroid size.

However, adenomas are usually darker than normal with a colour similar to that of the capsule of the liver. They are very soft and pliable which helps to distinguish them from nodules of thyroid and on cut section are orange in colour, sometimes with foci of haemorrhage. Cystic degeneration is also occasionally seen. Adenomas tend to be spherical whereas normal glands have a flattened appearance.

On histological examination parathyroid adenomas are composed of chief cells, oxyphil cells and transitional cells in varying proportions. The commonest type is predominantly chief cell, although adenomas composed mainly of oxyphil cells are seen in about 3% of cases. The cells are arranged in sheets and are embedded in a vascular stroma. These sheets either lack or have a reduced number of the stromal fat cells which are seen in normal parathyroid tissue, a point useful in diagnosis. In some cases, small areas of necrosis occur giving rise to a pseudo-follicular arrangement so that the lesion looks like thyroid tissue (*see Fig.* 16.12). A rim of normal but compressed parathyroid tissue indicates that the lesion is an adenoma rather than hyperplasia. A similar rim may, however, be present in a hyperplastic gland and many authorities therefore state that it is impossible to distinguish between adenoma and hyperplasia by histological examination of one gland only.

The chief cells of an adenoma are usually larger than the normal chief cells and may show nuclear pleomorphism; some cells are multinucleate. These features may be confused with a carcinoma, although in adenomas mitotic figures are rare. Groups of cells may show cytoplasmic vacuolation giving a clear cell appearance in some areas, although these cells are thought not to be the true 'water clear' cells discussed later.

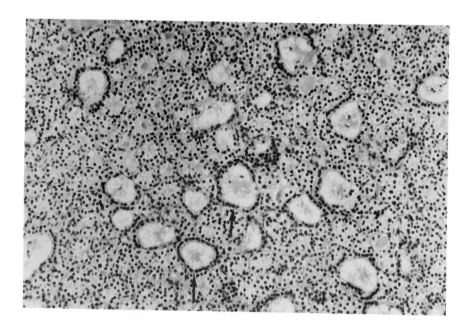

Fig. 16.12. Parathyroid adenoma; some pseudofollicles are seen (arrows). (H and E × 75)

Parathyroid hyperplasia

In this condition all four glands are enlarged. Each gland may be affected in total or in part. Unlike secondary hyperparathyroidism (*see* p. 475) no known stimulus of the hyperplasia can be detected. Some cases are associated with the multiple endocrine adenomatosis syndromes. The common form is hyperplasia of chief cells. Less frequently, clear cell hyperplasia is encountered.

A diagnosis of parathyroid hyperplasia at the time of surgery is simplified when all four glands are markedly enlarged. In many cases, however, the glands are either minimally enlarged or else there is asymmetrical hyperplasia. This last variety is obviously very easily confused with one or more adenoma(s). On cut section, the glands are yellow, tan or red and may show cystic degeneration.

Histologically, sheets of chief cells are seen with variable numbers of oxyphil cells. As with adenomas, there is classically a reduction in the number of stromal fat cells, although nuclear pleomorphism is less commonly seen. In early cases only isolated nodules of the gland may be hyperplastic leaving some normal parenchyma which can be mistaken for the rim of normal tissue seen in some adenomas. As stated earlier, many pathologists will not attempt to distinguish between an adenoma and a hyperplasia by the examination of one gland only.

Clear cell hyperplasia also causes hyperparathyroidism but it usually exhibits greater enlargement of the glands than the more usual chief cell hyperplasia. Microscopically the condition is characterized by one cell type. These have clear cytoplasm and distinct cell borders and are known as 'water clear' cells or 'Wasserhelle' cells.

Parathyroid carcinoma

Parathyroid carcinoma is a rare cause of hyperparathyroidism. They tend to be firmer than adenomas and may be adherent to or infiltrating into surrounding structures. These features give a clue to malignancy at the time of operation.

Parathyroid carcinomas may be difficult to distinguish from adenomas histologically as the latter often have considerable nuclear pleomorphism. However, in carcinomas, thick bands of fibrous tissue are often seen and the cells tend to be arranged in a trabecular pattern. The presence of capsular and blood vessel invasion and numerous mitotic figures also helps in the diagnosis.

Spread is usually to regional lymph nodes and less often by the blood stream to bone and viscera. After resection of the tumour, recurrences can be detected by a recurrence of hypercalcaemia. Bone metastases are associated with massive local bone reabsorption which can be appreciated on X-ray. Death is usually as a result of hypercalcaemia rather than due to metastatic deposits.

Intra-operative diagnosis of hyperparathyroidism

During a neck exploration for hyperparathyroidism, the surgeon may ask the pathologist one of the following questions:

1. *Is this tissue parathyroid?* In some cases the surgeon is not sure whether or not a particular nodule of tissue is parathyroid. A small biopsy is sent for frozen section and the pathologist can usually answer this question.

2. *Is this normal or abnormal parathyroid tissue?* If the surgeon finds all four glands enlarged the diagnosis is clearly hyperplasia. If he finds one enlarged and the others normal the diagnosis is clearly a single adenoma. A difficult situation may arise, however, in which one or more glands is/are enlarged and the remainder are borderline normal. This could be one or more adenomas, or alternatively asymmetrical hyperplasia. This problem may be answered by taking a biopsy of the borderline normal gland and asking whether it is normal or abnormal parathyroid tissue since, in hyperplasia, all four glands are abnormal. Some pathologists may be prepared to answer this question at the time of frozen section on the basis that abnormal parathyroid tissue (adenoma or hyperplasia) has less fat content (as seen on a fat stain) than normal tissue. Pathologists in non-specialized centres may, however, not be prepared to answer this question and in this case a Wang Test can be carried out in theatre (Wang and Rieder 1978). The principle is that normal parathyroid tissue is less dense (due to its greater fat content) than abnormal parathyroid tissue. Slivers of an obviously abnormal and a borderline normal gland are placed in mannitol which is gradually diluted with water until the specimens sink. Slivers from two hyperplastic glands will sink at the same rate whereas slivers of a normal and an abnormal gland will sink at different rates.

3. *Is this hyperplasia or adenoma?* Most pathologists will not attempt to answer this question when sent only one gland for frozen section examination.

Multiple Endocrine Adenomatosis

Wermer in 1954 described a familial syndrome in which patients developed pituitary, pancreatic islet cell and parathyroid adenomas. The parathyroid condition was subsequently shown to be a hyperplasia affecting all four glands and not adenomas. This syndrome is now termed multiple endocrine adenomatosis type 1 (MEA 1).

In 1961 Sipple described patients who developed phaeochromocytomas, medullary carcinomas of the thyroid and parathyroid hyperplasia. This is termed MEA 2. It was subsequently shown that these patients exhibit one of two phenotypes: MEA 2A who have a normal appearance and MEA 2B who have submucosal neuromas and tend to be Marfanoid. Parathyroid hyperplasia is seen only in MEA 2A.

The most important point in dealing with the hyperparathyroidism in MEA patients is to assume that all four parathyroids are involved so that asymmetrical hyperplasia is not confused with multiple adenomas. Recurrence of hyperparathyroidism is common in MEA patients and some surgeons therefore advocate total parathyroidectomy and auto-transplantation of a portion of the parathyroid into forearm muscle so that further surgical access is easy.

Secondary Hyperparathyroidism

Hypocalcaemia stimulates the parathyroid glands with resultant hyperplastic change and attempted return of the serum calcium to normal. This is termed secondary hyperparathyroidism. The hypocalcaemia may be caused by malabsorption or vitamin D deficiency but the commonest cause is chronic renal failure. Chronic renal failure causes phosphate retention which in turn lowers serum calcium. In addition, the damaged kidney may not be capable of metabolizing inactive vitamin D into the active form (1,25-dihydroxycholecalciferol). Additional factors include skeletal resistance to parathormone and impaired renal degradation of parathormone. The pathological changes in the parathyroids are similar to those seen in primary hyperparathyroidism due to hyperplasia. The patients may eventually develop severe bone disease with generalized pain in the lower back and legs. Sudden onset of severe bone pain is caused by pathological fractures.

Some patients are controlled medically but intractable cases require surgery.

Tertiary Hyperparathyroidism

In most cases of successful renal transplantation, the PTH levels return to normal within 1–4 months. In about 20% of cases, however, the PTH levels remain elevated for unknown reasons and this is termed persistent secondary hyperparathyroidism or tertiary hyperparathyroidism (Sicard and Wells 1983).

The condition may eventually require surgery which is either subtotal parathyroidectomy or total parathyroidectomy with auto-transplantation of a fragment of parathyroid tissue into the forearm.

Hypoparathyroidism

Clinically, patients with hypoparathyroidism develop increased excitability of nervous tissue. This is manifest as carpopedal spasm and eventually tetany. The patients may develop changes in the teeth and nails, and calcification of the basal ganglia and soft tissues may occur.

The commonest cause is inadvertent removal or damage to the parathyroids during thyroidectomy. It may also occur after surgical treatment of hyperparathyroidism. Usually, the deficiency of PTH in these cases is temporary, and is due to trauma, oedema or interference with blood supply of the remaining parathyroid tissue; rarely, it is permanent.

Pseudohypoparathyroidism

This is a very rare condition of unknown aetiology transmitted as an autosomal dominant trait with incomplete penetration. It is twice as common in females as in males. It is characterized by parathyroid glands which are normal or hyperplastic but there is apparent failure of the tissue to respond to PTH. Clinical features include mental deficiency, epilepsy, and tetany associated with short stature.

Parathyroid Cysts

These are rare and are occasionally associated with primary hyperparathyroidism. They more commonly present as cystic neck masses without hypercalcaemia.

Parathyroid cysts may be located as far cephalad as the angle of the mandible and as caudal as the mediastinum. They may contain thymic, lymphoid and muscle tissue and metaplastic bone.

ADRENAL GLANDS

Normal Structure

Each adrenal gland measures about 5 cm × 1 cm and weighs about 5 gm (the medulla being one-tenth the total weight). They are yellow in colour. The right gland, which is pyramidal in shape, surmounts the upper pole of the right kidney. It lies between the inferior vena cava and the right crus of the diaphragm, in contact with the bare area of the liver. The left gland is crescentic and lies on the medial border of the left kidney. Its lower pole is covered by the tail of the pancreas and it lies on the left diaphragmatic crus.

Each gland is supplied by three arteries, branches of the aorta, phrenic and renal arteries. The glands drain by single veins; the right into the vena cava and the left into the ipsilateral renal vein.

Histologically, the cortex has three distinct zones. The outer zona glomerulosa consists of nests of cells and is continuous with the columns of cells which form the middle zone or zona fasciculata. These columns are separated by venous sinuses. The innermost layer is the zona reticularis where the cells are interlaced in a network. All three zones secrete steroid hormones. The enzymes for aldosterone biosynthesis are limited to the zona glomerulosa, while the enzymes for cortisol and sex hormone synthesis are in the inner zones. The cells of the zona fasciculata are lipid-laden and are known as clear cells. Those in the zona reticularis have eosinophilic granular cells and are known as compact cells.

The adrenal medulla is of ectodermal origin and originates from cells which have migrated from the neural crest. It consists of interlacing cords of densely innervated granule-containing cells which are closely related to venous sinuses. There are two main cell types: (1) adrenaline secreting with large granules, and (2) noradrenaline secreting with smaller, very dense granules. The cell type secreting dopamine is unknown. The cells of the adrenal medulla form part of the APUD system (*see* p. 108).

Paraganglia are small groups of cells resembling those in the adrenal medulla found near the thoracic and abdominal sympathetic ganglia.

Normal Physiology

Adrenal cortex

The hormones of the cortex are derived from cholesterol. The C19 steroids have androgenic activity, while the C21 steroids have mineralocorticoid or glucocorticoid activity. The mineralocorticoids have their major effect on sodium and potassium excretion, while the glucocorticoids have their major effect on glucose and protein metabolism.

The physiological effects of the glucocorticoids include increased protein catabolism and increased hepatic gluconeogenesis (blood glucose therefore rises).

They are essential for vascular integrity. They promote salt and water retention and potassium excretion. Of surgical importance, they inhibit fibroblastic activity, decrease local swelling and block the systemic effects of bacterial toxins. The decreased local inflammatory reaction is due to inhibition of the release of arachidonic acid from tissue phospholipids. Also, by stabilizing lysosomal membranes, glucocorticoids inhibit the breakdown of lysosomes which occurs in inflamed tissue.

Both the basal secretion of glucocorticoids and the increased secretion provoked by stress are controlled by ACTH from the anterior pituitary. ACTH secretion is controlled by the hypothalamic hormone corticotrophin releasing factor (CRF).

Aldosterone and other steroids with mineralocorticoid activity increase the reabsorption of sodium from urine, saliva and gastric juice. Increased amounts of Na^+ are exchanged for K^+ and H^+ in the renal tubules. Various stimuli such as sodium loss, low sodium intake, surgery, trauma, haemorrhage or high K^+ intake increase aldosterone secretion. Control of aldosterone secretion is by the renin–angiotensin system, the serum level of potassium and the anterior pituitary. Renin is secreted from the juxtaglomerular cells which surround the afferent arterioles of the renal glomeruli. Renin acts on angiotensinogen (a circulating α_2-globulin) to release angiotensin I which subsequently forms the octapeptide angiotensin II, which in turn increases the secretion of aldosterone. A change in extracellular fluid volume alters afferent arteriolar pressure and changes renin secretion. This system is termed the 'renin–angiotensin–aldosterone (RAA) axis'.

Secretion of adrenal androgens is controlled by ACTH and not by gonadotrophins. Adrenal androgens account for about 20% of total androgen activity.

Adrenal medulla

The adrenal medulla can be thought of as a sympathetic ganglion in which the post-ganglionic fibres have lost their axons and become secreting cells. They secrete when stimulated by sympathetic preganglionic nerve fibres which reach the gland via the splanchnic nerves.

The medulla secretes the catecholamines adrenaline and noradrenaline. Noradrenaline is produced in larger quantities than adrenaline. They have a short half-life of about two minutes and are degraded to various metabolites including vanillylmandelic acid (VMA), which are excreted in the urine along with a small amount of free catecholamines.

Catecholamines increase glycogenolysis in liver and skeletal muscle, mobilize free fatty acids and generally stimulate the metabolic rate. They increase the force and rate of myocardial contraction. Noradrenaline produces vasoconstriction in most organs, while adrenaline dilates the blood vessels in skeletal muscle and liver.

THE ADRENAL CORTEX

In pathological states the adrenal cortex may produce excessive glucocorticoids (hypercortisolism or Cushing's syndrome), mineralocorticoids (hyperaldosteronism), androgens or oestrogens. Each of these may be produced by adrenal hyperplasia, adenoma or carcinoma. Alternatively the adrenal cortex may be hypofunctional, and this is either acute or chronic.

Cushing's Syndrome

Cushing's syndrome refers to the clinical manifestations of glucocorticoid excess, irrespective of the specific aetiology. The causes of spontaneous Cushing's syndrome are given in *Table* 16.3. In the ectopic ACTH syndrome, the ACTH is produced by tumours, such as bronchial carcinoma and pancreatic carcinoma. In addition to these, ectopic CRF production has recently been documented and this causes both pituitary and bilateral adrenal hyperplasia. Cushing's syndrome may also be secondary to pharmacological doses of corticosteroid or ACTH (iatrogenic Cushing's syndrome).

Table 16.3. Aetiology of spontaneous (non-iatrogenic) Cushing's syndrome (Huff 1977)

	(%)
ACTH dependent:	
Cushing's disease	68
Ectopic ACTH syndrome	15
ACTH independent:	
Adrenal adenoma	9
Adrenal carcinoma	8

Cushing's syndrome affects women more often than men (except in the subgroup due to bronchial carcinoma) and the peak incidence occurs in patients aged 20–40 years.

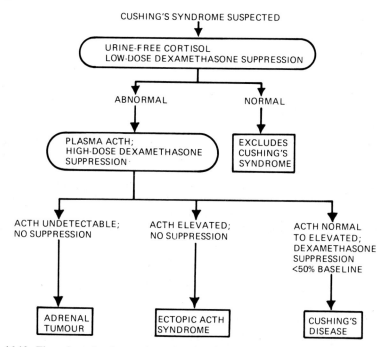

Fig. 16.13. Flow chart showing a scheme for the diagnosis of suspected Cushing's syndrome. (Adapted from Baxter and Tyrrell 1981.)

Clinical presentations include facial and truncal obesity, muscle weakness, osteoporosis, electrolyte disturbance (hypokalaemic alkalosis), hypertension, amenorrhoea, hirsutism and carbohydrate intolerance.

The diagnosis and differential diagnosis of Cushing's syndrome is shown schematically in *Fig.* 16.13. Essentially, the initial step is to make a diagnosis of Cushing's syndrome by the low dose dexamethasone suppression test and the measurement of urinary cortisol in a 24 hour collection. The next step is to determine the specific aetiology by measuring plasma ACTH levels and by using the high dose dexamethasone test. A low dose of dexamethasone will suppress the hypothalamic–pituitary–adrenal axis in most normal people (resulting in a low plasma cortisol) but not in patients with Cushing's syndrome. A high dose of dexamethasone will suppress the hypothalamic–pituitary–adrenal axis in patients with pituitary-dependent Cushing's syndrome (Cushing's disease) but not in patients with the ectopic ACTH syndrome, or in those with an autonomously functioning adrenal tumour. Details of these tests and of the pitfalls which may be encountered will be found in the standard texts of endocrinology.

Cushing's disease

Cushing's disease is pituitary-dependent adrenocortical hyperplasia. In nearly all cases, an adenoma of the pituitary is found, although it may be small and not detectable clinically or radiologically (microadenoma). Persistent abnormalities of the hypothalamic–pituitary axis have been described in a few of those cases in which an adenoma has not been found. Pathological changes occur in the pituitary, the adrenals and in the organs affected by excessive hormonal output.

Pituitary findings

Tyrrell *et al.* (1978) carried out 18 successful trans-sphenoidal explorations of the pituitary in cases of presumed Cushing's disease and found adenomas in 15. Inadequate specimens were obtained in the remaining three, although all of these had correction of the syndrome postoperatively. The pathological diagnoses were chromophobe adenoma (10), basophil adenoma (2) and basophil/chromophobe adenoma (3). Six of the 18 patients had normal preoperative sella tomographs and no patient had generalized sella enlargement on plain X-ray. Currently, CT scanning would be used to assess the sella, although a normal CT scan does not exclude the possibility of a microadenoma. Most similar studies have presented comparable data and good results have also been reported in children (Styne *et al.* 1984). It is now realized that 93–95% of those cases of Cushing's syndrome which are associated with bilateral adrenal hyperplasia (excepting those due to ectopic ACTH production) are due to a pituitary adenoma or microadenoma.

In addition to the finding of tumour in the pituitary, Cushing's disease, like other causes of Cushing's syndrome, causes Crooke's hyaline degeneration of the basophils in the pituitary due to the high levels of circulating cortisol. The cytoplasm of the basophils is filled with a basophilic hyaline substance.

Adrenal findings

The adrenal glands increase in size and may weigh 6–12 g each instead of the usual 4–6 g. The cut surface of the gland will show either diffuse or nodular hyperplasia. The cortex in diffuse hyperplasia shows two layers: an inner brown area equivalent to the zona reticularis and an outer yellow zone equivalent to the zona fasciculata. In the nodular form this pattern is distorted by nodules of varying sizes.

Microscopic examination confirms the thickening of the adrenal cortex with sheets of compact cells of the zona reticularis in the inner layer and columns of clear cells arranged in a zona fasciculata pattern in the outer layer (*see Fig.* 16.14). The nodules contain either clear or compact cells or a mixture of both. The fact that these nodules are associated with hyperplastic adjacent cortex distinguishes them from functioning adenomas and non-functioning nodules. The zona glomerulosa is largely unaffected.

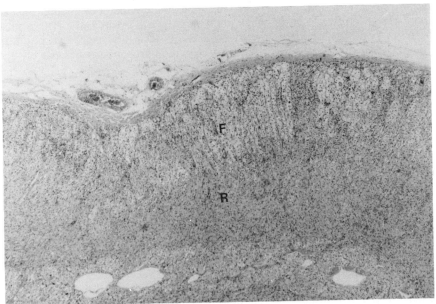

Fig. 16.14. Adrenocortical hyperplasia showing the zona fasciculata (F) and the zona reticularis (R). (H and E × 7)

Prognosis

If untreated, Cushing's disease is often fatal due either to the complications of hypercortisolism or to the underlying pituitary tumour.

An improvement in operative mortality and morbidity has taken place with the change of treatment from bilateral adrenalectomy to pituitary surgery.

A proportion of cases treated primarily by bilateral adrenalectomy develop a clinically obvious rapidly growing pituitary adenoma with associated skin pigmentation. This is known as Nelson's syndrome.

Cushing's syndrome due to adrenal adenoma

Once the cause of Cushing's syndrome is known to be an adrenal tumour (by using the investigations outlined on p. 480), various localizing procedures, such as CT scan and venous sampling, are used to determine the affected side.

Adenomas are rounded tumours, 2–4 cm in diameter and weighing between 10 and 70 g, although occasionally they may be much larger. The cut surface is yellow or brown, possibly with some necrosis or haemorrhage. The surrounding adrenal is classically atrophied since ACTH production is suppressed by the cortisol over-production. Rarely functional adenomas appear dark brown or black, the so-called 'black' adenoma.

The adenoma is composed of clear cells (similar to the zona fasciculata) in clusters and columns with well demarcated areas of compact cells similar to those seen in the zona reticularis also present. The fact that the surrounding cortex is atrophied is important in distinguishing an adenoma from nodular hyperplasia (when the surrounding cortex is hyperplastic). Adenomas sometimes show nuclear pleomorphism, in which case they may be exceedingly difficult to distinguish from carcinomas (see below). In the black adenoma, the cell cytoplasm contains many lipofuscin granules. Treatment is by surgical removal and since the pituitary–adrenal axis is suppressed, patients must be given cortisone for periods of up to two years postoperatively.

Cushing's syndrome due to adrenal carcinoma

Adrenal carcinoma is rare and accounts for only 0·02% of all cancers. The most common presentation is with abdominal symptoms such as pain and there may be a palpable mass. In Nader et al.'s (1983) large series of adrenal carcinomas, only one-third showed evidence of Cushing's syndrome. Many were non-functional and a few secreted aldosterone or sex hormones.

Grossly, the tumours are bulky and bosselated. The normal adrenal is usually completely replaced by tumour. The cut surface has a variegated appearance with yellow and brown areas. Haemorrhage and necrosis are much in evidence. The weight of the tumour is helpful in the distinction from adenoma and any tumour over 100 g should be treated with suspicion.

The tumour may be divided into undifferentiated and well differentiated types (Nader et al. 1983). The undifferentiated tumours have sheets of cells often with obvious invasion of surrounding tissues. The nuclei are pleomorphic with frequent bizarre forms and mitotic figures are present. The diagnosis in these cases is readily apparent. The differentiated type consists of sheets and cords of clear and compact cells and is exceedingly difficult to distinguish from adenoma, especially as the latter may show pleomorphic cells. One study showed that experienced pathologists frequently disagreed on the diagnosis (O'Hare et al. 1979). The most important indicators of malignancy in these cases are the large size of the tumour, vascular and capsular invasion, necrosis, high mitotic rate and the presence of broad fibrous bands of stroma.

Cell culture techniques have been shown to be useful in differentiating adrenal carcinomas from adenomas, in that cells from adenomas respond to ACTH, whereas those from carcinomas do not. This test is not in general use.

In Nader et al.'s (1983) series, most had distant metastases at the time of presentation, commonly to lung and liver. The five year survival rate for the whole series was 30%.

Hyperaldosteronism

Hyperaldosteronism is either primary or secondary. Primary hyperaldosteronism

(Conn's syndrome) is due to autonomous oversecretion of aldosterone by the adrenal. This suppresses the RAA axis and, therefore, plasma renin is low. Secondary hyperaldosteronism is usually caused by overproduction of renin and hence angiotensin II. This occurs if renal blood flow is reduced, as in renal artery stenosis or in malignant hypertension. Other causes include congestive heart failure, cirrhosis of the liver and the nephrotic syndrome. A primary renin secreting tumour of the kidney has also been described. In secondary hyperaldosteronism, the plasma renin is high and therefore assay of plasma renin distinguishes between primary and secondary hyperaldosteronism.

Primary hyperaldosteronism has a peak incidence in the third and fourth decades and accounts for about 2% of cases of hypertension. It may be caused by adrenocortical hyperplasia (23%), adrenal adenoma (75%) or adrenal carcinoma (2%).

The diagnosis of primary hyperaldosteronism can be made biochemically by a low serum potassium, a high supine plasma aldosterone and a failure of aldosterone suppression after saline infusion in the presence of a low or normal plasma renin.

The aetiology of primary hyperaldosteronism can be determined by a series of investigations, including serum 18-hydroxycorticosterone (greatly increased in adenoma; normal or slightly increased in hyperplasia) and CT scanning. However, the most useful investigation is bilateral simultaneous adrenal venous aldosterone estimation which distinguishes between hyperplasia and tumour and locates a tumour.

Primary hyperaldosteronism due to adrenal hyperplasia

The size of the adrenals is variable in the absence of a tumour and in many cases may be normal. Microscopically, there is hyperplasia of the zona glomerulosa (i.e. the zone where aldosterone is usually produced) which may be diffuse or nodular. The aetiology is unknown.

Primary hyperaldosteronism due to adrenal adenoma

These are usually less than 4 cm in diameter and are typically yellow on cut section (*see Fig.* 16.15). Microscopically, they consist of clear and compact cells. The former may predominate and may be arranged in clusters similar in structure to those seen in the zona glomerulosa. The surrounding cortex, unlike cortisol secreting adenomas, may be normal or hyperplastic. As with cortisol secreting adenomas, nuclear pleomorphism may cause difficulty in differentiating the lesion from a carcinoma.

Primary hyperaldosteronism due to adrenal carcinoma

Aldosterone secreting carcinomas are similar to cortisol producing and non-functioning carcinomas. They are exceedingly rare. Some cases of aldosterone-secreting carcinomas are distinguished by having a yellow cut surface and microscopically by cells arranged in a zona glomerulosa type of pattern.

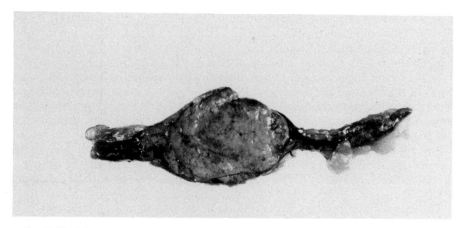

Fig. 16.15. Adrenal adenoma. This patient had Conn's syndrome.

Overproduction of Sex Steroid Hormones

This may occur as a congenital disorder in which case there is adrenal hyperplasia and overproduction of male sex hormones due to an enzyme defect. Adults may have adrenal adenomas or carcinomas, either of which may be virilizing (androgen producing) or feminizing (oestrogen producing). Occasionally, latent congenital adrenal hyperplasia may present in adult life.

Congenital adrenal hyperplasia

The most common defect to cause this condition is a deficiency of the enzyme 21-hydroxylase; this accounts for 90% of cases. This enzyme is essential for cortisol production and if absent, or present only in reduced amounts, there is an accumulation of intermediate metabolites. Since cortisol production is low, ACTH is produced in increased amounts and this stimulates the adrenal to produce more intermediate metabolites such as 17-hydroxyprogesterone. An outlet for these intermediate metabolites is via androstenedione to testosterone with resultant virilization. The enzyme 21-hydroxylase is also necessary for aldosterone production and if it is completely absent no aldosterone is produced and the patient loses salt in addition to the simple virilization (salt-losing congenital adrenal hyperplasia).

In untreated cases, each adrenal is enlarged, weighs up to 30 g and is classically brown on cut section. Microscopically, there is gross widening of the zonae reticularis and fasciculata. In untreated cases, bizarre giant cell forms are seen.

Female children with congenital adrenal hyperplasia develop enlargement of the external genitalia (pseudo-hermaphrodite) and later have primary amenorrhoea and failure of breast development. Males develop premature secondary sexual characteristics.

Overproduction of sex hormones due to adrenal adenoma

Adenomas of the adrenal cause virilization much more commonly than feminization. They vary in size and are characteristically associated with a normal contralateral adrenal as ACTH production is unaffected. Microscopically, they consist mainly of compact cells which resemble the zona reticularis. Nuclear pleomorphism may cause great difficulty in distinguishing benign from malignant tumours.

Overproduction of sex hormones due to adrenal carcinoma

Carcinomas identical to the adrenal carcinomas described earlier may be virilizing or feminizing depending on whether they secrete androgens or oestrogens. The pathological features are similar to those described earlier, although they have a tendency to be brown in colour on cut section and to have a greater number of compact cells similar to those of the zona reticularis. In King and Lack's (1979) study of 49 adrenal carcinomas, virilization was present in seven women and feminization with gynaecomastia was seen in three men.

Hypofunction of the Adrenal Cortex

Although the treatment of hypofunction of the adrenal cortex is mainly by medical means, surgeons may encounter this condition as a cause of serious postoperative complications. Hypofunction of the adrenal cortex is either acute or chronic. The chronic form is either primary or secondary.

Acute adrenal insufficiency

Adrenal haemorrhage occurring in the neonatal period will cause sudden loss of function. In children and adults a bacteraemic infection usually by meningococcus causes a coagulation defect with haemorrhage into the skin and adrenals. This manifests as widespread purpura and circulatory collapse (the Waterhouse–Friderichsen syndrome). Staphylococcus, Pneumococcus and *Haemophilus influenzae* may also be responsible.

Primary adrenal haemorrhage may be caused by anticoagulant therapy and can occur in association with postpartum haemorrhage.

Traumatic necrosis of the adrenal may follow surgery, especially nephrectomy. Occasionally after severe chest or abdominal trauma, adrenal necrosis is seen up to a week later (Sevitt 1955). One speculative aetiology is that a sudden pressure rise in the inferior vena cava due to the trauma causes rupture of the central venules of the adrenal. Adrenal haemorrhage and infarction may also complicate retrograde venous angiography.

Primary chronic adrenal insufficiency (Addison's disease)

This is adrenal insufficiency resulting from disease of the adrenal itself. The commonest cause is idiopathic atrophy characterized by a lymphocytic infiltration in the adrenal cortex and circulating anti-adrenal antibodies. Other less common causes include tuberculosis, metastatic deposits in the adrenals (especially from oat cell carcinoma of the lung), sarcoidosis and amyloid. The clinical features are weakness, nausea, vomiting, hypotension and pigmentation.

In cases of stress due to surgery, trauma or infection the chronic insufficiency may become acute with hypoglycaemia and circulatory collapse.

Secondary chronic adrenal insufficiency

This is adrenal insufficiency secondary to hypothalamic–pituitary axis disease, such as occurs with tumour, irradiation or infarction.

ACTH levels are low and therefore pigmentation is not seen. The adrenal cortex is reduced in size and microscopically it consists mainly of zona glomerulosa—the aldosterone secreting part which is less affected by ACTH deficiency.

THE ADRENAL MEDULLA

Adrenal Medullary Hyperplasia

It has recently been recognized that in multiple endocrine adenomatosis type 2A, phaeochromocytomas and medullay carcinomas of the thyroid are preceded by a phase of hyperplasia of the adrenal medulla and parafollicular C-cells of the thyroid respectively. Adrenal medullary hyperplasia is now a recognized entity and has been reported as the cause of paroxysmal symptoms similar to those occurring with a phaeochromocytoma. It is now thought that this condition explains those cases without tumour in which phaeochromocytomas have been strongly suspected on symptomatic and pharmacological grounds.

Clinical diagnosis is difficult although Delellis et al. (1976) found that a raised urinary adrenaline to noradrenaline ratio indicated the condition. Medullary hyperplasia may not be obvious in an operative specimen and the pathological diagnosis may require special morphometric measurements.

Tumours of the Adrenal Medulla

The adrenal medulla cells are derived from neural crest cells which migrate into the adrenal cortex in fetal life. These differentiate either via phaeochromoblasts into phaeochromocytes (also called chromaffin cells as they have catecholamine-containing granules which stain with chromate compounds) or via neuroblasts into sympathetic ganglion cells (non-chromaffin cells). Tumours of the adrenal medulla are therefore either chromaffin tumours (phaeochromocytoma) or non-chromaffin tumours.

A further population of phaeochromocytes migrates via the sympathetic nervous system to occupy mainly paravertebral and retroperitoneal sites and the organ of Zuckerkandl, where they form the chromaffin paraganglia. These are the origins of extra-adrenal phaeochromocytomas.

Neuroblastomas, ganglioneuroblastomas and ganglioneuromas are derived from the non-chromaffin part of the sympathetic nervous system. As neuroblasts develop into mature ganglion cells they pass through different stages of development and it is thought that these different tumours arise from the cells occurring during the various stages. Neuroblastomas therefore arise from the most primitive cells, ganglioneuromas from the most mature cells and ganglioneuroblastomas from intermediate cells. All these cell types are capable of secreting catecholamines. One study reported elevated urinary levels of VMA in 90% of children with neuroblastomas, ganglioneuroblastomas and ganglioneuromas (Editorial 1975).

Phaeochromocytoma

These rare tumours account for less than 1% of all cases of hypertension and have an annual incidence of approximately one per million persons. They arise either *de novo* or in association with MEA type 2A or 2B, in which case they may be preceded by adrenal medullary hyperplasia. Phaeochromocytomas secrete catecholamines and both adrenaline and noradrenaline can usually be detected in the blood and urine in increased quantities. Also, metabolites such as vanillylmandelic acid (VMA) can be detected in the urine. Whereas adrenal medullary tumours secrete both adrenaline and noradrenaline, extra-adrenal tumours secrete mainly noradrenaline. Bilateral tumours occur in 10% of patients, although up to half of those occurring in patients with an MEA syndrome are bilateral.

Between 10% and 20% of phaeochromocytomas occur outside the adrenal medulla. In Modlin et al.'s (1979) series of 72 cases, 13 were outside the adrenal medulla, most commonly in the perirenal region, the organ of Zuckerkandl and the bladder wall. Of their 72 cases, 98% had hypertension and 86% had paroxysms of palpitations, sweating, headache and anxiety. Urinary VMA was elevated in nearly all cases when it was measured.

Biochemical diagnosis in phaeochromocytoma is achieved by demonstrating raised serum catecholamines and raised urinary catecholamines and catecholamine metabolites. Recently, suppression tests using clonidine have been used as some patients with essential hypertension have mildly raised catecholamines.

Since phaeochromocytoma is a rare cause of hypertension, some authorities consider it to be unnecessary to screen all hypertensives. However, hypertensive patients who have symptoms suggestive of phaeochromocytoma, or variable hypertension, or increased serum calcium, or a thyroid swelling, or a family history should be investigated.

Selective venous sampling with assay of adrenaline and noradrenaline is successful in up to 97% of cases in diagnosing and localizing tumours (Allison et al. 1983). CT scanning is very useful in localizing phaeochromocytomas and recently Ackery et al. (1984) have shown that radioisotope imaging using iodine-131-meta-iodobenzyguanidine (^{131}I-MIBG) is also of value.

Morphology

Phaeochromocytomas vary greatly in size but average 100 g in weight. The tumour is soft and encapsulated by either fibrous tissue or attenuated adrenal cortex. The cut surface is grey and may contain haemorrhagic areas. The specimen should be sent to the laboratory fresh, without fixative, where a piece of tissue is placed in a dichromate solution. The tumour turns dark brown/black due to oxidation of adrenaline/noradrenaline and this confirms the diagnosis (*see Fig.* 16.16). Electron microscopy demonstrates adrenaline- and noradrenaline-containing granules.

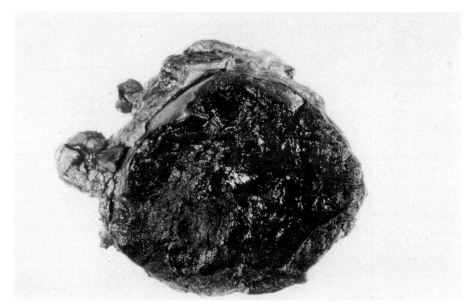

Fig. 16.16. Phaeochromocytoma. The dark colour is because the specimen was dipped in chromate solution (*see* text).

The histological appearance in many cases is similar to that of the normal adrenal medulla with clusters of phaeochromocytes separated by a very vascular stroma (*see Fig.* 16.17). The cytoplasm is granular and is stained brown if a fixative containing dichromate is used. Cellular pleomorphism and even vascular invasion can be seen in benign lesions and therefore the most widely accepted criterion of malignancy is the demonstration of metastases.

Prognosis

If a diagnosis of malignancy is restricted to those cases with proven metastases then 95% are benign.

Careful preoperative and intra-operative management, particularly with α blockade, has reduced the operative mortality to about 2%. Of Modlin *et al.*'s (1979) patients, two-thirds were alive 10 years after resection. Only one of their five malignant cases died in the follow-up period. Malignant phaeochromocytomas are very slow growing and long-term survival is often possible if the blood pressure can be controlled by α and β blockade.

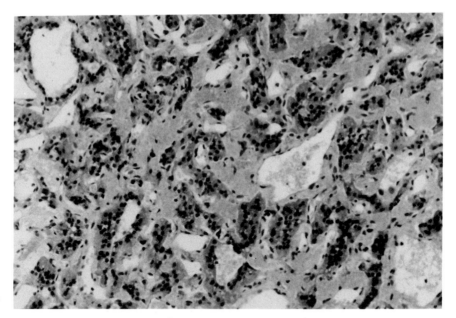

Fig. 16.17. Phaeochromocytoma. (H and E × 150)

Neuroblastoma

This is a common malignancy of childhood with up to 80% occurring before the age of five years. Cases may be congenital and several series have been reported in which the tumour has presented in adult life (Lopez *et al.* 1980). Clinically the child presents with weight loss and general poor health. An abdominal mass may be palpable. Urinary VMA is a useful screening test.

Morphology

The most common site of origin is the adrenal medulla, although it can arise in association with any part of the sympathetic chain from the neck to the pelvis. The tumour is soft and lobular. The cut surface is grey; haemorrhage and necrosis are sometimes present.

Microscopically the cells are typically small and round with hyperchromatic nuclei and little cytoplasm; they are similar to lymphocytes but larger (*see Fig.* 16.18). They are arranged in sheets, often without any recognizable pattern and separated by a very delicate stroma. If rosettes (circles of cells with a central meshwork of neurofibrils) are present, they distinguish the tumour from other 'small blue cell tumours' of childhood (Ewing's sarcoma, malignant lymphoma and embryonal rhabdomyosarcoma). The presence of rosettes and larger cells with more cytoplasm are signs of differentiation and improve the prognosis. Even the slightest signs of differentiation, such as increase in nuclear size, presence of visible cytoplasm and cytoplasmic processes, are of prognostic value (Makinen 1972).

Unfortunately it is rarely possible to remove a primary neuroblastoma completely because it is a very vascular and infiltrative tumour.

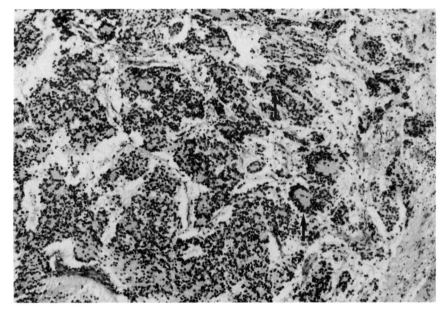

Fig. 16.18. Neuroblastoma. Some rosettes are seen (arrowed). (H and E × 30)

Spread and prognosis

Spread occurs in the early stages directly into adjacent organs and lymph nodes. Blood spread occurs very frequently to liver, lungs and bones. Metastases to the skull and orbit with exophthalmos is termed a Hutchinson-type neuroblastoma, whereas metastases to liver is termed a Pepper-type neuroblastoma.

The overall prognosis for children with neuroblastomas is exceedingly poor with only about 10% surviving two years. However, there are several situations in which prognosis may be greatly improved: (1) The tumour may undergo spontaneous regression, possibly by an immunological mechanism. This is more likely in patients under one year old and these children, therefore, have a much improved prognosis compared with those in the older age groups. (2) The tumour may mature into a ganglioneuroblastoma or a ganglioneuroma. (3) Tumours arising in the thorax have a better prognosis. (4) Patients with a particular pattern of metastases to the liver, skin and lymph nodes have an improved prognosis (for unknown reasons). (5) Occasionally, treatment of the primary tumour may stimulate regression of metastases.

Ganglioneuroblastoma

This is a rare tumour arising in the adrenal medulla or, more commonly, in extra-adrenal sites such as the retroperitoneum and mediastinum. It occurs in older children and adults and, although it has a much better prognosis than a neuroblastoma, it does, however, give rise to metastases. They may secrete catecholamines and a raised urinary VMA level may be found.

Grossly, the tumour contains soft neuroblastoma-like areas and firmer ganglioneuroma areas. Microscopically, mature ganglion cells and nerve fibres are seen interspaced with immature neuroblastoma-type tissue. One of the regulatory peptides, neuropeptide Y (NPY), is normally found in high concentrations in the human central nervous system. It has been found in high concentrations in extracts from these tumours and also in the plasma of patients with phaeochromocytoma and ganglioneuroblastoma. This may provide a future screening test (Adrian *et al.* 1983).

Ganglioneuroma

These tumours may occur in childhood or in adults. Although they also secrete catecholamines, normally there are no symptoms and presentation is by palpation or the radiological finding of a mass; the tumour is benign.

Grossly, it appears as a firm encapsulated mass, white or grey on cut section. Microscopically bundles of ganglion cells are seen among many nerve fibres. The presence of neuroblastoma areas must be excluded by examination of many sections of the tumour.

Myelolipoma of the Adrenal

This is a rare non-functioning benign tumour which arises in either the cortex or medulla of the adrenal gland. It is composed of adipose and haemopoietic tissue and varies in size from several millimetres to over 20 cm. The tumour is well demarcated from the surrounding adrenal by a false capsule. The lesion is composed of large vacuolated fat cells, between which are areas resembling bone marrow cells. They are benign and are frequently symptomless. Occasionally they present with pain, swelling or haematuria (Filobbas and Seddon 1980).

References

Ackery D. M., Tippett P. A., Condon B. R., Sutton H. E., Wyeth P. (1984) New approach to the localisation of phaeochromocytoma: imaging with iodine-131-meta-iodobenzylguanidine. *Br. Med. J.* **288**, 1587–91.

Adrian T. E., Allen J. M., Terenghi G. *et al.* (1983) Neuropeptide Y in phaeochromocytomas and ganglioneuroblastomas. *Lancet* **2**, 540–2.

Allison D. J., Brown M. J., Jones D. H., Timmis J. B. (1983) Role of venous sampling in locating a phaeochromocytoma. *Br. Med. J.* **286**, 1122–4.

Baxter J. D., Tyrrell J. B. (1981) The adrenal cortex. In: Felig P., Baxter J. D., Broadus A. E., Frohman L. A. (eds.) *Endocrinology and Metabolism.* New York, McGraw-Hill.

Boonstra C. E., Jackson C. E. (1971) Serum calcium survey for hyperparathyroidism: results in 50 000 clinic patients. *Am. J. Clin. Pathol.* **55**, 523–6.

Burke J. S., Butler J. J., Fuller L. M. (1977) Malignant lymphomas of the thyroid: a clinical pathologic study of 35 patients, including ultrastructural observations. *Cancer* **39**, 1587–602.

Chong G. C., Beahrs O. H., Sizemore G. W., Woolner L. H. (1975) Medullary carcinoma of the thyroid gland. *Cancer* **35**, 695–704.

Cole W. H., Majarakis J. D., Slaughter D. P. (1949) Incidence of carcinoma of thyroid in nodular goitre. *J. Clin. Endocrinol.* **9**, 1007–11.

Delellis R. A., Wolfe H. J., Gagel R. F. *et al.* (1976) Adrenal medullary hyperplasia. A morphometric analysis in patients with familial medullary thyroid carcinoma. *Am. J. Pathol.* **83**, 177–190.

Editorial (1975) Neuroblastoma. *Lancet* **1**, 379–80.

Filobbas S. A., Seddon J. A. (1980) Myelolipoma of the adrenal. *Br. J. Surg.* **67**, 147–8.

Hamburger J. (1983) The autonomously functioning thyroid adenoma. Clinical considerations. *N. Engl. J. Med.* **309**, 1512–13.

Hazard J. B., Hawk W. A., Crile G. (1959) Medullary (solid) carcinoma of the thyroid: a clinicopathologic entity. *J. Clin. Endocrinol.* **19**, 153–61.

Hazard J. B., Kenyon R. (1954) Atypical adenoma of the thyroid. *A.M.A. Arch. Pathol.* **58**, 554–63.

Holm L.-E., Blomgren H., Löwhagen T. (1985) Cancer risks in patients with chronic lymphocytic thyroidits. *N. Engl. J. Med.* **312**, 601–4.

Huff T. A. (1977) Clinical syndromes related to disorders of adenocorticotrophic hormone. In: Allen M. B., Makesh V. B. (eds.) *The Pituitary: A Current Review*, pp. 153–68. New York, Academic Press.

Kendall-Taylor P., Atkinson S., Halcombe M. (1984) A specific IgG in Graves' ophthalmopathy and its relation to retro-orbital and thyroid autoimmunity. *Br. Med. J.* **288**, 1183–6.

King D. R., Lack E. E. (1979) Adrenal cortical carcinoma. A clinical and pathologic study of 49 cases. *Cancer* **44**, 239–44.

Lopez R., Karakousis C., Rao U. (1980) Treatment of adult neuroblastoma. *Cancer* **45**, 840–4.

Löwhagen T., Granberg P.-O., Lundell G., Skinnari P., Sundblad R., Willems J.-S. (1979) Aspiration biopsy cytology (ABC) in nodules of the thyroid gland suspected to be malignant. In: Economou S. G. (ed.) *Surgical Clinics of North America: Endocrine Surgery*, Vol. 59, No. 1, pp. 3–18. Philadelphia, W. B. Saunders.

Makinen J. (1972) Microscopic patterns as a guide to prognosis of neuroblastoma in childhood. *Cancer* **29**, 1637–46.

Mazzaferri E. L., Oertel J. E. (1983) The pathology and prognosis of thyroid cancer. In: Kaplan E. L. (ed.) *Surgery of the Thyroid and Parathyroid Glands*, pp. 18–39. Edinburgh, Churchill Livingstone.

Mazzaferri E. L., Young R. L. (1981) Papillary thyroid carcinoma: a 10 year follow-up report of the impact of therapy in 576 patients. *Am. J. Med.* **70**, 511–18.

Modlin I. M., Farndon J. R., Shepherd A. *et al.* (1979) Phaeochromocytomas in 72 patients: clinical and diagnostic features, treatment and long-term results. *Br. J. Surg.* **66**, 456–65.

Nader S., Hickey R. C., Sellin R. V., Samaan N. A. (1983) Adrenal cortical carcinoma. A study of 77 cases. *Cancer* **52**, 707–11.

O'Hare M. J., Monaghan P., Neville A. M. (1979) The pathology of adrenocortical neoplasia; a correlated structural and functional approach to the diagnosis of malignant disease. *Human Pathol.* **10**, 137–54.

Okita N., Row V. V., Volpe R. (1981) Suppressor T lymphocyte deficiency in Graves' disease and Hashimoto's thyroiditis. *J. Clin. Endocrinol. Metab.* **52**, 528–33.

Sevitt S. (1955) Post-traumatic adrenal apoplexy. *J. Clin. Pathol.* **8**, 185–94.

Sicard G. A., Wells S. A. (1983) Surgical treatment of secondary hyperparathyroidism. In: Kaplan E. L. (ed.) *Surgery of the Thyroid and Parathyroid Glands*. Edinburgh, Churchill Livingstone.

Silverberg S. G. (1983) *Principles and Practice of Surgical Pathology*. New York, John Wiley and Sons.

Sipple J. H. (1961) The association of phaeochromocytoma with carcinoma of the thyroid gland. *Am. J. Med.* **31**, 163–6.

Sokal J. E. (1960) The incidence of thyroid cancer and the problem of malignancy in nodular goitre. In: Astwood E. B. (ed.) *Clinical Endocrinology*, pp. 223–65. New York, Grune and Stratton.

Styne D. M., Grumbach M. M., Kaplan S. L., Wilson C. B., Conte F. A. (1984) Treatment of Cushing's disease in childhood and adolescence by transsphenoidal microadenomectomy. *N. Engl. J. Med.* **310**, 889–93.

Thomas C. G., Buckwalter J. A. (1973) Poorly differentiated neoplasms of the thyroid gland. *Ann. Surg.* **177**, 632–42.

Tyrrell J. B., Brooks R. M., Fitzgerald P. A., Cofoid P. B., Forsham P. H., Wilson C. B. (1978) Cushing's disease. Selective transsphenoidal resection of pituitary microadenomas *N. Engl. J. Med.* **298**, 753–58.

Wade J. S. H. (1983) The management of malignant thyroid tumours. *Br. J. Surg.* **70**, 253–5.

Wang C. A., Rieder S. V. (1978) A density test for the intraoperative differentiation of parathyroid hyperplasia from neoplasia. *Ann. Surg.* **187**, 63–7.

Wermer P. (1954) Genetic aspects of adenomatoses of endocrine glands. *Am. J. Med.* **16**, 363–71.

Chapter 17

The Skin

Normal Structure

Skin is composed of the dermis (corium), a connective tissue layer of mesenchymal origin, and the epidermis, of ectodermal origin. Deep to the dermis is loose connective tissue which forms the superficial fascia. The epidermis is the primary barrier to mechanical damage, fluid loss and invasion by micro-organisms, and when damaged it has a high capacity for regeneration. The epidermis also produces the skin appendages, namely hairs, nails and sweat and sebaceous glands. The dermis gives the skin mechanical strength because of its high content of collagen and elastic fibres. Its cellular components combat infection and repair deep wounds.

Thin, hair bearing skin with sebaceous glands covers most of the body surface, but thick skin without hair and sebaceous glands covers the palms, soles and flexor surfaces of the digits.

The vascular supply of the skin is confined to the dermis; the epidermis depends on diffusion of nutrients from the capillaries of the superficial areas of dermis.

Histologically, the epidermis is composed of keratinizing stratified squamous epithelium. The cells are continually lost from the surface and are replaced by cell division in the deeper layers.

The epidermis consists of several well-defined layers (*see Fig.* 17.1). The basal cell layer (stratum basale) lies on the basal lamina which is in contact with the dermis. It produces the upper layers by mitosis and differentiation. Occasional melanocytes of neural crest origin and pale staining Langerhans' cells, which may have a phagocytic function, are located in this area. Next to the basal cell layer is the prickle cell layer (also termed squamous cell layer or stratum spinosum) which

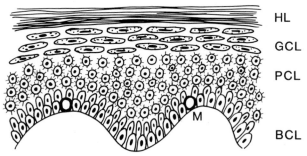

Fig. 17.1 Diagrammatic representation of normal epidermis: HL—horny layer; GCL—granular cell layer; PCL—prickle cell layer; BCL—basal cell layer; M—melanocyte.

is of variable thickness. These cells are metabolically active and in pathological states such as psoriasis, the prickle cell layer becomes widened by hyperplasia. This change is known as acanthosis. Superficial to the prickle cell layer is the granular layer where the cells begin to degenerate. Keratohyaline granules are seen in the cell cytoplasm and the nuclei shrink and disappear. The next layer is the horny layer (stratum corneum or keratin layer) which is composed of cell remnants and keratin.

The dermis varies in thickness in different parts of the body. It consists of fibrous tissue arranged into deep reticular and superficial papillary layers. The deep layer consists of strong fibrous tissue containing elastic fibres. In many areas of the body the elastic fibres are arranged into parallel bands which constitute the relaxed skin tension lines; surgical incisions along these lines heal with minimum scar tissue. The papillary layer contains papillae which project perpendicularly into the undersurface of the epidermis. Each papilla consists of bundles of fibrillar tissue with a capillary loop.

The main skin appendages are sweat glands, hairs and sebaceous glands. Sweat glands are of two types. In most areas of the skin they are simple coiled tubular glands which secrete an odourless fluid, important in the regulation of body temperature, directly onto the skin surface. In the axillae and genital regions, apocrine sweat glands are found. These secrete a viscous odoriferous secretion into hair follicles and hence onto the skin surface.

A hair follicle with its sebaceous glands and arrector pili muscle together form a pilosebaceous apparatus. Hairs are found in all parts of the body except the palms and soles, flexor aspects of the fingers and toes, parts of the genitalia and the mucocutaneous junctions of the lips. The hair follicle is an invagination of the epidermis and the hair bulb is a terminal expansion of the hair follicle where hair growth takes place. The sebaceous glands secrete into ducts which open into the associated hair follicles. The greasy sebum produced has protective qualities and prevents loss of water from the epidermis. It also has some bactericidal activity.

The skin of the finger tips, toes, nail beds, palms and ears contains special arteriovenous anastomoses which bypass the usual capillaries. These anastomoses are known as Sucquet–Hoyer canals and each connects an artery with a nearby vein. The canal has a narrow lumen and a thick wall which contains modified smooth muscle cells or glomus cells. The structure is termed a glomus and has a rich nerve fibre network; it is involved in temperature regulation.

Skin Infection

Bacterial

Impetigo

Impetigo most commonly affects children and is due to infection with Staphylococcus, Streptococcus, or both. Initially vesicles are present, particularly on the face around the mouth. These rapidly break down to form the characteristic yellow crusting lesions.

Folliculitis

Folliculitis is an infection of hair follicles most often due to *Staph. aureus* infection.

The hair follicle becomes filled with pus and if this cannot discharge onto the surface, the wall of the follicle breaks down allowing spread into the surrounding dermis, thus forming a furuncle or boil. Histologically, there is an intense inflammatory reaction in the dermis together with a foreign body granulomatous reaction to the hair. Involvement of several adjacent follicles causes a large boggy mass termed a carbuncle.

Scalded skin syndrome

This occurs in children as a result of Staphylococcal infection. The Staphylococcus (mainly phage type 71) produces a toxin which causes epidermal splitting. Clinically there is superficial peeling of the skin together with erythema and pain.

Viral

Verruca vulgaris

This is the common wart and it can occur anywhere on the skin or mucous membranes. It is due to infection by one of the human papilloma viruses. Common areas of involvement are the hands and face where they appear as an elevated lesion with a rough keratinized surface. On the soles of the feet they are depressed into the skin to form plantar warts.

Histologically, hyperplasia of the epithelium and hyperkeratosis are seen. Many of the epidermal cells are large and vacuolated, giving an empty appearance. Basophilic viral inclusion bodies are seen in the cornified cells of the epidermis.

Verruca plana

The plane wart occurs as a smooth topped papule and is caused by one of the human papilloma viruses. Histologically, there is hyperplasia of the epidermis but no inclusion bodies are seen.

Condylomata acuminata

Condylomata acuminata or genital warts occur as multiple, cauliflower-like, exophytic lesions in the perineal and vulval regions and on the glans penis. They are also caused by one of the human papilloma viruses. Histologically, there is hyperplasia of the epidermis and characteristically the cells are swollen and pale due to intracellular oedema. Numerous mitotic figures may be present due to the rapid rate of growth and in sections which are cut obliquely the lesion has occasionally been mistaken for squamous carcinoma.

Giant condylomata of Buschke and Loewenstein

This entity is possibly due to a viral infection and appears as a very large genital wart. Its importance is that it often recurs after excision and in some cases it may become malignant.

Molluscum contagiosum

Molluscum contagiosum is a common lesion caused by a pox virus. Clinically, it is seen most commonly in children on the skin or mucous membranes. The typical clinical appearance of clusters of pearly pink elevated papules, each with a central punctum, is diagnostic in many cases and biopsy may be avoided. Single lesions in adults may, however, require biopsy. Histologically, there is thickening of the epidermis. Individual cells of the epidermis contain characteristic inclusion bodies; towards the base of the epidermis these are strongly eosinophilic but they become more basophilic near the surface and finally are cast off onto the surface as the dense basophilic molluscum bodies which are histologically diagnostic (*see Fig.* 17.2).

Most lesions involute and disappear after about two months.

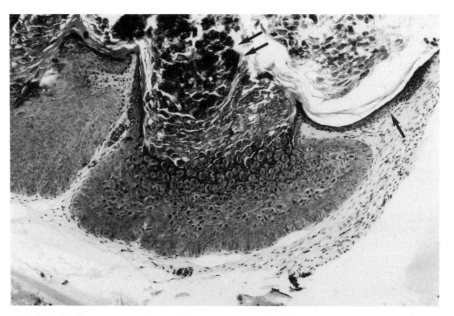

Fig. 17.2. Molluscum contagiosum. One arrow, normal epidermis; two arrows, molluscum bodies. (H and E × 75)

Skin Cysts

The two common types of skin cysts are the epidermal inclusion cyst and the pilar (tricholemmal) cyst. The term sebaceous cyst is often used by pathologists to describe pilar cysts and clinicians often refer to all simple skin cysts as sebaceous cysts since pilar and epidermal cysts are clinically indistinguishable. The term sebaceous cyst should, therefore, be used with qualification.

Simple skin cysts may rupture, in which case they may stimulate a considerable inflammatory reaction due to leakage of keratin. Alternatively, they may become infected and ulcerated. Excision may be required for either of these complications or if they are unsightly or of nuisance value on combing the hair.

At the time of excision, the entire capsule should be removed to prevent recurrence.

Epidermal inclusion cysts

These may arise spontaneously or follow trauma in which case they are due to implantation of the epidermis into the dermis. Clinically, they are smooth, dome-shaped swellings which are fixed to the undersurface of the epidermis. A central keratin filled punctum may be seen. Epidermal inclusion cysts are seen most often on the face, scalp, neck and trunk.

Histologically, the cyst lining consists of keratinizing squamous epithelium in which a granular cell layer is present (i.e. it is similar to normal epidermis). The cyst contains keratin (*see Fig.* 17.3).

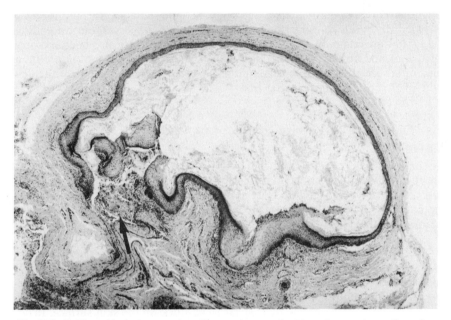

Fig. 17.3. Epidermal inclusion cyst. A small area of rupture has given rise to a giant cell reaction to keratin (arrow). (H and E × 7)

Pilar cysts

Most pilar cysts occur on the scalp. In some patients they may be inherited as an autosomal dominant trait in which case they are frequently multiple.

Clinically, they are identical to epidermal inclusion cysts. Histologically, the cyst is lined by swollen cells which resemble the normal lining of hair follicles. The contained material is amorphous and does not show the layering characteristic of an epidermal inclusion cyst.

Dermoid cysts

These are found most commonly on the head and neck, especially around the eyes. They are probably the result of sequestration of skin into the dermis around embryological lines of closure.

Histologically, they are similar to epidermal inclusion cysts with the important difference that skin appendages, such as hair follicles and sweat glands, are seen in the wall.

Unlike dermoid cysts of the ovary, they are composed only of mature ectoderm and are not of germ cell origin.

Ganglions

These are subcutaneous cystic swellings which invariably have a connection with a joint or occasionally a tendon sheath and can be regarded as synovial hernias. They are probably degenerative in origin, although some authorities have suggested that they are benign tumours of tendon sheath or joint capsule. Ganglions contain viscous fluid and may be unilobulated or multilobulated. Histologically, the cyst wall is composed of fibrous tissue without an epithelial lining. They are common on the dorsum of the wrist but may also be found on the finger, foot and ankle. Cosmetic effects, pain and nerve compression are indications for surgery. Recurrence is common if excision is incomplete or if the defect in the joint capsule is not closed.

Benign Tumours of the Epidermis

Skin tag

The simple skin tag or fibro-epithelial polyp is not a true epithelial neoplasm. They appear as soft filiform projections or as pedunculated bag-like structures on the neck, axilla, trunk and thighs. They are particularly common in elderly patients. Histologically, they are composed of a fibrovascular core with overlying simple squamous epithelium.

Basal cell papilloma (seborrhoeic keratosis)

This is a very common benign tumour occurring in middle-aged and elderly patients as tan-coloured plaques on the skin. The surface tends to be greasy and irregular. They are superficial and appear to be stuck on the skin surface. In some cases pigmentation is marked and confusion with a malignant melanoma is possible.

Histologically, the lesion is a proliferation of cells which are similar to the basal cells of the epidermis. Within these sheets of cells are cysts filled with keratin (horn cysts) which are characteristic of the lesion. The base is fairly flat and level with the base of the surrounding normal epidermis (thus giving the superficial, stuck-on appearance) (see Fig. 17.4).

The irritated basal cell papilloma is a well recognized variant. The irritation may be due to infection or trauma and results in the formation of whorls of squamous cells within the sheets of basal cells. In some cases this may be misdiagnosed as squamous carcinoma, although the presence of horn cysts indicates the true nature of the condition.

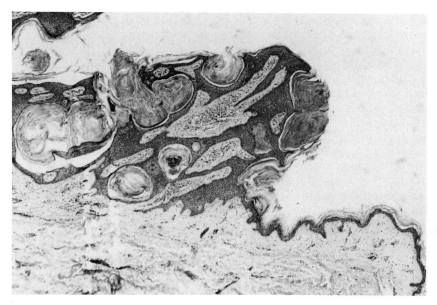

Fig. 17.4. Basal cell papilloma (seborrhoeic keratosis). Note that the base of the lesion is at the same level as the base of the epidermis, thus accounting for the characteristic 'stuck on' gross appearance. (H and E × 30)

Basal cell papillomas do not require treatment unless they are unsightly or become painful due to irritation. On rare occasions, multiple basal cell papillomas may be an indication of internal malignancy.

Keratoacanthoma

The importance of keratoacanthoma is that it may be confused macroscopically and microscopically with a squamous cell carcinoma. Keratoacanthomas are rapidly growing but self-limiting benign tumours which occur most commonly on skin exposed to sunlight, especially the face. Patients are usually middle-aged. If not excised, the tumour goes through a phase of rapid growth, lasting 6–8 weeks, followed by a period of resolution lasting also about 6–8 weeks. There may be a short static period between these two phases. Any lesion diagnosed as keratoacanthoma clinically which lasts more than three months without showing signs of resolution should be regarded as a squamous carcinoma and excised without further delay.

The cause is unknown; a viral aetiology has been suggested but not proven. It is thought most likely that they arise from hair follicles.

Grossly, a keratoacanthoma appears as a small red lump which quickly grows into a pale dome-shaped mass with a typical central keratin plug which is eventually extruded as the lesion regresses.

Histological examination at low magnification shows a roughly symmetrical exophytic cup-shaped lesion containing a central core of keratin. The surrounding normal epithelium is raised around it to form a characteristic shoulder, important for the diagnosis. Tongues of squamous epithelium push into the dermis from the base and sides. These squamous cells are large and have glassy cytoplasm and, although mitotic figures are commonly seen, pleomorphism is not a feature. The distinction from a squamous carcinoma is made by virtue of the shoulder of surrounding epithelium, the cup-shaped symmetry and the lack of pleomorphism.

It is important to excise the lesion completely in order to appreciate these features and make the diagnosis. A curette of the lesion may show only infiltrating strands of squamous cells which are indistinguishable from squamous carcinoma and this may lead to the wrong diagnosis.

The relationship between keratoacanthoma and squamous carcinoma is unknown. Some authorities claim that transition from keratoacanthoma to squamous carcinoma is common, while others claim the reverse. However, it is postulated that keratoacanthomas regress by virtue of the host immunological reaction and if this defence is defective, as in the immunosuppressed patient, the lesion may become chronic and locally aggressive.

Pre-malignant Conditions of the Epidermis

Actinic keratosis

This appears as a focal area of redness or scaling on exposed solar damaged skin. It is a common condition affecting mainly fair-skinned individuals. Histologically, there are three characteristic features: (1) alternating columns of parakeratosis (retention of nuclei in the keratin layer) and hyperkeratosis on the skin surface; (2) dysplastic cells in an atrophic epithelium which can amount to severe dysplasia or carcinoma-in-situ, and (3) solar (actinic) damage in the dermis. Although dysplasia is present, the natural history of actinic keratosis is long and very few cases progress to invasive squamous carcinoma.

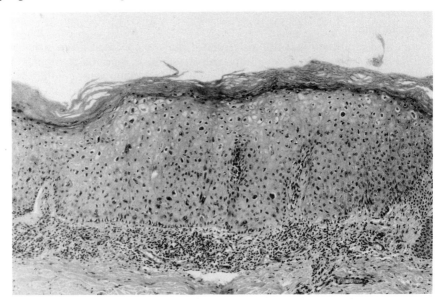

Fig. 17.5. Bowen's disease of the epidermis. (H and E × 75)

Bowen's disease

This is an in situ (intra-epidermal) squamous carcinoma. Clinically it appears as a reddened, scaly, slightly raised plaque. It can be confused with actinic keratosis or with a localized patch of psoriasis, although the latter two conditions have thicker and more adherent scales.

Histologically, the normal layering of squamous epithelium is completely lost and replaced by atypical cells (see Fig. 17.5). Some of these atypical cells are pale and very large. Dysplasia may extend into hair follicles—an important point, since it makes topical therapy less effective. If infiltrating carcinoma occurs, it does so after a long time (15–20 years). About 5% of cases show evidence of invasion at the time of removal. There is some evidence that Bowen's disease is associated with internal malignancy in the respiratory or gastrointestinal tract.

Arsenical and tar keratoses

These are similar to actinic keratosis. In arsenical keratosis, much of the body surface may be affected and multiple squamous carcinomas may develop.

Cutaneous horn

Usually found in the elderly, the horn may be associated with surrounding inflammatory changes. Carcinomatous change has been rarely reported. However, a squamous carcinoma can masquerade as a cutaneous horn and many surgeons advocate excision of all cutaneous horns with histological examination of the base.

Malignant Tumours of the Epidermis

Squamous cell carcinoma

In the UK, squamous cell carcinomas (epitheliomas) tend to affect middle-aged and elderly patients. In countries with sunny climates, such as Australia, the peak incidence is at a younger age and the condition tends to occur in people of Northern European stock.

Carcinoma may arise *de novo* or there may be underlying factors such as actinic keratosis (due to chronic exposure to sunlight), Bowen's disease, radiation injury, chronic ulceration or sinus formation, contact with chemicals such as organic hydrocarbons and the ingestion of arsenicals.

Morphology

Squamous carcinomas tend to occur on the exposed parts of the skin, such as the nose, ear, lip, forehead, etc., although they do occur on non-exposed parts relatively more frequently than basal cell carcinomas. Grossly, the early lesion often appears as an area of keratosis which when picked off leaves a small oozing ulcer. Later, the lesion becomes more widely ulcerated and the edges become raised and indurated. Features of one of the underlying conditions mentioned above may be seen in the surrounding tissue. Occasionally, squamous carcinoma may appear as an inflammatory area, similar to a carbuncle, and these so-called inflammatory squamous carcinomas are poorly differentiated histologically. The regional lymph nodes may be enlarged due to either metastases or to infection in the malignant ulcer.

Histologically, tongues of squamous cells breach the basement membrane of the epidermis and invade the dermis. In well differentiated cases, the cells are easily recognized as squamous and have a pale-coloured nucleus and eosinophilic cytoplasm. Intercellular bridges, characteristic of squamous cells, can be seen on light microscopy (*see Fig.* 17.6). The cells tend to form circular islands with central keratinization (keratin pearls). Less well differentiated tumours are composed of small dark cells with poor keratin pearl formation.

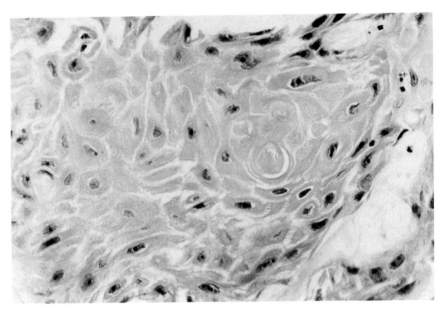

Fig. 17.6. Squamous cell carcinoma showing intercellular bridges. (H and E × 300)

Several histological variants are recognized:

1. The spindle cell squamous carcinoma is a variant of the poorly differentiated squamous carcinoma. Spindle cells are seen arising from the epidermis but usually some evidence of squamous differentiation can be identified in part of the lesion.
2. Verrucous carcinomas are slowly growing squamous lesions occurring in the mouth, on the genitalia and occasionally elsewhere on the skin. They are fungating tumours which invade deeply and extensively but only rarely metastasize.

Spread and prognosis

The TNM staging system for squamous cell carcinoma of the skin is shown in *Table* 17.1.

Table 17.1. TNM staging system for squamous carcinoma of the skin

Tis	Pre-invasive carcinoma (carcinoma-in-situ)
T0	No evidence of primary tumour
T1	Tumour 2 cm or less in its largest dimension, strictly superficial or exophytic
T2	Tumour more than 2 cm but not more than 5 cm in its largest dimension or with minimal infiltration of the dermis, irrespective of size
T3	Tumour more than 5 cm in its largest dimension or with deep infiltration of the dermis, irrespective of size
T4	Tumour with extension to other structures such as cartilage, muscle or bone
N0	No evidence of regional lymph node involvement
N1	Evidence of involvement of movable homolateral regional lymph nodes
N2	Evidence of involvement of movable contralateral or bilateral regional lymph nodes
N3	Evidence of involvement of fixed regional lymph nodes
M0	No evidence of distant metastases
M1	Evidence of distant metastases

Distant metastases from squamous carcinomas are unusual and occur in only 3% of cutaneous lesions, although they are said to be more common in carcinomas arising in ulcers, burns or scars (up to 30%). About 11% of mucocutaneous lesions metastasize (Moller *et al* 1979). Those arising on the pinna, vulva or penis tend to be more aggressive than those elsewhere. Pathological features which determine the likelihood of metastases are histological grade (well, moderately or poorly differentiated), depth of invasion, bulk of tumour and vascular invasion.

Treatment of early lesions can be with surgical excision or radiotherapy with excellent results (90% five year survival). Those with lymph node involvement require more extensive surgery with block dissection of local lymph nodes. Radiation should be avoided for lesions on the pinna (risk of radionecrosis) and scalp (hair loss). If the lesion is excised, at least 1 cm of margin must be removed.

Basal cell carcinoma

This is the commonest malignant skin tumour. As with squamous carcinoma, it occurs in middle-aged and elderly patients in temperate climates, although the peak age incidence is lower in sunny climates.

The most important aetiological factor is sunlight, although cases have been described following arsenic ingestion and occasionally injury. Patients with the rare basal cell naevus syndrome (autosomal dominant) develop multiple basal cell carcinomas.

The cell of origin is unknown although the most likely candidates are the basal cells of the epidermis or the epithelium of hair follicles.

Morphology

The common appearance is a raised nodule with a characteristic waxy appearance, on the surface of which tiny vessels are seen (*see Fig.* 17.7). Central regression may cause depression or umbilication of the surface and later a true ulcer with typical rolled, pearly edges is seen (rodent ulcer). Several variants are recognized on gross examination: (1) the pigmented type may be confused with a malignant melanoma although the characteristic surface vessels are not seen in the latter; (2) some undergo cystic change; (3) multifocal basal cell carcinomas may present as a diffuse erythematous scaly patch; (4) sclerosing types are seen as white fibrous plaques; (5) the so-called cicatrizing or field-fire type has a central white scarred zone, surrounded by a red scaly peripheral zone.

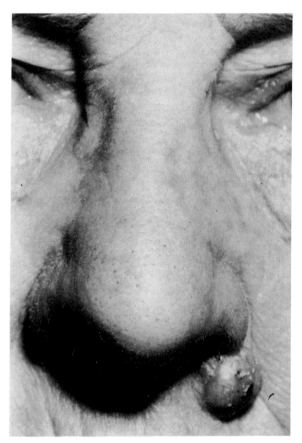

Fig. 17.7. Basal cell carcinoma. Tiny vessels can just be seen on the surface.

Microscopically, the classical basal cell carcinoma shows islands of basal cells arising from the overlying epidermis. The basal cells have ovoid darkly staining nuclei and little cytoplasm. They tend to line up in a regular fashion at the periphery of the islands of tumour cells to form palisading which is typical of the tumour (*see Fig.* 17.8). Between the islands of tumour cells is a fibrous tissue stroma. Several histological variants are recognized: (1) the cystic type in which the spaces are due to central degeneration of cells; (2) the pigmented type in which pigment is seen within macrophages in the stroma; (3) the multifocal type which

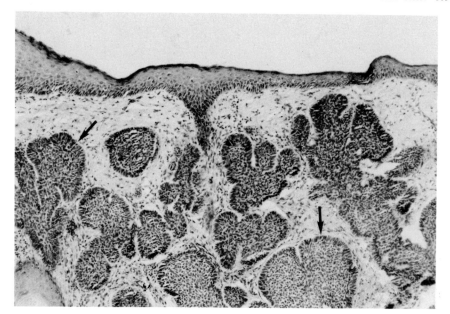

Fig. 17.8. Basal cell carcinoma. Note the palisading around the nests of tumour cells (arrows). (H and E × 30)

shows multiple, widely dispersed buds of tumour arising at many points along the dermal–epidermal junction; (4) the sclerosing (morphea) type which has sparsely placed strands of tumour cells infiltrating deeply and surrounded by dense fibrous stroma; (5) the infiltrating type which shows wide and deep infiltration. In addition to these sub-types, some tumours exhibit areas of differentiation into squamous, sebaceous or other cell types.

A further sub-type, important because of its aggressive behaviour, is the metatypical basal cell carcinoma. In this condition, nests of plump polygonal cells with little peripheral palisading are seen. These tumours are also known as basi-squamous tumours, although this term may lead to confusion with the ordinary basal cell carcinoma which has simple squamous differentiation.

Spread and prognosis

Local invasion of bone or cartilage may be seen in neglected cases. Metastases from a basal cell carcinoma are exceedingly rare and when they do occur they are likely to be from a metatypical (basi-squamous) type.

Local recurrence of basal cell carcinoma is more likely in the infiltrating, multifocal and sclerosing types than in the more common varieties.

When assessing the limit of excision histologically, it is important to include the fibrous stroma as part of the tumour. One study found a recurrence rate of 5·7% when the margins were clear and 24·4% when they were involved (Taylor and Barisoni 1973). Clear margins of at least 5 mm are advisable.

Treatment by surgical excision or radiotherapy gives good results. Cryotherapy and topical 5-fluorouracil have also been used for multiple lesions. An absolute indication for surgery is the recurrence of a previously irradiated tumour.

Disorders of Melanocytes

It is widely accepted that cutaneous melanocytes originate in the neural crest and migrate to their position in the basal layer of the epidermis during embryological life. Here, they are seen as cells with dark nuclei and clear cytoplasm. Their function is to produce melanin which they pass on to the surrounding epithelial cells in order to protect them from ultraviolet light. Abnormalities of melanocytes may give rise to a series of benign and malignant conditions.

The benign lesions have a characteristic natural history. Firstly, there is proliferation of melanocytes at the dermal–epidermal junction to form 'junctional activity'. Then melanocytes 'drop off' the epidermis into the dermis where they become known as naevus cells. At this stage there is both a junctional component and a dermal component and the lesion is termed a compound naevus. Next, the junctional activity ceases, leaving only a dermal component—the intradermal naevus (*see Fig.* 17.9). Finally, the naevus cells disappear and become incorporated

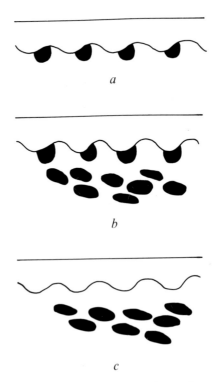

Fig. 17.9. Schematic representation of the three main types of naevus: *a*, junctional: *b*, compound; *c*, intradermal (*see* text).

into the fibrous tissue of the dermis. Distinct varieties of benign naevi, arising from epidermal melanocytes, are the spindle-cell (Spitz) naevus and the halo naevus.

During embryological migration, some melanocytes do not reach the epidermis and remain within the dermis. These melanocytes give rise to the Mongolian spot and to the blue naevus.

Congenital naevi are present at or shortly after birth and have certain features which distinguish them from acquired naevi and these will be described later.

Dysplastic naevi are an important subgroup discussed later.

Junctional naevus

These are the common moles in prepubertal children, appearing as flat, hairless, well-defined brown patches. On close inspection the normal skin markings are present and this distinguishes them from melanomas.

Histologically, the lesion is characterized by a focal proliferation of melanocytes which still remain in contact with the epidermis. This is known as junctional activity. These lesions usually evolve into compound and then intradermal naevi and very few become malignant.

Compound naevus

These are seen commonly in adolescents as dark brown or black, elevated or nodular lesions. They may be hair-bearing and the nodularity may lead to confusion with a malignant melanoma.

Histologically, as well as junctional activity, nests of naevus cells are seen in the dermis. The cells become smaller as they progress more deeply into the dermis. This is known as 'maturation' and when seen in a naevus it is strong evidence that it is benign. Most of these develop into intradermal naevi and very few undergo malignant change.

Intradermal naevus

This is the mature mole of adults. Grossly, the appearance is variable. It can be flat, raised, nodular or pedunculated. It may be pigmented or non-pigmented and hairs may or may not be seen (*see Fig.* 17.10).

Histologically, there is no junctional activity and naevus cells are seen only in the dermis. They form nests in the superficial part of the lesion and in the deeper parts they become more diffuse. Intradermal naevi virtually never undergo malignant change.

Spindle cell (Spitz) naevus

This lesion is also known as a juvenile melanoma which is an unsatisfactory term as it can occur in adults and is benign.

Grossly, it appears as a raised lesion, often on the face. It is a characteristic reddish-brown colour.

The great importance of this variety of naevus is that it can easily be confused histologically with malignant melanoma.

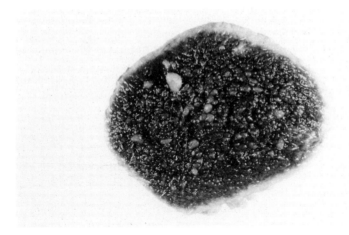

Fig. 17.10. Intradermal naevus. A raised warty pigmented hair bearing lesion.

It is a variant of the compound naevus and has both junctional activity and intradermal components. Bundles of spindle-shaped melanocytes are seen in the dermis. Other naevus cells which resemble epithelial cells are also seen. Although mitotic figures are common, the lesion does not show the irregular or nodular invading edge of a malignant melanoma.

Halo naevus

The classic clinical appearance is of a brown naevus surrounded by an area of skin depigmentation (the halo). The depigmented area appears to be due to immunological destruction of melanocytes. Histologically, therefore, the appearance is of a compound or intradermal naevus with a heavy lymphocytic infiltration. Since a lymphocytic infiltrate is a feature of malignant melanoma, it is important that the surgeon informs the pathologist of the clinical appearance.

Blue naevus

The blue naevus is a small pigmented tumour derived from dermal melanocytes and confined to the dermis. On histological examination, the lesion is seen to be wedge-shaped with the apex pointing deeply. High power microscopic examination shows spindle-shaped melanocytes and numerous deeply pigmented melanophages which contain coarsely clumped granules of melanin.

A variant, the cellular blue naevus, occurs frequently on the wrists and buttocks as a raised pink, often amelanotic nodule. It is composed of bundles of densely packed spindle-shaped cells. Malignant transformation is very rare.

Congenital naevus

These vary widely in size from a small spot to a large area (giant congenital naevus) which may be in the bathing trunk distribution. They may be melanotic or amelanotic and in the later stages they become hairy (giant hairy naevus). Histologically, there are usually abnormal skin appendages present in addition to the naevus cells, suggesting that the condition is a hamartoma. The superficial part of the naevus is similar to an acquired compound naevus as described above. The distinguishing feature of the congenital naevus is that deep in the dermis the naevus cells form nests in the sheaths of hair follicles and in association with sebaceous glands and ducts.

Congenital naevi are said to be more prone to undergo malignant change than other naevi (*see* later).

Dysplastic naevus (Greene *et al.* 1985)

Certain patients have naevi which are atypical both clinically and histologically. These dysplastic naevi may occur familially or non-familially and their importance is that affected patients have an increased risk of developing malignant melanomas.

Dysplastic naevi differ clinically from normal naevi in that they are larger, more irregular in shape, indistinctly bordered and variably pigmented. They are commonest on the trunk but tend also to occur in unusual sites such as the scalp, buttocks and breast.

Histologically, the melanocytes at the dermal–epidermal junction are large and atypical and a lymphocytic infiltrate is seen in the dermis.

Patients with the familial form have a family history of atypical moles and malignant melanomas (B–K mole syndrome or familial atypical mole/malignant melanoma syndrome). They have a cumulative lifetime incidence of melanoma approaching 100% and it is estimated that 5–10% of all malignant melanomas occur in patients who have a family history of the disease. Patients with the sporadic form of the disease are at less risk from developing malignant melanoma.

Patients with atypical moles should be carefully followed up and any moles which change in appearance should be excised.

Malignant melanoma

A melanoma is a malignant tumour of melanocytes. It accounts for 1–3% of all malignant tumours and the incidence is increasing throughout the world (Editorial 1985). This rise is confined to cutaneous malignant melanoma; the incidence of extracutaneous melanomas is probably constant. The reported incidence is highest in Queensland (35/100 000). In Australia, the incidence in males and females is equal and in most of Europe males predominate (2 : 1) (although in the UK an excess in females has been reported). The incidence increases with advancing age although the condition has been reported in babies. Melanomas are multiple in 1–4% of patients. They tend to occur on the trunk in males and on the legs in females. Several factors have been implicated in the aetiology and pathogenesis.

1. ULTRAVIOLET LIGHT: There is much evidence that exposure to sunlight increases the incidence of melanoma. Lentigo maligna melanoma (*see* below) tends to occur on the exposed skin of the face due to the cumulative effect of sunlight over many

years. Short, intermittent exposure to sunlight may predispose to the other varieties.

2. PRE-EXISTING NAEVUS: The relationship between a pre-existing mole or naevus and a malignant melanoma is uncertain. Since malignant melanomas are rare and naevi are very common, it follows that moles rarely undergo malignant change although, conversely, evidence of a pre-existing mole can be identified in about 20% of malignant melanomas. In junctional and compound naevi, melanocytes are still undergoing active cell division in the junctional area and these are thought to be the most likely types of naevi to undergo malignant change. Intradermal naevi which have no junctional component almost never undergo malignant change.

The features of a mole which suggest malignant transformation are given in *Table* 17.2.

Table 17.2. Changes in a mole which suggest malignant transformation (adapted from Davis 1982)

Size	— enlargement
Outline	— becomes irregular (indented and notched)
Colour	— becomes darker, then there is irregularity of colour with various shades of brown, black, pink, etc.
Elevation	— becomes thicker and nodular
Surface	— normal skin markings are lost
Surroundings	— lumps in surrounding tissue may be satellite tumours
Symptoms	— tingling, serous discharge, recurrent minor bleeding

Morphology

The vast majority of melanomas arise from the melanocytes in the basal zone of the epidermis. Melanomas characteristically have two phases of growth which overlap: (1) the radial growth phase, and (2) the vertical growth phase. In the initial or radial phase, the atypical melanocytes spread radially within the epidermis where they can take up one of two patterns: (1) lentiginous, in which case there is a diffuse replacement of the basal layer of the epithelium by melanocytes, and (2) aggregated, in which nests of atypical melanocytes are seen at various points along the dermal–epidermal junction. While the malignant melanocytes are confined to the epidermis, the lesion is said to be pre-invasive, pre-malignant or Clark level 1 (*see Fig.* 17.15 later). The vertical phase is characterized by invasion of the dermis as the lesion then becomes an invasive malignant melanoma. A dense lymphocytic infiltrate occurs, probably as a result of an immunological reaction to the invading cells. Several sub-types are recognized.

LENTIGO MALIGNA MELANOMA: The common clinical presentation of the pre-invasive stage of this lesion is a pigmented (blue or black) irregular flat lesion, most often on the face of an elderly patient. This is termed lentigo maligna or Hutchinson's melanotic freckle (*see Fig.* 17.11). In an unknown proportion, invasive melanoma occurs and the lesion is then termed lentigo maligna melanoma.

Grossly, the onset of invasive malignancy is seen as nodularity and an increased irregularity of outline.

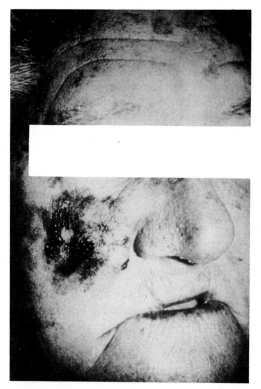

Fig. 17.11. Lentigo maligna.

Histologically, lentigo maligna is seen as a diffuse continuous replacement of the basal layer of the epidermis by atypical melanocytes. Lentigo maligna melanoma is characterized by dermal invasion of melanocytes occurring in an area of lentigo maligna. This is associated with a dense lymphocytic infiltration and the epidermis is generally thinned and atrophic. There is associated solar damage in the dermis. About 7% of malignant melanomas are of this type. Lymph node metastases are rare and occur late.

SUPERFICIAL SPREADING MELANOMA: This is the commonest variety of melanoma (64%). They are seen as skin nodules with a variegated colour and irregular edge. Intermittent itch is a common symptom (*see Fig.* 17.12).

The radial phase of this variety shows nests of atypical melanocytes at the dermal–epidermal junction and, also, melanocytes invading upwards into the epidermis. Thus, superficial spreading melanoma can be distinguished histologically from lentigo maligna melanoma by examination of the surrounding epidermis in most cases. When only the radial phase is present, the lesion is an '*in situ* superficial spreading melanoma'. When invasion of the dermis occurs, the lesion becomes an invasive superficial spreading melanoma.

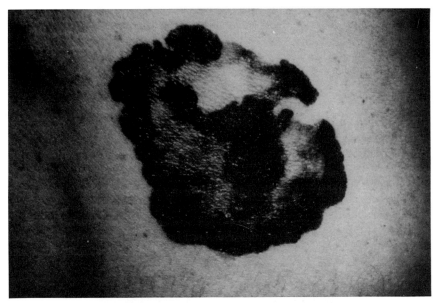

Fig. 17.12. Superficial spreading melanoma. Note the irregular edge and variegated appearance.

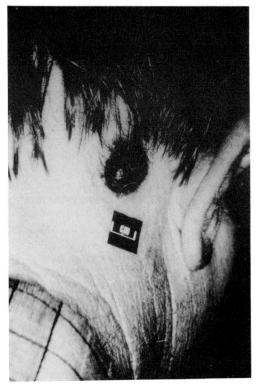

Fig. 17.13. Nodular melanoma.

NODULAR MELANOMA: This accounts for about 28% of all cases of melanoma. It presents as a palpable lump in the skin (*see Fig.* 17.13) which can be melanotic or amelanotic (although usually some pigment is present at the base and this can be seen clinically). There is a very short radial growth phase and therefore a history of an enlarging pigmented mole is not usually obtained. Itch and bleeding are frequent and ulceration occurs early.

Histologically, the malignant melanocytes are seen invading upwards into the epidermis, causing ulceration, and downwards into the dermis. No *in-situ* change is seen in the surrounding epidermis and this distinguishes the lesion from the previous two types. Lymph node metastases occur more frequently in the nodular than in the superficial spreading type.

ACRAL LENTIGINOUS MELANOMA: These occur in sites of thick epidermis, especially the soles of the feet (*see Fig.* 17.14). The radial phase may have characteristics of both lentigo maligna melanoma and superficial spreading melanoma. The basal layer of the epidermis is replaced by large atypical melanocytes and these tend to spread upwards into the epidermis and downwards into the dermis. It has a bad prognosis.

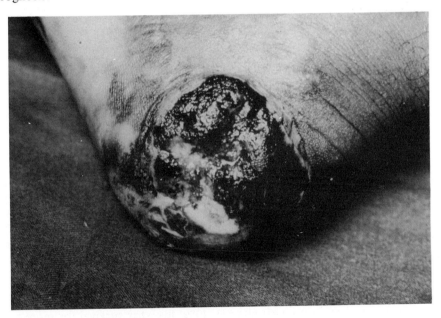

Fig. 17.14. Acral lentiginous melanoma.

RARE VARIETIES: A proportion of malignant melanomas do not have the typical features of one of the above sub-types and they remain unclassified. A desmoplastic melanoma is a distinct variety in which there is a massive desmoplastic reaction with fibroblastic proliferation in the dermis. It has a poor prognosis. Neurotrophic melanomas have an unusual predilection to infiltrate nerves. Masses of spindle-shaped cells tend to blend with the peripheral nerves giving a picture which is occasionally similar to a traumatic neuroma.

Spread and staging

Spread is initially to the regional lymph nodes. Cutaneous metastatic deposits may be seen between the tumour and the regional lymph nodes (in-transit lesions). The incidence of regional nodal metastases rises with the depth of invasion of the primary tumour. Nodal metastases are found in 29%, 42% and 58% of patients with Clark levels 3, 4 and 5 respectively. Later, haematogenous spread takes place to the liver, lung and brain.

The clinical staging of melanoma, based largely on the presence or absence of metastases, is given in *Table* 17.3.

Table 17.3. Staging of malignant melanoma (adapted from Adam and Efron 1983)

Stage I
 —localized melanoma, without metastasis to distant or regional nodes
 —multiple primary melanomas
 —locally recurrent melanoma within 4 cm of the primary site

Stage II
 —metastasis limited to regional lymph nodes
 —primary melanoma present or removed with simultaneous metastasis
 —primary melanoma controlled with subsequent metastasis
 —locally recurrent melanoma with metastasis
 —in-transit metastasis beyond 4 cm from the primary site

Stage III
 —disseminated melanoma
 —visceral and/or multiple lymphatic metastases
 —multiple cutaneous and/or subcutaneous metastases

Prognosis

The most important factor in determining the prognosis of melanoma is the tumour thickness (measured from the granular cell layer of the epidermis to the deepest, easily identifiable tumour cell). Breslow (1970) showed that the thickness, measured in this way, is inversely proportional to the five year survival rate. The Clark level of invasion (*see Fig.* 17.15) is also reported by pathologists. This has greater inter-observer variation than the Breslow thickness.

The ten year survival rates for Stage I disease, according to tumour thickness, are given in *Table* 17.4.

For clinical Stage II, the survival rate depends on the number of involved nodes (five year survival for one involved node, 40%; five year survival for more than three nodes, 15%).

When assessing the prognostic importance of other factors it is essential to make a statistical adjustment for tumour thickness. Factors of independent prognostic significance include sex (women have a better prognosis) and age (patients under 50 years old do better). Mackie and Young (1984) found that lesions on the back, upper arms, neck, shoulders, palms, soles and midline do worse than those at other sites. The presence of a pre-existing naevus may be associated with a better prognosis. All of these factors are of little significance when compared with tumour thickness.

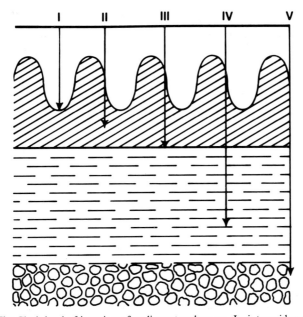

Fig. 17.15. The Clark level of invasion of malignant melanoma. I—intraepidermal; II—papillary dermis; III—interface between papillary and reticular dermis; IV—reticular dermis; V—subcutaneous fat. (Adapted from MacKie 1984.)

Table 17.4. Prognosis of Stage I malignant melanoma according to tumour thickness

Tumour thickness	10-year survival
< 0·75 mm	98–99%
0·75–1·50 mm	90%
1·5–3·0 mm	70%
3·0–4·5 mm	60%
> 4·5 mm	30%

Vascular Lesions of the Skin

Vascular ectasias

These lesions are localized dilatations of preformed vessels. They are, therefore, not true tumours.

Naevus flammeus (salmon patch)

This is the common birth mark. It is seen as a flat pink, red or purple patch, most often on the face and neck of new born infants. Fifty per cent of infants have a birth mark and most have resolved by one year, although remnants may be seen in adult life. Histologically, there is simple dilatation of the vessels of the dermis.

Port wine stain

The port wine stain is a variant of the naevus flammeus which starts as a flat red patch, often on the face, involving areas of the trigeminal distribution. However, instead of regressing, it grows with the child, becoming elevated and unsightly. Histologically, there is, however, only dilatation of the vessels and none of the proliferation of vessels seen in haemangiomas (which are considered to be true benign neoplasms). They show no tendency to regress. Some may be associated with the Sturge–Weber syndrome (port wine stains over the trigeminal distribution, vascular malformations of the leptomeninges and intracerebral calcification).

Spider naevus

This is the name given to a small cutaneous arteriole from which small vessels radiate. Pressure causes blanching and release of pressure allows refilling which characteristically takes place in a radial direction. They are a common finding in pregnancy and in patients with liver failure.

Haemangiomas

Haemangiomas are benign vascular tumours; several types are seen in the skin.

Capillary haemangioma

Capillary haemangiomas are the commonest variety of haemangioma and they usually appear in the first year of life. They are seen as elevated purple or red soft nodules, often on the head or neck. Histologically, they are composed of lobules of proliferating capillaries.

Juvenile haemangioma

A juvenile haemangioma is a clinical variant of the capillary haemangioma in which there is a characteristic natural history. It begins as a flat lesion in the first few weeks of life and undergoes a rapid growth phase which lasts several months, by which time the lesion is elevated and protruding (the strawberry naevus). This is followed by regression, the majority having involuted to leave a small brown spot by the age of seven years. Histologically, in the proliferating phase, numerous capillaries with plump endothelial lining cells are seen. The endothelial cells may be so swollen that the vascular channels are obliterated. Later, the endothelium becomes flattened and the lesion resembles an ordinary capillary haemangioma as described above.

Cavernous haemangioma

These are less common than the capillary haemangiomas, although they also occur in childhood, especially on the head and neck. Their gross appearance depends on the location within the skin. Superficial lesions are blue puffy masses, whereas the deep ones may not impart any abnormal colour to the skin. Histologically, dilated thin walled vessels with flattened endothelial linings are seen. They are usually present at birth, or appear soon after, and are more common in female infants. They may infiltrate adjacent structures.

Cavernous haemangiomas do not usually regress and therefore, if unsightly, they require treatment.

Pyogenic granuloma

Pyogenic granulomas were originally considered to be infective lesions although they are now thought to represent a variant of capillary haemangioma. They develop rapidly, reaching a size of 1–2 cm within a few weeks. In one-third of cases there is a history of trauma. The gross appearance is of a polypoid red friable mass which is ulcerated and bleeds easily. The common sites are the mucous membrane of the mouth, especially the tongue, the fingers and the face. They can occur at any age.

Histologically, they are exophytic growths which have the structure of a capillary haemangioma. The superficial part, near the area of ulceration, is heavily inflamed and has the appearance of granulation tissue. The base of the lesion is well circumscribed and this helps to differentiate it from angiosarcoma and Kaposi's sarcoma, both of which have infiltrating edges with tongues of tumour invading between collagen bundles.

Glomus Tumour

Glomus tumours are derived from the glomus body (see p. 494).

The classical clinical presentation of a glomus tumour is as a haemorrhagic spot under a finger or toe-nail which gives paroxysms of severe pain. Those occurring elsewhere appear as small, subcutaneous nodules. In some instances, nothing is seen grossly and the diagnosis depends on histological examination of the painful area of skin. The patient who complains of severe pain localized to one spot on the finger but with no visible abnormalities should not, therefore, be dismissed until a glomus tumour has been excluded.

Histologically, branching blood vessels are seen between which are the proliferating glomus cells. These are round or cuboidal cells with sharply defined cell bodies and central pale staining nuclei. Surgical excision is the treatment of choice.

Skin Appendage Tumours

The two main skin appendages are the pilosebaceous units and the eccrine sweat glands. The eccrine sweat glands and any of the parts of the pilosebaceous unit may give rise to tumours, the majority of which are benign. Clinically, the benign forms often present as a lump under the skin which may be quiescent for many years and then suddenly expand and ulcerate. Only the common skin appendage tumours will be described.

Benign skin appendage tumours

Hair follicle origin

PILOMATRICOMA: A pilomatricoma is also known as a calcifying epithelioma of Malherbe. It is a well recognized common entity which occurs as a subcutaneous, often calcified, nodule located on the face or scalp of young people. Histologically, it consists of a mass of small darkly staining cells which enlarge towards the centre of the lesion and lose their nuclei to become the ghost cells which are characteristic of the condition. They eventually calcify.

Eccrine gland origin

SYRINGOMA: These are benign lesions which appear as small (1–2 mm) papules on the face (especially the lower eyelids) and abdomen. They usually appear at puberty and are often multiple.

Histologically, they consist of clumps of duct-like structures in the dermis. The ducts are lined by a double cell layer.

Apocrine gland origin

HIDRADENOMA PAPILLIFERUM: This is a benign lesion specific to the vulva and perineum where it occurs as a subcutaneous nodule. Histologically, the cysts have many branching villous processes which are covered by a double cell layer.

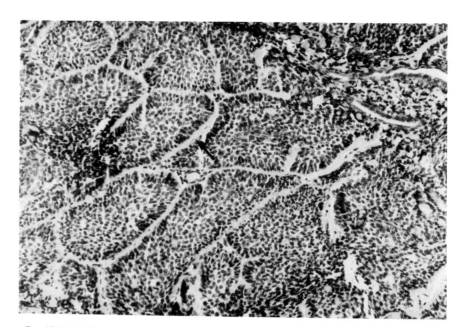

Fig. 17.16. Cylindroma. Note the thick basement membranes around the nests of tumour cells (arrow). (H and E × 75)

CYLINDROMA: These typically occur on the scalp where they may be multiple. Several large cylindromas may virtually cover the scalp and this has been given the descriptive term 'turban tumour'. Multiple tumours may be inherited in an autosomal dominant fashion. The condition is unrelated to adenoid cystic carcinoma of the salivary gland or bronchus, both of which have also been termed cylindromas in the past.

Histologically, the lesion appears as nests of darkly staining cells surrounded by characteristic thick eosinophilic basement membranes (*see Fig.* 17.16).

Malignant skin appendage tumours

Malignant hair follicle tumours are extremely rare, only a few cases having been reported.

Apocrine carcinomas are also rare but have been described in the axilla, on the areola of the nipple and on the vulva. They may be associated with extra-mammary Paget's disease of the skin.

Eccrine carcinomas may arise *de novo* or in a pre-existing benign lesion. Metastases occur commonly (over two-thirds of cases).

Sebaceous carcinomas occur most often around the eyelids although they are rare at all sites. Histologically, in the better differentiated types, areas of sebaceous differentiation are seen.

Merkel Cell Carcinoma

Merkel cells are found in normal epidermis where they may play a role in transforming mechanical stimuli into neural stimuli. Electron microscopy shows that they contain dense core granules and therefore they may be part of the diffuse neuroendocrine system.

Merkel cell carcinomas are rare tumours usually occurring in elderly patients, especially females. Clinically, they present as a nodule, often red or blue-red in colour. Histologically, they consist of trabeculae or sheets of uniform cells with a high mitotic rate. They may be confused with a cutaneous lymphoma or with a secondary deposit from an oat cell carcinoma of lung.

The tumour often recurs locally and metastasizes.

Burns

Temperatures above 40 °C cause burns of the human skin. Burns are responsible for approximately 400–500 deaths annually in the United Kingdom.

Aetiology and pathogenesis

The aetiological agents responsible for burns may be thermal, electrical or chemical. Thermal burns are the commonest with scalding of children with hot liquids and ignition of clothing in adults being typical.

Heat of low intensity (up to 45 °C) causes damage by several mechanisms, including accelerated metabolism of cells, inactivation of thermolabile enzymes and vascular injury. With increasing temperatures, protein is denatured. Up to 45 °C the changes are probably reversible but beyond this temperature, the denaturation exceeds the cells' ability to repair the damage.

Morphology

A superficial (first degree) burn involves the epidermis only and causes redness and oedema of the skin. In a few days the outer injured cells desquamate and the skin heals without scarring. The water barrier of the skin is not damaged and therefore areas of superficial burns are not included when calculating intravenous fluid replacement.

Second degree burns extend into the dermis. By definition, some epithelial elements remain and these proliferate and produce healing. Since epithelial destruction is incomplete, second degree burns may also be termed partial thickness burns and they can be subdivided into superficial and deep. In superficial partial thickness burns, some islands of the basal layer of the epidermis survive as well as skin appendages and therefore healing is relatively fast, taking 10–21 days. In deep partial thickness burns (deep dermal burns), the epidermis is completely destroyed together with the upper dermis. The only epithelial elements to remain are the linings of the hair follicles and sweat glands. Healing of deep dermal burns takes over 30 days and, if not treated with skin grafting, there may be scarring.

Second degree burns are erythematous, weeping and painful. The accumulation of fluid results in bullae. Pin prick sensation may be lost in deep dermal burns, but pressure sensation remains.

In full thickness (third degree) burns, the epidermis and dermis are both destroyed. The skin is white and inelastic or charred in adults, although in children the surface may be dark red. The surface is insensitive and dry and thrombosis of superficial vessels can be seen. The skin appendages are destroyed and therefore the burn cannot heal by re-epithelialization.

A fourth degree burn is one in which there is damage to subcutaneous tissue such as fat, bone and muscle.

Jackson (1953) demonstrated that the intensity of damage in a burn is greatest in the centre and least at the periphery. He therefore distinguishes three zones (*see Fig.* 17.17), although often one of these will predominate to the exclusion of others.

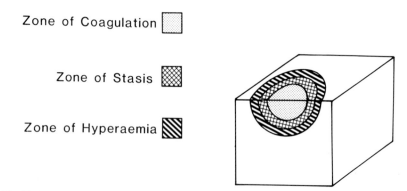

Zone of Coagulation

Zone of Stasis

Zone of Hyperaemia

Fig. 17.17. Three zones of a burn as described by Jackson (1953) (*see* text).

The central zone is coagulated and usually white. There is no circulation and the capillaries are coagulated with associated vessel thrombosis. Surrounding this is a 'zone of stasis'. The capillaries in this zone are initially dilated, but after several minutes or hours, the circulation ceases and the capillaries become stuffed with red cells. Cell death then occurs and this gives a mottled pink and white appearance. The outer zone shows hyperaemia only and does not blister although it may or may not desquamate.

Histologically, in skin which has been subjected to low intensity heat, the cells show both nuclear and cytoplasmic swelling which is the result of deranged membrane permeability. With more intense heat, the cells show nuclear pyknosis and granular coagulation of the cytoplasm. The dermis appears as an amorphous gel.

At the margin of the burn, an inflammatory response appears. There is an increase in vascular permeability with leakage of blood constituents. The increased vascular permeability is accompanied by rapid fluid loss and cell margination and emigration. Neutrophils migrate into the tissues followed by monocytes and macrophages.

Complications

FLUID LOSS: Plasma leaks from damaged capillaries into the adjacent tissues and on to the surface. If the epidermis is lost, the fluid evaporates and this is associated with body cooling due to loss of latent heat. The loss of fluid is greatly reduced by the application of a skin graft to the burn surface. Damage to cell membranes causes an increase in intracellular sodium and water with the result that further fluid is lost from the extracellular fluid (the sick cell syndrome). Fluid loss is maximal in the first 48 hours.

CARDIOVASCULAR: The fluid loss results in a drop in blood volume with consequent haemodynamic problems. A myocardial depressant factor may also be present. Apart from the haemodynamic effects of fluid shift and loss, red cell survival is decreased, red cells are lost through increased capillary permeability and the bone marrow is depressed. Platelets are initially decreased in number but, later, thrombocytosis occurs. Diffuse intravascular coagulation is occasionally a problem.

RESPIRATORY: The lungs may be directly damaged by inhalation of fumes at the time of the injury. Injury to the laryngeal and tracheobronchial mucosa may cause intense oedema with airway obstruction. Damage to the pulmonary parenchyma may lead to the adult respiratory distress syndrome (see p. 397) and to secondary infection.

The fall in cardiac output causes a ventilation/perfusion imbalance which exacerbates blood gas abnormalities. If the chest wall is burned, eschar formation may cause restriction of ventilatory movement.

SEPSIS: After the first day, the burn wound is colonized by large numbers of bacteria. These at first involve the devitalized debris on the surface of the wound, but later they spread to infect adjacent viable tissue, and this may lead to rapid spread of infection in the subcutaneous fat. Staphylococcus and Streptococcus are common infecting organisms. Gram-negative bacilli such as Pseudomonas may cause endotoxic shock.

Burns patients are prone to bacterial infection, not just because of damage to the epithelial barrier, but also because of immunological defects. T-suppressor cells appear to be activated and macrophages have an impaired phagocytic function probably due to a loss of their ability to produce fibronectin which facilitates attachment of bacteria to the cell membrane prior to phagocytosis (Robbins *et al.* 1984).

RENAL: Hypovolaemic shock may cause acute renal failure (*see* p. 224) which may be exacerbated by myoglobin release. Diffuse intravascular coagulation may also affect renal function.

GASTROINTESTINAL: The hypovolaemia causes splanchnic vasoconstriction and this contributes to the paralytic ileus which commonly is associated with major burns. Acute gastric dilatation (*see* p. 77) may exacerbate the state of shock. Acute gastric erosions or ulcers (Curling's ulcers) may cause bleeding or perforation (*see* p. 55).

Prognosis

The prognosis depends on the age of the patient and on the surface area of the burn and is shown in *Fig.* 17.18.

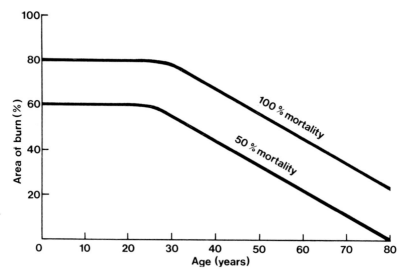

Fig. 17.18. Mortality in burns patients, according to the percentage area involved and the age. (Reproduced with permission from the publishers from Muir 1978.)

References

Adam Y. G., Efron G. (1983) Cutaneous malignant melanoma: current views on pathogenesis, diagnoses, and surgical management. *Surgery* **93**, 481–94.

Breslow A. (1970) Thickness, cross-sectional areas and depth of invasion in the prognosis of cutaneous melanoma. *Ann. Surg.* **172**, 902–8.

Davis N. C. (1982) Malignant melanoma: clinical presentation and differential diagnosis. In: Emmett A. J., O'Rourke M. G. E. (eds.) *Malignant Skin Tumours.* Edinburgh, Churchill Livingstone.

Editorial (1985) More on melanoma. *Lancet* **1**, 201–2.

Greene M. H., Clark W. H., Tucker M. A. *et al.* (1985) Acquired precursors of cutaneous malignant melanoma. *N. Engl. J. Med.* **312**, 91–7.

Jackson D. MacG. (1953) The diagnosis and depth of burning. *Br. J. Surg.* **40**, 588–96.

MacKie R. M. (1984) *Milne's Dermatopathology.* London, Edward Arnold.

MacKie R. M., Young D. (1984) Human malignant melanoma. *Int. J. Dermatol.* **23**, 433–43.

Moller R., Reymann F., Hou-Jensen K. (1979) Metastases in dermatological patients with squamous cell carcinoma. *Arch. Dermatol.* **115**, 703–5.

Muir I. F. K. (1978) Current problems in the treatment of burns. In: Hadfield J., Hobsley M. (eds.) *Current Surgical Practice,* Vol. 2. London, Edward Arnold.

Robbins S. L., Cotran R. S., Kumar V. (1984) *Pathological Basis of Disease,* 3rd ed. Philadelphia, W. B. Saunders.

Taylor G. A., Barisoni D. (1973) Ten years' experience in the surgical treatment of basal cell carcinoma. A study of factors associated with recurrence. *Br. J. Surg.* **60**, 522–5.

Chapter 18

The Soft Tissues

Abnormalities of the soft tissues will be considered in four sections. Firstly, there is a series of tumour-like conditions such as the fibromatoses and proliferative myositis. Secondly, there is a group of benign tumours of soft tissue which are truly neoplastic, such as the common lipoma. Thirdly, there is a group of tumours which are generally very slow growing but which may eventually metastasize and these are discussed under the heading of tumours of intermediate malignant potential. Finally, there are the unequivocally malignant sarcomas of soft tissues.

Tumour-like Conditions of Soft Tissues

The fibromatoses

Fibromatoses are described by Enzinger and Weiss (1983) as 'a broad group of benign fibrous tissue proliferations of similar microscope appearance that are intermediate between benign fibrous lesions and fibrosarcomas', i.e. they tend to recur but they never metastasize. Several clinical entities are seen.

PALMAR FIBROMATOSIS (DUPUYTREN'S CONTRACTURE): This is a common form of fibromatosis which affects the superficial fascia of the palm of the hand. The patient initially develops firm nodules in the palm and later fibrous cords develop between these nodules and in the fingers (especially the fourth and fifth fingers) causing flexion of the MP and PIP joints. The DIP joint is not involved (*see Fig.* 18.1). Palmar fibromatosis is often associated with other forms of fibromatosis in the same patient. There is some evidence that the lesion is commoner in diabetics, epileptics and possibly alcoholics, than in the general population.

PLANTAR FIBROMATOSIS: This is similar to palmar fibromatosis and affects the fascia of the foot.

PENILE FIBROMATOSIS (PEYRONIE'S DISEASE): This presents as a fibrous subcutaneous thickening in the shaft of the penis which causes curving. It may affect the fascial covering of the penis or the corpus cavernosum. Patients may complain of symptoms on passing urine and during intercourse (*see* p. 286).

ABDOMINAL FIBROMATOSIS (ABDOMINAL DESMOID): The abdominal desmoid tumour arises most commonly from the rectus sheath as an abdominal wall tumour. It has a strong predilection to affect young women during pregnancy or in the first year

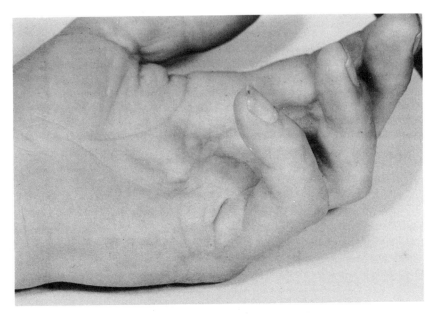

Fig. 18.1. Dupuytren's contracture.

thereafter. Being an abdominal wall (rather than intra-abdominal) tumour it is still palpable after tensing the rectus muscle. Since the tumour is locally invasive, it tends to recur and the frequency of recurrence depends on the adequacy of excision.

EXTRA-ABDOMINAL FIBROMATOSIS (EXTRA-ABDOMINAL DESMOID): This is a condition similar to the abdominal desmoid. It arises from the fascia especially around the shoulder girdle and on the chest, back and thigh. The tumour tends to be poorly circumscribed and widely infiltrates the surrounding muscle. Recurrence after surgery occurs in up to 60% of cases.

Histologically, the fibromatoses are composed of a proliferation of spindle-shaped fibroblasts. Although in early lesions there may be considerable cellularity and some mitotic figures, the cells are generally uniform in size and shape and no abnormal mitoses are seen. The edge of the lesion does, however, tend to infiltrate the surrounding tissues and may affect subcutaneous fat in palmar and plantar fibromatoses, making dissection difficult. Desmoid tumours characteristically infiltrate the surrounding skeletal muscle, making wide excision necessary.

Nodular fasciitis

Nodular fasciitis (sometimes termed pseudosarcomatous fasciitis) is a relatively common condition presenting as a nodule which is sometimes painful. It grows rapidly over a period of one or two weeks and commonly affects young adults. The common sites are the forearm, chest wall and back, where it may arise from the subcutaneous tissue.

Histologically, it consists of short interlacing bundles of mature fibroblasts which show a high number of mitotic figures, all of which are normal in configuration. The cellularity and number of mitotic figures may suggest a fibrosarcoma and thus it is important that the surgeon gives the pathologist an accurate history.

The cause of the condition is unknown although it is likely to be reactive rather than neoplastic. Recurrence after excision is rare.

Proliferative myositis and proliferative fasciitis

The presentation is a firm subcutaneous or intramuscular nodule, most commonly on the arms or legs of elderly patients. The nodule grows rapidly over a period of several weeks. A history of trauma is frequently given.

Histologically, the two conditions are similar. There is proliferation of fibroblasts, many of which show mitotic figures, and the lesion infiltrates fat or muscle, although complete replacement of these tissues does not occur. The features may be mistaken for malignancy. The lesion is, however, benign and very rarely recurs after excision.

Keloid

Keloid is an overgrowth of scar tissue which extends beyond the site of the original wound. Exuberant scar tissue confined to the wound is termed a hypertrophic scar and is not keloid. Young adults are commonly affected, there being a predilection for dark skinned races. Keloid may arise after surgical excision, trauma, vaccination, furuncles, etc. Some arise spontaneously, although these are probably the result of trivial injury.

Scar tissue extends outwards from the original site of the injury in claw-like elevations of the skin. Histologically, the typical feature is the presence of thick glassy eosinophilic bands of collagen fibres set in hyalinized scar tissue.

Keloids do not regress and may require surgical removal. Radiotherapy and local steroid injection following surgery are recommended by some surgeons.

Retroperitoneal fibrosis

This is a rare condition characterized by the deposition of fibrous tissue in the retroperitoneal space.

In less than 10% of cases there is an associated tumour such as carcinoid, lymphoma or stomach neoplasm. Associations with scleroderma, mediastinal fibrosis, Riedel's thyroiditis, orbital pseudotumour and sclerosing cholangitis have been reported.

There is a well documented, although rare, association with several beta-blocking drugs (Bullimore 1980; McCluskey et al. 1980). Methysergide is also associated with retroperitoneal fibrosis and other drugs such as hydralazine and methyldopa have been implicated. Although a similar type of fibrosis has been noted near inflammatory aortic aneurysms (see p. 364) and in the vicinity of urine leaking from an obstructed kidney, current views on the pathogenesis imply an immunological stimulation of collagen production.

Usually males are affected in later middle-age and presentation is usually due to ureteric obstruction which may cause loin pain, renal colic and occasionally renal failure. There may be a nephrotic syndrome due to renal vein obstruction. Inferior vena cava obstruction causes bilateral leg oedema and occasionally varicocoele formation. If the lumbar nerve roots are involved, pain in the appropriate distribution is a symptom. Systemic symptoms of malaise, weight loss and pyrexia occur. In one-quarter of patients a mass may be palpated rectally.

Intravenous pyelography shows the ureters to be deviated medially in the middle third with proximal dilatation. There may be hydronephrosis (*see* p. 240).

The fibrous tissue forms a thick plaque over the bodies of the lower lumbar vertebrae. It usually extends from the aortic bifurcation to the renal vessels and spreads laterally over the psoas muscles. The mesentery is usually free of fibrosis. Occasionally, the fibrosis extends upwards into the mediastinum. The ureters, aorta, major veins and the nerve plexuses may all be involved.

Microscopically, there is dense fibrous tissue with an inflammatory cell infiltration.

Ultrasound and CT scanning may be useful for monitoring treatment. Surgery may be required for diagnosis, biopsy and ureterolysis. Provided there is no associated malignancy and no permanent renal damage, the prognosis is good.

Benign Tumours of Soft Tissue

Fibrous histiocytoma (dermatofibroma)

The terms fibrous histiocytoma, dermatofibroma and sclerosing haemangioma are now considered synonymous. The condition is a common benign lesion presenting as a subcutaneous or a pedunculated nodule, most commonly on the limbs. Rarely the origin is in deeper tissue.

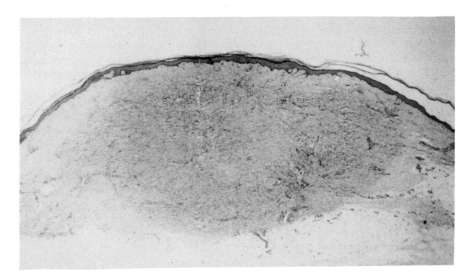

Fig. 18.2. Dermatofibroma. A proliferation of cells in the dermis with ill-defined edges. (H and E × 8·5)

Microscopically, low power examination reveals a proliferation of cells in the dermis with an ill-defined edge which merges into the normal surrounding dermis (*see Fig.* 18.2). The lesion is composed of uniform spindle-shaped cells arranged in criss-crossing bundles. A characteristic feature is arrangement of the cells radially around a central hub giving a cartwheel or so-called 'storiform' pattern. Scattered inflammatory cells, foam cells and giant cells may also be seen.

The cell of origin is unknown, although both fibroblasts and histiocytes have been suggested. Fibrous histiocytomas are benign although they may occasionally recur after excision.

Benign tumours of fat

Lipomas are benign tumours consisting of mature fat cells. They are rare up to the age of 20 years but become very common in adult life. Superficial (cutaneous) lipomas occur in any part of the body although they are most frequent on the head and neck. Deep-seated lipomas may be found in the deeper tissues of the limbs, mediastinum, retroperitoneum, etc. Lipomas occasionally cause pressure symptoms on adjacent organs.

Grossly, lipomas are thinly encapsulated fatty masses (*see Fig.* 18.3). Histologically, they are composed of mature fat cells.

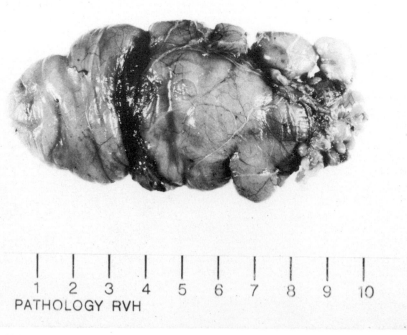

Fig. 18.3. Simple lipoma.

Lipomas only occasionally recur after excision. Several reports of malignant change in lipomas have been recorded, although Enzinger and Weiss (1983) regarded them as unconvincing.

Several variants of lipoma are recognized.

ANGIOLIPOMAS: These occur as painful nodules, most frequently on the limbs of young adults. Histologically, numerous blood vessels mingle with the fat.

SPINDLE-CELL LIPOMAS: These are most common around the shoulder. Part of the fat is replaced by regularly orientated spindle-cells.

PLEOMORPHIC LIPOMAS: These consist histologically of fat cells, spindle cells and bizarre giant cells. The giant cells are characterized by radially orientated nuclei which give them the appearance of the petals of a flower (floret giant cells). They are occasionally misdiagnosed as liposarcomas.

INTRA- AND INTERMUSCULAR LIPOMAS: These variants occur as large deep-seated tumours which infiltrate and replace muscle. Histologically the tumour is composed of mature fat cells identical to those seen in an ordinary lipoma. The fat cells are seen to be infiltrating between and replacing muscle cells. The infiltrating pattern may lead to confusion with a liposarcoma and liposarcomas may have very well differentiated areas identical to a lipoma, thus adding to the confusion. These tumours must, therefore, be examined extensively before a definite diagnosis can be made.

INTRANEURAL LIPOMAS: This type of lipoma is intimately intermingled with the fibres of a nerve. Nearly all cases involve the median nerve at the wrist and cause neurological symptoms in the hand. At the time of surgery it is important to recognize this condition since attempts at surgical removal may leave severe neurological deficit in the hand.

Leiomyomas

Leiomyomas are benign tumours of smooth muscle. They are most common in the uterus but are also found in the gastrointestinal tract, skin and deep soft tissues.

Leiomyomas of the skin most often arise from the arrector pili muscle and lie in the dermis. They are often multiple, appearing as subcutaneous nodules which may give rise to spontaneous pain. Histologically, bundles of well orientated regular spindle cells are seen. Angiomyomas (vascular leiomyomas) form variants which occur as painful nodules, usually in the lower legs. Histologically, thick walled blood vessels course through the smooth muscle. These tumours are benign although multiple lesions may be difficult to excise completely.

Leiomyomas occurring in the deep tissues of the limbs or in the retroperitoneum may be very large and difficult to distinguish from leiomyosarcomas which are more common in these deep sites (*see* later).

Rhabdomyomas

Rhabdomyomas are rare benign tumours of skeletal muscle. They are much less common than rhabdomyosarcomas. In adults, rhabdomyomas occur as painless masses, usually in the region of the head and neck. Histologically, they are composed of deeply eosinophilic cells, some of which show the cross striations typical of skeletal muscle. The lesion is entirely benign and malignant transformation has not been described. Rhabdomyomas occurring in young children may show a histological pattern difficult to distinguish from rhabdomyosarcoma. One rare variant of rhabdomyoma occurs in the heart and, as the tumour cells contain vacuoles full of glycogen, it is sometimes termed a 'glycogen tumour'.

Benign tumours of vascular origin

Haemangiomas, pyogenic granulomas, vascular ectasias and glomus tumours have been dealt with in Chapter 17.

Lymphangioma

The vast majority of lymphangiomas present within the first years of life and about half are present at birth. They probably result from the failure of a group of lymphatic vessels to communicate with the main lymphatic system. Common sites are the axillae, neck, head and occasionally the internal organs such as lung and spleen. The lesion is a soft fluctuant mass which expands and becomes tense when the infant cries. They can easily become infected but since they are soft and compressible, pressure symptoms on adjacent organs are unusual. When adults are affected, the lesion is most commonly in the abdominal cavity or skin.

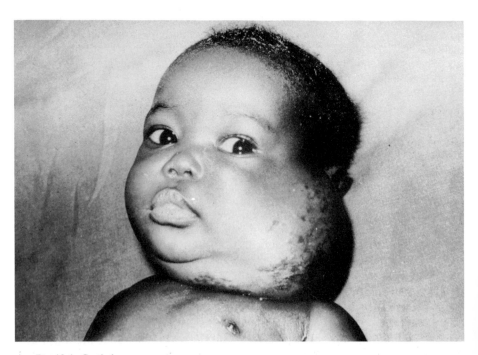

Fig. 18.4. Cystic hygroma.

Grossly, lymphangiomas are composed of large interconnecting cysts (*see Fig.* 18.4) (cystic hygroma or cystic lymphangioma) or a sponge-like mass (cavernous lymphangioma). Many examples contain areas of both patterns.

Microscopically, the cystic spaces and channels are lined by endothelium and they are often filled with proteinaceous fluid containing a few lymphocytes. Aggregates of lymphocytes are usually seen in the stroma between the channels, a point which helps distinguish these lesions from haemangiomas.

Lymphangiomas do not usually regress and therefore most require surgical removal. Those in the region of the shoulder may extend into the mediastinum and therefore a chest X-ray is essential prior to excision. Lymphangiomas have a tendency to insinuate themselves into tissue planes, making excision difficult.

Haemangiolymphangioma

Some children present with a mixed lesion (often on lip or skin) which histologically shows a mixture of lymph-filled and blood-filled spaces. They usually behave clinically as lymphangiomas. Occasionally they regress spontaneously. Surgical excision is indicated for those lesions causing cosmetic problems.

Giant cell tumours of tendon sheath

These are benign tumours found in close association with tendon sheaths. They are most commonly found on the fingers where they present as a mass attached to deep structures but not to skin. Grossly, they have a lobulated appearance. Histologically, they consist of sheets of regular polygonal cells, with a scattering of multinucleate giant cells. Although completely benign, they may recur following excision.

Soft Tissue Tumours of Intermediate Malignant Potential

Dermatofibrosarcoma protuberans

This is a tumour which presents as a nodular mass in the skin of adult patients. It shows a similarity to both benign fibrous histiocytoma and malignant fibrous histiocytoma. Although locally aggressive, it rarely metastasizes and is therefore considered to be of intermediate malignancy.

Histologically, the tumour is seen to infiltrate the dermis and subcutaneous tissue at its edges. It is composed of closely packed bundles of spindle-shaped cells, arranged in a cartwheel or 'storiform' pattern. Mitotic figures are seen but there is little nuclear pleomorphism.

The tumour has a strong tendency to recur locally and recurrence may take place many years after initial excision. If metastases do occur, they usually arise from recurrent tumours. The recurrence may show a progression towards fibrosarcoma.

Wide local excision is recommended. Excision of isolated pulmonary metastases may also be carried out in view of the low grade of malignancy.

Atypical fibroxanthoma

This is a relatively uncommon tumour of skin, occurring either in the head and neck region of elderly patients or in the limbs of young patients. It presents as a nodule or as an ulcer which may resemble a squamous or basal cell carcinoma grossly.

Histologically, the tumour is exceedingly bizarre, showing randomly placed pleomorphic cells with numerous mitotic figures. It may therefore be easily mistaken for a primary or secondary malignant tumour.

Despite the bizarre appearance, the prognosis is excellent with virtually no metastases and few recurrences after surgery.

Haemangiopericytoma

Haemangiopericytomas are tumours of pericytes. They may be benign or malignant. Clinically they occur in adults (rarely in children) as slow growing tumours which may pulsate due to their vascularity. Some are associated with hypoglycaemia. The common sites of origin are the thigh, pelvic cavity and retroperitoneum. They usually present as a painless mass situated deep in muscle.

Grossly, the cut surface of the tumour shows vascularity and areas of haemorrhage. Histologically, the neoplastic pericytes are seen as closely packed spindle cells which surround endothelial lined vascular channels (*see Fig.* 18.5). Malignant haemangiopericytomas are diagnosed by the presence of numerous mitotic figures, pleomorphism of cells, necrosis and haemorrhage.

Benign haemangiopericytomas outnumber malignant ones, although prediction of clinical behaviour from histological features may be difficult.

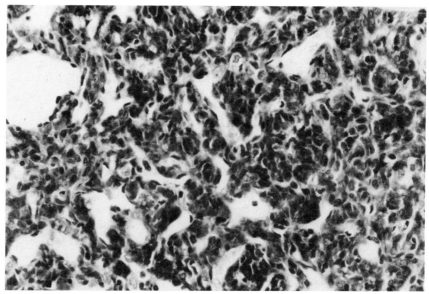

Fig. 18.5. Haemangiopericytoma. Many vascular channels between which are pericytes. (H and E × 150)

Malignant Tumours of Soft Tissues (Soft Tissue Sarcomas)

Soft tissue sarcomas are relatively rare tumours, the prevalence in the USA being 2/100 000. The aetiology is essentially unknown although viral induced sarcomas are well described in animal models. The relationship between viral infection and human sarcomas is not known. Prior irradiation may be a factor in the induction of some sarcomas (e.g. fibrosarcoma following irradiation for breast cancer) which develop in the irradiated site or at the edge of a radiation field. Recently, there has been interest in the chemical induction of sarcomas, particularly with herbicides and with Agent Orange, a defoliant which was used in Vietnam. The evidence for a direct aetiological link between various chemicals and sarcomas is still unclear but there is some data showing that exposure to phenoxy acids increases the risk of sarcoma by six times and that exposure to chlorophenols increases the risk by threefold (Eriksson *et al.* 1981). Patients with immune deficiency have a predisposition to develop Kaposi's sarcoma. Childhood rhabdomyosarcoma may have a familial basis.

The staging and histological grading of soft tissue sarcomas is shown in *Table* 18.1. CT scanning is useful in staging and angiography is useful to determine the involvement of fascial planes and whether or not vital structures are affected.

Table 18.1. Staging and histological grading of soft tissue sarcomas

*TNM classification**	
T0	No evidence of primary tumour.
T1	Tumour of 5 cm or less in its greatest dimension and without extension to bone, major blood vessel or major nerve.
T2	Tumour more than 5 cm in greatest dimension but without extension to bone, major blood vessel or major nerve.
T3	Tumour with extension to bone, major vessel and nerve.
Tx	Not assessed.
N0	Regional nodes not involved.
N1	Regional nodes involved.
Nx	Not assessed.
M0	No distant metastases.
M1	Distant metastases.
Mx	Not assessed.
Histopathological grading	
G1	High degree of differentiation.
G2	Medium degree of differentiation.
G3	Low degree of differentiation (undifferentiated).
Gx	Not assessed

* TNM system does not apply to Kaposi's sarcoma, dermatofibrosarcoma, desmoid tumour and sarcomas arising from dura, brain or hollow viscera.

Overall the most common age group is 50–70 years but they can occur at all ages. The most common soft tissue sarcoma in children is a rhabdomyosarcoma. Liposarcoma is the most common type in adults and most adult tumours are located in the extremities, usually the legs (*see Fig.* 18.6). Most present as a local mass and spread by direct invasion of adjacent structures and by blood, often to lung. Lymph node metastases are relatively uncommon.

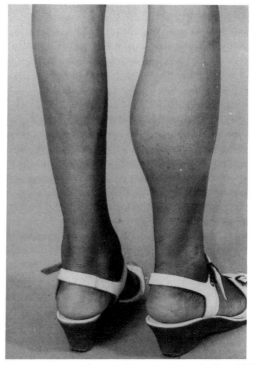

Fig. 18.6. Soft tissue sarcoma presenting as a deep-seated mass in the calf. Histology in this case showed a liposarcoma.

Site appears to be a prognostic factor, the more proximal lesions having a worse prognosis than distal lesions, although this may be related to resectability (Brennan 1984). Tumours greater than 5 cm have a worse prognosis than smaller lesions and one series found that in the extremities, lesions greater than 5 cm have a 46% five year survival compared with 63% five year survival in lesions less than 5 cm (Shiu *et al.* 1975). Currently, the prognosis of soft tissue sarcomas does not vary greatly between the various histological types.

Fine needle aspiration cytology is of little use in these tumours as it is very difficult to make a precise diagnosis. A core needle biopsy is occasionally adequate but an incisional biopsy is preferable. Frozen section tends to be unreliable and it is desirable to await paraffin section before commencing definitive therapy. Frozen section may, however, be used to determine whether or not a margin is tumour-free during surgery. The site of the incisional biopsy must be chosen with care so as not to compromise the future *en-bloc* resection.

Malignant fibrous histiocytoma

This tumour was formerly considered to be rare but it is now realized that many lesions formerly classified as fibrosarcomas or other soft tissue sarcomas are malignant fibrous histiocytomas. Malignant fibrous histiocytoma is in fact the most common soft tissue sarcoma of elderly patients.

Clinically, they present as a firm or soft tissue mass, arising most commonly in the muscles of the lower limb or in the retroperitoneum.

They are thought to arise from primitive mesenchymal cells which may differentiate towards both histiocytes (tissue macrophages) and fibroblasts.

Histologically, the typical findings are areas of fibroblast-like cells showing a cartwheel or 'storiform' pattern, interspaced with areas of more pleomorphic cells. The latter areas contain rounded histiocytic cells, inflammatory cells and, in particular, giant cells. Abnormal mitotic figures are common; several variants containing myxoid elements or prominent giant cells or inflammatory areas are recognized.

Local spread along fascial planes is a common finding. This may only be visible microscopically and therefore surgical excision should be wide. Between a fifth and a half of these tumours metastasize and this is mainly via the blood stream. An important point regarding prognosis is that superficial lesions in the skin have a much lower incidence of metastases than those arising in deep tissues such as muscle.

Fibrosarcomas

Fibrosarcomas are defined as malignant tumours of fibroblasts. The tumours are most common in middle-aged adults and they can arise from fibrous tissue anywhere in the body. The most frequently affected sites are the thigh (especially around the knee), trunk, forearms, lower legs, paranasal sinuses and retroperitoneum.

Clinically, they present as deep seated tumour masses which only cause pain if very large. Grossly the tumour is a fleshy mass which, in some cases, has an ill-defined capsule.

Histologically, the principal feature is the presence of spindle shaped cells resembling fibroblasts with no evidence of differentiation into any other soft tissue elements such as fat, muscle, etc. The cells tend to be arranged in long fasicles which interlace to give the 'herring bone' pattern typical of this tumour.

Local spread may result in nodules of tumour around the main mass. Metastatic spread via the blood stream is to the lungs, bone and liver.

Wide surgical excision is the treatment of choice. Encapsulated tumours which are enucleated in the mistaken belief that they are benign result in recurrence because of satellite nodules of tumour. In the case of limb tumours, the proximal margin of excision should be greater than the distal as the tumour tends to spread upwards along the neurovascular bundles.

Overall, a five year survival rate of approximately 50% may be obtained. Those patients with histologically high grade tumours, as indicated by cellular pleomorphism and mitotic activity, have the worst prognosis.

Liposarcoma

Whereas malignant fibrous histiocytoma is the commonest soft tissue sarcoma in elderly patients, liposarcoma is the commonest in adults of all ages. They are rare in children.

They arise, not from mature fatty tissue, but from primitive mesenchymal cells. Therefore, they do not necessarily occur in adipose tissue but do in fact more commonly arise from deeper tissues such as the deep fascia.

Clinically, they present as a slow-growing deep seated mass. The most common site is the thigh, followed by the retroperitoneum and other parts of the limbs.

Grossly, the tumour may have a gelatinous appearance (*see Fig.* 18.7) and if it contains a lot of mature fat it can be yellow in colour. Others are white and fleshy and indistinguishable from other soft tissue sarcomas.

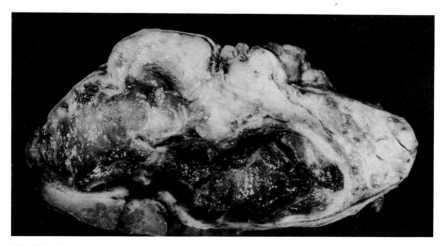

Fig. 18.7. Liposarcoma showing a gelatinous appearance.

Histologically, the diagnosis of liposarcoma is based on the identification of lipoblasts which appear as multi- or univacuolated cells due to their fat content. The lipoblasts may be seen in a background of a myxoid matrix (myxoid liposarcoma) or of cells resembling mature fat (well differentiated liposarcoma), and both of these types indicate a good prognosis. Alternatively, the background may consist of densely packed rounded cells (round cell liposarcoma) or of giant cells and pleomorphic cells (pleomorphic liposarcomas), and both of these types indicate a bad prognosis.

The tumour tends to metastasize via the blood stream to lung and liver, lymph node metastases being rare. The myxoid variety characteristically metastasizes to serosal surfaces such as the pleura.

Prognosis depends on site and histological type. Those in the retroperitoneum have a worse prognosis than those in the limbs, probably due to the larger size at the time of diagnosis. Five year survival rate for well differentiated and myxoid types is up to 80% whereas the figure for the round cell and pleomorphic types is only 30%.

Treatment is by wide excision to include satellite nodules and microscopic spread (as determined by frozen section); radiotherapy may sometimes be used after excision.

Leiomyosarcoma

Leiomyosarcomas are malignant tumours of smooth muscle. Leiomyosarcomas of soft tissue (as opposed to those arising in the gastrointestinal tract) are most common in the retroperitoneum. They also occur in the limbs, skin, subcutaneous tissue and elsewhere. Occasional cases arise in the inferior vena cava and other vascular channels. They are relatively uncommon soft tissue sarcomas.

Clinically the majority of retroperitoneal leiomyosarcomas occur in women and produce symptoms similar to those found with other large retroperitoneal masses (i.e. a palpable mass, ureteric obstruction, weight loss and general poor health). Tumours arising in the inferior vena cava may cause a Budd-Chiari type syndrome or leg oedema.

Histologically, leiomyosarcomas tend to be spindle cell tumours. The cell nuclei are characteristically blunt ended or cigar shaped and myofibrils can be identified by special stains. Some lesions are less well differentiated and contain pleomorphic cells and giant cells.

The main histological problem with any smooth muscle tumour is to determine whether it is benign or malignant. Enzinger and Weiss (1983) consider there to be a spectrum of tumours from benign to malignant and state that a high mitotic rate is the single most important indicator of malignancy.

In general, retroperitoneal leiomyosarcomas are aggressive tumours with a very poor prognosis (five year survival rates range from zero to 30%), whereas cutaneous leiomyosarcomas, because of their early diagnosis, have a better prognosis.

Rhabdomyosarcomas

Rhabdomyosarcomas are usually described as malignant tumours of striated muscle although they are more likely to arise from primitive mesenchymal cells which have a capacity to differentiate into rhabdomyoblasts (precursors of striated muscle).

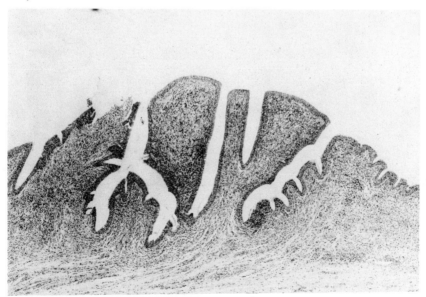

Fig. 18.8. Botryoid variant of embryonal rhabdomyosarcoma of bladder, showing the typical polypoid appearance. (H and E × 7)

Rhabdomyosarcomas are the commonest soft tissue sarcomas of children, adolescents and young adults. They are rare over the age of 45 years. The commonest site of origin is in the head (especially the orbits, sinuses and nasal cavity), followed by the retroperitoneum, genito-urinary tract (especially the urinary bladder, prostate, vagina and paratesticular area) and the limbs.

Grossly, the tumours are similar to other soft tissue sarcomas, being large infiltrating tumours which vary from soft to firm and fleshy depending on the degree of cellularity. The botryoid type of embryonal rhabdomyosarcoma which occurs most commonly in the urinary bladder and vagina does, however, have a typical polypoid or grape-like gross appearance, the sarcoma botryoides (*see Fig.* 18.8).

Histologically, several types are recognized. The embryonal rhabdomyosarcoma occurs in children and shows widespread areas of small round hyperchromatic cells, interspersed between which are rhabdomyoblasts. Rhabdomyoblasts are large cells which appear round on cross-section or strap-like on longitudinal section; the cytoplasm is deeply eosinophilic and may contain cross-striations similar to those seen in skeletal muscle (*see Fig.* 18.9). In the botryoid variant of embryonal rhabdomyosarcoma, which also occurs in children, histological examination of the typically polypoid areas shows that they are composed of mucoid material and cells. The alveolar type occurs in adolescence and histologically shows a fibrous meshwork in the spaces (alveoli) of which are the tumour cells. The pleomorphic type is found in adults and histologically is composed of bizarre pleomorphic cells with occasional rhabdomyoblasts.

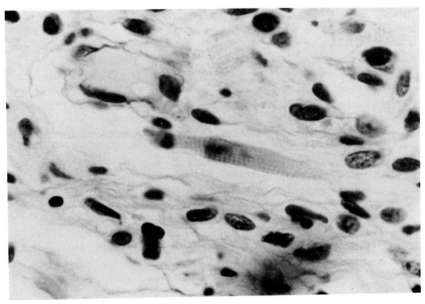

Fig. 18.9. Rhabdomyoblast, showing cross striations, in an embryonal rhabdomyosarcoma. (H and E × 750)

Rhabdomyosarcomas are aggressive and rapidly destroy local tissue including bone. They spread by blood (to lung, liver, bone, etc.) and by lymphatics. The prognosis, which used to be exceedingly poor with surgery only, is now much improved with a combination of surgery, radiotherapy and cyclical chemotherapy. A five year survival rate of up to 80% for early disease may now be achieved.

Angiosarcomas

Angiosarcomas are rare soft tissue sarcomas. Enzinger and Weiss (1983) use the term 'angiosarcoma' to include haemangiosarcoma and lymphangiosarcoma as these may be difficult or impossible to separate morphologically. Unlike other soft tissue sarcomas, they tend to occur superficially in the skin rather than in the deep soft tissue. They commonly affect elderly patients, the common sites being the head and neck, especially the scalp. The breasts and liver may also be affected.

Chronic lymphoedema (e.g. congenital or after mastectomy as in the Stewart–Treves syndrome) is associated with the development of angiosarcoma. Some occur after radiotherapy and hepatic angiosarcomas have been described after the administration of various chemicals (see p. 170).

The typical clinical features of cutaneous angiosarcoma are the presence in the skin of red or blue blister-like areas which occasionally cause pain and may bleed spontaneously. Satellite nodules are common and metastases occur via both lymphatics and blood.

Grossly, on sectioning, haemorrhagic areas or actual blood filled spaces may be seen. Histologically, there is a proliferation of intercommunicating vascular channels. The endothelial cells are hyperchromatic and tend to be piled up. Unlike simple haemangiomas, the vascular channels at the edge of the lesion tend to infiltrate and split the surrounding tissue. Poorly differentiated tumours may show only poorly defined vascular channels and can be confused with carcinoma or other sarcomas.

Cutaneous angiosarcomas are associated with a good prognosis if they are identified at an early stage and treated by a wide excision. The Stewart–Treves syndrome has a poor prognosis.

Kaposi's sarcoma

Kaposi's sarcoma is seen in one of three situations: (1) as a tumour endemic in Africa, (2) as a rare sporadic tumour outside Africa, and (3) as a complication of the acquired immunodeficiency syndrome (AIDS) (see also p. 424).

The African Kaposi's sarcoma had a geographical distribution similar to that of Burkitt's lymphoma. For this reason, a virus has been implicated in the aetiology, although the human T-cell lymphotropic virus type III (HTLV-III), which has been suggested as the cause of AIDS is not associated with African Kaposi's sarcoma (Biggar et al. 1984). The African Kaposi's sarcoma occurs mainly in men and has a peak incidence in the fourth decade.

Kaposi's sarcoma rarely occurs outside Africa on a sporadic basis not associated with AIDS. The patients are usually elderly males and many develop a lympho-reticular malignancy.

About one-third of patients with AIDS present with a Kaposi's sarcoma. AIDS is a disease in which there is an acquired defect in cell-mediated immunity. It is likely to be due to a virus which is spread by close contact (usually sexual). The main groups at risk are homosexuals, intravenous drug abusers, people from the Caribbean and haemophiliacs. AIDS is currently attributed to an infection with HTLV-III (Editorial 1985). It appears to attack T-cells which are responsible for cell-mediated immunity. AIDS is considered to be one of several related conditions caused by the HTLV-III, the others being persistent generalized lymphadenopathy and various combinations of fatigue, weight loss, diarrhoea and oral candidiasis. AIDS patients present clinically with generalized lymphadenopathy, opportunistic infections (especially due to *Pneumocystis carinii*) or Kaposi's sarcoma. Some may also develop non-Hodgkin's lymphoma.

Grossly, Kaposi's sarcoma starts as multiple cutaneous lesions, usually in the distal parts of the lower extremities. These lesions are blue-red nodules which increase in size and coalesce to form plaques and polypoid growths. In the African form there is often visceral and lymph node involvement at an early stage.

Histologically, the early lesions consist of a proliferation of capillaries in the dermis. These capillaries are surrounded by spindle cells and many polymorphs and red blood cells are seen. At this stage, the lesion may be confused with granulation tissue. Later, as the tumour matures, it becomes more cellular and consists of spindle cell areas. The inflammatory cells are lost, but characteristic slit-like spaces containing red blood cells are seen within the spindle cell areas.

The prognosis of non-African sporadic Kaposi's sarcoma is relatively good. It is slowly progressive and only about 20% of patients die of the disease, although they may develop a second malignancy. The endemic African type and the AIDS associated Kaposi's sarcoma both have a worse prognosis. About 40% of patients with the AIDS associated Kaposi's sarcoma die within one year.

Synovial sarcoma

Synovial sarcomas are malignant tumours which occur most commonly in the limbs of adolescents and young adults, especially around the knee. They arise in close association with tendons, tendon sheaths, joint capsules and bursas, but are rarely found inside joint cavities.

The presentation is as a firm slowly growing, often painful, mass. A misdiagnosis of synovitis or arthritis may be made.

Grossly, they are circumscribed masses, often with cyst formation.

Histologically, the main feature is a biphasic pattern, that is, both epithelial-like elements and spindle cell elements are present. The epithelial cells may be in cords or nests or they may line cleft-like spaces. The spindle cells form compact masses around the epithelial components. Sometimes only one component is present (monophasic synovial sarcoma). This may be difficult to distinguish from fibrosarcoma if only the spindle cell element is present, or from secondary carcinoma if only the epithelial element is present.

Recurrence after excision is common and the five year survival is in the region of 50%.

References

Biggar R. J., Melbye M., Kestems L. *et al.* (1984) Kaposi's sarcoma in Zaire is not associated with HTLV-III infection. *N. Engl. J. Med.* **311**, 1051–2.

Brennan M. F. (1984) The management of soft tissue sarcomas. *Br. J. Surg.* **71**, 964–7.

Bullimore D. W. (1980) Retroperitoneal fibrosis associated with atenolol [letter]. *Br. Med. J.* **281**, 564.

Editorial (1985) AIDS and health professions. *Br. Med. J.* **290**, 583–4.

Enzinger F. M., Weiss S. W. (1983) *Soft Tissue Tumours.* St Louis, C. V. Mosby.

Eriksson M., Hardell L., Berg N. O., Moller T., Axelson O. (1981) Soft tissue sarcomas and exposure to chemical substances: a case-reference study. *Br. J. Indust. Med.* **38**, 27–33.

McCluskey D. R., Donaldson R. A., McGeown M. G. (1980) Oxprenolol and retroperitoneal fibrosis. *Br. Med. J.* **281**, 1459–60.

Shiu M. H., Castro E. B., Hajdu S. I., Fortner J. G. (1975) Surgical treatment of 297 soft tissue sarcomas of the lower extremity. *Ann. Surg.* **182**, 597–602.

Chapter 19

The Bones and Joints

H. Kerr Graham

Introduction

The common disease processes affecting bones and joints will be more clearly understood by an awareness of the gross anatomy, ultrastructure and physiology of the tissues concerned. Of particular importance are the variations in bone structure and blood supply with age, which may play an important role in the outcome of specific diseases.

Anatomy of long bones

Long bones are cylinders of compact bone, which have expanded ends filled with spongy or cancellous bone. The trabeculae of cancellous bone are not arranged in a random fashion, but in such a way as to resist the forces applied to the bone (Wolff's Law). The long bones of children have a growth plate at each end, where longitudinal growth occurs. The growth plate, or physis, divides the bone into three indistinct compartments. The epiphysis is the region above the growth plate, the metaphysis is the region below the growth plate, merging with the diaphysis between the growth zones (*see Fig.* 19.1). Disease processes may show a predilection for a specific compartment. Most of the cortical surface is covered by periosteum, which varies in thickness with age and consists of an outer fibrous layer and an inner cambial layer. The latter is responsible for the circumferential growth of bone in childhood. This propensity is less obvious in the adult unless reactivated by infection or trauma. The thick vascular periosteum of the child has few Sharpey's fibres, and is much more easily stripped from bone surgically, or by disease process, than that of the adult.

Bone as a tissue—cellular components

Osteoblasts are derived from pleuripotential fetal mesenchymal cells and are responsible for the synthesis of bone matrix. This consists of a collagen framework, or osteoid, which is later mineralized. The resulting combination of protein and mineral has the ability to resist both compressive and bending stresses. Osteoblasts are rich in alkaline phosphatase, one of the enzymes required for mineralization. Rapid bone turnover, such as occurs in childhood or in Paget's disease, is characterized by an elevated serum alkaline phosphatase. Once osteoblasts become embedded in matrix, they become osteocytes which are surrounded by bone tissue fluid and are in contact via canaliculi with other cells. Between the general extracellular fluid and the bone tissue fluid is a cellular envelope of osteoblasts, limiting

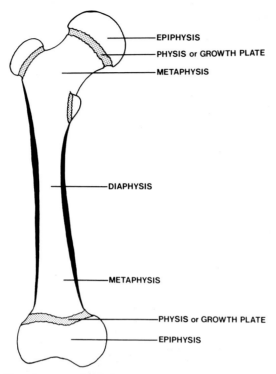

EPIPHYSIS

PHYSIS or GROWTH PLATE

METAPHYSIS

DIAPHYSIS

METAPHYSIS

PHYSIS or GROWTH PLATE

EPIPHYSIS

Fig. 19.1. Typical long bone—anatomical zones.

the bone fluid to a separate compartment (Owen *et al.* 1972). The bone surface area available for metabolic exchange across this envelope is enormous and has been estimated to be $1300 \, m^2$ (Rasmussen and Bordier 1974). This points to the second vital function of bone in providing a large accessible reservoir for mineral homeostasis. Recent studies using radio-isotope tracers (such as ^{18}F) have suggested that plasma filtration across the bone cell envelope may be equal in magnitude to that of the kidney.

Osteoclasts are large multinucleated cells, usually prominent in areas of high bone turnover during growth or repair, but rarely seen in sections of normal bone. They may arise from either mesenchymal cells or from the blood monocyte line. Lying in Howship's lacunae, they reabsorb adjacent bone releasing calcium, phosphate and hydroxyproline. Thus, in Paget's disease, increased bone turnover is reflected in elevated urinary hydroxyproline, derived from breakdown of collagen by osteoclasts.

Bone is a living, dynamic tissue, responding to the organism's need for mechanical support. Formation and reabsorption are continuous and usually coupled so that there is little net change in bone mass. The mechanism of this coupling process is thought to be electrical. Bassett and Becker (1962) have observed that bone under compression develops a positive electrical potential, and under tension a negative potential. Clinicians have attempted to exploit the relationship between electrical effects and bone formation by applying electromagnetic fields to fractures complicated by non-union (electrical osteogenesis).

Blood supply of bone (*see Fig.* 19.2)

The blood supply of a child's long bone has four components.

1. The principal nutrient artery is a branch of a major axial artery and enters the cortex via a strong fascial attachment. In the medullary canal it divides into ascending and descending vessels which ramify to form the endosteal circulation; this supplies most of the bone.
2. The metaphysis is supplied by multiple small vessels from a periarticular plexus. These penetrate the cortex and enlarge within the cancellous bone. There are anastomoses with the diaphyseal system which are not active in the normal bone but can be rapidly utilized if the principal nutrient vessels are disrupted by fracture or by surgery.
3. The epiphysis is supplied by many small delicate vessels which penetrate the non-articular cortex and form a series of arcades directed towards the growth plate. Prior to the development of the growth plate, free anastomoses occur between epiphyseal and metaphyseal circulations in the infant long bone. The mature growth plate acts as a barrier between the two systems and this has

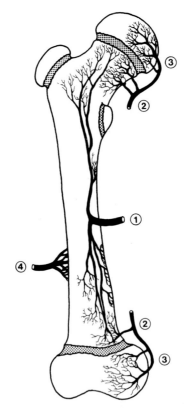

Fig. 19.2. Typical long bone—blood supply: 1. Principal nutrient artery. 2. Metaphyseal. 3. Epiphyseal. 4. Periosteal vessels.

important implications in the localization of infection in haematogenous osteomyelitis. At skeletal maturity, when the growth plate fuses, free anastomoses are restored.

4. Periosteal vessels normally make only a small contribution to diaphyseal blood supply. They enter bone at strong fascial attachments, such as the linea aspera of the femur, and supply only the outer one-third of the cortex at that site (Rhinelander 1980). However, if the endosteal supply is disturbed, the cortex becomes increasingly dependent on the periosteal circulation.

The main cortical circulation is therefore centrifugal from the endosteal surface outwards. At operation, following stripping of the periosteum, multiple small collections of venous blood oozing from the cortical surface can be seen. This circulatory arrangement is of importance in fracture healing and the choice of implants for internal fixation. Intramedullary reaming destroys the diaphyseal endosteal circulation which is then supplied by opening up of the anastomoses from the metaphyseal system. If the cavity is filled with a metal implant and bone cement, regeneration of vessels cannot occur. In the metaphysis, blood supply is maintained by the separate metaphyseal plexus but in the diaphysis, prolonged devascularization of bone may occur (Rhinelander 1980). Intramedullary nails should, theoretically, be chosen to have a small contact area with the inner cortex to allow rapid regeneration of the endosteal circulation. Broad plates tightly applied to the external surface block the normal centrifugal efflux of blood. The effect is minimized by the fact that usually less than one-third of the circumference is so covered. Cerclage wires have little effect on bone blood supply, provided they are narrow, as there is little external longitudinal blood supply to be disrupted. Broad cerclage devices may block venous drainage in the way a plate does, but if kept raised from the bone surface, are less deleterious.

Bone and Joint Infections

Acute haematogenous osteomyelitis

The metaphysis of long bones is the commonest site for acute haematogenous osteomyelitis, especially the lower femur, upper tibia, upper humerus and lower radius. The susceptibility of the metaphysis may be due to frequent exposure to minor trauma and the sluggish blood flow in its large thin walled veins. A minor injury to the metaphysis increases the local blood supply. If a transient bacteraemia occurs during such a period, the bacteria may settle in the metaphysis and initiate the acute infection. The bacteraemia may originate from skin infections, dental sepsis or nasopharyngeal infection. Previously healthy individuals in the first two decades of life are most commonly affected. In adults, a predisposing cause such as diabetes mellitus, intravenous drug abuse, systemic steroid administration, rheumatoid arthritis and sickle cell anaemia is much more likely. Since the infection frequently originates in cutaneous sites, *Staphylococcus aureus* may be identified in 90% of isolates. The remaining 10% of isolates include Gram-negative organisms such as *Haemophilus influenzae, E. coli, Proteus pyocyaneus* and Salmonella. *Streptococcus pyogenes* is less common than it was previously, owing to the widespread use of penicillin.

Morphology

In a typical case, *Staph. aureus* from a minor skin infection settles in the metaphyseal area of the long bone and, in this favourable environment, rapidly multiplies. An acute inflammatory reaction ensues with the production of an exudate containing inflammatory cells. Initially neutrophils, and later monocytes, are seen in great numbers. In the rigid confines of bone, the swelling typical of soft tissue inflammation cannot easily take place and the intra-osseous pressure rises, leading to venous obstruction and thrombosis. If unrelieved, further pressure effects may lead to widespread arterial thrombosis and infarction of medullary contents and bone. During this time, from about the first to third day, the diaphyseal cortex becomes increasingly dependent on its periosteal blood supply. Spontaneous decompression may occur by the exudate passing through the Volkmann's canals of the cortex into the subperiosteal space. Juvenile periosteum has few Sharpey's fibres and is easily stripped by the inflammatory exudate from the underlying bone, leaving large areas of cortex bereft of any blood supply and liable to infarction and sequestrum formation. Small sequestra can be removed by osteoclast activity, but large pieces of dead bone may overcome this mechanism and chronic infection is then likely. Reactive bone (involucrum) is formed by the periosteum around the sequestrated bone, especially in young children (*see Fig.* 19.3). In time, this may provide the main support for the limb. In infants, before the growth plate is mature, spread into the epiphysis may occur, leading to epiphyseal damage or destruction and the exudate may decompress into the joint causing septic arthritis. The older child is less susceptible to this complication as the epiphyseal and metaphyseal circulations are separated by the growth plate. However, in a situation where the metaphysis is intracapsular, such as the hip joint, septic arthritis may still occur.

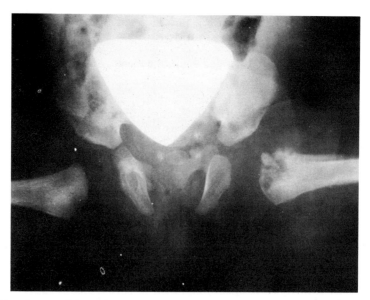

Fig. 19.3. Osteomyelitis in the proximal femur of a child. Note the osteolytic area in the metaphysis, a small sequestrum and the sub-periosteal new bone.

Clinical features

The typical patient is a child with rapid onset of fever, malaise and bone pain. The earliest physical sign is metaphyseal tenderness. The ESR is elevated in a large percentage of cases, but the white cell count less commonly so. A mild anaemia may be present and blood culture is positive in about half of cases. Early intensive treatment with anti-staphylococcal drugs (fusidic acid and flucloxacillin) is recommended until the results of cultures are available. The place of early surgery has been debated (Blockey 1980), but there are advantages in providing material for culture, and in relieving tension by incision of subperiosteal abscesses, or by drilling the metaphyseal medulla (Mollan and Piggot 1977).

Prompt diagnosis is vital as early treatment is likely to produce complete resolution in the majority of cases. Conversely, delay in diagnosis greatly increases the risk of complications, especially chronicity. Chronic infection is usually associated with persistent sequestra, cavities, fibrosis and poor blood supply. Even if infection is eradicated, long-term follow-up is required to assess damage to the growth plate which may cause severe shortening of the limb in later years. Destruction of the joint surface may result in premature degenerative arthritis.

Primary subacute osteomyelitis

The clinico-pathological features of bone infections depend on the interaction between host defences and the virulence of the infective organism. If host defences are high, or if the virulence of the bacteria is low, the disease may run a subacute course. Two eponymous types are described, although a variety of other presentations may be seen.

Brodie's abscess

This is a small abscess surrounded by sclerotic bone. It is commonly diaphyseal in site, and produces chronic bone pain. The diagnosis is often delayed. It must be differentiated from osteoid osteoma which it can closely resemble clinically and radiologically. At operation, the cavity contains pus and organisms may be cultured, compared with the osteoid osteoma which contains neoplastic osteoid.

Garré's sclerosing non-suppurative osteomyelitis

The scar tissue produced by healing bone is bone. In some cases, diffuse low grade infection leads to greatly thickened cortical and cancellous bone, similar in appearance to Pagetic bone. Clinical features of infection may be absent, apart from chronic bone pain.

Chronic osteomyelitis

The most common cause of chronic osteomyelitis is incomplete resolution of acute osteomyelitis. There are many patients with chronic disease, dating from the pre-antibiotic era, still alive. Other causes include compound fractures and following implant surgery. Sepsis rates average 1–2% after total hip replacement, but this still results in an appreciable number of patients with chronic bone infection. The presence of metal implants and acrylic bone cement makes eradication of infection difficult, probably because of inhibition of host defences and the relative avascularity of adjacent tissue.

The essential difference between the acute and the chronic process is the development of dense avascular scar tissue and bone, with an associated chronic inflammatory reaction in the latter. These areas may harbour organisms for years, and may at intervals cause acute flare-ups with the discharge of pus along sinus tracks from openings in the bone called cloacae. Because the organisms are located in relatively avascular areas, systemic antibiotics cannot readily reach them and radical excisional surgery may be required.

If all avascular infected tissue can be removed, the lesions will heal. In children, the removal of large sequestra must be carefully timed, so that the involucrum has formed a strong enough support for the limb, otherwise pathological fracture and limb shortening may occur. Microscopically, the presence of lymphocytes and plasma cells indicates chronic infection.

Two late complications of chronic infection are described, but are now rarely seen owing to improved early treatment: (1) amyloid disease (leading to death from uraemia), and (2) cutaneous malignancy in sinus tracks. Both squamous cell carcinoma and fibrosarcoma have been described.

A useful advance in the administration of chemotherapeutic agents has been the introduction of beads of methylmethacrylate bone cement impregnated with heat-stable antibiotics, usually gentamicin. As the antibiotic elutes from the beads in an osteomyelitic cavity, a high concentration is reached which could not be achieved by systemic therapy (Carlsson *et al.* 1978).

Septic arthritis

Purulent arthritis is caused by the presence of pyogenic organisms proliferating in the joint cavity. The same bacteriological spectrum is seen as in osteomyelitis in the older child. However, under the age of two years *Haemophilus influenzae* is more often found than *Staphylococcus aureus*. In children, many cases are secondary to osteomyelitis and the hip and knee are most commonly involved. Adult patients usually have a predisposing chronic joint condition, such as rheumatoid arthritis. Infection by direct spread or by blood-borne organisms is also seen. The clinical and pathological outcome is determined by the interaction of host resistance and the virulence of the organism, as modified by antibiotic treatment.

Three stages may be described, although in reality they merge together. In the first stage there is a serous effusion from the synovial membrane producing an excess of clear fluid in the joint. This effusion may be reabsorbed or, if defences are overwhelmed, become serofibrinous. During this second stage, the synovium is inflamed and the fluid becomes turbid owing to the presence of bacteria, leucocytes and fibrin. Fibrinous deposits may mature to fibrous adhesions and so resolution may be incomplete. In virulent infections, the third stage of purulent arthritis quickly supervenes as the joint capsule becomes distended with a collection of pus. Proteolytic enzymes released from dead bacteria and leucocytes cause necrosis of cartilage and synovium. If the acute chondrolysis affects more than the most superficial layer, permanent joint damage is inevitable, with irregularity, stiffness and ankylosis in severe cases. Rising pressure in the joint may cause further complications.

1. Tamponade of the circulation may lead to infarction and sequestration of the epiphysis. Absence of the epiphysis on X-ray may also be due to reversible decalcification.
2. Softening and stretching of the supporting ligaments can cause dislocation of the joint. This is common in the hip and may be avoided by splintage in abduction. If dislocation occurs, the prognosis is poor.
3. If the full thickness of cartilage becomes necrotic and detached, the underlying bone may be exposed. Direct spread of infection will then cause a local or more generalized osteomyelitis.
4. The capsule may perforate, leading to a periarticular soft tissue abscess.

The prognosis depends on the stage at which the infection is eradicated, either by natural processes or by therapeutic efforts. Early treatment of septic arthritis is vital and the essentials are early diagnosis, appropriate antibiotics, joint aspiration or drainage and immobilization of both joint and patient.

Tuberculosis

The incidence of tuberculosis has declined in most developed countries, largely because of improved socio-economic conditions, with additional help from health care programmes such as BCG immunization and mass miniature chest radiography. It remains a major cause of death and deformity in the Third World.

Bone and joint tuberculosis is usually secondary to disease elsewhere, usually in the lungs. Haematogenous spread from a pulmonary focus has a predilection for cells of the reticulo-endothelial system. In the skeleton, tubercle bacilli settle in a favourable area, such as the metaphysis, the synovium and the subchondral bone of the epiphysis. The initial response is ingestion by polymorphonuclear leucocytes, which are unable to lyse the bacteria and die releasing live bacilli. Lymphocytes, monocytes and multinucleated histiocytes (Langhans' giant cells) now appear and surround the focus of infection to form a granuloma. As the granuloma enlarges and fuses with others, a small white nodule or tubercle may be seen macroscopically.

Tuberculous osteomyelitis

Involvement of a long bone in the absence of joint involvement is unusual. The metaphysis is the most common site. The centre of the lesion may undergo caseous necrosis and fibrosis of the periphery occurs which, because of its avascularity, inhibits chemotherapeutic penetration. Thrombosis and ischaemic sequestration of bone occurs. Live bacilli may be harboured for years in such areas and cause acute flare-ups of infection at times of lowered resistance. Generalized bone changes, such as osteoporosis or osteosclerosis, may be seen.

Tuberculous arthritis

Tuberculous follicles may invade from the metaphysis across the growth plate, a feature rarely seen in pyogenic infections, or, alternatively, infection may originate in the synovium. Fibrinous deposits spread from the periphery of the joint, across the cartilage surfaces as a dense pannus and this may lead to adhesions or ankylosis. Proteolytic enzymes are absent and the articular cartilage is preserved until directly undermined by subchondral granulomas.

Untreated, the disease runs a chronic course with destruction of all the joint tissues. Healing may occur by joint contracture or ankylosis, but is inhibited by the presence of abscesses or large amounts of debris.

The complications of bone and joint tuberculosis include ankylosis of joints (often in poor functional position), instability (leading to subluxation or dislocation), osteoporosis and pathological fracture.

Tuberculous spondylitis (Pott's disease)

Often a whole segment of the vertebral column is involved, most commonly thoracic, sometimes lumbar and rarely cervical. As each intercostal artery supplies half of the vertebrae on either side of an intervertebral disc, haematogenous infection follows this pattern. Infection in the subchondral bone of the end plates undermines the nutrition of the disc, which becomes necrotic and is later sequestrated. Several complications may arise.

1. ABSCESS FORMATION: Cold abscesses formed by caseous material, necrotic disc and bone fragments, leucocytes and bacilli may 'burrow' along tissue planes to present at distant sites. In the lumbar spine the abscess may remain within the psoas sheath and present as a lump in the groin.

2. DEFORMITY: If three or more contiguous vertebral bodies are involved, collapse may lead to a severe kyphosis. In childhood, growth disturbance anteriorly with continued growth of posterior elements may cause severe deformity even when the disease is quiescent.

3. PARAPLEGIA: In spinal tuberculosis, paraplegia may be caused by many mechanisms. In active disease, the cord may be involved directly, following penetration of the meninges. Most commonly, pressure from an extradural abscess is responsible. Even when the disease is inactive, progressive deformity may cause bony encroachment of the spinal canal with subsequent paraplegia. Occasionally, deformity leads to a sudden spinal subluxation with an acute spinal cord compression. Chronic fibrosis and ischaemia may also result in direct damage to the cord and explain the unrewarding results from decompression surgery.

Aspects of treatment of tuberculous bone and joint disease

In the early vascular stage, combination chemotherapy will cure 85% of patients (MRC 1976). If there are large amounts of sequestra, abscess material and debris, surgery may be required. The essentials are to resect avascular material, leaving a vascular bed for bone grafting and to assist drug penetration. Badly damaged joints may require arthrodesis or, occasionally, arthroplasty.

Syphilis

This is now less common than in the pre-pencillin era. Bone and joint involvement occurs in both acquired and congenital infections.

Congenital syphilis

1. PARROT'S SYPHILITIC OSTEOCHONDRITIS: The spirochaete (*Treponema pallidum*) lodges near the growth plate during the fifth or sixth month of pregnancy and produces an epiphysitis or metaphysitis. Syphilitic granulation tissue is produced following the initial acute inflammatory response and is characterized by lymphocytic infiltration. Endochondral ossification is disrupted and deformity and even separation of the epiphysis may occur.

2. CLUTTON'S JOINTS: These are symmetrical painless effusions of the knee joints seen in children between 8 and 16 years who usually have other stigmata of congenital syphilis.

Acquired syphilis

Non-gummatous osteomyelitis or arthritis may occur but are rare. The more common lesions are due to the process of gummatous inflammation.

The gumma microscopically consists of lymphocytes and plasma cells in relation to the walls of small arterioles. The resultant vasculitis causes infarction and coagulative necrosis. This may produce an arthritis or synovitis, depending on the location. In the diaphysis of a long bone, it is seen radiologically as a circumscribed 'punched out' lesion, and must be distinguished from secondary tumour deposits.

CHARCOT'S JOINTS: These are not specific to syphilis, but rather represent the end-stage painless destruction of a weight-bearing joint, unprotected by afferent stimuli. In syphilis, it occurs in the tertiary stage in association with locomotor ataxia (tabes dorsalis).

PERIOSTITIS: This may occur in both congenital and acquired forms of the disease and at any age. However, its most florid results may be seen in older children. The tibia is the most commonly affected bone and may show patchy or diffuse involvement. Subperiosteal inflammation leads to widespread new bone formation on the surface of the original cortex. The X-ray appearances may show an 'onion peel' appearance and this is clinically manifested by deformed long bones, such as 'sabre tibia'.

Brucellosis

Three main species of the genus Brucella infect domestic animals; *Br. melitensis* (goats and sheep), *Br. abortus* (cattle) and *Br. suis* (pigs). Brucellosis is a typical zoonosis in that infection is acquired by direct contact with infected farm animals or their products, but is not passed from man to man. Entry to the body is via skin, conjunctiva, alimentary tract or respiratory tract.

The bacteria spread and multiply in the lymphatic system and cause a febrile illness with vague symptoms of lassitude, sweating, headaches, etc. Later, in about 10% of cases, there is bone and joint involvement. In young patients, an acute peripheral arthritis may occur which usually resolves completely. In adults, the vertebral column is the most common site. A chronic granulomatous infection, similar in many respects to tuberculosis, is seen. The granulomas may become caseous or encapsulated by fibrous sheaths. As tissue hypersensitivity to the brucella antigens develops, caseous necrosis and abscess formation occurs, mainly in the bone itself, unlike tuberculosis. Paravertebral abscess is uncommon.

Tumours

Primary bone tumours are comparatively rare, in contrast to secondary deposits which become increasingly frequent in patients over the age of 50 years. Diagnosis of bone lesions depends on information from three main areas: (1) history and

Table 19.1. Primary bone tumours (modified from the 1972 WHO classification)

1. *Bone forming tumours*

Benign	*Malignant*
1. Osteoma	1. Osteosarcoma
2. Osteoid osteoma	2. Parosteal osteosarcoma
3. Osteoblastoma	

2. *Cartilage forming tumours*

Benign	*Malignant*
1. Chondroma	1. Chondrosarcoma
2. Osteochondroma	
3. Chondroblastoma	
4. Chondromyxoid fibroma	

3. *Giant cell tumours*
Wide spectrum of behaviour, benign–malignant

4. *Marrow tumours*

Malignant
1. Ewing's sarcoma
2. Myeloma
3. Malignant lymphoma

5. *Vascular tumours*

Benign	*Intermediate*	*Malignant*
1. Haemangioma	1. Haemangioendothelioma	1. Angiosarcoma
2. Lymphangioma	2. Haemangiopericytoma	
3. Glomus tumour		

6. *Other connective tissue tumours*

Benign	*Malignant*
1. Desmoplastic fibroma	1. Fibrosarcoma
2. Lipoma	2. Liposarcoma
	3. Undifferentiated sarcoma

7. *Other tumours*

Benign
1. Chordoma
2. Adamantinoma

8. *Unclassified tumours*

9. *Tumour-like lesions*
1. Solitary bone cyst
2. Aneurysmal bone cyst
3. Metaphyseal fibrous defect
4. Fibrous dysplasia
5. Eosinophilic granuloma
6. Brown tumour of hyperparathyroidism

clinical findings, (2) radiology and (3) pathology. To consider information from only one or two of these disciplines makes the task more difficult for the clinician, not to say dangerous for the patient, in that the wrong conclusion may be reached with disastrous consequences.

Good quality plain X-rays may yield vital information in deciding whether a lesion is behaving in a benign or malignant fashion. In a smaller number of cases, ancillary investigations may be helpful, such as tomography, isotope bone scanning and computerized tomography. Because of the improvement in these non-invasive techniques, angiography has fewer indications. CT scanning is most useful in demonstrating soft tissue involvement in malignant tumours. It is also much more sensitive than conventional radiography in delineating pulmonary metastases at an early stage.

There are many classifications of bone tumours based on differing criteria. The 1972 WHO classification is based on the differentiation shown by the tumour cells and the type of intercellular substance they produce (*see Table* 19.1). In addition to true tumours, a group of tumour-like lesions is included.

Benign Bone Forming Tumours

Osteoma

The common clinical term is 'ivory exostosis', which aptly describes the small, hard lesion, arising from bones of intramembranous ossification (skull and face). Radiologically, it appears as a well defined bone mass. Histologically, osteomas of the calvarium are composed of mature, lamellar bone, whereas those of the facial bones are composed of immature bone. The lesion may be excised if causing pressure symptoms. It does not recur following excision and does not undergo malignant change. Osteomas of the frontal bone are associated with Gardner's syndrome. (*See* p. 117.)

Osteoid osteoma

This is a relatively common lesion, consisting of a nidus of new bone, vascular channels and osteoid surrounded by an area of sclerosis. The nidus is usually less than 1 cm in diameter (*see Fig.* 19.4). It most commonly presents in the second and third decades of life. The lower limb is more commonly affected, particularly the femur and tibia.

Patients complain of chronic pain, which may be present at night and disturb sleep. Many cases are relieved by aspirin, perhaps because of its anti-inflammatory effect which reduces vascularity.

The typical radiological appearance is of a small lucent nidus surrounded by an area of sclerosis. Tomograms or a bone scan (in which the lesion shows up as a 'hot spot') may be helpful. Radiologically, the differential diagnosis is from Brodie's abscess.

Microscopically, the central nidus shows many small spicules of immature bone, lined by osteoblasts and osteoclasts. The stroma between these spicules is characteristically very vascular. The central nidus is surrounded by sclerotic cortical bone.

Treatment is by complete excision of the lesion, preferably under X-ray control; a complete cure is expected.

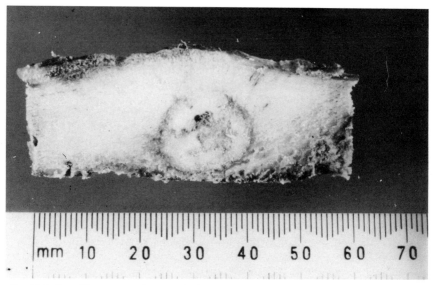

Fig. 19.4. Osteoid osteoma—the central nidus is 5 mm in diameter.

Osteoblastoma

There is some controversy as to whether this is a separate entity from the osteoid osteoma or merely a larger tumour of the same pathological type. It occurs most commonly in the first two decades but may be found at all ages. The main sites are vertebral column, femur, tibia and skull. The main symptoms are pain (not at night and not relieved by aspirin) and, occasionally, swelling in peripheral areas.

On X-ray, a lucent lesion with some mottling (depending on the degree of mineralization of the tumour osteoid) surrounded by a narrow margin of sclerosis is seen. A reddish vascular lesion, similar to a large osteoid osteoma, is typical but it is usually more than 2 cm in size.

Histologically, it is similar to an osteoid osteoma, although the pattern is less regular. Occasionally, osteoblastomas show more aggressive behaviour than osteoid osteomas and may be difficult to distinguish from osteosarcomas. Treatment is by curettage or local excision and bone grafting. Local recurrence is rare, but malignant change has been reported.

Malignant Bone Forming Tumours

Osteosarcoma

The WHO definition is 'a malignant tumour characterized by the direct formation of bone or osteoid by the tumour cells'.

Clinical features

More than 50% of cases occur in the second decade and there is a small second peak in old age, the result of sarcomatous change in Paget's disease. In decreasing order, the commonest sites are lower femur, upper tibia and upper humerus (together totalling 80% of all cases). Bone pain and swelling are the presenting features, with later cases demonstrating malaise, weight loss and anaemia. The serum alkaline phosphatase may be elevated and return to normal following excisional surgery; it may rise again when widespread metastases occur.

Radiology

The appearances are very variable ranging from lytic to sclerotic. Most cases display cortical perforation (with a soft tissue mass) and new bone formation but the classic Codman's triangle (periosteal new bone) and 'sun ray spiculation' are not always seen. Also, other lesions, including infection, may produce a similar appearance. Hence the need for biopsy in all cases in which this tumour is suspected, especially before radical surgery. The biopsy incision should be carefully placed with the possibility of further major surgery in mind.

Morphology

These tumours tend to be large metaphyseal lesions often filling the medulla. The cortex is perforated at one or more points causing periosteal elevation and soft tissue penetration (*see Fig.* 19.5). The typical white gritty appearances are due to

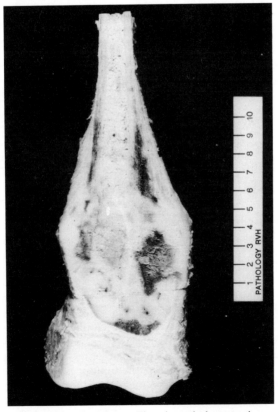

Fig. 19.5. Osteosarcoma of the distal femur. There is cortical penetration, periosteal elevation and extension into the soft tissues.

new bone formation, but bluish areas of cartilage and reddish areas of haemorrhage are also common.

The diagnostic histological feature is the production of osteoid or woven bone by malignant stromal cells (*see Fig.* 19.6). However, cartilage, myxoid and fibrous tissue are also produced from the pleuripotential mesenchymal tumour cells. The stromal cells are anaplastic, that is, they have bizarre nuclei and prominent nucleoli: many atypical mitotic figures are seen. Some areas may show undifferentiated spindle cells which are not producing ground substance. Normal looking osteoclasts may be seen and they represent a reactive change. Metastasis is usually by the haematogenous route and lymph node involvement is rare.

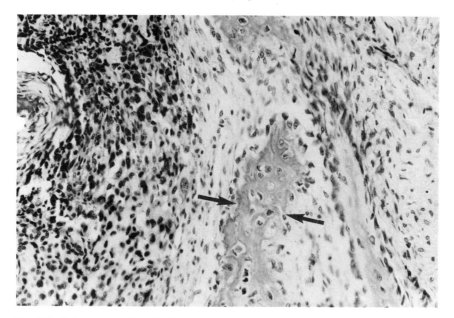

Fig. 19.6. Osteosarcoma. Note the formation of osteoid (arrows). (H and E × 75)

Prognosis and aspects of treatment

At the time of diagnosis, up to 80% of patients have pulmonary metastases either microscopic or overt. Until recently, radical ablative surgery has had poor results. Only 20% of patients were disease-free at 3 years and 50% showed pulmonary metastases by 6 months from diagnosis (Price *et al.* 1973). These dismal figures have been improved upon since the introduction of adjuvant chemotherapy in the early 1970s. The principal agents used are high dose methotrexate (with citrovorum 'rescue'), vincristine, adriamycin and cyclophosphamide.

By this attack on metastases, the disease-free interval has been lengthened. Surgery has become more conservative with either less radical amputation or limb preserving procedures. In suitable cases, the tumour is excised *en bloc* with a cuff of soft tissue and a custom-made large metal prosthesis is inserted (Scales 1983). Some patients with a small number of pulmonary metastases are now offered pulmonary wedge resection. Marcove *et al.* (1975) reported 45% 3 year survival in patients with pulmonary metastases treated by aggressive multiple thoracotomies.

Parosteal osteosarcoma

This is a more highly differentiated tumour arising from the periosteum and associated connective tissue. It occurs most commonly between the ages of 20 and 40 years with a preponderance of female cases. The usual sites are the lower femur and upper humerus, where it presents as a hard mass on the surface of the bone. Radiological appearances are characteristic with a large dense juxtacortical mass of new bone. Histologically, masses of woven new bone are seen arising in a fibrosarcomatous stroma.

Treatment is by *en bloc* resection or local amputation and the 5 year survival rate is over 60%.

Osteosarcoma arising in Paget's disease

Most patients are elderly with polyostotic Paget's disease of long duration. Many histological types are seen but all are anaplastic. Only a few survivors have been recorded even after radical amputation. It occurs in about 1% of all Paget's cases and in up to 10% of cases with extensive disease. Multicentric tumours may be seen in some patients.

Irradiation sarcoma

Sarcoma may develop in an irradiated bone after a long latent period. The risk appears to be dose related with a threshold of 1500 to 3000 rads. Most are histologically similar to conventional osteosarcoma and have a similar prognosis.

Benign Cartilage Forming Tumours

Chondroma

This rather common tumour occurs mainly in the small tubular bones of the hands and feet. It is usually centrally situated, in which case it is termed an 'enchondroma', but it may also be seen in relation to the outer cortex and periosteum ('ecchondroma'). The usual modes of presentation are either as a painful swelling or as a pathological fracture.

On X-ray, a well-defined lucent area with spicules of calcification is seen. It may be centrally located but if eccentric, the overlying cortex becomes thinned and liable to fracture. It is usually single. Multiple lesions are found in Ollier's disease, or in combination with soft tissue haemangiomas (Maffucci's syndrome).

Grossly, the lesion consists of bluish lobules of hyaline cartilage with variable grittiness. Microscopically, nests of proliferating cartilage cells are seen in a cartilaginous matrix. Areas of myxoid change, necrosis and endochondral ossification are seen. The cells have small dark uniform nuclei. Malignant transformation is rare in solitary lesions, but occurs in 25% to 50% of patients with Ollier's disease. Treatment is by curettage and bone grafting.

Osteochondroma (osteocartilaginous exostosis)

This is the commonest benign tumour of bone and is considered by some authorities to be a hamartoma. It consists of a cartilage capped bony projection on the surface of any bone which develops by endochondral ossification. The commonest sites are the metaphysis of long bones, particularly the lower femur and upper humerus. Approximately 80% of patients present in the first two decades of life and there is no significant difference in sex incidence. It usually presents as a painless swelling but may eventually produce pressure symptoms.

On X-ray, it appears as a well defined bony outgrowth, which often appears smaller than it feels on examination because the cartilage cap is radiolucent.

Grossly, the lesion is a pedunculated or sessile bony protuberance covered by periosteum and capped by hyaline cartilage. It is usually single, but a familial form occurs, in which the tumours are multiple (diaphysial aclasis).

Histologically, a cartilage cap is seen overlying poorly organized cancellous bone and areas of endochondral ossification (*see Fig. 19.7*).

Pressure effects on overlying muscles or tendons may lead to bursa formation. Rarely, nerve compression occurs. In 1–2% of lesions, malignant transformation occurs in later life as a peripheral chondrosarcoma. Malignant change occurs in up to 10% of patients with diaphysial aclasis.

Treatment is by local excision for pressure symptoms or when suspicion of malignant change arises. Asymptomatic lesions may be followed radiologically.

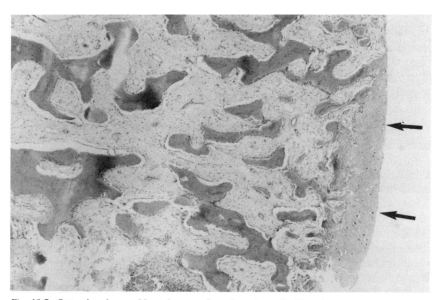

Fig. 19.7. Osteochondroma. Note the cap of cartilage (arrow). (H and E × 30)

Chondroblastoma (epiphyseal chondroblastoma)

This benign tumour of cartilaginous origin arises in the epiphysis of a long bone (femur, tibia and humerus) and rarely crosses the growth plate into the metaphysis. The majority of cases occur in teenage boys, before skeletal maturity.

Radiologically, it appears as a clear or stippled area of bony rarefaction with a sclerotic margin.

Grossly, the appearances may vary but many are greyish tumours with gritty areas of calcification.

Histologically, small round or polyhedral cells make up much of the tumour with a variable number of multinucleated giant cells. Focal areas of chondroid matrix are seen with individual cells surrounded by lines of calcification ('chicken wire' calcification). Lichtenstein (1977) considers it to represent an accessory epiphyseal cartilage centre.

Treatment is by curettage and bone grafting. Recurrence and malignant transformation may rarely occur. The differential diagnosis is from giant cell tumour and chondrosarcoma.

Chondromyxoid fibroma

This rare benign cartilage forming tumour contains areas of myxoid and chondroid intercellular matrix. It occurs between the ages of 10 and 30 years with an equal sex distribution. The usual site is in the lower limb, particularly the lower femur and upper tibia. The presentation is with chronic pain and, occasionally, swelling.

Radiologically, it appears as an oval radiolucency in the metaphyseal area, surrounded by a sclerotic rim.

Grossly, it appears as a white or yellow firm rubbery tumour.

Histologically, lobules of myxoid matrix containing few cells are interspersed with more densely cellular areas. The latter contain spindle cells and a few giant cells.

Treatment is by curettage, although there is a significant rate of recurrence, especially in younger patients. Some surgeons, therefore, advocate *en bloc* resection. Malignant transformation to chondrosarcoma has been recorded.

Malignant Cartilage Forming Tumours

Chondrosarcoma

This is a very variable tumour in terms of clinical and pathological features, as well as biological behaviour. Primary or central chondrosarcomas arise from the medullary cavity of long bones. Secondary chondrosarcomas arise from benign cartilage tumours, particularly if multiple (multiple endochondromatosis—Ollier's disease; and multiple osteochondromata—diaphysial aclasis). Rarely, chondro-sarcoma arises in Paget's disease or following radiation. Chondrosarcoma is a tumour of young adults, the majority of patients being 20–50 years old. Most arise in the metaphysis of long limb bones (femur, tibia, humerus), but pelvis, scapula and ribs may also be affected. The usual history is of pain and swelling. Presentation is often delayed, especially with those peripheral tumours arising from osteochondromas. Radiologically, a mottled partially calcified area is seen. Extensive stippled calcification gives appearances similar to a bone infarct. Cortical penetration may be present, indicating malignancy, but the pronounced periosteal reaction associated with osteosarcoma is usually absent.

Grossly, the tumour is lobulated and has the bluish-white appearance of cartilage. Areas of calcification and necrosis may be seen. Myxoid areas show a gelatinous appearance.

Histologically, chondrosarcomas vary greatly in their degree of differentiation. Low grade tumours show proliferating cartilage and are difficult to distinguish from enchondromas. Increased cellularity, nuclear hyperchromatism and pleomorphism and binucleated cells all point towards malignancy (*see Fig.* 19.8). Clinical features help in the distinction. Lesions which are large, central rather than peripheral and showing bone destruction on X-ray are viewed with suspicion. High grade lesions show anaplastic cellular features with spindle cell areas. Low grade chondrosarcomas may undergo malignant transformation into highly malignant osteosarcomas or fibrosarcomas and this change may not be recognized in a limited biopsy.

Treatment is by surgical excision, the extent of which depends on the histological grade and the anatomical site. Low grade early tumours are suitable for *en bloc* resection and prosthetic replacement. Anaplastic tumours may require amputation. The five year survival figures vary enormously from 20% to 80% depending on the type of tumour.

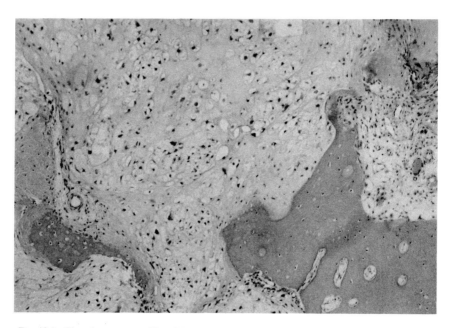

Fig. 19.8. Chondrosarcoma. (H and E × 30)

Giant cell tumour (Osteoclastoma)

Many aspects of this tumour are controversial because of its variable biological behaviour. Many other bone lesions which contain giant cells may be confused with giant cell tumours, e.g. chondroblastoma, chondromyxoid fibroma, aneurysmal bone cyst, non-ossifying fibroma, and the brown tumour of hyperthyroidism.

The usual age of presentation is between 20 and 40 years and there is a slight male preponderance. The location is usually epiphyseal, extending up to the subchondral bone and into the metaphysis. The most commonly affected sites are lower femur, upper tibia and lower radius. Pain and swelling are the usual presenting features, sometimes with restriction of movement of the neighbouring joint.

The tumour appears as a radiolucent area at one end of a long bone in a skeletally mature individual. The subchondral bone cortex may be thinned out but it remains intact unless a fracture has occurred or frank malignancy has supervened. A trabeculated 'soap bubble' appearance may be seen on X-ray.

Grossly, it is a soft grey tumour showing areas of haemorrhage. Histologically, there is a vascular stroma of mononuclear spindle cells, liberally interspersed with multinucleated giant cells. Schajowicz (1961) has shown the similarity between these giant cells and osteoclasts. Histological grading has not been helpful in predicting biological behaviour. Approximately one-third remain benign, one-third become locally invasive and one-third metastasize.

Treatment is surgical. Curettage is followed by a high recurrence rate and *en bloc* resection is better. Reconstruction may be by metal prostheses or osteocartilaginous allografts. Cryosurgery has been advocated by Marcove *et al.* (1973). Others have used curettage and filling of the cavity with acrylic bone cement (Persson and Wouters 1976).

Marrow Tumours

Ewing's sarcoma

This is a highly malignant primary sarcoma of bone, affecting young people and carrying a poor prognosis. In 1921, Ewing attributed its origin to the vascular endothelium of bone marrow, although this theory of histiogenesis is not universally accepted (Schajowicz and Araujo 1983).

The 5–20 year old age group is most commonly affected, with a preponderance of male patients. It affects the diaphyseal region of long bones (femur, tibia, humerus) and less commonly, flat bones such as the pelvis. The local lesion produces pain and often a lump. There are often marked constitutional effects such as fever, anaemia, a raised ESR and leucocytosis. On X-ray, a lucent area of bone destruction may be seen surrounded by lamellae of periosteal new bone ('onion peel'). This sign is not pathognomonic and is not always present. The clinical and radiological pictures may closely resemble osteomyelitis (pyogenic, tuberculous or even syphilitic). Grossly, it is a soft greyish tumour arising in the medulla. It may be red from haemorrhage and necrosis. At post-mortem examination, often many bones are affected, but it is not clear whether this represents metastatic spread or multicentric tumour.

Histologically, dense fields of small round cells are seen with uniform dark nuclei; the cell wall is often indistinct. The cells contain glycogen which can be demonstrated by PAS staining. This feature may help to distinguish Ewing's sarcoma from 'the small blue cell tumours of childhood', such as metastatic neuroblastoma, lymphoma and embryonal rhabdomyosarcoma. Early spread to the lungs and other bones occurs. Until recently, the prognosis was considered to be uniformly dismal. Recent use of chemotherapy combined with radiotherapy and local surgical resection has improved short term control of the disease.

Myeloma

Multiple myeloma is the commonest primary malignant tumour of bone. The cell of origin is the plasma cell and the usual sites are the bones which contain red marrow in adult life; vertebrae, ribs, skull and pelvis. Occasionally, there is only a single deposit (solitary plasmacytoma) but the majority progress to the state of multiple myelomatosis after a variable time interval. The majority of tumours are functional in that they secrete a monoclonal immunoglobulin. The large quantities of this circulating protein may be responsible for some of the complications of the disease such as amyloid deposition and renal failure.

The usual patient affected is in the 50–70 year old age group, with a slight predominance of male cases. Bone deposits may cause pain or pathological fracture. Back pain and sciatica are common presenting features. There may be marked constitutional symptoms such as lassitude, malaise and weight loss. Anaemia, hypercalcaemia and uraemia are frequently noted. The characteristic 'M' band on the serum protein electrophoresis is due to production of a specific immunoglobulin by the tumour cells.

The ESR is raised (often over 100 mm/hr) and the urine may show Bence-Jones protein (light chain subunits of the circulating immunoglobulin). Multiple lytic areas show up as 'punched out' lesions. Occasionally, diffuse osteoporosis is the only radiological sign.

Grossly, multiple soft grey or red tumours are found throughout the affected bone. Histologically, sheets of regular round cells are seen, similar in appearance to normal plasma cells. Fields of immature or atypical forms may also be seen. The nuclei show typical 'clock face' stippling caused by peripheral chromatin aggregation.

Occasionally, single lesions are amenable to surgery or radiotherapy. Diffuse myelomatosis responds best to combination chemotherapy which often relieves symptoms and may prolong life.

Vascular Tumours

All of these tumours are rare and of little clinical importance. They are listed (with short notes) to complete the classification.

Benign

HAEMANGIOMA: The vertebral bodies are the commonest site and the tumour is a rare cause of backache. The majority of cases are incidental X-ray or post-mortem findings. Following biopsy, haemorrhage may be profuse. Diffuse haemangiomas may be responsible for rare cases of massive osteolysis or 'disappearing bone disease'.

GLOMUS TUMOUR: These are very rare and are similar to those found in soft tissues. The usual site is a terminal phalanx where they cause exquisite pain.

Intermediate

HAEMANGIOENDOTHELIOMA AND HAEMANGIOPERICYTOMA: These are rare vascular tumours with variable biological behaviour. They may be multicentric and appear as vascular spaces lined by endothelial cells.

Malignant

ANGIOSARCOMA: This is a rare, highly malignant tumour arising from vascular endothelial cells. It grows rapidly, producing local bone destruction, and it metastasizes early to the lungs and other organs. Histologically, atypical vascular endothelial cells are seen in an anaplastic stroma.

Other Connective Tissue Tumours

Benign

DESMOPLASTIC FIBROMA: This is a rare tumour in bone and is similar to soft tissue desmoid tumours (*see* p. 525). Histologically, it is difficult to distinguish from fibrosarcoma.

LIPOMA: This is also very rare in bone and similar grossly and histologically to the soft tissue equivalent (*see* p. 528).

Malignant

FIBROSARCOMA: This may arise primarily from the connective tissue of the medullary cavity, but many are secondary to pre-existing benign conditions such as Paget's disease, giant cell tumour or fibrous dysplasia. Some appear after irradiation of bone. The usual age is between 30 and 60 years and the typical site is the metaphyseal area of femur and tibia. The histological picture varies from relatively well differentiated fibroblasts to an anaplastic picture. Treatment is surgical and the extent of resection depends on the histological grade (*en bloc* resection for differentiated lesions, amputation for anaplastic tumours).

LIPOSARCOMA: This is an extremely rare tumour of bone and only a few cases have been reported.

Other Tumours

Chordoma

This is a rare, slow growing tumour, arising from notochordal remnants. It is found only in the axial skeleton, sometimes proximally (spheno-occipital 10%), but more commonly distally (sacrococcygeal 70%). It rarely metastasizes, but is locally invasive, involving bone and soft tissues. Sacrococcygeal tumours usually present with a picture suggestive of nerve root compression, such as sciatic pain, paraesthesia, numbness or weakness.

Grossly, chordomas appear lobulated and well encapsulated. They range in colour from grey to blue and have a gelatinous texture.

Histologically, cords of polyhedral cells are seen containing intracellular mucin. Distinction from mucin secreting adenocarcinoma of the rectosigmoid may be difficult.

Treatment is by surgical excision when possible. Alternatively, good palliation may be achieved with radiotherapy.

Adamantinoma

This is a very rare tumour of long bones, resembling ameloblastoma of the mandible. Patients with long bone lesions are usually between 15 and 30 years of age. Clinically, it is a slow growing tumour, affecting the tibial diaphysis in 90% of cases. It may produce pain and swelling and the history is usually long.

Radiologically, it appears as a multicystic osteolytic lesion, which expands and thins the cortex ('soap bubble appearance').

Histologically, spindle shaped collagen producing cells are seen, alternating with nests of epithelioid cells. Late metastatic spread to the lungs may occur in 10% of cases. Local *en bloc* resection is usually curative.

Tumour-like Lesions

The importance of these lesions is that although they are not tumours, they may be mistaken as such and treated inappropriately.

Solitary bone cyst (simple or unicameral bone cyst)

These are seen in children but are rare after skeletal maturity. The usual site is the proximal metaphysis of femur or humerus. Some cysts are found as incidental

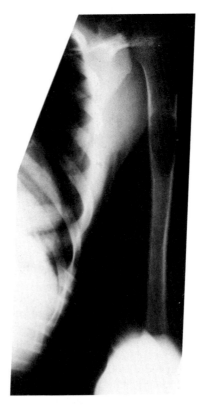

Fig. 19.9a. Simple (unicameral) bone cyst of the humerus which presented with a pathological fracture.

X-ray findings; others present as a pathological fracture (*see Fig.* 19.9*a, b*). Radiologically, they are seen as lucent areas in the metaphysis which expand and thin the cortex. In children, they are typically juxta-epiphysial in situation. Serial radiographs may show migration away from the epiphysial plate from the effect of growth.

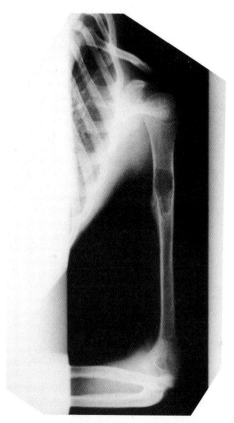

Fig. 19.9*b*. On follow-up, fracture healing is apparent.

The lesion is a single (unicameral) cavity, filled with clear fluid or blood (after fracture). The wall is composed of vascular connective tissue which may show giant cells. They are so rare in adults that spontaneous resolution probably occurs in the majority of cases. Pathological fracture may trigger the healing process. Penetration of the wall by a trocar and injection of steroid has given good results (Scaglietti *et al.* 1979). Curettage and bone grafting may be required in some cases if fracture appears a serious risk.

Aneurysmal bone cyst (multilocular haematic bone cyst)

This is a solitary, expansile lesion of bone, containing irregular blood filled spaces. Lichtenstein (1977) has suggested that the cause might be an intra-osseous arterio-venous shunt. Aneurysmal bone cysts occur mainly between the ages of 10 and 30 years, in either the metaphysis of long bones or vertebral bodies. The presentation is a painful swelling, increasing in size. On X-ray, an eccentrically placed radiolucency is seen with thinning of the overlying cortex and a fine trabecular pattern. Serial radiographs may show rapid expansion. The gross lesion shows a blood filled cavity divided by fibrous or bony septa. Histological examination shows blood filled cystic spaces separated by septa. The septa contain multinucleated giant cells, osteoid or immature bone. The presence of giant cells may lead to confusion with giant cell tumour. Treatment by excision and grafting gives good results but there is an appreciable incidence of local recurrence.

Metaphyseal fibrous defect (non-ossifying fibroma)

This is a common lesion seen in the metaphyseal region of the long bones of children and young adults. It is often discovered as an incidental finding on X-ray, but occasionally causes pain or pathological fracture.

Radiologically, it is seen as an eccentrically placed radiolucency with a sclerotic margin. Grossly, it is composed of friable soft tissue.

The lesion is characterized by whorls of regular spindle shaped connective tissue cells, interspersed with haemosiderin pigment and multinucleated giant cells.

There is a strong tendency to spontaneous healing and treatment is required only for symptomatic lesions or when there is risk of pathological fracture.

Fibrous dysplasia

This is a slow growing hamartomatous lesion, consisting of bone and fibrous tissue. It is probably developmental in origin, rather than a bone tumour, although the pattern of inheritance is not known.

Fibrous dysplasia is a relatively common lesion and is an important differential in the diagnosis of isolated lytic lesions of bone.

The commonest presentation is as an incidental finding on X-ray. Symptoms of pain, deformity or pathological fracture present in childhood or adolescence. Usually only one bone is affected (monostotic), but there is a rare polyostotic form which may be associated with patchy skin pigmentation and precocious puberty in girls (Albright's syndrome). The craniofacial skeleton, ribs and long bones are the usual sites. In long bones, the diaphysis or metaphysis is affected, but the epiphysis is spared. Malignant change (fibrosarcoma) is rare. Grossly, a fusiform expansion of the bone is seen with thinning of the cortex and replacement of cancellous bone by white, gritty tissue. Repeated minor fractures in the upper third of the femur may cause progressive collapse into varus deformity ('shepherd's crook' appearance) (*see Fig.* 19.10).

Histologically, irregular areas of woven bone are seen in a fibrous stroma. Areas of giant cells or fracture callus are sometimes present and may cause diagnostic confusion. On X-ray, the usual appearance is a radiolucent area with a 'ground glass' appearance. Fracture and deformity are commonly seen. The clinical course is variable. Some lesions may heal spontaneously, but others progress and may require treatment. Excision biopsy and bone grafting may be appropriate for small lesions. Osteotomy and intramedullary fixation may be required for deformity.

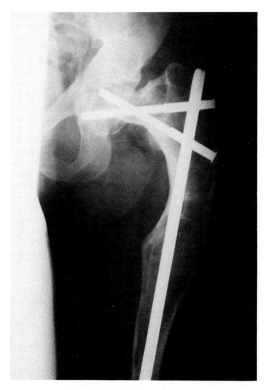

Fig. 19.10. Fibrous dysplasia with pathological fracture of the femoral neck and 'shepherd's crook' deformity of the proximal femur.

Eosinophilic granuloma

The term histiocytosis X includes three conditions which demonstrate similar lesions in bone—eosinophilic granuloma, Hand–Schüller–Christian disease, and Letterer–Siwe disease (Lichtenstein 1977). The biological behaviour and the presence of eosinophils suggests an allergic response rather than a neoplasm. Eosinophilic granuloma presents most commonly to the surgeon as an isolated lytic lesion of bone. The most common age of presentation is childhood or adolescence. The sites affected are the skull and long bones.

Clinically, the presentation is local bone pain and tenderness or, more rarely, pathological fracture. It may be found as an incidental X-ray finding, or as a 'punched-out' radiolucent area. The overlying cortex may be thinned and expanded with a periosteal reaction. Ewing's sarcoma and osteomyelitis are important differential diagnoses.

Grossly, tissue curetted from an eosinophilic granuloma is soft reddish material, sometimes flecked with yellow. Histologically, eosinophils, plasma cells and multinucleated giant cells are seen. Biopsy is often required for diagnosis and following this most lesions heal.

Brown tumours of hyperparathyroidism
See p. 585.

Disorders of the Hip in Children

Congenital dislocation of the hip (CDH)

Genetic and environmental factors are believed to play a role in the development of CDH. A familial incidence varying between 6% and 36% has been reported (Wynne-Davies 1970). The inherited factor may be increased laxity of the joint capsule or acetabular dysplasia. Environmental factors may be pre-natal or post-natal. CDH is more common in breech presentation, caesarian delivery and first born children. Females are more commonly affected than males, in a ratio of 4 : 1, and in 25% of patients the condition is bilateral. The position of the hips after birth may be important. In races which swaddle their infants (hips extended and adducted), such as the Lapps and North American Indians, the incidence of CDH is high. The Bantu, who nurse infants on the mother's back (hips abducted and flexed), have a much lower incidence of the condition. Genetic factors may also play a part in these racial differences.

The age of presentation of CDH depends on the effectiveness of neonatal screening. In the hands of skilled examiners, almost all cases may be diagnosed in infancy using the Ortolani and Barlow tests. However, most screening programmes have a significant failure rate, with many cases undetected until the child demonstrates a limp on beginning to walk.

Grossly, the early development of the hips is relatively normal. Most of the pathological features are secondary changes induced by the position of dislocation.

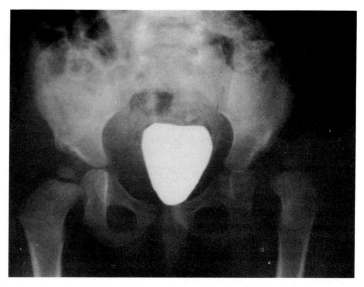

Fig. 19.11. Congenital dislocation of the left hip. There is poor acetabular development.

In the acetabulum, the fibrocartilaginous labrum becomes inverted and the ligamentum teres and pulvinar fat pad enlarge. The bony acetabulum fails to develop properly, remaining shallow and facing anterolaterally (*see Fig.* 19.11). These features are probably related to the absence of normal femoral head contact pressure. The capsule stretches and infolds to form an 'hour-glass constriction' between the femoral head and acetabulum (*see Fig.* 19.12). In time, the soft tissues become adaptively shortened. The femoral neck is often excessively anteverted in relation to the shaft. The bony nucleus of the capital epiphysis appears later and remains smaller than that on the unaffected side. Contrast arthrography is useful in outlining the cartilaginous epiphysis and soft tissue obstructions to reduction in the acetabulum.

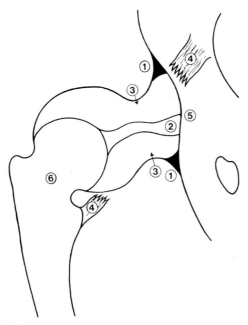

Fig. 19.12. Diagrammatic representation of the main features of CDH (after Apley 1973): 1. Inverted labrum. 2. Hypertrophied ligamentum teres. 3. 'Hour-glass' constriction of capsule. 4. Tight psoas tendon. 5. Shallow acetabulum. 6. Anteverted femoral neck.

The principle of treatment is to reduce the dislocation and maintain the reduction until the hip is stable.

Early diagnosis is of the greatest importance. In the neonate, three months treatment in an abduction splint will result in a normal hip in many patients. In older children, reduction is often more difficult and complications are more frequent. The blood supply of the epiphysis is vulnerable to pressure from forced abduction in the presence of soft tissue contractures and obstructions in the acetabulum. Avascular necrosis of the epiphysis may cause deformity of the developing femoral head. Damage to the epiphyseal plate may result in growth arrest.

Perthes' disease

Perthes' disease is a childhood hip condition of uncertain aetiology. Predisposing factors have been described from epidemiological studies. These include low social class, children with older parents, low birth weight, children born late in the family and trauma to the hip. Boys are affected four times more frequently than girls and in 12% of patients, the condition is bilateral. The age of onset is usually between 3 and 10 years.

The clinical presentation is a healthy child with a painful irritable hip and a limp. Pain may not last long, but restriction of hip movements persists, particularly abduction in flexion and internal rotation.

One theory of the pathogenesis of Perthes' disease is the 'tamponade' effect of a joint effusion. During childhood, the blood supply of the epiphysis is from medial and lateral retinacular vessels. The intracapsular course of these vessels renders them susceptible to closure by the pressure of a joint effusion. Minor trauma or viral illness may initiate such an effusion and the resultant 'tamponade' may lead to avascular necrosis of the epiphysis.

Following infarction of the epiphysis, histological examination reveals death of marrow cells, as well as of osteocytes and osteoblasts. The articular cartilage is nourished by synovial fluid and continues to grow. During this stage, the bony epiphysis is radiologically normal, but there is an increased 'joint space' (more accurately, increased 'cartilage space'). This is followed by a repair phase in which there is ingrowth of vascular granulation tissue. New bone is laid down on the dead trabeculae by the process of 'creeping substitution', or more accurately, 'creeping apposition'. Radiologically, this stage may show increased bone density of the epiphysis. However, some necrotic trabeculae may not be able to withstand the pressures of weight bearing. Collapse and fragmentation may follow. These crushed areas are reabsorbed and produce permanent deformity. Metaphyseal changes are seen in severe cases with radiolucent or cystic areas on X-ray (*see Fig.* 19.13).

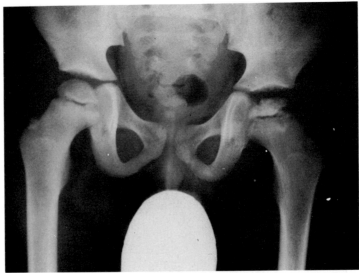

Fig. 19.13. Perthes' disease of left hip. There is collapse and increased density of the epiphysis, and a metaphyseal cyst.

The end stage of severe Perthes' disease is flattening and irregularity of the femoral head. As this may lead to premature degenerative arthritis, treatment is aimed at preserving the shape of the capital epiphysis. In the early acute phase, bed rest and skin traction are advised until pain and muscle spasm are relieved. Thereafter, management is controversial. Most forms of treatment are based on the principle of containing the femoral head in the acetabulum during the healing phase. It has been suggested that the cartilage is in a plastic state during the active phase of the disease. The aim of containment is to keep the epiphysis covered by acetabulum during this stage, in the hope of improving the final shape of the femoral head. This may be achieved by conservative means (abduction splintage) or by surgery. Surgical options are pelvic or femoral osteotomy. The selection of patients for surgical treatment is important as 60% of patients will achieve a good result without operation. Selection may be based on a number of radiological features indicating 'the head at risk' of deformity, collapse and a poor result (Catterall 1982).

Slipped upper femoral epiphysis

The growth plates are potential areas of weakness in the long bones of children. Forces that would produce a fracture or dislocation after bony maturity result in an epiphyseal separation in the younger patient. The upper femoral epiphysis is unique in that displacement or 'slipping' may be produced by normal weight bearing forces or trivial trauma. In 70% of cases, the process is gradual, but in 30% the presentation is acute. Clinical features are pain in the hip or knee, associated with a limp. There is a history of minor trauma in about half of the patients and boys are affected slightly more frequently than girls. The peak age of onset coincides with the adolescent growth spurt—15 years in boys and 13 years in girls. In 60% of cases, the patient is obese with delayed sexual development. A few cases are associated with endocrine disorders, such as hypothyroidism (Puri et al. 1985). Diagnosis may be delayed as the knee is often X-rayed on the first visit to hospital. When the hip is X-rayed, the early changes may be difficult to see on the anteroposterior film. The lateral radiograph is the most sensitive way of diagnosing early degrees of slipping (see Fig. 19.14).

Grossly, the capital epiphysis slips posteriorly, tearing the anterior periosteum off the femoral neck, together with the associated retinacular vessels. The posterior periosteum is elevated and new bone formation leads to a posterior 'beak' on the femoral neck. The anterior portion of the neck undergoes partial resorption and the overall effect is posterior bowing of the neck. Histological examination reveals a wide, irregular growth plate with disturbed endochondral ossification. Focal areas of haemorrhage may be seen between the growth plate and metaphysis.

Complications are often, but not exclusively, the result of treatment. Manipulative reduction may tear the remaining posterior retinacular vessels and cause avascular necrosis of the femoral head. Subsequent bony collapse will lead to secondary osteoarthritis. Acute chondrolysis refers to cartilage necrosis affecting both femoral epiphysis and acetabulum. It is more frequent in Negroes, following prolonged immobilization, and penetration of the joint by fixation pins. Some patients have elevated immunoglobulins and C3 complement levels, suggesting an autoimmune basis.

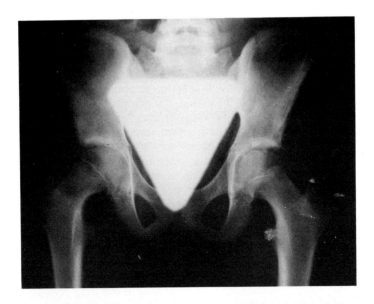

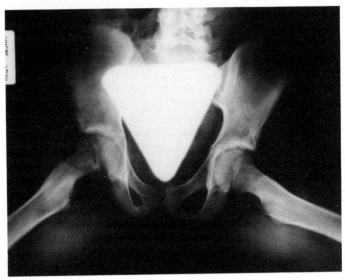

Fig. 19.14 Slipped upper femoral epiphysis of the right hip (AP projection *top*). Slipped upper femoral epiphysis of the right hip (lateral view *bottom*). Minor degrees of slip are more easily appreciated on a lateral projection.

Treatment depends on the degree of slip and the state of the growth plate. The most common procedure is pinning *in situ* (to prevent further slipping). In hips with more than 50 degrees of slip, open reduction or late corrective osteotomy may be advised. Both procedures are difficult and have a significant complication rate.

Inherited Dysplasias of Bone

There is a large number of genetic disorders which have skeletal manifestations. The nature of the basic defect is not understood in many of these disorders and this leads to difficulties in classification.

In conditions such as the mucopolysaccharidoses, in which the pathogenesis is known, the basic defect is biochemical. It is probable that other bone dysplasias will be found to have enzyme defects leading to a biochemical abnormality. In the absence of more definitive criteria, a classification based on clinical features is useful.

Examples of some of the types of inherited bone dysplasias follow.

Bone dysplasia with dwarfism

Short limb dwarfism (achondroplasia)

This is the commonest form of dwarfism and is apparent at birth. The classical type of achondroplasia is inherited on an autosomal dominant basis. Since these patients have problems in reproduction, 85% of cases in the population may be the result of spontaneous mutations.

Clinically, the limbs are disproportionately short, with the proximal segment particularly affected. Increased subcutaneous tissue and shortened phalanges lead to the characteristic trident appearance of the fingers. The abdomen is prominent with a lumbar lordosis and hip flexion contractures are present.

Radiological features include irregular metaphyseal development in the limb bones (with normal epiphyses) and lumbar spinal stenosis. Histologically, there is abnormal endochondral ossification in long bones, with masses of cartilage cells, which fail to orientate correctly. Surgery may be required for signs of spinal cord compression in the narrow spinal canal. Varus deformity of the knees may be corrected by osteotomy to prevent degenerative arthritis.

Proportionate dwarfism

The lysosomal storage diseases (mucopolysaccharidoses) are the result of enzyme deficiencies leading to the accumulation of mucopolysaccharides such as dermatan, keratin and heparin sulphate. The central nervous system, heart and reticulo-endothelial system are most seriously affected. At least ten and probably more syndromes exist (Bullough and Vigorita 1984).

MPS-I (Hurler's syndrome) is inherited as an autosomal recessive gene. Infants appear normal until the age of one year. Mental retardation is progressive and severe. By the age of two years, the characteristic facies has developed with enlarged tongue and corneal clouding. Visceral deposits lead to hepatosplenomegaly. Joint stiffness may be marked and the hips are frequently dislocated. Death from pulmonary disease is usual before the age of 10 years.

Radiological features include thoracolumbar kyphosis (due to anterior wedging of the vertebrae), coxa valga and hip dysplasia. The phalanges have irregular epiphyses and the metacarpals are conical at the proximal end.

Histological examination of the affected tissues shows the accumulation of abnormal metabolites. Histochemical studies of cultured fibroblasts may identify the particular enzyme defect, but specific therapy is not yet available.

MPS-II (Hunter's syndrome) is inherited as an X-linked recessive trait and is therefore only seen in males. Clinically, mild and severe forms are recognized. The severe form resembles MPS-I but with a later age of onset (2 to 4 years) and longer survival (20 to 40 years).

In the mild form, there may be no mental impairment and survival to adulthood is usual.

Bone dysplasia without dwarfism

This includes a large number of disorders which may be classified according to the region of the bone affected (such as multiple epiphyseal dysplasia or multiple metaphyseal dysplasia); other dysplasias in this group may be grouped according to a generalized change in bone density.

Increased bone density (osteopetrosis)

This is a rare bone dysplasia in which the bones show increased density on X-ray. There are at least two clinical types—an adult (tarda) form (autosomal dominant) and a severe infantile type (autosomal recessive).

Although bone density is increased, the tarda form may present with repeated fractures. Cranial nerve palsies occur from compression in the basal foramina of the skull. In the infantile form, stillbirth is common. Surviving infants have anaemia, hepatosplenomegaly and die from overwhelming infection, aplastic anaemia or haemorrhage.

Radiologically, the signs are of increased bone density and the medullary canal may be obliterated. Areas of normal bone often alternate with more dense bone, giving a characteristic banded appearance. In the spine, this is referred to as a 'rugger jersey' appearance.

On gross inspection, the metaphyses of the long bones are flared with an 'Erlenmeyer flask' deformity. In children, central diaphyseal thickening may suggest a 'bone within a bone', the 'endobone' appearance.

Histologically, there is abnormal remodelling. Although osteoclasts are seen in normal numbers on light microscopy, they lack their normal 'ruffled border' on electron microscopy. This suggests loss of remodelling activity. In the severe infantile types, steroids and bone marrow transplantation may prolong life. In adults, pathological fractures are treated by conventional means.

Decreased bone density (osteogenesis imperfecta)

This term includes several clinical syndromes characterized by increased fragility of bone. The severe congenital form presents at birth with multiple fractures and is of autosomal recessive inheritance. There is a high incidence of stillbirth and survivors show severe dwarfing. Osteogenesis imperfecta tarda is seen more commonly in clinical practice, presenting in early childhood with multiple pathological fractures.

There is evidence of a generalized connective tissue disorder affecting collagen. Patients may have blue sclerae, generalized joint laxity, otosclerosis and poor dentition. Deficient skin collagen leads to excessive bruising and poor healing of surgical scars.

Radiologically, the skull shows a broad vault with multiple ossification centres or wormian bones. In the long bones, generalized osteoporosis, fractures and deformity are seen.

Grossly, the long bones show 'eggshell' cortices with old and recent fractures (*see Fig.* 19.15). The epiphyses appear large in relation to the rest of the bone and may be irregular from the effects of repeated trauma. Histologically, the lamellar pattern of the bone matrix may be abnormal, with a hypercellular appearance due to the relative deficiency of matrix.

Management of fractures is difficult because immobilization results in further weakening of bone due to disuse osteoporosis. This increases the tendency to fracture from trivial trauma in the rehabilitation period. Patients should be treated in weight bearing casts whenever possible. Bones that are badly deformed and subject to frequent refracture may be straightened and stabilized by multilevel osteotomy and intramedullary fixation (fragmentation and rodding) (Williams 1965).

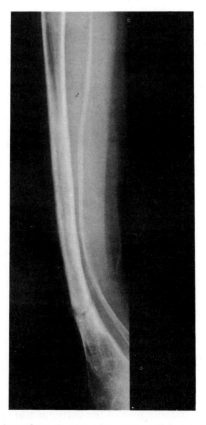

Fig. 19.15. Osteogenesis imperfecta. Bowing of the tibia and fibula, with a recent pathological fracture.

Osteoarthrosis (OA)

OA is a common degenerative joint disease arising in articular cartilage and sometimes progressing to destruction of the weight bearing surfaces of the joint.

The articulating bone ends making up a synovial joint are covered by articular cartilage, permitting the smooth gliding of one articular surface over another. The resilience of articular cartilage under repeated loading is due to the remarkable qualities of the constituent matrix and cells (matrix: proteoglycan 15%, collagen 15%, water 70%; cells: chondrocytes). There are no blood vessels or nerves.

The proteoglycan molecule consists of a hyaluronic acid core with protein side chains, linked to sulphated mucopolysaccharides (chondroitin and keratin sulphate). The collagen of articular cartilage consists of three α-1 chains in a triple helix formation. The collagen fibres form a three-dimensional lattice with the proteoglycan firmly attached within the framework. Proteoglycan is a hydrophilic colloid and binds many water molecules. Normally there is an equilibrium between the oncotic pressure within the cartilage and the external mechanical pressure. If the load is increased, deformation takes place, water leaves the matrix, the oncotic pressure rises and a new equilibrium is established. The collagen network withstands tensile stress and the proteoglycans withstand compressive stress.

The matrix is synthesized and maintained by chondrocytes which are embedded in the cartilage. They have a low metabolic rate and rely on diffusion from the synovial fluid for nutrition. Under normal conditions, chondrocytes have limited powers of reduplication and only when the matrix is disrupted is a significant number of new chondrocytes seen.

The subchondral bone is light and cancellous. It is more elastic than compact bone and better able to absorb stress.

In the normal joint, a balance exists between the destructive effects of stress and the ability of chondrocytes to remodel cartilage and maintain the matrix. In degenerative joint disease, this balance is tipped in favour of breakdown rather than repair. However, OA is not always progressive and in some joints, spontaneous clinical and radiological improvement occurs.

Aetiology

It has been customary to divide OA into primary or idiopathic (when no cause is known) and secondary (when it follows a definite abnormality). The concept of idiopathic OA has been seriously questioned by Solomon (1976) who studied 327 cases of degenerative joint disease and found an identifiable cause in all but 27 cases. It is useful to consider OA as the result of abnormal stress or abnormal cartilage.

ABNORMAL STRESS: This may be initiated by a variety of mechanical factors: (1) joint incongruity, for example Perthes' disease, intra-articular fracture and slipped upper femoral epiphysis; (2) uneven loading, for example congenital dislocation of the hip, varus deformity of the knee, anterior cruciate deficient knee and obesity.

ABNORMAL CARTILAGE: If the integrity of the cartilage itself is weakened, degeneration may occur even if the stress on the joint is normal. There is evidence for decreasing tensile strength of collagen with age, perhaps due to increased cross-linking of collagen. Pannus formation such as occurs in rheumatoid disease and tuberculosis may inhibit cartilage nutrition. Pyogenic infection releases toxins which directly attack the articular cartilage, and crystal disease such as gout may cause depolymerization of proteoglycan. Abnormal synovial fluid may affect cartilage nutrition, for example repeated haemarthroses of haemophilia. Finally, minor changes in the ultrastructure of cartilage may affect its long-term performance. These may have a genetic basis or be part of a syndrome of generalized skeletal dysplasia.

Pathogenesis

One of the earliest changes is an increase in water content, followed by depletion of proteoglycans. This is seen in human OA and in a canine model (the anterior cruciate deficient knee) (McDevitt *et al.* 1977). The proteoglycan molecules are strongly hydrophilic and the mechanical integrity of the collagen network may be a factor limiting the uptake of water. The collagen fibre network is fatigue prone and the tensile strength falls with age (Freeman 1975). One hypothesis of cartilage failure is that disruption of the collagen fibre network leads to a failure to restrict the oncotic pressure of proteoglycans, resulting in an increase in water content and swelling of the cartilage layers which, in turn, leads to decreased resilience under stress. A spiral of collagen breakdown, proteoglycan loss and decreased mechanical integrity ensues. Synovitis is probably a reactive phenomenon to debris in the joint rather than an initiating factor.

Morphology

These ultrastructural changes are manifested grossly as fibrillation of the cartilage surface. The cartilage appears granular, velvety or irregular compared with the smooth shiny appearance of normal cartilage. Fibrillation may remain static for many years in some joints but in others it may progress rapidly to fissure formation. These are deeper splits into the basal layers of the cartilage and subchondral bone. Shearing forces may now cause loss of flakes of cartilage exposing subchondral bone (*see Fig.* 19.16).

Microscopically, clusters of chondrocytes may be seen in relation to fissures in an attempt at repair. The ability of articular cartilage to repair itself is limited due to the absence of direct blood supply and the low cell-to-matrix ratio. If a full thickness defect occurs, vascular granulation tissue may gain access from the rich plexus in the subchondral bone and repair the defect with fibrocartilage.

With the loss of cartilage, the unprotected exposed subchondral bone now becomes the direct weight bearing surface, leading to microfracture, collapse and irregularity. Surviving osteoblasts increase bone formation to resist the new stresses producing sclerosis. Progressive remodelling and ossification of cartilage at the periphery causes osteophyte formation. Cysts are seen in the subchondral area on X-ray. These are really pseudocysts as they are usually filled with myxomatous fibrous tissue rather than fluid. They were formerly thought to represent synovial fluid entering the bone under excessive pressure, but a more probable explanation is that they represent areas of bone necrosis.

Inflammatory changes in soft tissue are usually much less marked than in rheumatoid disease. The degree of synovitis is variable from one subject to another and may represent a response to varying amounts of wear debris deposited in the synovium. Histologically, the early changes include perivascular cellular response and the presence of foreign body giant cells. Later, fibrosis of capsule and ligaments occurs leading to contracture and fixed deformity. Destruction of the supporting ligaments may lead to instability and accelerate the degenerative process.

Radiological features correspond to the pathological features already described. Early changes are joint space narrowing and 'squaring' of the lateral joint margins. Subchondral sclerosis, pseudocysts and marginal osteophytes are frequently seen at a later stage.

Clinically, the main symptoms are pain, stiffness and deformity. Many patients are helped by conservative measures, including analgesics, rest, heat and physiotherapy. Much of the orthopaedic surgeon's time is spent in the operative treatment of this common condition by osteotomy, arthrodesis and arthroplasty.

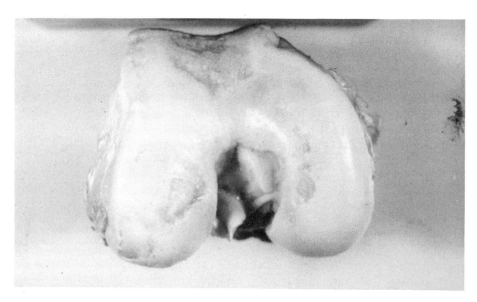

Fig. 19.16. Osteoarthritis of the knee: there are areas of full thickness cartilage loss with exposure of subchondral bone affecting both femoral condyles. In the surrounding area there is fibrillation and fissuring.

Rheumatoid Arthritis (RA)

Rheumatoid disease is a systemic disorder in which a symmetrical chronic polyarthritis is the main feature. Many organs may be affected, including heart, lungs, skin and eyes. The effects of the disease on joints and tendons is due to a chronic inflammatory synovitis. This synovitis is non-specific and the many forms of chronic polyarthritis are classified according to clinical and laboratory criteria.

Rheumatoid disease is common, affecting about 3% of the population. The peak age of onset is the fourth decade of life, although any age may be affected. It is three times more common in women than in men.

Clinical features

Clinical features include a symmetrical polyarthritis of the small joints of the hands and feet, associated with systemic symptoms such as malaise, fatigue, weight loss and fever. Other patterns of joint involvement include a monoarticular form or asymmetrical involvement of weight bearing joints. There is no specific test for RA and diagnostic criteria are therefore clinical. Rheumatoid factor, an IgM immunoglobulin, is present in 80% of cases, but is also found in other diseases and in 5% of the normal population. Twenty per cent of patients with a typical clinical form of rheumatoid arthritis are seronegative. The clinical course and severity of the disease are very variable.

Aetiology and pathogenesis

The inner surface of diarthroidal joints, except that part covered in cartilage, is lined by synovial membrane. It is also present as an enveloping sheath around the long flexor and extensor tendons. It consists of an inner cellular layer supported by a fibrous connective tissue layer. At the articular margin, it inserts into the periosteum of the subchondral bone. The surface is smooth and moist, arranged with a few folds and villi. The synovial cells are divided into two categories according to their ultrastructural appearance on electron microscopy. Type A cells look like macrophages and function as phagocytes of joint debris. Type B cells have large amounts of rough endoplasmic reticulum and secrete hyaluronic acid. Synovial fluid is a clear viscous fluid with a yellowish tinge. It is a dialysate of plasma with the addition of hyaluronate. This confers an ability to lubricate the joint and protect articular cartilage.

The precise cause of rheumatoid disease has not yet been established. Genetic and immunological factors are well recognized, but the initiating agent remains elusive. Various bacterial and viral agents have been suggested. In summary, the disease may result from the effect of an initiating factor in a genetically susceptible individual, leading to immunological overactivity. Genetic susceptibility is suggested by the familial tendency and the frequency of certain histocompatibility antigens (HLA-DW4, HLA-CW3) in affected patients.

Evidence of immune overactivity includes the presence of rheumatoid factor (an IgM immunoglobulin active against IgG), synovial infiltration by lymphocytes and plasma cells and low complement levels in synovial fluid. Thoracic duct cannulation and removal of circulating lymphocytes may cause a remission of the disease and reinfusion of lymphocytes causes a relapse.

The sequence of events may start with an unidentified antigen reaching the synovium. Following phagocytosis by the type A synovial cells, antigen may be released into the synovial fluid. B-lymphocytes are stimulated and transform into antibody-secreting plasma cells. Antigen–antibody complexes initiate a full scale inflammatory reaction with the recruitment of T-lymphocytes and the activation of complement and kinin systems.

Morphology

Proliferative phase

Macroscopically, there is marked proliferation of villi and folds of synovial membrane. This is due to the proliferation of synoviocytes. The increased surface area is in part responsible for the accompanying joint effusion. The synovial fluid appears turbid because of the greatly increased number of cells (polymorphs, lymphocytes and plasma cells). There is a marked reduction in the level of hyaluronate, which results in loss of viscosity. This may affect joint lubrication and cartilage nutrition. Fibrin is produced, lining the synovium and extending onto the articular surface. This appears to inhibit cell nutrition as cell necrosis is often seen underneath such deposits. Cellular infiltrates are often marked. Polymorphs are seen only in the early phase, but remain in the synovial fluid for a longer period.

Maturation/repair phase

At a later stage, mesenchymal transformation of synovial cells takes place, with the proliferation of fibroblasts and collagen synthesis. This is seen macroscopically as a tough adherent membrane or 'pannus'. This does not directly attack cartilage but may cause damage by inhibiting nutrition from the synovial fluid by close adherence. Synovial villi may become thickened with fibrous cores which later become hyalinized. Fragments of these become detached and coated in fibrin, producing the characteristic 'rice bodies'.

End stage

This phase is characterized by permanent damage to the joint and secondary degenerative changes. Unlike osteoarthrosis, there is little reparative activity.

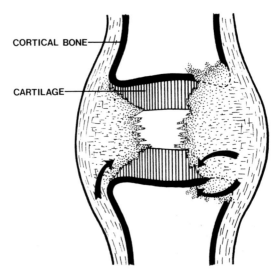

Fig. 19.17. Rheumatoid arthritis: on the left, early synovial proliferation and cartilage destruction; on the right, full thickness loss of cartilage and bone (marginal erosions).

Cartilage is damaged by the effects of pannus and proteolytic enzymes released from polymorphs. This occurs first at the synovial-cartilage junctions or joint recesses. In time, cartilage necrosis spreads centripetally towards the centre of the joint. Exposed subchondral bone is reabsorbed, giving rise to the characteristic marginal erosion seen on X-ray (*see Fig.* 19.17). Pseudocysts form in the osteoporotic subchondral bone due to increased hydrodynamic pressure. Very high pressures may occur in rheumatoid joints due to the presence of an effusion and the decreased compliance of a chronically inflamed synovium and capsule.

When most of the synovium and cartilage have been eroded and covered in pannus, fibrous ankylosis may occur. Rarely, dystrophic calcification may lead to bony ankylosis.

Ligaments and capsular destruction may lead to joint subluxation or frank dislocation. The resultant increased mechanical pressure on articular cartilage may accelerate secondary osteoarthritic degeneration. In the late stages, acute inflammation may subside, leaving a joint with degenerative changes anatomically indistinguishable from OA.

Other soft tissue changes

Baker's cyst

Raised intra-articular pressure may lead to distension of a bursa with the formation of a large extra-articular fluid collection. The best known example is Baker's cyst in the popliteal fossa. Arthrography has demonstrated a valve-like mechanism whereby fluid may enter the cyst on flexion but reflux does not occur on extension. The cyst wall is formed from fibrous connective tissue with a synovial lining which may be involved with varying degrees of synovitis.

Tendon sheaths

The long flexor and extensor tendons are surrounded by a layer of synovium to enhance their gliding functions. In some areas, particularly the digital fibrous sheaths, there is little room for expansion. Inflammatory synovitis may cause swelling and impede the nutrition of the tendon by a pressure effect. In combination with direct inflammatory infiltration, this may lead to tendon weakening and spontaneous rupture. If synovitis becomes chronic, inflammatory adhesions may mature into fibrous bands which restrict tendon gliding. Intra-articular ligaments, such as the cruciates and long head of biceps, may undergo similar erosion and spontaneous rupture.

Subcutaneous nodules

These are found in 20% of patients with seropositive rheumatoid disease. They consist of firm, grey nodules found in subcutaneous sites, especially overlying bone. Histologically, they are seen to have a necrotic centre surrounded by a characteristic palisade of histiocytes and giant cells. The outermost layers are composed of fibrous tissue which provide attachment to adjacent tissues. Mechanical pressure effects are felt to be an initiating factor, but the essential process is of immune complex deposition (IgM rheumatoid factor plus IgG) in relation to small blood vessels. Complement activation and vasculitis then ensue.

Many other changes are seen in this systemic disease, including skin and muscle atrophy and parenchymal tissue involvement (heart, lung, kidneys and eyes).

Aspects of treatment

In the light of the above discussion, some general principles are given below.

Conservative

DRUGS: Non-steroidal anti-inflammatory drugs are widely used because they give symptomatic relief from the symptoms of early synovitis (pain, swelling and stiffness). They probably have little effect on the course of the disease. Disease-modifying drugs, such as gold and D-penicillamine are given to modify the disease process rather than simply suppress symptoms. Corticosteroids, both systemically and locally, have a role to play in controlling the inflammation of RA, but there is a high price to pay in terms of side effects, particularly osteoporosis, skin atrophy and muscle wasting.

GENERAL MEASURES: Rest probably reduces fluid production and secondary intra-articular pressure. Splintage may selectively 'rest' a joint in an otherwise active patient. Physiotherapy helps to retain a maximum range of joint motion.

Surgery

SYNOVECTOMY: With improved drug control and implant surgery, the role of synovectomy has decreased.

TENDON SURGERY: Synovectomy of the long flexor and extensor tendons of the hand may prevent rupture. Secondary repair is, however, necessary in many cases.

JOINT EXCISION: This simple measure is effective in a few restricted sites, e.g. head of radius or distal ulna. This may relieve pain and increase movement.

ARTHRODESIS: This is rarely used primarily, but rather as a salvage following failure of arthroplasty.

OSTEOTOMY: This has a role to play in 'burnt out' cases where secondary osteoarthritis has supervened.

REPLACEMENT ARTHROPLASTY: This is the most widely used technique whereby joint surfaces are excised and replaced by implants. The present state of joint arthroplasty may be summarized as well established (hip, knee and small joints of the hand), early evaluation (elbow) and experimental (shoulder, ankle).

Ankylosing Spondylitis

Ankylosing spondylitis is the most familiar of a group of disorders termed 'seronegative spondyloarthropathies'. Patients are seronegative for rheumatoid factor, but 95% carry the HLA-B27 antigen. The other disorders in the group are psoriatic arthritis, Reiter's disease, enteropathic arthritis, panarticular juvenile

RA, Behçet's syndrome and possibly others. Acute anterior uveitis may occur in patients with evidence of spondyloarthropathy or as an isolated finding in patients who are HLA-B27 positive.

The aetiology is unknown, although it may represent an abnormal immune response, in genetically predisposed individuals, to infectious agents or their products.

Clinically, the patients at first suffer from lower backache and early morning stiffness. The sacroiliac joints are first involved, followed by the spine (leading to restriction of chest movements) and peripheral joints. Eventually, bony ankylosis leads to joint immobility.

Grossly, in the spine, bony ankylosis of the vertebral joints produces a continuous immobile bony column ('bamboo spine'), usually with a kyphosis. Within the intervertebral disc, the annulus fibrosis becomes ossified while the central portion of the disc remains unossified. Characteristically the spinal ligaments are ossified. Bony ankylosis of the costovertebral joints further reduces chest movement and involvement of peripheral joints such as the hips and knees produces severe loss of function.

Histologically there are inflammatory changes at the insertion of ligaments and tendons into bone ('enthesitis') as well as in the synovial membranes of affected joints. The articular cartilage becomes covered by pannus and active endochondral ossification is seen across the articular cartilage or intervertebral disc.

Metabolic Bone Disease

The most obvious function of bone is that of mechanical support and protection. Although it may appear to be a solid, static tissue, bone is constantly undergoing remodelling to meet the changing requirements of growth and activity. A less obvious function is that of providing a large reservoir for mineral homeostasis. The body of the average 70 kg man contains approximately 1 kg of calcium, 99% of which is found in the skeleton. The small amount in the soft tissues is vital for many biochemical and physiological processes, including muscle contraction, nerve conduction, blood clotting and cellular secretion. Hence, plasma calcium is rigidly controlled as these processes require a stable concentration of calcium ions. Complex mechanisms have evolved to maintain plasma calcium within narrow limits. This involves the action of three main hormones—parathormone (PTH), vitamin D (1,25-dihydroxycholecalciferol) and calcitonin (CT)—acting on three major target organs, namely kidney, bone and gut.

Parathyroid hormone (parathormone PTH)

Parathyroid hormone is an 84 amino acid polypeptide, secreted by the chief cells of the parathyroid gland. The chief cells respond to the concentration of calcium ions in the blood by increasing or decreasing secretion of PTH, i.e. a closed loop, negative feedback system. The actions of PTH are in defence of plasma calcium. Osteoclastic reabsorption of bone is stimulated, releasing Ca^{2+} ions into the bloodstream. In the kidney, calcium reabsorption is increased and phosphate reabsorption is decreased (the 'phosphaturic' effect).

PTH circulates in several forms—intact molecule, N terminal fragment and C terminal fragment. Biological activity resides in the N terminal. Measurement of

PTH by radioimmunoassay gives varying results depending on which of these forms the antibody is raised against.

Vitamin D

This is a fat soluble vitamin which is found in dairy foods and is also produced by the action of ultraviolet light on 7-dehydrocholesterol in the skin. The physiologically active metabolite, 1,25-dihydroxycholecalciferol (1,25-DHCC), is produced by hydroxylation in the 25 position in the liver and in the 1 position in the kidney. The 1-hydroxylase enzyme responsible for the final renal hydroxylation is controlled by PTH. The principal effect of vitamin D in mineral metabolism is to facilitate intestinal calcium absorption. In bone, vitamin D is necessary for normal mineralization of osteoid.

Calcitonin (CT)

This is a 32 amino acid polypeptide, secreted by the chief cells of the thyroid gland in response to a rise in plasma calcium. The actions of CT oppose those of PTH. Osteoclastic bone reabsorption is inhibited. Plasma calcium levels are usually unaffected, except by pharmacological doses which may cause hypocalcaemia. The physiological role of CT is not completely understood—it may prevent post-prandial hypercalcaemia by diverting absorbed calcium rapidly into bone tissue fluid (Norimatsu et al. 1982). A specific deficiency or hypersecretion syndrome has not been described. Although greatly elevated levels are found in patients with medullary carcinoma of the thyroid, the hormone in these cases is biologically inactive.

Other hormones

Other hormones play a secondary role in calcium balance. Glucocorticoids inhibit Ca^{2+} and PO_4^{3-} absorption by an anti-vitamin D effect and enhance renal excretion of these ions. Cellular activity in bone is decreased and the result is osteoporosis. Oestrogens stimulate calcium absorption and reduce the effect of PTH on bone. Post-menopausal bone loss is largely due to oestrogen deficiency. Hyperthyroidism increases bone turnover, but there is a net loss of mineral resulting in hypercalcaemia, hypercalciuria and osteoporosis.

Hyperparathyroidism (osteitis fibrosa cystica)

Hyperparathyroidism is caused by excessive secretion of PTH by the parathyroid glands. It may be classified as primary, secondary or tertiary.

Primary hyperparathyroidism is most frequently due to an adenoma of one of the four parathyroid glands. The classical presentation used to be stones (renal calculi), bones (bone pain and osteoporosis), abdominal groans (peptic ulcer, pancreatitis) and psychic moans (depression, psychosis). At the present time, the most common presentation is mild asymptomatic hypercalcaemia, identified by routine biochemical screening. Severe symptoms are now uncommon as the disease is diagnosed at an earlier stage. Non-specific symptoms of hypercalcaemia include malaise, lethargy, depression and nausea.

It is a common disorder affecting perhaps 1 in 2000 of the population. Middle-aged and elderly women are most commonly affected. In rare cases, it may be familial and associated with multiple endocrine adenomatosis (Chapter 16).

Biochemical tests show hypercalcaemia, hypophosphataemia and the alkaline phosphatase may be elevated if there is bone involvement. PTH may be elevated or within the normal range. The PTH level must be interpreted with a simultaneous measurement of serum calcium. It will be inappropriately high, for the serum calcium, even though it is within the 'normal range'.

The radiological features of bone involvement (osteitis fibrosa cystica) are subperiosteal erosions affecting the radial border of the middle phalanges of the hand, the symphysis pubis, sacro-iliac joints and the distal clavicles. There may be generalized diffuse osteopenia. In the skull, demineralization shows a granular 'salt and pepper' appearance. True bone cysts may be seen as well as isolated osteolytic lesions, the so-called 'brown tumour' of hyperparathyroidism.

Histological examination shows a greatly increased number of osteoclasts of the periosteal and endosteal surfaces of bone. There is marked 'tunnelling' or 'dissecting' reabsorption of trabeculae and replacement by fibrous tissue. 'Brown tumours' contain numerous giant cells in a fibrous stroma. The brown colour is due to haemosiderin deposits from old haemorrhage. Bone cysts are fluid-filled cavities lined by fibrous tissue.

Treatment of primary hyperparathyroidism is by surgical removal of the adenoma or hyperplastic glands. The generalized histological and radiological features in bone quickly regress. Postoperative hypocalcaemia is common in patients with extensive skeletal involvement because of the phenomenon of 'bone hunger'. Calcium returns to bone as the skeletal lesions heal faster than it can be absorbed from the intestine. Brown tumours heal completely, but bone cysts remain.

Osteoporosis

Generalized decrease in bone density or osteopenia may be due to osteoporosis, osteomalacia or inherited bone dysplasia.

Osteopenia may be defined as the clinical state in which there is a reduction in bone mass below that which normally characterizes the skeleton for the particular age, sex and race of an individual (Avioli 1977). Throughout life, bone is constantly being deposited and reabsorbed. In the growing child, the net balance is in favour of deposition so that growth occurs. From shortly after skeletal maturity, there is a net loss from the skeleton as reabsorption exceeds formation by a small amount. In women, this process becomes much more rapid after the menopause. The process is symptomless in most individuals for long periods and in the vast majority never becomes clinically apparent. The determinants of this are the bone density at skeletal maturity, the rate of subsequent loss and the age to which the individual lives.

BONE DENSITY AT SKELETAL MATURITY: Males have a higher bone mass per kg body weight than females. Negroes have a heavier skeleton at all ages than Caucasians.

RATES OF LOSS: The degree of physical activity may have an effect, as a sedentary life style is associated with a faster loss than an active one. Males and females lose

Table 19.2. Classification of osteoporosis

Primary
Post-menopausal or senile osteoporosis
Juvenile idiopathic osteoporosis

Secondary

Endocrine	Malignant disease
—Cushing's disease	—Carcinomatosis
—Hyperparathyroidism	—Myelomatosis
—Hyperthyroidism	—Lymphoma
—Acromegaly	
—Hypogonadism	Chronic disease
	—Rheumatoid arthritis
Mechanical	—TB
—Immobilization	—Renal disease
—Disuse	—Ankylosing spondylitis
—Weightlessness	
	Inherited disorders
Drugs	—Osteogenesis imperfecta
—Corticosteroids	—Vitamin D resistant rickets
—Alcohol	—Marfan's syndrome
—Heparin	—Down's syndrome

Nutritional
—Generalized malnutrition or scurvy

bone at roughly equal rates until the menopause, when the rate of loss increases in the female.

AGE OF INDIVIDUAL: Osteoporosis becomes clinically apparent with increasing frequency in older populations.

Physiological osteoporosis occurs in all individuals as a natural ageing process. Pathological osteoporosis occurs when bone loss becomes clinically apparent. This may be subdivided into primary (idiopathic) and secondary (*see Table* 19.2).

The majority of patients are over 60, but in those with secondary causes, the age at presentation may be much younger. Females are much more often affected than males.

Presenting features are bone pain, loss of height or pathological fracture. Blood biochemistry and haematology are usually normal, although there is some evidence for 1,25-DHCC deficiency. Between 30% and 50% of bone must be lost before it is seen on a plain X-ray film as loss of density. More sophisticated measurements are available as research techniques but are not in general use, e.g. photon absorption densitometry, neutron activation analysis and computerized axial tomography.

The axial skeleton is usually first involved, especially the lower dorsal and lumbar areas. In vertebral bodies, trabecular bone is lost, leaving a thinned out texture. The loss of structural integrity leads to microfracture and wedging forwards. If this happens over many vertebrae, a generalized kyphosis is the result (Widow's hump). Biconcave expansion of vertebral discs into the vertebral body is characteristic, the so-called 'codfish' appearance. Weakening of tubular bones causes increased rate of fracture in well defined sites, such as distal radius and neck of femur.

Histologically, there is a reduction in trabecular bone mass with a normal ratio of mineral to organic matrix identified. Biopsy is sometimes necessary to rule out carcinomatosis or myelomatosis.

Treatment is generally unsatisfactory except in those cases with an obvious cause. Oestrogen replacement given to post-menopausal females will prevent bone loss, but the long-term safety is not fully established. Once bone has been lost, it is very difficult to build it up again. Fluoride, in combination with calcium and vitamin D, has been shown to be of benefit. In the elderly patient, osteomalacia often coexists and this should be excluded as it is more easily treated.

Osteomalacia

Osteomalacia is characterized by osteopenia and inadequate mineralization of bone matrix. This may be due to calcium deficiency, hypophosphataemia or defects in the vitamin D metabolic pathway. These include inadequate dietary intake, lack of exposure to sunlight, malabsorption, hepatic disease and renal disease.

The clinical features in the adult may be insidious and the condition often remains undiagnosed for many years or is misdiagnosed as osteoporosis. Bone pain, backache and proximal myopathy predominate. Serum calcium and phosphate are low or normal, but the alkaline phosphatase is elevated.

Radiological features include osteopenia, biconcave vertebral bodies ('codfish' vertebrae), bowing of long bones and a 'trefoil' pelvis, due to indentation by hip joints and sacrum. These gross deformities are uncommon, but Looser zones (pseudofractures) are frequently seen. These are ribbon-like zones of rarefaction seen in the diaphyses of long bones and the pelvis. Histologically, these areas are cortical fractures which heal by fibrous tissue and poorly mineralized callus.

Histological examination of osteomalacic bone shows a marked increase in the ratio of unmineralized matrix or osteoid to mineralized bone.

Treatment depends on aetiology, but includes improved diet, exposure to sunlight and vitamin D supplements. Synthetic analogues of vitamin D metabolites, such as 1-alpha-hydroxycholecalciferol, may be useful.

Rickets

Rickets is the childhood manifestation of defective bone mineralization. Because of rapid bone growth in children, the effects are often more florid and deformity more severe than osteomalacia in adult patients. The aetiological factors are similar in the two conditions, but renal causes assume a greater importance in children. Classical rickets was due to vitamin D deficiency but is now rare in Western society since the introduction of preventive measures. Renal rickets is now more commonly seen and is divided into tubular and glomerular types.

Renal tubular rickets due to familial hypophosphataemia is now probably the commonest cause. This is an X-linked dominant disorder which presents in the second year of life with deformity, short stature and characteristic facies. Impaired renal tubular reabsorption of phosphate leads to hypophosphataemia. Calcium levels are normal but bone mineralization is defective. The serum alkaline phosphatase is elevated, but the level must be interpreted according to age.

Renal glomerular osteodystrophy includes rickets due to different forms of chronic renal failure. Uraemia and phosphate retention are associated with a depression of serum calcium. This is due to defective calcium absorption and 1,25-DHCC deficiency (1-hydroxylase is deficient in renal failure). The effects include rickets, secondary hyperparathyroidism (due to hypocalcaemia) or tertiary hyperparathyroidism, soft tissue calcification and osteoporosis (due to hyperphosphataemia).

In infants, the rapidly growing skull bones may show thinning and softening with frontal bossing and posterior flattening (craniotabes). At the age of one year, bilateral indentation of the chest wall gives rise to Harrison's sulcus at the line of attachment of the diaphragm. Swelling of the costochondral junctions of the ribs is termed the 'rachitic rosary'. In long bones, the growth plate is widened, metaphyses are flared into a cup shape and the diaphyses are bowed. Weight bearing accentuates lower limb deformity, with bow legs or knock knees. Pseudo-fractures (Looser zones) are uncommon. Epiphyseal slipping occurs in chronic renal failure, particularly affecting the upper femoral epiphysis.

Histologically, the growth plate shows the proliferating cartilage cells to be irregular and disorganized. The calcified zone fails to develop properly and there are large amounts of unmineralized bone throughout the skeleton.

Treatment is directed at the cause. Hypophosphataemic rickets respond to phosphate and vitamin D supplements. Chronic renal failure with renal glomerular osteodystrophy may require haemodialysis or transplantation. Epiphyseal slipping may require internal fixation. Persistent deformity after medical treatment may require corrective osteotomy.

Paget's disease

This is a chronic bone dystrophy which is difficult to classify as the cause is not known. It is not a true metabolic disease as the lesions are focal rather than generalized. The old term 'osteitis deformans' suggests an inflammatory basis. Recent work has shown the presence of intranuclear viral inclusion bodies in osteoclasts from Pagetic bone. A 'slow virus' syndrome has been postulated, perhaps from measles infection in childhood (Singer and Mills 1983).

There are great variations in the incidence of Paget's disease in different races. It is common in the UK, Australia and Germany but rare in most of Asia, Africa and Scandinavia. It is characterized by increased bone turnover with high rates of both formation and reabsorption. New bone is disorganized rather than lamellar in pattern.

Clinical features

Paget's disease becomes increasingly common over the age of 50 years; the sex incidence is equal. Some patients have only one bone affected (monostotic Paget's disease). This affected bone tends to enlarge, become deformed and liable to pathological fracture. Chronic bone pain is the commonest symptom but in many patients, monostotic Paget's disease is an incidental X-ray finding. Generalized Paget's disease may lead to an increased hat size. If the base of the skull is involved, neural foramina may become narrowed, leading to entrapment neuropathy and cranial nerve palsies. This may produce deafness or blindness.

The upper limbs may be extensively involved but result in few symptoms. In the lower limbs, weight bearing accentuates the progression of deformity, such as anterior bowing of the tibia. Involvement of subchondral bone leads to erosive arthritis. In the lumbar spine, kyphosis is common. Spinal stenosis may occur with progressive neurological deficit. Pagetic bone is very vascular and in generalized Paget's disease, a high output cardiovascular state exists. This has been quoted as a cause of high output cardiac failure, although it rarely, if ever, occurs. Blood calcium and phosphate levels are usually normal, unless the patient is immobilized, in which case severe hypercalcaemia may develop. Alkaline phosphatase levels are elevated reflecting increased osteoblastic activity. The urinary excretion of hydroxyproline is also increased, indicating increased osteoclastic activity. These indices provide a good monitor of disease activity and response to therapy.

Radiology

In the early stages, the skull shows patchy areas of osteolysis, termed osteoporosis circumscripta. The frontal and occipital bones show diffuse enlargement with a 'cotton wool' appearance. Indentation of the softened base of the skull by the cervical spine causes platybasia. The limb bones may show lytic or sclerotic areas, depending on the stage of the disease. The cortex is usually thickened with loss of corticomedullary differentiation. The convex cortex may show fine cracks or microfractures and the whole bone may be bowed (*see Fig.* 19.18).

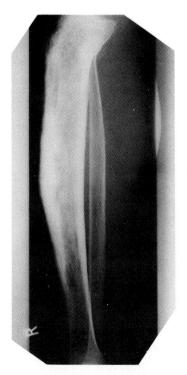

Fig. 19.18. Paget's disease affecting the tibia.

Morphology

The increased osteoclastic activity has been accurately described as 'irrational'. The repair process is abnormal so that the result is a bone with increased mass, but structurally weak and deformed.

The initial osteolytic phase is seen histologically as greatly increased random osteoclastic activity with large reabsorption cavities. The spaces are filled with vascular mesenchymal tissue in which osteoblastic repair commences. The new bone is irregular and often removed by fresh osteoclastic activity. Repeated cycles of reabsorption and formation lead to a disorganized microanatomy described as 'mosaic'. Later osteoblastic activity predominates and thick trabeculae are formed with a pattern that is neither cortical nor cancellous in its architecture.

Complications

Apart from nerve entrapment, arthritis, spinal stenosis and cardiac failure, the main complications are fracture and the development of sarcoma.

Fracture usually follows multiple microfractures and commonly affects the femoral neck and shaft. There is a significant rate of non-union and treatment may be difficult. Pagetic bone may be technically difficult to work with during internal fixation procedures.

Osteosarcoma in the elderly is almost always secondary to Paget's disease. The incidence is quoted as 1% of all Paget's cases, but it is up to 10% in those patients who have generalized skeletal involvement over many years. Synchronous tumours may develop in multiple sites. The patient complains of increased pain in a bone already deformed by Paget's disease, and diagnosis is often delayed. The alkaline phosphate level may rise to massive levels. X-rays show an osteolytic area of new bone destruction.

Histologically, the tumour is not a typical osteogenic sarcoma but may show a mixed pattern of osteosarcoma, fibrosarcoma, chondrosarcoma and giant cell sarcoma, i.e. a mixed mesenchymal pattern. The tumours usually grow rapidly and metastasize early. There are few survivors six months from diagnosis.

Treatment

In the early stages, simple analgesics such as aspirin may be helpful. Calcitonin is a most helpful agent as it directly suppresses osteoclastic activity. Biochemical response to treatment is measured by an early fall in urinary hydroxyproline and, later, the serum alkaline phosphatase. Resistance may develop due to antibody formation. The diphosphonate group of drugs decrease bone turnover by slowing down the growth and dissolution of pyrophosphate crystals.

Surgery may be indicated in the treatment of fractures, deformity or secondary arthritis.

The Fat Embolism Syndrome

The fat embolism syndrome (FES) is a clinical syndrome of acute respiratory insufficiency associated with the embolization of marrow tissue fat or intravascular lipids to the lungs in patients who have suffered musculoskeletal trauma. Fat globules are found in the microvasculature of the lungs in almost all patients who die after trauma. A similar picture may be seen after death from other conditions, including pancreatitis, diabetes, osteomyelitis, burns and sepsis. This fat embolism (FE) is usually silent and is an incidental post-mortem finding. In contrast to this, the clinical syndrome (FES) seen in 10–20% of patients after long bone fracture, is characterized by pulmonary fat embolism and the passage of embolic fat to the systemic circulation.

Clinical features include respiratory distress (tachypnoea, dyspnoea), a petechial rash, diminished level of consciousness, pyrexia, tachycardia, jaundice and the presence of fat in the retinal vessels. Anaemia and thrombocytopenia are frequently observed and suggest coagulopathy. The mainstay of diagnosis is blood gas analysis. Serious hypoxaemia, defined as PaO_2 less than 60 mmHg, is considered to be diagnostic of FES, in a patient with evidence of embolic fat, and in the absence of other causes of hypoxia (Moylan et al. 1976).

There are two main theories of pathogenesis in FES—mechanical and biochemical. The mechanical theory postulates the release of neutral fat from damaged marrow adipocytes following trauma. Due to a rise in marrow pressure, fat droplets enter the low pressure venous sinusoids and are carried to the pulmonary veins where they are trapped by the lung filter at the capillary level. In some cases, fat droplets pass through the lung capillary bed via patent arteriovenous shunts and cause systemic embolization. The biochemical theory postulates that stress-induced metabolic changes alter the stability of intravascular fat. Catecholamines may be partially responsible for a loss of chylomicron emulsion stability. Whatever the source, neutral fat entering the lung capillaries is converted by pulmonary lipase to free fatty acids (FFA) which are toxic in low concentrations to cell membranes (Nixon and Brock-Utne 1978).

Grossly, the lungs are oedematous and in some cases there is reddish consolidation due to interstitial haemorrhage. In patients surviving the first few days, secondary bacterial infection is common.

Histologically, sections stained with a fat stain such as oil red O show many sausage shaped globules of fat in the alveolar capillaries. Some fat escapes into the alveolar spaces and this is the source of sputum fat. Many small vessels are blocked by aggregates of fat, fibrin, platelets and granulocytes. The features are of chemical pneumonitis with oedema, interstitial haemorrhage, destruction of surfactant and micro-atelectasis.

Progressive interstitial fluid accumulation results in extensive alveolar collapse and segmental consolidation. These changes are reversible, but in some patients hyaline membranes appear, followed by fibroblast proliferation and replacement of alveoli by fibrous scar tissue. These permanent changes may be due to oxygen toxicity and the effect of mechanical ventilation.

The factors responsible for the enhanced passage of emboli through the lungs may include the total amount of embolic fat and the capacity of the lung filter. This capacity is probably age-related as children rarely develop FES whereas it is common in the elderly especially if there is pre-existing lung disease.

The release of vasoactive amines such as serotonin from platelets causes pulmonary vasoconstriction and raised pulmonary vascular resistance. The subsequent rise in pulmonary artery pressure may also increase the passage of emboli through the pulmonary filter bed. Embolic fat in the systemic circulation may cause multiple 'micro-infarcts' in the viscera. In the skin and conjunctiva, a petechial rash may be seen in 50% of cases.

The most serious effects are in the brain where, grossly, a widespread petechial eruption is seen, principally affecting white matter (*see Fig.* 19.19). Histologically, small vessels are blocked by fat with secondary areas of haemorrhagic necrosis. If the patient survives, neurological deficits usually recover completely.

In heart and kidney, fat embolism is usually clinically silent.

Treatment of FES is first directed at prevention by prompt effective immobilization of long bone fractures. Early recognition by monitoring blood gas levels in patients at risk of FES is important. Graduated oxygen administration is the only form of treatment of proven value. Early intubation and mechanical respiration may often produce dramatic improvement. The positive end-expiratory pressure technique (PEEP) may improve aeration of the lungs by opening collapsed alveoli and decreasing intrapulmonary shunting.

Corticosteroids have been used on the basis that they may stabilize lysosomal and capillary membranes, decreasing capillary leakage. Heparin, low molecular weight dextran, clofibrate and intravenous alcohol have all been tried in FES but their usefulness has not been proven by controlled clinical trials (Gossling and Donohue 1979).

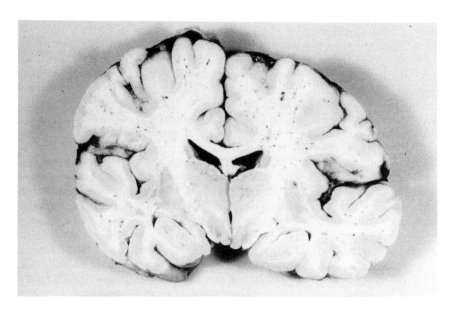

Fig. 19.19. Fat embolism syndrome—petechial haemorrhages are seen in the white matter.

Aseptic Bone Necrosis

Aseptic or avascular necrosis of bone (AVN) is being increasingly recognized as a cause of disability. Trauma is the commonest cause, particularly fracture of the neck of femur, scaphoid or talus, where anatomical peculiarities of blood supply are important factors. AVN may also be a feature of bone infection and Perthes' disease, as already described. There remains a mixed group of disorders associated with bone necrosis in which the pathogenesis is uncertain. Some cases are associated with the finding of raised intra-osseous pressure and venous hypertension. The large thin-walled venous sinuses of the medulla are poorly supported as they are surrounded mainly by fat cells. Swelling of these cells in response to various noxious stimuli may occlude the venous drainage of bone producing infarction. The causes include corticosteroids, alcoholism, Caisson disease, haemoglobinopathies (such as sickle cell disease), gout and Gaucher's disease.

The clinical features of juxta-articular lesions are bone pain and tenderness, with stiffness of associated joints. Medullary lesions are often symptomless and present as incidental findings on X-ray.

Dead bone cannot be distinguished from living on initial X-rays. Later, however, the principal feature of AVN is increased bone density. This may be 'apparent' due to osteoporosis of surrounding living bone, for example, fracture of the carpal scaphoid immobilized in a plaster cast. Real increase in bone density is due to reactive new bone formation on dead trabeculae or trabecular fracture and compaction. Articular cartilage receives its nutrition from synovial fluid and so the joint space is preserved until secondary degeneration supervenes.

Grossly, a recent bone infarct appears as a yellow, opaque area surrounded by a reddish zone of hyperaemia. Histological examination confirms necrosis of osteocytes and marrow cells with the ingrowth of vascular granulation tissue from the periphery. At a later stage the necrotic trabeculae are seen to be ensheathed by new bone by the process of 'creeping substitution'.

If diagnosis is made at a very early stage before bone failure, relief of venous hypertension by drilling of the bone (forage) would appear to be logical (Ficat and Ariet 1980). Unfortunately, most patients are seen with secondary degenerative arthritis and many require osteotomy or replacement arthroplasty.

Lumbar Disc Degeneration and Prolapse

The intervertebral disc is a fibrocartilaginous structure, which provides strong fixation between vertebral bodies and yet permits movement. The central part of the disc, or nucleus pulposus, consists of a hydrophilic protein–polysaccharide gel. It has visco-elastic properties, and acts to resist and redistribute compression forces. The peripheral part of the disc, or annulus fibrosus, consists of concentric fibrous lamellae, surrounding the nucleus and uniting the vertebral bodies. During spinal movements the fibres resist tension forces. In the normal disc, a balance exists between compression forces (gravity and muscle tone) and the visco-elastic recoil of the nucleus pulposus.

Large forces are transmitted through the lower lumbar discs. Average figures for a 70 kg man range from 100 kg when standing, 50 kg bending forwards, to 220 kg when lifting a 50 kg weight (Nachemson and Morris 1964). With age, the high water content of the nucleus gradually falls, resulting in a reduced load bearing capacity. Multiple fissures develop in the annulus fibrosus parallel to the surface of the vertebral bodies. Herniations of nuclear material develop in all directions through the annular tears (*see Fig.* 19.20). The effects of these herniations depend on their direction and size. Schmorl's nodes are herniations of disc material into the cancellous bone of the vertebral bodies. These are frequently seen on X-ray as small radiolucent areas surrounded by bony sclerosis.

Of much more importance clinically are posterior or posterolateral protrusions which may compress nerve roots or the cauda equina. Four stages may be described, though these are not easily differentiated clinically or radiologically. Stage one is a contained disc lesion and refers to the early stage of annular degeneration without significant herniation of the nucleus and may be compared to a 'sprained ligament'. This is probably a common cause of back pain (lumbago). Referred leg pain (sciatica) may also occur from nerve root irritation by local inflammatory reaction. There are usually no neurological signs and radiculography (myelography) is negative. The second stage is that of disc protrusion. Nuclear material extrudes, partially through the annulus, giving rise to a localized bulge which may cause pressure on nerve roots. Such a patient is likely to have motor and sensory deficits and reflex changes in addition to back pain and sciatica. The radiculogram is usually positive and at operation a smooth pearl-like swelling is found beneath the nerve root.

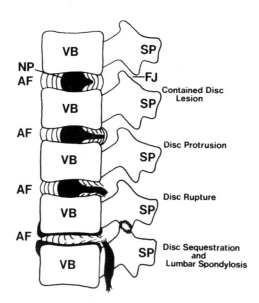

Fig. 19.20. Lumbar disc degeneration: VB—vertebral body; SP—spinous process; FJ—facet joint; AF—annulus fibrosus; NP—nucleus pulposus.

Disc rupture refers to the third stage when partial extrusion of nuclear contents occurs outside the annulus. Disc sequestration is the fourth and final stage, when the disc contents lie free in the spinal canal, often at some distance from the disc space and the torn annulus. These last two stages may be impossible to distinguish clinically or radiologically. Symptoms and signs may be more dramatic with sensory loss and motor weakness (foot drop in low lesions, quadriceps weakness in high lesions). A large central prolapse may cause urinary retention and sacral sensory loss from cauda equina compression.

In acute disc lesions, there may be no abnormality seen on plain X-ray films. In younger patients, muscle spasm may cause loss of lumbar lordosis and a sciatic scoliosis. Chronic disc degeneration is seen as loss of the disc space height and marginal osteophyte formation (spondylosis). Radiologically, secondary changes occur in the facet joints and may result in further nerve root irritation in the lateral recesses of the spinal canal and in the intervertebral foramina ('bony sciatica').

Treatment may be conservative or operative. The mainstay of conservative treatment is rest, often with pelvic traction. The place of physiotherapy, spinal manipulation and lumbo-sacral supports are less clearly defined. Epidural injections of local anaesthesia and corticosteroid may be of benefit. Direct injection of the disc with chymopapain, a proteolytic enzyme preparation, is being evaluated.

Surgery may be indicated as an emergency to remove a large central prolapse with cauda equina compression and urinary retention. More commonly, surgery is indicated for more minor neurological complications or failure of conservative treatment. Accurate radiological localization of the disc lesion is essential as this is not possible on clinical grounds alone. Radiculography with water soluble contrast media and CT scanning are the most useful techniques.

References

Apley A. G., (1973) *A System of Orthopaedics and Fractures.* 4th ed. London, Butterworth.

Avioli L, V. (1977) Osteoporosis: Pathogenesis and therapy. In: Avioli L. V., Krane S. M. (eds.) *Metabolic Bone Disease,* Vol. I. New York, Academic Press.

Bassett C. A. L., Becker R. O. (1962) Generation of electric potentials by bone in response to mechanical stress. *Science* 137, 1063–4.

Blockey N. J. (1980) Management of bone and joint infections. In: Owen R., Goodfellow J., Bullough P. (eds.) *Scientific Foundations of Orthopaedics and Traumatology,* pp. 481–91. London, Heinemann.

Bullough P. G., Vigorita V. J. (1984) Diseases resulting from disturbances in the breakdown and formation of bone. In: Bullough P. G., Vigorita V. I. (eds.) *Atlas of Orthopaedic Pathology.* London, Gower Medical.

Carlsson A., Josefsson G., Lindberg L. (1978) Revision with gentamicin-impregnated cement for deep infection in total hip arthroplasties. *J. Bone Joint Surg.* 60(A), 1059–64.

Catterall A. (1982) *Legg–Calvé–Perthes' Disease.* Edinburgh, Churchill Livingstone.

Ficat R. P., Arlet J. (1980) *Ischaemia and Necrosis of Bone.* Baltimore, Williams and Wilkins.

Freeman M. A. R. (1975) The fatigue of cartilage in the pathogenesis of osteoarthrosis. *Acta Orthop. Scand.* 46, 323–8.

Gossling H. R., Donohue T. A. (1979) The fat embolism syndrome. *J.A.M.A.* 241, 2740–2.

Lichtenstein L. (1977) *Bone Tumours.* 5th ed. St Louis, C. V. Mosby.

McDevitt C. A., Gilbertson E. M. M., Muir H. (1977) An experimental model of osteoarthritis: early morphological and biochemical changes. *J. Bone Joint Surg.* 59(B), 24–35.

Marcove R. C., Lyden J. P., Huvos A. G. *et al.* (1973) Giant cell tumours treated by cryosurgery. *J. Bone Joint Surg.* 55(A), 1633–43.

Marcove R., Martin N., Rosen G. (1975) The treatment of pulmonary metastasis in osteogenic sarcoma. *Clin. Orthop.* 111, 65–70.

Medical Research Council Working Party on Tuberculosis of the Spine (1976) A 5 year assessment of controlled trials of in-patient and out-patient treatment and of plaster of Paris jackets for tuberculosis of the spine in children on standard chemotherapy. *J. Bone Joint Surg.* 58(B), 399–411.

Mollan R. A. B., Piggot J. (1977) Acute osteomyelitis in children. *J. Bone Joint Surg.* 59(B), 2–7.

Moylan J. A., Birnbaum M., Katz A., Everson M. A. (1976) Fat emboli syndrome. *J. Trauma* **16**(5), 341–7.

Nachemson A., Morris J. M. (1964) *In vivo* measurement of intradiscal pressure. *J. Bone Joint Surg.* **46**(A), 1077–92.

Nixon J. R., Brock-Utne J. G. (1978) Free fatty acid and arterial oxygen changes following major injury—a correlation between hypoxaemia and increased free fatty acid levels. *J. Trauma* **18**(1), 23–6.

Norimatsu H., Yamamoto T., Ozawa H., Talmage R. V. (1982) Changes in calcium phosphate on bone surfaces and in living cells after the administration of parathyroid hormone or calcitonin. *Clin. Orthop.* **164**, 271–8.

Owen M., Melick R., Triffit J. (1972) Plasma proteins and bone tissue fluid. In: Ninth Symposium on Calcified Tissue Abstracts. Vienna, Verlag Der Weiner Medizinischen Akedemic.

Persson B. M., Wouters H. W. (1976) Curettage and acrylic cementation in surgery of giant cell tumour of the bone. *Clin. Orthop.* **120**, 125–33.

Price C. H. G., Ross F. G. M. (eds.) (1973) Bone, certain aspects of neoplasia. Proceedings of the 24th symposium of the Colston research society.

Puri R., Smith C. S., Malhoyra D., Williams A. J., Owen R., Harris F. (1985) Slipped upper femoral epiphysis and primary juvenile hypothyroidism. *J. Bone Joint Surg.* **67**(B), 14–19.

Rasmussen H., Bordier P. (1974) *The Physiologic and Cellular Basis of Metabolic Bone Disease*. Baltimore, Williams and Wilkins.

Rhinelander F. W. (1980) The blood supply of the limb bones. In: Owen R., Goodfellow J., Bullough P. (eds.) *Scientific Foundations of Orthopaedics and Traumatology,* pp. 126–51. London, Heinemann.

Scaglietti O., Marchetti P. G., Bartolozzi P. (1979) The effects of methylprednisolone acetate in the treatment of bone cysts. Results of three years follow-up. *J. Bone Joint Surg.* **61**(B), 200–4.

Scales J. T. (1983) Bone and joint replacement for the preservation of limbs. *Br. J. Hosp. Med.* **30**, 220–32.

Schajowicz F. (1961) Giant cell tumour of bone (osteoclastoma). A pathological and histological study. *J. Bone Joint Surg.* **43**(A), 1–29.

Schajowicz J., Araujo E. H. S. (1983) Cysts and tumours of the musculoskeletal system. In: Harris N. H. (ed.) *Postgraduate Textbook of Clinical Orthopaedics,* Ch. 20. Bristol, Wright PSG.

Singer F. R., Mills B. G. (1983) What is the aetiology of Paget's disease and can we cure it? In: Frame B., Potts J. J. (eds.) *Clinical Disorders of Bone and Mineral Metabolism.* Amsterdam, Excerpta Medica.

Solomon L. (1976) Patterns of osteoarthritis of the hip. *J. Bone Joint Surg.* **58**(B), 176–83.

Williams P. F. (1965) Fragmentation and rodding in osteogenesis imperfecta. *J. Bone Joint Surg.* **47**(B), 23–31.

Wynne-Davies R. (1973) *Heritable Disorders in Orthopaedic Practice.* Oxford, Blackwell Scientific Publications.

Chapter 20

The Nervous System

Normal Structure (*see Fig.* 20.1)

Traditionally the brain is divided into forebrain, midbrain and hindbrain.

The forebrain includes the cerebral cortex, basal ganglia, lateral ventricles, thalamus, hypothalamus and third ventricle.

The cerebral cortex, basal ganglia and lateral ventricles form the cerebral hemispheres, each of which has four lobes: (1) The frontal lobe is the cortical area in front of the central sulcus of Rolando. It includes the motor cortex (pre-central gyrus), the pre-motor cortex, the eye motor field, Broca's speech area and the pre-frontal cortex which is involved in emotional behaviour, 'intelligence' and autonomic control. (2) The parietal lobe includes the somatic sensory cortex and the parietal association cortex which is concerned with the recognition of somatic sensory stimuli. (3) The temporal lobe contains the higher auditory and olfactory

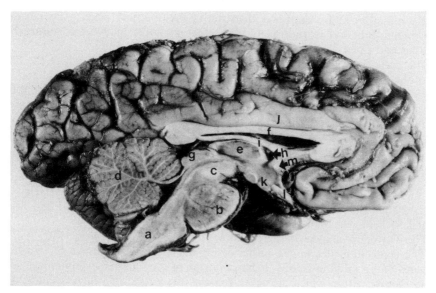

Fig. 20.1. Sagittal section of normal brain: *a.* medulla; *b.* pons; *c.* midbrain; *d.* cerebellum; *e.* thalamus; *f.* corpus callosum; *g.* corpora quadrigemina; *h.* interventricular foramen; *i.* column of fornix; *j.* cingulate gyrus; *k.* hypothalamus; *l.* optic chiasma; *m.* anterior commissure.

597

centres. Memory also resides in the temporal cortex.(4) The occipital lobe contains the visual cortex and the occipital association cortex which is involved in the recognition of visual stimuli.

Four basal ganglia are situated deep in each cerebral hemisphere and consist of the caudate nucleus, lentiform nucleus (divided into globus pallidus and putamen), claustrum and amygdala. The basal ganglia connect with the cerebral cortex and thalamus and efferent fibres pass to the hypothalamus, red nucleus, substantia nigra and olivary nucleus. They are part of the extrapyramidal system which is concerned with muscle tone, righting reflexes and regulation of unconscious muscle actions. Lesions of the basal ganglia may result in Parkinsonism, Wilson's disease, chorea or athetosis.

The thalamus and hypothalamus together form the diencephalon. The thalamus consists of two parts, each of which forms a lateral wall of the third ventricle and connects with its fellow via the massa intermedia. Posteriorly each part has three eminences, the pulvinar and the medial and lateral geniculate bodies. The thalamus is essentially a relay station for sensory pathways to the cerebral cortex. It can appreciate temperature, crude touch and pain, even when the sensory cortex is destroyed.

The hypothalamus forms the floor of the third ventricle. It includes the tuber cinereum, the infundibular stalk (which connects with the posterior lobe of pituitary), the mamillary bodies and the posterior perforated substances. The hypothalamus is involved with autonomic nervous system control, cardiovascular regulation, temperature regulation, food intake and water balance (via anti-diuretic hormone), gastrointestinal activity, sleep–waking activity (as part of the reticular activating system) and emotional responses.

The efferent fibres of the olfactory (Ist) cranial nerve pass upwards from the olfactory nasal mucosa, pierce the cribiform plate of the ethmoid bone and synapse in the olfactory bulb. The fibres then run in the olfactory tract to the cortex of the uncus. Bilateral disruption of the olfactory fibres may occur during head injuries and cause anosmia.

The optic (IInd) nerves pass backwards to the optic chiasma where the fibres from the medial half of the retina cross to run with the fibres from the lateral half of the opposite retina in the optic tract to the lateral geniculate body. From here the optic radiation passes backwards to the visual cortex. The optic nerve may be involved by gliomas or compressed by meningiomas. The optic chiasma may be compressed by pituitary tumours.

The midbrain (mesencephalon) connects with the pons and cerebrum. It consists of the cerebral peduncles which have descending and ascending fibre tracts, and the corpora quadrigemina which are concerned with motor co-ordination through optic and auditory reflexes. It also contains the nuclei of the IIIrd and IVth cranial nerves. The aqueduct of Sylvius which joins the third and fourth ventricles lies in the midbrain.

The hindbrain includes the cerebellum, pons, medulla and fourth ventricle.

The cerebellum lies in the posterior cranial fossa and consists of two hemispheres and a midline vermis. It has a cortex of grey matter overlying a mass of white matter within which are several nuclei, the largest of which is the dentate. The cerebellum connects to the brainstem via three cerebellar peduncles. It receives input from all the sensory organs and via the motor centres it regulates equilibrium, muscle tone and posture.

The pons forms part of the floor of the fourth ventricle and is connected to the cerebellum via the middle cerebellar peduncle. The pons plays a role in the regulation of respiration and contains the nuclei of the Vth, VIth, VIIth and VIIIth cranial nerves.

The medulla is continuous with the spinal cord through the foramen magnum. It receives the inferior cerebellar peduncle and anteriorly are the pyramids. The nuclei of the IXth, Xth, XIth and XIIth cranial nerves reside in the medulla and all the spinal cord tracts are represented. The centres for control of cardiac and respiratory function also lie in the medulla.

The pituitary gland consists of a vascular and cellular anterior lobe and a less vascular posterior lobe. The latter is connected with the tuber cinereum via the pituitary stalk. The optic chiasma lies above, the cavernous sinuses lie laterally and the body of sphenoid bone is inferior (providing one of the routes of surgical exposure). The pituitary fossa is roofed by a fold of dura, the diaphragma sellae.

The spinal cord extends from the foramen magnum to about the L1–L2 intervertebral disc; it is on average 46 cm long. The tapering lower end is termed the 'conus medullaris', from which the filum terminale extends down as far as the coccyx. Cross-section of the spinal cord shows the H-shaped grey matter surrounded by the white matter which contains the ascending and descending tracts.

Circulation of cerebrospinal fluid (CSF)

CSF is formed by the choroid plexus of the lateral, third and fourth ventricles. The two large lateral ventricles produce most of the CSF which flows into the third ventricle via the interventricular foramina of Monro. From the narrow third ventricle the CSF passes through the aqueduct of Sylvius to the fourth ventricle which lies between the medulla/pons and cerebellum. The CSF escapes from the fourth ventricle into the subarachnoid space via the median and lateral openings, termed the foramina of Magendie and Luschka respectively.

The subarachnoid space is enlarged in four areas to form cisterns, the cisterna magna, the cisterna pontis, the interpeduncular cistern and the chiasmatic cistern. CSF is absorbed by the arachnoid villi which are mainly in the superior sagittal sinus. Some is absorbed by spinal villi and by lymphatics within nerve sheaths.

Blood supply of the brain

The brain is supplied by the internal carotid and vertebral arteries. These form an anastomosis around the optic chiasma and pituitary gland termed the circle of Willis (see Fig. 20.2).

The branches of the internal carotid arteries are the anterior cerebrals (which supply the medial aspects of the frontal and parietal lobes and the adjacent lateral surfaces), the middle cerebral arteries (which supply most of the lateral surfaces of the hemispheres), the ophthalmic arteries, the anterior choroidal arteries and the posterior communicating arteries.

The two vertebral arteries pass upwards through the foramen magnum towards the lower border of the pons where they fuse to form the basilar artery. Before doing so each gives off a posterior inferior cerebellar artery (which supplies part of the medulla and the lower cerebellum) and branches which unite to form the anterior spinal artery.

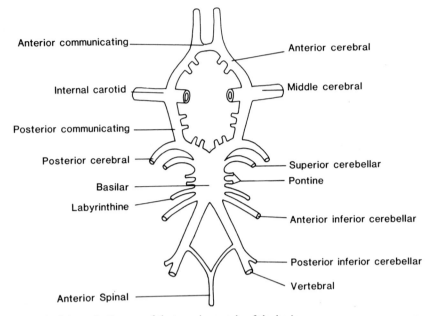

Anterior communicating

Anterior cerebral

Internal carotid

Middle cerebral

Posterior communicating

Posterior cerebral

Superior cerebellar

Basilar

Pontine

Labyrinthine

Anterior inferior cerebellar

Posterior inferior cerebellar

Vertebral

Anterior Spinal

Fig. 20.2. Schematic diagram of the vascular supply of the brain.

The basilar artery gives off anterior inferior cerebellar arteries, pontine branches, labyrinthine arteries, superior cerebellar arteries and posterior cerebral arteries (which supply the medial surfaces of the occipital lobes).

Meninges

The dura mater is a strong fibrous membrane which lines the cranial vault and the cranial fossae and extends down the spinal canal to the second sacral vertebra. The dura is prolonged over the nerve roots in the spinal canal. All the venous sinuses, except the inferior sagittal and the straight sinuses, lie between the periosteum and fibrous dura and are held permanently open by the unyielding dura.

The arachnoid mater is closely applied to the inner surface of the dura. The spinal subarachnoid space is large and communicates through the foramen magnum with the subarachnoid space of the posterior cranial fossa.

The pia mater invests the brain and cord closely and contains blood vessels. Traditionally it is said to extend into the depths of the fissures and sulci of the brain although recent work has questioned this.

Histology

The central nervous system is composed of neurones and neuroglial cells. The cell bodies of neurones reside in grey matter or in ganglia. Entering the cell body are numerous processes known as dendrites, which provide the major input of information. Leaving each cell body is a single axon or nerve fibre which traverses the white matter.

The non-neuronal cells of the CNS are the neuroglia which occupy the space between the neurones. They are of four types: (1) Astrocytes are cells with numerous star-like processes. Some of these processes envelop capillaries while others from the same astrocyte come in close contact with adjacent neurones. They probably have a role in metabolic exchange between blood and neuronal tissue. (2) Oligodendrocytes have a number of short branched processes. They are responsible for the myelination of axons and are the predominant neuroglial cell in the white matter. (3) Microglia are small cells with highly branched processes which become large phagocytic cells in response to injury. (4) Ependymal cells form the lining of the ventricular system and spinal canal.

The cerebrum has an outer layer of grey matter, arranged in a variable number of layers, and the deep hemisphere consists mainly of white matter. The cerebellar cortex is grey matter and consists of an outer (molecular layer) and an inner granular layer. The central core of the cerebellum is white matter. The spinal cord has an inner butterfly shaped region of grey matter and an outer layer of white matter; the arrangement is therefore opposite to that of the cerebrum and cerebellum.

Peripheral nerves

The peripheral nerves contain the afferent and efferent nerve fibres of both the somatic and autonomic nervous systems. The cell bodies of the nerve fibres lie either in the central nervous system (e.g. the anterior horn cells of the spinal cord) or in ganglia.

Cross-section of a peripheral nerve shows that each individual nerve fibre with its Schwann cell is encased in a layer of connective tissue, the endoneurium. Several such nerve fibres together form a fascicle and each fascicle is surrounded by a connective tissue layer known as the perineurium. If several fascicles are present in one nerve fibre, they are bound together and surrounded by an outer layer termed the epineurium.

Cerebral Biopsy

Cerebral biopsy is obviously of great importance in diagnosis and treatment of space-occupying lesions of the CNS. This procedure is normally carried out after exact anatomical localization of the lesion by appropriate neuro-imaging has been done. Cerebral biopsy, however, also has a role in establishing the diagnosis in certain diffuse cerebral lesions which cannot be diagnosed by other means. This procedure is not to be undertaken lightly, in that, occasionally, epilepsy can be a late complication.

The value of cortical biopsy in children suffering from various genetic disorders, including the lysosomal enzyme deficiency diseases, is well established, but biopsy should only be undertaken when diagnosis by various haematological and skin fibroblast analyses has failed. In such cases, though an exact diagnosis may not be made, the disease process may be categorized as genetic or otherwise.

In the adult, cerebral biopsy is indicated in various diffuse inflammatory or demyelinating processes where exact diagnosis influences therapy. Such conditions include herpes simplex encephalitis, progressive multifocal leucoencephalitis, inflammatory disorders of unknown aetiology, e.g. arteritis and sarcoidosis, and infective disorders where the infective agent has not been isolated from the cerebrospinal fluid. Diagnosis of various diffuse neoplastic processes, e.g. the reticuloses, has also been made in this way.

Cortical biopsy is rarely undertaken in cases of dementia because of the possibility of contamination of surgical instruments by the Creutzfeldt–Jakob agent. Strict criteria, however, have been laid down for the selection of cases of dementia for biopsy and for the sterilization of instruments in these cases. The procedure, therefore, is occasionally of value in dementia of unknown cause where an exact diagnosis may have practical importance.

Congenital Abnormalities

Craniosynostosis

Craniosynostosis is an abnormality of one or more of the skull sutures leading to premature fusion and consequently to skull deformity. The incidence is probably about 1 in 20 000 births in the UK. Initially there is a reduction in the number of interdigitations along the suture lines, followed by thickening of the bone edges and, finally, fusion. The most common form of the disease affects the sagittal suture and this causes narrowing of the skull with concomitant elongation to compensate for brain growth (scaphocephaly). Bilateral coronal suture synostosis causes broadening of the skull (brachycephaly). This may be associated with syndactyly (Apert's syndrome) or maxillary deformity (Crouzon's syndrome). Unilateral coronal suture closure causes flattening of the frontal bone and orbit (plagiocephaly).

Craniosynostosis produces a rise in intracranial pressure with resultant neurological deficit if no corrective measures are undertaken.

Hypertelorism

This is an abnormally large distance between the medial walls of the orbits. It may occur as a single defect or more commonly it is associated with other craniofacial abnormalities.

Encephalocoele

Encephalocoeles are herniations of meninges and brain tissue through a skull defect. Females are more often affected than males and the lesion is most common in the occipital region although frontal encephalocoeles also occur. They vary greatly in size and prognosis, the large lesions with incomplete skin covering being frequently fatal.

Spina bifida dorsalis

The aetiology of this condition is unknown although ingestion of blighted potatoes, nitrites and nitrates by the mother have been implicated. The incidence of neural tube defects varies throughout the world and is especially high in Northern Ireland where spina bifida cystica affects 4·5/1000 live births. The incidence in the USA is low and Negroes are less commonly affected than Caucasians. The condition is twice as common in females compared with males. If parents have one child with a neural tube defèct, the chance of the neXt child being affected is 1 in 20–25. The children of older parents and late birth order children have a relatively high risk.

Spina bifida occulta

This is a failure of fusion of the posterior vertebral arches, most commonly in the lumbosacral region. There may be associated abnormalities of the overlying skin, such as dimpling, pigmentation or a patch of hair. An associated intraspinal lipoma may be present in the spinal canal.

The condition is frequently asymptomatic although neurological symptoms affecting the bladder and lower legs may develop in adult life. In some cases this is due to abnormal tethering of the filum terminale to the sacrum with resultant dysfunction of the conus medullaris.

Spina bifida cystica

This is a more severe defect as meningeal and neural tissue may both be involved. Several types are recognized: (1) A myelocoele is a severe malformation in which the neural tube has failed to close. The open spinal cord is covered by granulation tissue which is continuous peripherally with skin. Leakage of cerebrospinal fluid and infection invariably occur. (2) A meningomyelocoele is a herniation of both meninges and neural tissue through a bony defect in the vertebrae. It consists of a sac of dura and arachnoid with spinal cord elements in the sac wall. (3) A meningocoele is a herniation of meninges only through a bony defect.

Clinically infants with myelocoeles and meningomyelocoeles have poor neurological function in the lower limbs, rectum and bladder. A large proportion have the Arnold–Chiari malformation and develop hydrocephalus.

Arnold–Chiari malformation

The Arnold–Chiari malformation is the name given to a series of deformities affecting mainly the medulla oblongata and cerebellum. The type I Chiari malformation consists of elongation of the medulla and herniation of the cerebellar tonsils through the foramen magnum. It rarely causes hydrocephalus. The commonest presentation of the Chiari type I is with syringomyelia which is not usually diagnosed until adult life. Occasionally syringobulbia, headache and cranial nerve palsies are presentations (Williams 1981). The type II Chiari deformity is a herniation of the cerebellar tonsils and vermis through the foramen magnum together with elongation of the medulla which becomes S-shaped (*see Fig.* 20.3). This is associated with hydrocephalus. If, in addition, the patient has spina bifida cystica, the condition is termed a Chiari type III deformity.

The cause of the hydrocephalus varies and may be due to either: (1) displacement of the exits of the fourth ventricle below the foramen magnum, in which case the CSF cannot get back up into the cranial cavity since the foramen magnum is blocked by the medulla and cerebellum; or (2) an associated narrowing of the aqueduct of Sylvius.

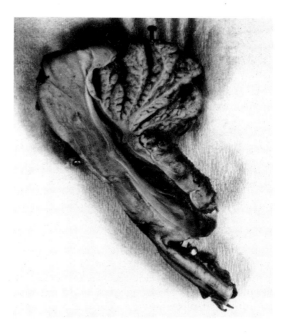

Fig. 20.3. Arnold–Chiari malformation. (Photograph kindly provided by Dr Scholtz and reproduced with the permission of Springer-Verlag.)

Hydrocephalus

In theory, hydrocephalus may be due to over-secretion of CSF, obstruction to the flow of CSF or failure of CSF absorption. In practice, the majority are obstructive. They can be classified as non-communicating, in which case the obstruction is within the ventricular system and CSF cannot pass into the subarachnoid space, or communicating, in which case the obstruction is outside the ventricular system and there is communication between the subarachnoid space and the ventricular system. In the latter case, CSF can escape from the ventricular system into the cisterna magna but cannot reach the supratentorial subarachnoid space where absorption occurs.

Hydrocephalus in the new-born or occurring early in life may be due to a malformation, an inflammatory condition or a tumour. The common malformations are stenosis or forking of the aqueduct of Sylvius, the Arnold–Chiari malformation (*see* above) and the Dandy–Walker syndrome, which is an occlusion of the foramina of the fourth ventricle. Inflammatory conditions include meningitis and subarachnoid haemorrhage, both of which cause fibrosis of the subarachnoid space and consequently a communicating type of hydrocephalus. Obstruction by tumour is very rare in neonates.

The clinical features of enlarging head and bulging fontanelle are well known. Papilloedema is unusual in infants under 6 months of age. Epilepsy, 'sunset eyes' and mental retardation are other features.

Various shunting procedures may be used and CT scanning is useful to monitor the response to treatment. Only one-quarter of the patients reach adult life, deaths being due to the hydrocephalus *per se*, meningitis or chest infection. In some patients, a natural arrest occurs at about age 1–2 years.

After infancy, obstructive hydrocephalus is frequently due to a tumour in the posterior fossa, midbrain or third ventricle. Occasionally stenosis of the aqueduct of Sylvius due to gliosis in the periaqueductal grey matter (which is associated with neurofibromatosis) or forking of the aqueduct present at this stage. Subarachnoid haemorrhage and meningitis may cause subarachnoid adhesions with resultant hydrocephalus, and occasionally no cause is found.

If the hydrocephalus develops slowly, the inner skull table becomes eroded and diverticula of the ventricles form. Chronic papilloedema and headache are frequent symptoms and the skull X-ray may show a 'beaten silver appearance' in the late stages.

Diastematomyelia

This is an embryological malformation involving a vertical division of a variable length of the spinal cord into two hemicords. The cords may be separated by dura, cartilage, fibrous tissue or bone. The condition is compatible with normal function.

Infection

The infections of the central nervous system which most commonly involve the surgeon are bacterial meningitis and abscess formation.

Bacterial meningitis

Bacterial meningitis can occur at any age. The predominant organism in each age group is: *Escherichia coli* in neonates; *Haemophilus influenzae* in infants and children; *Neisseria meningitidis* in teenagers and young adults; and *Streptococcus pneumoniae* in elderly patients.

N. meningitidis is a Gram-negative diplococcus and is the commonest cause of bacterial meningitis in the UK. It is found in the nasopharynx in up to 10% of the healthy population and is frequently responsible for epidemics of meningitis. The infection is associated with a skin rash and in some cases the septicaemia may lead to adrenal haemorrhage and circulatory collapse (the Waterhouse–Friderichsen syndrome). *E. coli* has a predilection for neonates who have neural tube defects. *H. influenzae* occurs as a commensal in the upper respiratory tract. Its encapsulated form is more virulent than its non-encapsulated form and it tends to cause a systemic infection complicated by meningitis. *S. pneumoniae* causes meningitis in older patients, especially as a complication of open trauma.

Meningitis may result from haematogenous or local spread of organisms. Local spread may be from skull fractures, ear infections, paranasal sinus infections, etc. Insertion of ventricular shunts and other neurosurgical operations may also predispose to meningitis.

The CSF is devoid of factors needed for bacterial clearance and is described as an 'immunological vacuum'. Therefore, when bacteria attack the meninges this 'closed sanctuary' provides them with a period during which they can multiply.

The clinical features of pyrexia, headache, vomiting and nuchal rigidity are well known. Diagnosis is confirmed by lumbar puncture and CSF analysis. Typically, the CSF appears cloudy. Polymorphs are present, the protein level is raised and the sugar level is decreased (to about one-half or less of blood sugar level). Viral meningitis differs from bacterial meningitis by having a CSF lymphocytosis, normal or slightly increased protein concentration and normal or slightly increased sugar content. Tuberculous and fungal meningitis are also associated with a CSF lymphocytosis, although in both viral and tuberculous meningitis there may be an early polymorph leucocytosis in the CSF.

Macroscopic examination of the brain at autopsy shows a fibrinous exudate and pus formation on the surface. The arachnoid is the most prominently affected part of the meninges. The inflammatory process may involve the ventricular system (ventriculitis) and can be carried into the cerebral substance along the perivascular spaces of Virchow–Robin.

Microscopic examination shows the presence of an acute inflammatory exudate of the meninges consisting mainly of polymorphs (*see Fig.* 20.4).

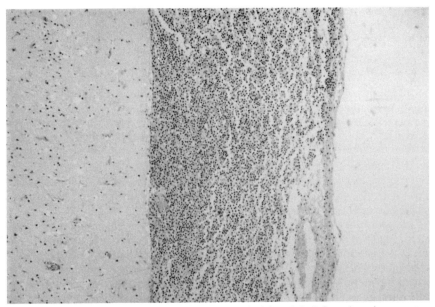

Fig. 20.4. Acute meningitis. Cerebral substance is to the left and the inflamed meninges are to the right. (H and E × 75)

The main complications of meningitis are as follows: (1) Cerebral infarction is due to thrombosis of a vessel as it crosses the pus-filled subarachnoid space. Veins are less resistant to this complication than arteries and when thrombosis occurs, haemorrhagic 'venous' infarcts are produced. (2) Hydrocephalus is due to fibrosis of the subarachnoid space, and may occur late in the disease process, being either communicating or non-communicating.

The mainstay of the treatment of meningitis is antibiotic therapy. Passage of antibiotics through the blood–CSF barrier depends on the relative lipid solubility, the pH and the molecular structure of the antibiotic. The inflammatory response increases the diffusion of some antibiotics and not others. Patients who develop meningitis after neurosurgery frequently have organisms which are antibiotic resistant.

Brain abscess

The incidence of brain abscess has fallen since the introduction of effective antibiotic treatment for sinusitis, middle ear infection, mastoid infection, etc. Infection of the paranasal air sinuses, the middle ear or mastoid may spread directly to the brain causing frontal lobe, temporal lobe and cerebellar abscesses respectively. The organisms are those of the underlying condition (commonly *Bacteroides fragilis* and Streptococci in the ear; *Strep. pneumoniae, Strep. pyogenes* and *Haemophilus influenzae* in the sinuses). Generalized systemic infection may lead to haematogenous spread and consequent metastatic abscesses in the brain. Cyanotic congenital heart disease is especially associated with cerebral abscess, possibly due to the reduced filtration of blood by the lungs and to cerebral hypoxia which may increase susceptibility to infection. Cranial trauma, either surgical or accidental, and chronic lung disease both predispose to brain abscess. Recently the importance of Gram-negative anaerobic bacilli in post-traumatic cases has been recognized.

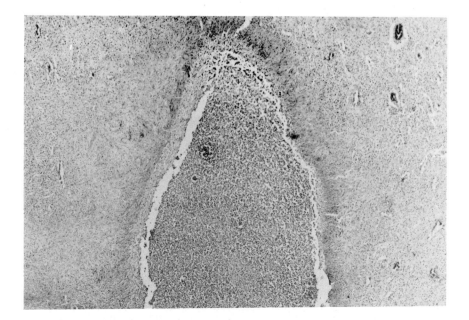

Fig. 20.5. Cerebral abscess with fibrosis and gliosis in the wall. (H and E × 30)

Clinically there is frequently evidence of a meningeal reaction followed by focal neurological signs. The abscess acts as a space-occupying lesion, causing a rise in intracranial pressure (ICP) and eventually uncal and tonsillar herniation (*see* p. 620).

Macroscopically, abscesses develop most commonly at the junction of grey and white matter. In the early stages there is an area of cellulitis and then central necrosis gives rise to an abscess cavity which becomes surrounded by a wall of fibrosis.

Histologically, the abscess cavity contains cell debris and polymorphs. Surrounding this is a zone of fibrous tissue. Formation of fibrous tissue in the brain is unusual and is fairly specific for bacterial infection. Surrounding the fibrous tissue is a zone of gliosis which is the usual cerebral response to injury (*see Fig.* 20.5).

Surgery with adequate drainage of the necrotic core is the definitive treatment as aspiration produces only temporary control. Steroids may control increased ICP but they decrease vascular permeability to antibiotics and their use is therefore controversial. The mortality is approximately 10% (Strong and Ingham 1983).

Other intracranial abscesses

Other abscesses within the cranial cavity may be extradural (due to spread from surrounding bones), subdural and subarachnoid (rare). Subdural abscess is usually the result of spread of infection from the skull bones, sinuses or ears. Pus may compress the underlying brain and cause thrombosis of the veins which traverse the subdural space. This in turn leads to haemorrhagic infarction of an area of cortex.

Spinal abscesses

Acute spinal abscesses are most commonly in the extradural location. The usual sequence of events is haematogenous spread of infection from a lesion such as a boil to a vertebral body, causing a focus of osteomyelitis, and an accumulation of extradural pus. The patient develops backache and root pain together with a systemic upset. Cord compression eventually develops. The commonest organism is Staphylococcus.

Intradural abscesses are rare.

Paravertebral abscesses occur in spinal tuberculosis. The infection usually starts in adjacent vertebrae and destroys the intervertebral discs with subsequent collapse and kyphosis. The area most often affected is the thoracic region and cord compression here causes signs and symptoms in the legs (Pott's paraplegia). Early cord compression is usually due to abscess formation whereas late cord compression is usually due to bone deformity.

Cerebral Vascular Disease

Transient ischaemic attacks

A transient ischaemic attack (TIA) is an episode of focal neurological disturbance lasting for less than 24 hours and followed by total recovery. TIAs may affect either the carotid or the vertebral/basilar territories. Those affecting the carotid territory are most commonly related to atheromatous plaques of the internal carotid artery in the region of the bifurcation of the common carotid artery. Usually the atheroma is most severe in the first 2 cm of the posterior wall of the internal carotid artery, extending into the distal common carotid artery. Atheromatous plaques also occur at the origins of the great vessels, at the siphon of the internal carotid in the cavernous sinus or at the proximal segments of the middle and anterior cerebral arteries. Symptoms include contralateral weakness and numbness together with ipsilateral monocular blindness. TIAs affecting the vertebral/basilar territory are frequently due to atheromatous plaques at the origin of the vertebral artery. In these cases there is vertigo, ataxia and diplopia and the symptoms may be related to extension or rotation of the neck.

TIAs can be caused by either a 'low flow' haemodynamic situation or by embolism. Rare causes of TIAs include polycythaemia rubra vera, cardiac arrhythmias and hypotension.

LOW FLOW: Low flow situations cause cerebral infarction or TIAs affecting the watershed areas between cerebral vascular territories. In the carotid circulation this requires a pressure drop in the artery distal to a stenotic lesion and usually a 70% reduction in carotid lumen diameter is needed leaving a residual lumen of less than 2 mm in diameter (*see Fig.* 20.6). Furthermore, the collateral circulation to the region must be impaired, usually because of an incomplete circle of Willis.

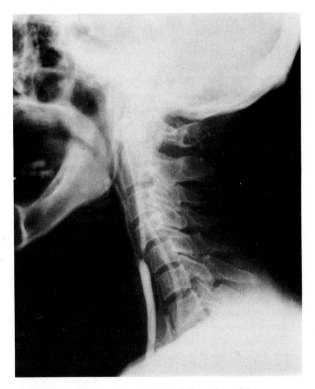

Fig. 20.6. Carotid angiogram showing stenosis at the bifurcation of the common carotid artery.

The cause of low flow ischaemic attacks is unclear. An intermittent occlusion of a severely stenotic lesion at the carotid bifurcation due to local mechanical factors may be a cause. Rarely, systemic haemodynamic factors may reduce flow to a critical level across the lesion (Kistler *et al.* 1984). Sudden changes in posture or steal phenomena may sometimes be responsible.

TIAs due to a low flow situation are characteristically fleeting and classically monocular blindness lasting one to two minutes is reported. If the TIA lasts longer than one hour, embolism is the usual cause.

EMBOLISM: When emboli arise from a stenotic or ulcerated internal carotid artery the symptoms usually relate to the occlusion of the middle cerebral artery and its branches. Less often the anterior cerebral artery is affected. The emboli are commonly composed of platelets and atheromatous debris. Ulceration of an atheromatous plaque exposes collagen which causes platelet aggregation, thus predisposing to emboli.

The importance of transient ischaemic attacks is the fact that they may go on to a complete stroke in the same anatomical territory. If they remain untreated, 40% of patients with TIAs go on to frank strokes within 5 years. In the best centres, carotid endarterectomy has a mortality of less than 2% and a postoperative stroke incidence of about 1–2%. Following surgery the long-term incidence of stroke is 0·5%/year compared with the natural history of untreated TIAs which is 5%/year (Loftus and Quest 1983).

Strokes

A stroke is a focal neurological defect of sudden onset due to a vascular lesion. A complete stroke is one in which there has been no progression in the neurological defect over a period of several hours. A stroke in evolution is one in which the neurological deficit is continuing to evolve over a period of hours. It may be due to progressive narrowing of an artery by thrombus, to the development of cerebral oedema or to obliteration of collateral vessels by thrombus propagation. About 85% of complete strokes are due to cerebral infarction and 15% are due to cerebral haemorrhage. In all age groups the incidence is about 200 per 100 000 per year. The incidence rises steadily with age to about 5000 per 100 000 in the over 85 year old group.

Hypertension is the most important risk factor associated with stroke as it promotes the formation of atheroma in the extra- and intracranial arteries and it damages the small penetrating blood vessels of the brain by causing deposition of lipid (lipohyalinization). Microaneurysms of Charcot–Bouchard may also be caused by hypertension (*see* p. 612). Both the systolic and the diastolic pressures are important. Several studies have shown that effective long-term control of hypertension decreases the incidence of both ischaemic and haemorrhagic stroke. Smoking, obesity and hyperlipidaemia also increase the risk of stroke.

Cerebral infarction

It is now realized that many cases of cerebral infarction occur as the result of extra-cranial cardiovascular disease. The cause may be occlusion (internal carotid or vertebral), embolism, or hypotension (which may occur as a complication of myocardial infarction or cardiac arrhythmia).

Emboli arising in the heart may consist of thrombus (from the left atrium in patients with atrial fibrillation, or from a mural thrombus after myocardial infarction) or debris (from rheumatic or calcified valves). Other emboli consist of platelets and fibrin which arise from atheromatous plaques in the aorta, or the carotid or vertebral arteries.

The effect of occlusion of the internal carotid or vertebral artery depends on the state of the remaining vessels and the efficiency of anastomoses between the remaining cerebral vessels.

Clinically, cerebral infarction causes a reduction in the level of consciousness and a neurological defect. In those cases in which occlusion of the internal carotid artery leads to infarction, there is dense contralateral hemiplegia, sensory loss and hemianopia. Occlusion of the middle cerebral artery causes a similar clinical picture. Perceptual deficits are common and speech disorders occur if the dominant lobe is involved. Paralysis is more pronounced in the arm than in the leg. The anterior cerebral artery supplies the frontal lobe (via Heubner's artery) and the anterior limb of the internal capsule; occlusion causes mental symptoms and paralysis which mainly affects the contralateral leg. The posterior cerebral arteries are the terminal branches of the basilar artery and are supplied by the basilar as opposed to the carotid system in most people. They supply the visual cortex, upper midbrain, superior cerebellar peduncles and the posterior limbs of the internal capsules. Most infarcts involve only part of this territory, the common clinical feature being contralateral hemianopia with sparing of the fixation point. Occlusions of the other cerebellar arteries cause various brain stem and cerebellar syndromes.

In cases of general cerebral hypoperfusion as occurs in shock, the watershed areas of the cerebral circulation, for example between the middle and anterior cerebral arteries, become infarcted giving rise to a so-called 'boundary zone infarction'.

Cerebral infarction which is not caused by atheromatous disease or emboli occurs occasionally, usually in the younger age groups. In early childhood, systemic infection with dehydration and malnutrition can predispose to cortical venous thrombosis. Cyanotic heart disease can produce septic emboli. A congenital vascular malformation, especially in the middle cerebral territory, may produce a spontaneous intracranial haemorrhage or infarction. Extension of an aortic dissection into the carotid system may cause a stroke. Various forms of arteritis can involve the vertebral, carotid, ophthalmic and central retinal arteries. Traumatic injury to the vessels of the neck and skull base, with rupture, thrombosis or dissection, can be due to a wide variety of penetrating and indirect injuries.

Grossly, cerebral infarctions pass through various phases according to their age. Initially the infarcts may appear haemorrhagic (see Fig. 20.7) and the surrounding area usually shows numerous petechial haemorrhages. After a few days the infarcted area becomes soft and oedematous and the infarct can be palpated as an area of a softening on the surface of the affected brain. In the early stages, surrounding cerebral oedema with swelling may cause an increase in intracranial pressure and resultant brain shifts (see p. 620). Eventually breakdown of the infarcted areas occurs and a fluid-filled cyst remains.

Histologically, in the initial period, the hypoxic neurones become eosinophilic and their nuclei become pyknotic. An infiltrate of polymorphs appears at the edge of the infarct after about a day. Within a week, macrophages invade the necrotic tissue where they phagocytose debris and become lipid-laden 'gitter cells'. Eventually an area of gliosis forms in the wall of the cystic cavity.

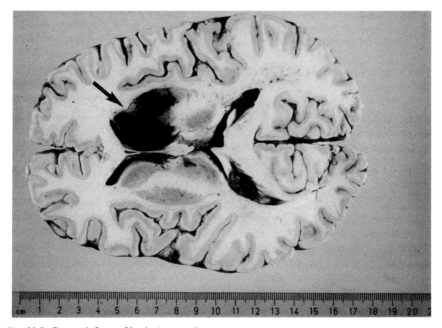

Fig. 20.7. Recent infarct of brain (arrowed).

Intracerebral haemorrhage

Hypertensive patients are especially at risk from intracerebral haemorrhage. The clinical syndrome is one of various neurological deficits, depending on the anatomical site, coma and reflex hypertension. Usually patients are over 50 years of age.

Hypertensive patients tend to develop microaneurysms (Charcot–Bouchard aneurysms) in the intracerebral branches of the major arteries, especially the lenticulo-striate branch of the middle cerebral artery. It is thought that these represent areas of weakness of the vessel walls which may be the origin of the haemorrhage. The lenticulo-striate artery supplies the putamen (part of the lentiform nucleus) which is the initial site of intracerebral haemorrhage in over 50% of cases; haemorrhage in this area frequently involves the closely related internal capsule. Other sites (cerebral cortex, thalamus, pons and cerebellar hemisphere) are involved in approximately equal proportions. Other lesions which predispose to intracerebral haemorrhage include berry aneurysms, vascular malformations, septic emboli, mycotic aneurysms, haemorrhage into an area of infarction, bleeding into intracranial tumours, trauma and bleeding diatheses.

Grossly, the haemorrhage tracts through the white matter and often ruptures into the ventricles. The rise in intracranial pressure may cause tentorial herniation and secondary midbrain haemorrhage.

Histologically, blood is seen separating nerve bundles. In the later stages of the process, the blood clot is invaded by macrophages and becomes organized. Eventually a fluid-filled cyst with a gliotic wall, similar to an old infarction, is seen.

The distinction between cerebral haemorrhage, infarction and tumour is aided by CT scanning. Most patients require medical support with adequate hydration, control of hypertension and control of the raised intracranial pressure which is secondary to both the mass lesion and the cerebral oedema. The operative management is controversial.

Subarachnoid haemorrhage

Subarachnoid haemorrhage (SAH) is due to rupture of a berry aneurysm in more than 50% of cases. In 25% no cause is found; rupture of a vessel (without aneurysm) in hypertensive patients accounts for 15%; arteriovenous malformations cause 5% and the remainder are due to such conditions as blood dyscrasias, tumours and trauma. Rarely, mycotic or traumatic aneurysms are the cause.

Clinically, subarachnoid haemorrhage may be complicated or uncomplicated. In uncomplicated SAH, bleeding is into the subarachnoid space only. Focal neurological signs, such as IIIrd nerve palsy may, however, occur due to the space-occupying effect of the aneurysm itself. In complicated SAH, bleeding also occurs into the brain with resultant focal neurological signs.

The patients develop sudden headache and neck stiffness, with or without neurological deficit and the level of consciousness may be lowered. The clinical state of the patient is important in determining the treatment and prognosis and it can be divided into grades ranging from grade I (slight headache and neck stiffness) to grade V (coma and decerebrate rigidity). Extracranial clinical complications include hypertension, electrocardiograph changes, glycosuria and neurogenic pulmonary oedema. The cardiac abnormalities are thought to be due to an increased production of catecholamines resulting from spasm of the hypothalamic arteries.

Patients with SAH are subject to a number of late complications. The most important of these is cerebral infarction which appears to be caused by vasospasm. The vasospasm is most marked in that part of the artery distal to an aneurysm and it occurs not immediately, but rather after an interval of 3–7 days. Surgical intervention at this time may worsen the situation. The cause of the vasospasm is unknown although there is some evidence that it is related to the presence of periarterial haematoma.

Communicating hydrocephalus may develop some weeks or months after the bleed; the presence of blood in the subarachnoid space causes arachnoiditis which impairs the absorption of CSF.

Other late complications include dementia and epilepsy.

Berry aneurysms

Berry aneurysms are found in 1–8% of routine autopsies. They may occur *de novo* or in association with conditions such as the Ehlers–Danlos syndrome, coarctation of the aorta and polycystic kidneys. Close relatives of affected patients are at increased risk. Patients with hypertension and hyperlipidaemia also have an increased incidence of berry aneurysm.

Table 20.1. Sites of berry aneurysms

	Percentage
Middle cerebral artery	19
Anterior cerebral and anterior communicating arteries	41
Internal carotid and posterior communicating arteries	37
Basilar artery circulation	3
	100

The pathogenesis of berry aneurysms is unknown. The site of predilection is at the points of branching of the cerebral arteries, which may be explained by the presence of gaps or holes in the smooth muscle of the media commonly found in these areas in all people. However, since berry aneurysms only occur in a small proportion of people there must be additional factors to account for their causation. One such factor is fragmentation of the internal elastic lamina which is found in the vicinity of berry aneurysms and which probably represents a degenerative change. The incidence at various sites is given in *Table* 20.1. In about 15% of cases they are multiple.

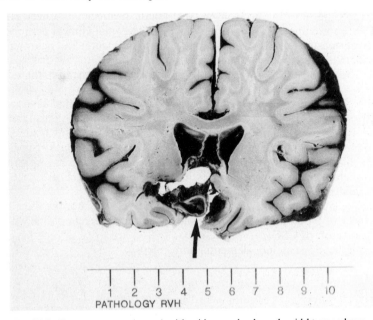

Fig. 20.8. Berry aneurysm (arrow) with widespread subarachnoid haemorrhage.

Grossly berry aneurysms (*see Fig.* 20.8) vary greatly in size and shape from small saccular forms to large multilobulated aneurysms. The larger ones tend to be filled with laminated blood clot which may give a false impression of small size on angiography. Aneurysms may fail to fill on angiography due to spasm, thrombosis or small size.

Giant aneurysms are above 2 cm (or above 2·5 cm in some series) and are rare. They tend to occur in three distinct locations: (1) the supraclinoid portion of the internal carotid artery; (2) the peripheral intracranial arteries, especially the middle cerebral; (3) the vessels of the posterior cerebral circulation. There are two theories to explain the origin of giant aneurysms. Firstly, that they are different from berry aneurysms and are truly congenital. Secondly, that a small aneurysm leaks, forming haematoma which later becomes organized and incorporated into the wall.

Intracavernous aneurysms are protected, as they enlarge, by the dural walls of the cavernous sinus. Rupture is unusual but if it does occur, a carotico-cavernous fistula results.

Following SAH from a berry aneurysm the greatest incidence of rebleeding occurs between the fifth and ninth day. Without surgery the mortality rate is 7% per week until six weeks have passed and thereafter 10% of the survivors who have been treated conservatively die per year. Hospital mortality from the first bleed is 14%, while mortality after the second bleed is 42%. However, many die before reaching hospital and the overall initial mortality without operation may be up to 40%.

Other aneurysms

Mycotic aneurysms are uncommon. The inflammatory reaction causes destruction of the internal elastic lamina and media, with resultant weakening and dilatation of the wall. Complications such as infarction or haematoma of the adjacent brain commonly occurs.

Fusiform dilatations of the internal carotid or basilar arteries are usually due to atheroma. Associated embolism or thrombosis may cause infarction of the relevant vascular territory and the aneurysm may cause direct compression on vital structures.

True traumatic aneurysms are also rare. Aneurysms of meningeal vessels, arterio-venous fistulas and false aneurysms have all been reported, following major cranial trauma. Traumatic aneurysms tend to occur on susceptible vessels such as the anterior cerebral artery in relation to the falx or the carotid artery near the tentorium. They have a high mortality (about 50%) if rupture occurs.

Head Injuries

Just over 4000 people died of head injury in England and Wales in 1983. Almost two-thirds of these were males, adolescents between 15 and 20 years old being especially at risk. The commonest cause is road traffic accident. Other causes include falls (particularly in the elderly), assault, industrial accidents and, in Northern Ireland, gunshot wounds.

Head injuries may be due to blunt force which often produces a closed head injury or to localized force which often produces a penetrating injury.

Head injury consequences have been classified into primary (impact) damage which occurs at the time of injury and secondary damage which occurs as a complication of the injury.

Blunt head injuries: primary brain damage

This produces either localized brain damage or a diffuse axonal injury.

Localized brain damage

The brainstem has a relatively fixed position due to the attachment of cranial nerves and blood vessels. The cerebral hemispheres are relatively unfixed. When the brain moves within the skull, as happens in a deceleration injury, it does so about an axis which is between the fixed and unfixed parts. Those areas of the brain which are the greatest distance from this axis move with the greatest velocity and therefore make the most forceful contact with the skull. Thus, localized brain damage is commonest in the frontal and temporal lobes, which may become contused or lacerated (*see Fig.* 20.9). A contusion is a haemorrhagic area which tends to be on the crest of a cerebral gyrus. Several areas of contusion may coalesce to form an intracranial haematoma. A laceration implies actual macroscopic tearing of the brain substance. Localized brain damage may be at the site of impact (*coup* injury) or away from the site of impact (*contre coup* injury). The classic example of this is a fall on the occiput resulting in contusion of both the occipital and frontal lobes due to the brain accelerating backwards and forwards within the cranial cavity.

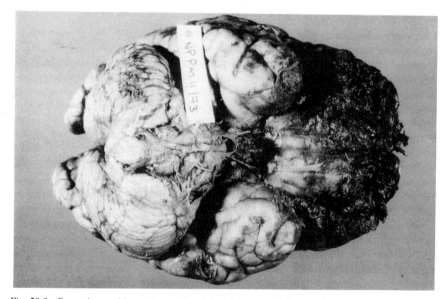

Fig. 20.9. Contusion and laceration of frontal and temporal lobes.

Diffuse white matter axonal injury

The rotational forces set up between the relatively fixed brainstem and the relatively unfixed cerebral hemispheres cause shearing forces within the brain substance which tear the axons of the white matter. Shearing forces are especially strong at the interface between areas of white and grey matter, due to their different densities.

This 'diffuse white matter axonal injury' is exceedingly important in primary brain damage (Strich 1956). Macroscopically the surface of the brain may appear normal. On cut section there are frequently small areas of haemorrhage especially in the brainstem and corpus callosum. These are bilateral, asymmetrical and associated with intraventricular bleeding. Later, small scars form and finally there may be a degree of cerebral atrophy. The torn axons retract and histologically characteristic axonal 'retraction balls' are found representing sites of axonal tearing (*see Fig.* 20.10). The distal nerve processes degenerate and a cellular reaction occurs forming microglial scars.

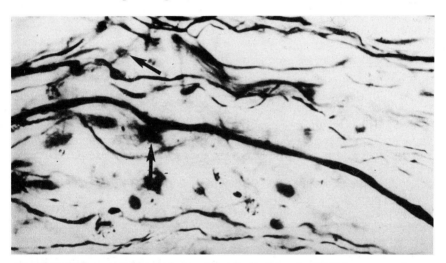

Fig. 20.10. Diffuse axonal injury showing 'retraction balls', some of which are arrowed

Clinically, primary brain damage presents with alteration of consciousness which may be monitored by the Glasgow coma scale (Teasdale and Jennett 1974). It is thought that the deeper the coma the more widespread is the diffuse axonal damage. It seems likely that even in relatively minor head injuries, diffuse axonal injury can occur. Oppenheimer (1968) has shown that microglial scars are present in patients who have recovered from short periods of unconsciousness and who later died from unrelated extracranial causes. Diffuse axonal injury is probably responsible for the cumulative effects of repeated mild concussion.

Blunt head injuries: secondary brain damage

Further clinical deterioration after primary brain damage is likely to be due to secondary brain damage. The factors responsible for secondary brain damage have been subdivided into intracranial and extracranial (Mendelow and Teasdale 1983).

Intracranial causes of secondary brain damage

HAEMATOMA: Extradural haematoma is classically associated with a skull fracture and tearing of the middle meningeal artery or vein. Since there is usually only mild primary brain damage, the patient often does not lose consciousness immediately, but rather has a 'lucid interval' of several minutes or hours before the onset of symptoms. Acute subdural haematoma is associated with greater primary brain damage and the patient is less likely to have a lucid interval. An acute intracerebral haematoma is suspected in patients who have focal signs and who fail to recover consciousness rapidly. Chronic subdural haematoma presents days or months after the original trauma with confusion, a fluctuating level of consciousness and focal neurological signs.

BRAIN SWELLING: An increase in brain volume may be due either to an increase in cerebral blood volume or to cerebral oedema (an increase in intra- or extracellular fluid volume). Brain swelling is usually associated with raised intracranial pressure.

Hypoxia and hypercapnia tend to increase cerebral blood volume by causing vascular dilatation. An obstructed airway raises central venous pressure and this adds to cerebral congestion.

Cerebral oedema can be produced by various mechanisms.

1. Vasogenic oedema is due to damage of cerebral vessel walls with a breakdown in the blood–brain barrier which allows passage of large osmotically active molecules into the extracellular space. This is responsible for the generalized cerebral oedema which occurs in head injury (*see Fig.* 20.11).
2. Cytotoxic oedema is due to accumulation of intracellular fluid in response to ischaemia and is responsible for the localized oedema around the areas of injury.
3. Hydrostatic oedema is due to an increase in cerebral venous pressure; an obstructed airway predisposes to this type of oedema.
4. Interstitial oedema around the ventricles occurs when there is obstruction to the flow of CSF.

The brain swelling causes compression of cerebral capillaries and further ischaemic damage to the brain. The raised intracranial pressure causes brain shifts (*see* p. 620) and eventually cerebral perfusion ceases and death ensues.

INFECTION: This is usually a later sequela than haematoma or brain swelling and either a brain abscess or meningitis can occur. Usually a compound skull fracture or fracture of the skull base gives a portal of entry for the organism. Meningitis may produce a communicating hydrocephalus and brain abscess may cause an elevated intracranial pressure and the other effects of a space occupying lesion.

SUBARACHNOID HAEMORRHAGE: This occurs commonly in severe head injuries. The effect of blood in the subarachnoid space can produce vasospasm with further ischaemic damage to the brain.

HYDROCEPHALUS: Blockage of the subarachnoid space by blood and debris causes early hydrocephalus in some cases.

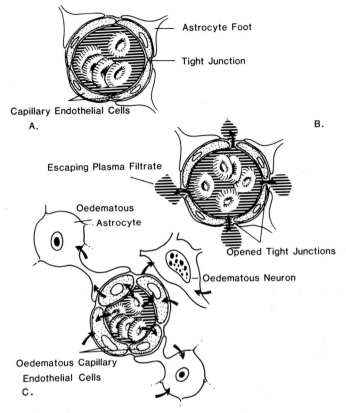

Astrocyte Foot

Tight Junction

Capillary Endothelial Cells

A.

B.

Escaping Plasma Filtrate

Oedematous
Astrocyte

Opened Tight Junctions

Oedematous Neuron

Oedematous Capillary
Endothelial Cells

C.

Fig. 20.11. Stages in the pathogenesis of vasogenic cerebral oedema. (Reproduced with kind permission from Fishman 1975.)

Extracranial causes of secondary brain damage

HYPOXIA: Hypoxia may occur as a consequence of brainstem damage which can produce an alteration in the pattern of respiration, pulmonary oedema and shunting. Alternatively, hypoxia may be due to chest injury or aspiration. Whatever the cause, hypoxia aggravates cerebral ischaemia.

HYPOTENSION: This may be due to blood loss, cardiac tamponade or spinal injury. Low systemic pressure, especially associated with an elevated intracranial pressure, markedly decreases the cerebral perfusion pressure and this added to hypoxia makes cerebral ischaemic damage considerably worse. Because neurones rely on glycolysis to produce energy, oxygen and glucose are essential and a diminished or interrupted supply produces cellular damage. Autopsy studies have revealed that hypoxic damage occurs in two settings: (1) in the territory of a major intracranial artery, such as the posterior cerebral artery, which may become occluded during transtentorial herniation; (2) ischaemic damage in the basal ganglia, hippocampus and cortical regions (i.e. at the boundaries of distribution between major vessels) in cases of generalized hypoperfusion.

Raised intracranial pressure and brain shifts (see Fig. 20.12)

The various forms of secondary brain damage tend to cause serious complications via a final common pathway of raised intracranial pressure and brain shift. Since the intracranial contents are within a rigid bony case, a small change in volume can lead to a large increase in intracranial pressure. This has the effect of interfering with cerebral blood flow and squeezing brain substance into areas of lower pressure. Brain shifts may complicate any intracranial space-occupying lesion.

If the pressure increase is above the tentorium, a shift of the cingulate gyrus may occur under the falx.

Alternatively, the brain may herniate from the supratentorial compartment to the posterior fossa via the tentorial hiatus (transtentorial herniation). Transtentorial herniation compresses the ipsilateral IIIrd cranial nerve causing dilatation of the pupil and ptosis. Brainstem distortion and ischaemia produces extensor (decerebrate) rigidity and this is associated with flame shaped (Duret) haemorrhages in the substance of the midbrain. Compression of the posterior cerebral artery causes infarction of the medial occipital cortex.

Displacement from the posterior fossa through the foramen magnum into the spinal canal (tonsilar herniation) is associated with a marked decrease in conscious level. Tonsillar herniation produces compression of the medulla with vasomotor and respiratory abnormalities and death.

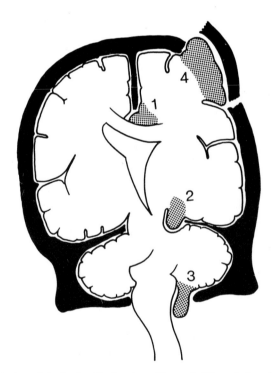

Fig. 20.12. Herniation of the brain; (1) cingulate; (2) uncal; (3) cerebellar; (4) transcalvarial. (Reproduced with permission from Fishman 1975.)

Finally, brain tissue may be pushed out through a compound fracture (transcalvarial herniation).

Late sequelae of head injuries

EPILEPSY: This is probably due to cortical scarring in most cases. It is associated with post-traumatic amnesia lasting over 24 hours, dural tears with compound depressed fractures and intracranial haematomas.

HYDROCEPHALUS: Late hydrocephalus may be due to loss of white matter (cerebral atrophy). Communicating hydrocephalus is most commonly due to obstruction of CSF flow by blood in the subarachnoid space (Beyerl and Black 1984).

Prognosis after closed head injury

A score of 8 or less on the Glasgow coma scale or post-traumatic amnesia greater than 24 hours (especially more than one week) indicates a severe head injury. If a severe head injury is associated with hypoxia and hypotension the prognosis is poor. One study correlated maximum intracranial pressure with prognosis and showed that if the pressure remained under 20 mmHg, then 27% did badly (i.e. the outcome was severe disability, a vegetative state or death); for 20–40 mmHg, 46% did badly; for 40–60 mmHg, 76% did badly. All patients with a maximal intracranial pressure of over 60 mmHg died (Miller and Becker 1982). Patients with intracranial haematoma do less well compared with those without and 55% and 27% respectively died in one series (Gentleman and Jennett 1981). If a patient has an intracranial haematoma and associated hypoxia or hypotension, mortality rises to over 70%.

Penetrating head injuries

With missile injuries to the head, the problems of indriven fragments of bullet, bone and clothing carry a risk of infection. A tangential bullet injury frequently causes 'gutter' fractures with bone fragments being driven in several directions intracranially. In addition to damage in the missile track, radial expansile forces cause temporary 'cavitation' of the brain with damage distant from the track. This cavitation phenomenon occurs particularly with high velocity missile injuries (Gordon 1975). The local effect of missile trauma depends on the site of the track and the degree of cavitation. Adequate debridement and early controlled ventilation to avoid hypoxia and straining and to reduce central venous pressure are necessary.

Late epilepsy occurs in up to 40% of cases. CSF leaks, meningitis and brain abscesses are other sequelae which occur more commonly with missile injury than with non-penetrating injury.

The prognosis for gunshot missile injuries depends on various factors but a clue can be obtained from the patient's state of consciousness on admission. In one series of 93 cases, of those who were alert on admission, 88% survived: of those who were drowsy, 66% survived; of those who only reacted to painful stimuli, 21% survived; and of those cases admitted in coma, none survived (Gordon 1975).

Peripheral Nerve Injuries

Neuronal response to injury

When an axon is transected, the cell body (in the anterior horn of the spinal cord or in a posterior root ganglion or in an autonomic ganglion (undergoes chromatolysis, seen as neuronal swelling accompanied by displacement of Nissl substance to the periphery of the cell. As a regenerative response, the neuronal cytoplasm increases in volume due to an increase in RNA which produces new polypeptides for regeneration of axoplasm. The axon distal to the transection undergoes Wallerian degeneration. If the axon is myelinated, the myelin sheath also degenerates forming globules of debris which are removed by macrophages. After 3–4 days, regenerative features are seen at the proximal end of the axon which begins to sprout.

Three types of neuronal injury have been described (Seddon 1943).

Neuropraxia is a physiological block in conduction without anatomical axonal interruption. It is caused by blunt injuries, high velocity missile injuries adjacent to the nerve, mild compression and ischaemia or excessive stretching of the nerve. An example is 'Saturday night palsy' which is due to drooping an arm over a chair with compression of the posterior cord of the brachial plexus or radial nerve. Macroscopically, the nerve appears normal and only segmental demyelination is seen on histology. Distally the nerve is normal and there is no Wallerian degeneration. Atrophy does not occur. Complete return of motor and sensory function occurs.

Axonotmesis is an anatomical disruption of the axon without serious interruption of the endoneuronal or perineuronal framework. Distal Wallerian degeneration occurs and clinically there is total motor and sensory loss. However, the regenerating axons are relatively unimpeded in their course and thus there is minimal straying of axons and a good return of function.

Neurotmesis is partial or complete division of the nerve with disruption of axons, myelin sheath and connective tissue support. If the nerve is transected completely, a proximal stump neuroma develops. This is composed of whorls of disorganized and branching axons with connective tissue and Schwann cells. The distal stump forms a nodule due to the proliferation of Schwann cells and connective tissue. If there is a gap between the stumps, it is filled by clot. Later, organization into connective tissue and ingrowth of Schwann cells occurs. Regenerating axons grow into this area and useless branching and re-routing occurs so that clinical recovery is poor.

Chronic injuries to peripheral nerves

These are caused by entrapment neuropathies. Predisposing factors include; (1) compression by narrowing of the compartment through which the nerve passes, for example the carpal tunnel syndrome; (2) repetitive stretching as nerves pass over an anomalous structure, such as a cervical rib; (3) impingement by narrowing of the normal boundaries of a compartment, as in the thoracic outlet syndromes; and (4) repeated dislocations, as in tardy ulnar paralysis.

The effects are expressed via pressure on and ischaemia of the nerve. The mildest changes are disturbance of axonoplasmic flow and disturbance of the blood–nerve barrier; not all fibres within a fascicle are uniformly affected. Further entrapment results in paranodal and segmental demyelination (although the axon still remains intact). Local remyelination rapidly returns function to normal after release of pressure.

Normal Pressure Hydrocephalus (*see Fig.* 20.13)

This is a syndrome in which chronic hydrocephalus is associated with progressive dementia, abnormalities of gait and urinary incontinence. A single reading of CSF pressure taken at lumbar puncture is normal, but continuous monitoring of patients shows that they have intermittent periods of raised intracranial pressure. These periods occur especially during sleep, when a slight hypercapnia leads to cerebral vasodilation. In some cases there is a past history of trauma or subarachnoid haemorrhage whereas other cases are idiopathic. It appears that the pressure/volume adaptive mechanisms are abnormal so that minor increases in volume result in an exaggerated increase in intracranial pressure.

Grossly there is dilatation of the ventricles and one study showed meningeal fibrosis and disruption of the ependymal lining of the ventricles (Di Rocco *et al.* 1977). In the idiopathic case there appears to be a functional block in CSF reabsorption.

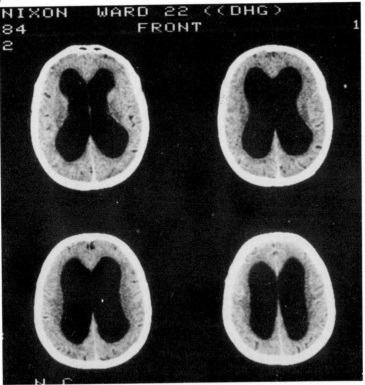

Fig. 20.13. CT scan in a case of normal pressure hydrocephalus showing dilatation of the ventricles.

The importance of recognizing normal pressure hydrocephalus is that it is a form of dementia which responds to surgical treatment (ventricular shunting).

Primary Intracranial Tumours

Epidemiology

Tumours of the central nervous system accounted for just under 2500 deaths in England and Wales during 1983. The incidence rate among adults is between four and ten per 100 000 (being highest in the sixth decade) and about two per 100 000 amongst children. Primary brain tumours are the sixth commonest cancer in adults and the second commonest in children. Meningiomas and neurilemmomas are more common in females than males whereas most other primary brain tumours are more common in males than females. Blacks have a lower incidence of brain tumours than whites.

Aetiology

The administration of ionizing radiation in childhood is associated with an increased risk of developing meningiomas up to 15 years later (Modan *et al.* 1974). There have also been several individual case reports of astrocytomas arising after radiotherapy, although the association is not proven. The use of barbiturates has been implicated in the development of brain tumours in animals although there is little other evidence for incriminating chemical substances. Follow-up studies of patients with previous head injury do not show an increased incidence of brain tumours. Some tumours occur on a hereditary basis, examples being acoustic neuromas occurring in von Recklinghausen's disease and haemangioblastomas of the cerebellum occurring in von Hippel–Lindau disease.

Classification

A primary intracranial tumour is one which arises from the brain itself or from other intracranial contents such as the meninges, cranial nerves and pituitary gland. Tumours of the brain itself may arise from neurones, from neuroglial cells or from blood vessels. Tumours of neurons and of neuroglial cells are together termed neuroepithelial tumours. The vast majority of these are derived from neuroglial cells (for example astrocytomas, oligodendrogliomas and ependymomas), whereas primary neuronal tumours (for example, gangliocytomas) are exceedingly rare within the central nervous system.

A classification of primary intracranial tumours based on the WHO (1979) system is given in *Table* 20.2.

Location

In children, about two-thirds of tumours are infratentorial. Approximately 60% of tumours in childhood are astrocytomas and these have a predilection for the cerebellum and brain stem. The next most common tumour in children is the medulloblastoma which arises in the midline of the cerebellum. Most of the remainder are ependymomas, which arise in the ventricular system, and craniopharyngiomas, which arise in the suprasellar region.

Table 20.2. Classification of primary intracranial tumours (adapted from the WHO classification 1979)

I	*Tumours of neuroepithelial tissue*
	—Astrocytic tumours
	—Oligodendroglial tumours
	—Ependymal and choroid plexus tumours
	—Pineal cell tumours
	—Neuronal tumours
	—Poorly differentiated and embryonal tumours
	(including glioblastoma and medulloblastoma)
II	*Tumours of nerve sheath cells*
	—Neurilemmoma (Schwannoma)
	—Neurofibroma
III	*Tumours of meningeal and related structures*
	—Meningioma
	—Meningeal sarcoma
	—Melanotic tumours
IV	*Primary malignant lymphomas*
V	*Tumours of blood vessel origin*
	—Haemangioblastoma
VI	*Germ cell tumours*
	—Teratoma
	—Other germ cell tumours
VII	*Other malformative tumours and tumour-like lesions*
	—Craniopharyngioma
	—Dermoid cyst
	—Colloid cyst of the third ventricle
VIII	*Vascular malformations*
	—Capillary telangiectasia
	—Cavernous angioma
	—Arteriovenous malformation
	—Sturge–Weber syndrome
IX	*Tumours of the anterior pituitary*
	—Adenoma
	—Carcinoma

In adults, about two-thirds of tumours are supratentorial. Compared with children, adults more commonly develop glioblastomas, pituitary adenomas, acoustic neuromas, haemangioblastomas, oligodendrogliomas and meningiomas. Glioblastomas and astrocytomas are relatively common in the frontal and temporal lobes, less frequent in the parietal lobes and uncommon in the occipital lobes. Haemangioblastomas are most common in the cerebellum although they also occur on the surface of the medulla and spinal cord. Oligodendrogliomas occur in the cerebral hemispheres and rarely in the posterior fossa. Meningiomas occur at any site on the brain surface.

Clinical features

The clinical features of brain tumours are due to both the local effects and the generalized effect of an intracranial mass.

The local effects, which include focal neurological deficits and epilepsy, are due to the destruction of brain tissue and surrounding oedema. The oedema is due to the breakdown of the blood–brain barrier which occurs in the vicinity of brain tumours (especially metastases). Epilepsy occurs in about one-fifth of all patients with brain tumours and is especially associated with slowly growing varieties such as oligodendrogliomas. In certain 'silent' areas, such as the non-dominant temporal lobe, the corpus callosum, the frontal lobe and the thalamus, neurological signs occur late in the disease process.

The main generalized effect is increased intracranial pressure which can be attributed to either the mass of the tumour with its surrounding oedema or to obstruction of the ventricular system. The rise in intracranial pressure occurs at a later stage in infants and the elderly than in young adults. In infants, this is due to the fact that the sutures are still open, whereas in the elderly, atrophy of the brain substance allows for greater expansion. Eventually, the rise in intracranial pressure produces brain shifts as discussed on p. 620.

Malignancy in central nervous system tumours

Tumours of the central nervous system in general do not metastasize and therefore the usual criteria for malignancy cannot be applied. In general the more rapidly growing tumours are the most likely to cause death quickly and therefore the malignant potential of CNS tumours depends to a large extent on the speed of growth and brain destruction. The aggression of individual neuroepithelial central nervous system tumours correlates with the histological grading system of Kernohan *et al.* (1949). In this system, tumours are divided into four grades ranging from grade I which is well differentiated with few mitoses to grade IV which is anaplastic with many mitoses. Therefore, brain tumours tend to be reported as a particular histological grade rather than as benign or malignant. It is, however, important to appreciate that the histological grade can vary in different areas of the same tumour and therefore the result of one biopsy may not be representative of the whole lesion.

Tumours of neuroepithelial tissue

Astrocytic tumours

ASTROCYTOMAS: These occur most commonly as well differentiated cerebral tumours of young adults. At the time of operation the involved hemisphere is rubbery in consistency and when incised the tissue characteristically stays open whereas normal brain falls together. An exploring cannula tends to be gripped by the tumour. On cut section the tumour is ill defined and merges imperceptibly into normal brain and when both white and grey matter are invaded there is loss of the usual definition between them. Infiltration of the brain causes enlargement and distortion of the involved hemisphere and the tumour may spread from one hemisphere to the other, across the corpus callosum. Cerebellar astrocytomas tend to be cystic. Those in the brainstem characteristically cause general enlargement of the region while maintaining the basic original shape.

Histologically, although mixed cell types occur, most are predominantly of one cell type. In fibrillary astrocytomas (*see Fig.* 20.14), the tumour cells contain

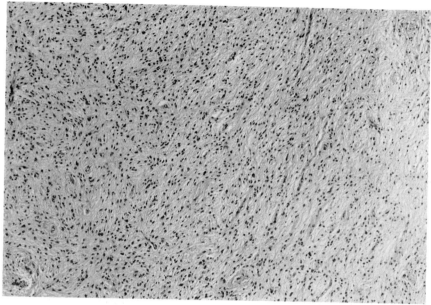

Fig. 20.14. Astrocytoma. (H and E × 30)

intracytoplasmic glial fibrils which can be demonstrated with an immuno-peroxidase technique. Gemistocytic astrocytomas are composed of plump cells with abundant eosinophilic cytoplasm. Protoplasmic astrocytomas (the rarest type) contain small darkly staining cells with very few glial fibrils. Pilocytic astrocytomas are considered as a separate variant (*see* below).

All these tumours are well differentiated and contain regularly shaped cells with few mitotic figures. They generally correspond to Kernohan's grade II.

The problem of distinction between astrocytoma and gliosis may arise at the time of brain biopsy of cerebral lesions. Gliosis in the brain occurs as a reaction to lesions such as infarction, abscess and tumour. It is characterized by a variety of cells including astrocytes, macrophages and inflammatory cells, whereas an astrocytoma contains one cell type. At the time of surgery, therefore, the finding of one cell type in a smear or on frozen section proves the diagnosis of tumour. The finding of a mixture of cells may suggest gliosis surrounding an abscess or infarction, although the possibility of an area of gliosis surrounding a tumour cannot be ruled out.

An important feature of astrocytomas is that they frequently undergo progressive loss of differentiation and eventually they may behave as glioblastomas (*see* below). In these cases the rate of growth is increased and the patient deteriorates rapidly.

PILOCYTIC ASTROCYTOMAS: These tumours are given a separate category as they are very well differentiated and have a better prognosis than other astrocytomas. They are composed of fusiform cells which have characteristically long wavy fibrillary processes which are hair-like (pilocytic). Intracytoplasmic eosinophilic club-shaped fibres (so-called Rosenthal fibres) are commonly found. Solid areas of tumours are interspaced with microcystic areas and histologically they are Kernohan grade I.

These tumours commonly occur in the optic nerve (optic nerve glioma) and as solid and cystic cerebellar astrocytomas. A well recognized sub-category is the pilocytic astrocytoma of juvenile type which occurs in children and adolescents. These classically occur in the cerebellum as a nodule of tumour in the wall of a cyst. They are well defined and can be completely resected, the prognosis being excellent after complete removal.

ANAPLASTIC ASTROCYTOMA: This is a tumour which contains areas of well differentiated astrocytoma together with anaplastic areas. It is histologically Kernohan grade III and its behaviour is between that of an astrocytoma and a glioblastoma multiforme. A small biopsy may not be sufficiently representative and can lead to an erroneous diagnosis of either astrocytoma or glioblastoma. They occur in the same sites as glioblastomas but have a better prognosis.

PROGNOSIS OF ASTROCYTOMAS: This depends on grading. Grade I tumours, most of which are cerebellar astrocytomas of childhood, have a three year survival of 66%. For grade II and III lesions the three year survival drops to about 15%. Occasional tumours are very slow growing and the patient may survive for up to 10 years.

Oligodendrogliomas

These account for about 3% of primary intracranial tumours. They occur at any age but have a slight predilection for the elderly. Characteristically they are slowly

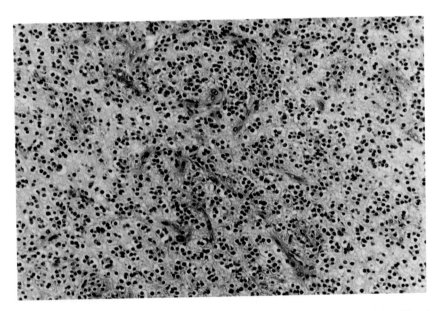

Fig. 20.15. Oligodendroglioma showing typical rounded cell nuclei and clear cytoplasm. (H and E × 180)

growing tumours of the cerebral hemispheres, although they have a tendency to undergo spontaneous haemorrhage. Typically, intracranial calcification is seen on X-ray.

Grossly, they are similar to astrocytomas, although they may be slightly better defined. There may be seeding of the immediate subarachnoid space and some are said to be of a slimy consistency.

Microscopically the cells have rounded nuclei, clear cytoplasm and distinct cell borders (see Fig. 20.15). Finely branched blood vessels are characteristic. The tumours are generally of Kernohan grade II and they behave in a similar fashion to grade II astrocytomas.

Tumours which contain oligodendroglial and astrocytic cells are classified as oligoastrocytomas. Tumours which have areas of anaplasia are termed anaplastic oligodendrogliomas, whereas totally anaplastic tumours behave as glioblastomas (see below).

Ependymal and choroid plexus tumours

EPENDYMOMAS: These tumours are more common in children (usually 8–15 years) than in adults and account for 3% of primary intracranial tumours. They arise from the ependymal cells which line the ventricles and characteristically project from the ventricular wall, especially in the fourth ventricle. In advanced cases there may be spread of tumour throughout the ventricular system and over the spinal cord. Although the lesions tend to be slow growing, blockage of the ventricular system may cause a sudden rise in intracranial pressure.

Grossly, they are red, cauliflower-like tumours. Histologically the characteristic feature is the presence of rosettes. Most ependymomas appear histologically non-aggressive, being of Kernohan grade I or II. An anaplastic aggressive subgroup with few rosettes does, however, occur.

Because it is commonly sited in the fourth ventricle, total removal is often impossible. They are relatively radiosensitive but recurrences many years later do occur.

CHOROID PLEXUS TUMOURS: These occur in the ventricular system more commonly in adults than in children. They present with raised intracranial pressure due either to obstruction of the ventricular system or possibly to oversecretion of CSF. They are rare, accounting for only 1% of intracranial tumours.

Grossly, they are papillary tumours which are attached to the ventricular wall although they do not invade the brain substance.

Histologically, the tumour is composed of papillae which are covered with cells similar to those of the normal choroid plexus (see Fig. 20.16).

An anaplastic variant, sometimes termed a choroid plexus carcinoma, does occur. It is more aggressive and invades the surrounding brain tissue.

Pineal tumours

Pineal tumours are rare. Pinealomas are tumours of pineal cells and pinealoblastomas are poorly differentiated tumours similar to medulloblastomas. Other tumours which arise in the area of the pineal include teratomas and dermoid cysts (see p. 637).

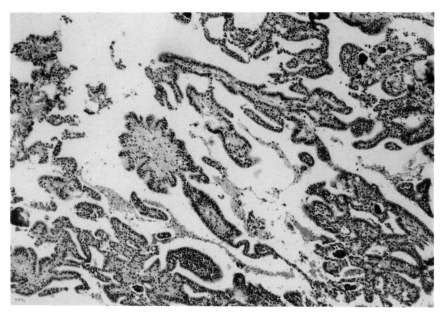

Fig. 20.16. Choroid plexus papilloma. (H and E × 30)

Neuronal tumours

Tumours of neuronal origin are very rare in the central nervous system. Gangliocytomas are composed of neoplastic ganglion cells and gangliogliomas are composed of a mixture of ganglion cells and glial cells. Neuroblastomas may occur and they are similar to those found in the adrenal gland.

Poorly differentiated and embryonal tumours

GLIOBLASTOMAS: These poorly differentiated tumours may arise *de novo* or may occur as a result of transformation in an astrocytoma or an oligodendroglioma, or rarely an ependymoma. They are the commonest primary tumours of adults, accounting for about 30% of all intracranial tumours. The majority occur in the cerebral hemispheres, especially the frontal and temporal lobes. Males are affected slightly more commonly than females.

Grossly, they have a variable appearance, hence the term glioblastoma multiforme (*see Fig.* 20.17). Haemorrhage gives the tumour a brown appearance and areas of necrosis are commonly seen.

Histologically, they are Kernohan grade IV. Poorly differentiated areas are seen together with cells resembling astrocytes and oligodendrocytes. Two characteristic histological features are necrotic areas with surrounding palisading of cells (*see Fig.* 20.18) and vascular endothelial proliferation. Treatment is palliative and the three year survival rate is only about 4%.

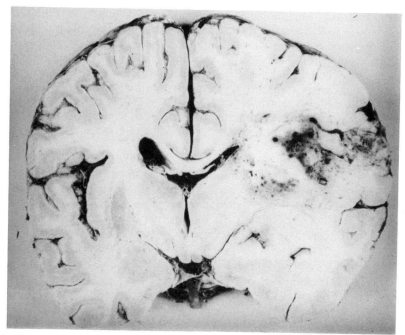

Fig. 20.17. Glioblastoma multiforme.

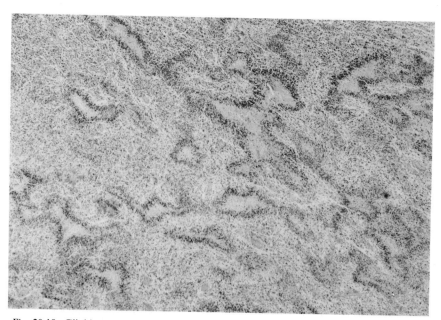

Fig. 20.18. Glioblastoma multiforme. The areas of necrosis with surrounding palisading are characteristic. (H and E × 30)

MEDULLOBLASTOMAS: Medulloblastomas occur predominantly in children and adolescents (age 6–10 years). They are more common in boys than girls. About one-third of intracranial tumours in childhood are medulloblastomas, although figures vary from series to series. They are highly malignant tumours which arise most commonly in the midline of the cerebellum. Clinically they present with ataxia, brainstem signs and morning vomiting. Hydrocephalus may result from obstruction of the fourth ventricle outlet.

Grossly, they are infiltrating tumours which form a soft purple mass. They have a tendency to seed rapidly throughout the subarachnoid space, making complete removal impossible.

Histologically they are highly cellular (*see Fig.* 20.19). The individual cells have darkly staining nuclei, scanty cytoplasm and tend to form sheets and pseudo-rosettes. Distant metastases occasionally occur to bones and lymph nodes. At operation as much tumour as possible is removed and radiation is then given to cover the entire CNS and spinal cord because of the seeding propensity. With surgery and radiotherapy, 25–40% are alive at 5 years.

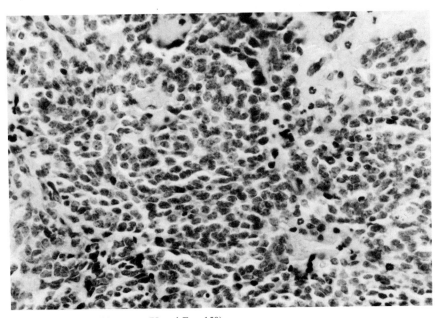

Fig. 20.19. Medulloblastoma. (H and E × 150)

Tumours of nerve sheath origin

Schwannomas

The cranial nerves, being peripheral nerves, are subject to peripheral nerve tumours, the most common of which is the schwannoma (also called neuri-lemmoma or neuroma). These are tumours of Schwann cells, which are the myelin producing cells of the nerve sheath, and are most common on the sensory cranial nerves, especially the vestibular division of the VIIIth (acoustic neuromas).

Patients with von Recklinghausen's disease tend to develop bilateral acoustic neuromas, frequently at a young age. Females are affected more often than males. Overall, schwannomas account for 10% of primary intracranial tumours.

The classical clinical presentation of acoustic neuroma is deafness, tinnitus and enlargement of the internal auditory meatus as seen on tomography of the temporal bone.

Grossly, the tumours are encapsulated and firm. The cut surface is lobulated and fleshy pink or yellow in appearance. Histologically, the tumour is diagnosed by the presence of Antoni A areas (cellular areas in which the nuclei are often arranged in parallel bundles) and Antoni B areas (hypocellular loosely packed areas).

Schwannomas are extremely slow growing. Using microsurgical techniques, total removal, frequently avoiding facial nerve palsy, is now possible. Malignancy may rarely develop.

Neurofibromas

Neurofibromas are tumours of Schwann cells together with other cellular elements. In contrast to schwannomas, they are more often multiple and more often malignant. Neurofibromas are rare intracranial tumours and, when they do occur, they are usually associated with von Recklinghausen's neurofibromatosis (*see* p. 641).

Tumours of meningeal and related structures

Meningiomas

These are relatively common accounting for about 15% of all primary intracranial tumours. Although seen in all age groups, they have a predilection for elderly females. Some cases occur in association with von Recklinghausen's disease.

Clinically, they present as a slowly growing space occupying lesion. A typical feature is the presence of thickening of the adjacent skull bone which may be either internal (endostosis) or external (exostosis). The vascular nature of the lesion is seen on angiography.

Meningiomas arise from the arachnoid. Most (90%) are supratentorial. Parasagittal lesions (25%) are related to the sagittal sinus; 20% occur on the convexity of the hemispheres; 20% arise from the sphenoidal wing and grow into both the anterior and middle cranial fossas; 10% occur in the olfactory groove and may involve the optic nerve producing the Foster Kennedy syndrome (ipsilateral optic atrophy with contralateral papilloedema); 10% are suprasellar arising from the tuberculum sellae and these may compress the optic chiasma. Other sites include the basilar groove, cerebello–pontine angle and tentorium. Occasionally, intraventricular meningiomas occur and they may also rarely occur in the cerebral substance, probably arising from perivascular mesenchyme. Multiple meningiomas are found in 10–15% of cases.

Grossly, they are encapsulated, firm, pink tumours which have a bosselated external appearance. They compress rather than invade the surrounding brain.

Histologically, several sub-types are recognized. Meningioendotheliomatous meningiomas are composed of uniform cells, the cytoplasm of which appears to form a syncytium. In fibrous meningiomas, the cells are similar to fibroblasts and form prominent whorls (*see Fig.* 20.20). Psammomatous meningiomas contain small spherical calcified bodies known as psammoma bodies. Some show a very prominent vascular pattern and are termed angiomatous meningiomas. Rarely, the pattern is identical to that of a haemangiopericytoma. Aggressive forms of meningioma do occur in which case anaplastic areas are seen, the so-called anaplastic meningioma. Those which resemble sarcomas are termed meningeal sarcomas.

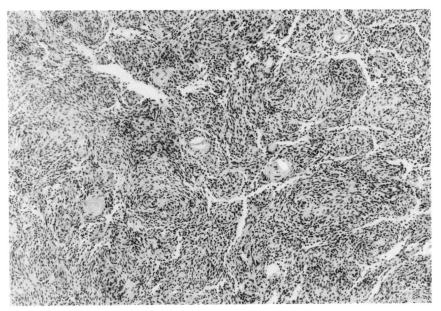

Fig. 20.20. Meningioma, fibrous type with whorls. (H and E × 30)

The tumour may invade the Haversian canals and veins of bone and this acts as a focus for later recurrence. The tumour may spread through bone to lie as a mushroom under the scalp. Occasionally they spread over the surface of the brain in which case they are termed meningioma *en-plaque*.

Although considered benign because of slow growth and absence of mitotic figures, their vascularity and frequent inaccessible site makes surgery difficult. Prognosis is good if the tumour can be totally removed but about 20% recur within five years (probably due to inadequate initial removal). Incomplete removal of the tumour may still be compatible with prolonged survival but if there is a sarcomatous component prognosis is worse.

Primary malignant lymphomas

Less than 1% of primary intracranial tumours are lymphomas and they usually present in adults. Morphologically, it may be impossible to distinguish between primary lymphoma and central nervous system invasion by lymphomas arising elsewhere. They have a predilection to affect the deeper subependymal parts of the brain and may either infiltrate the brain diffusely or else less commonly they form a discrete mass which can be identified on CT scan.

Histologically, the infiltrate is perivascular and tends to form concentric rings around blood vessels giving a pseudo-inflammatory appearance.

Tumours of blood vessel origin

Haemangioblastomas

These tumours occur in the cerebellum of patients aged usually 30–50 years, more commonly in men than women. They run a relatively benign course. Some examples are found outside the cerebellum, for example in the fourth ventricle and spinal cord. Clinically, they present with cerebellar signs and raised intracranial pressure. Some cases occur as part of the von Hippel–Lindau syndrome which also includes renal cell carcinoma and phaeochromocytoma. Some cases are associated with polycythaemia.

On gross examination the typical finding is a tumour nodule growing in the wall of a cyst which contains clear yellow fluid, although some are totally solid. The tumour tends to be yellow on cut section. Histologically, the typical feature is the presence of numerous vascular channels which are lined by plump endothelial cells and surrounded by lipid-laden, vacuolated stromal cells (*see Fig.* 20.21). Distinction from a metastatic renal cell carcinoma may be difficult although the latter has a more aggressive appearance with mitotic figures and necrosis.

If the lesion is cystic, only the tumour nodule needs to be removed. The solid types are vascular and if they rupture during removal, recurrence occurs in about 20%. The prognosis for cystic tumours is excellent.

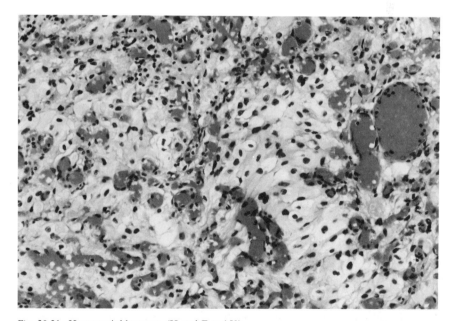

Fig. 20.21. Haemangioblastoma. (H and E × 150)

Germ cell tumours

Tumours of germ cell origin occur in the vicinity of the pineal and are the most common tumours in that region. Teratomas occur in young males. Germinomas are identical to testicular seminomas and ovarian dysgerminomas. Choriocarcinomas and yolk sac tumours have also been described.

Other malformative tumours and tumour-like conditions

Craniopharyngiomas

These tumours are seen both in children and adults. They arise from the squamous epithelium which is a vestigial remnant of Rathke's pouch and are most commonly suprasellar although they occasionally arise within the sella itself. Presentation is a space occupying lesion or as endocrine dysfunction due to pituitary or hypothalamic damage. Visual disturbance is caused by pressure on the optic chiasma. Calcification is seen in 75% of cases on X-ray.

Grossly, most (90%) craniopharyngiomas are cystic (*see Fig.* 20.22) and filled with a dark fluid which characteristically contains cholesterol crystals. These can be appreciated by polarized light and are useful diagnostically when cyst fluid is sent for intra-operative analysis. The cyst lining is commonly of squamous epithelium and the solid areas of the tumour consist of squamous and columnar epithelium embedded in a fibrous stroma.

Craniopharyngiomas are very slow growing. Radical removal should be attempted but the tumour may be adherent to the anterior cerebral arteries. Radiotherapy is also of benefit.

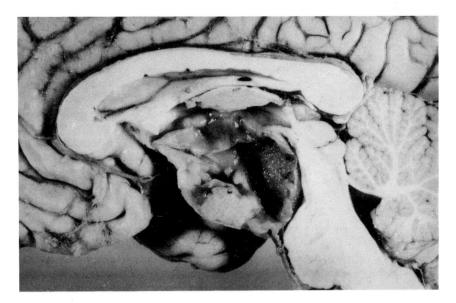

Fig. 20.22. Craniopharyngioma.

Dermoid cysts

These are benign cysts found most commonly in the pineal region. They are due to defective ectodermal closure. Histologically, the lining is of squamous epithelium and the walls contain skin appendages. Posterior fossa dermoids are midline and may have a sinus to the occipital region with the consequent risk of meningitis and brain abscess.

Colloid cysts (see Fig. 20.23)

These benign cysts occur in the third ventricle in the region of the foramina of Monro where they may cause an acute hydrocephalus and sometimes sudden death. They are thin-walled cysts containing proteinaceous fluid and are lined by cuboidal cells which resemble ependymal cells.

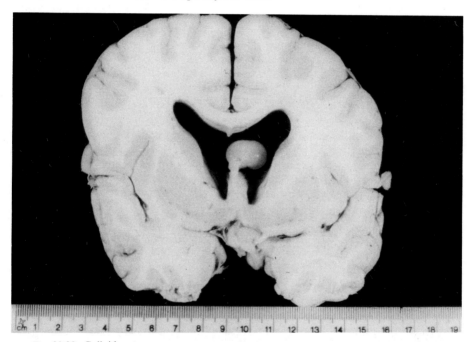

Fig. 20.23. Colloid cyst.

Vascular malformations

Capillary telangiectases are often incidental findings, although occasionally they may cause focal neurological signs and haemorrhage. Small blood vessels can be seen grossly on sections of brain and on microscopic examination the vessels are surrounded by normal brain tissue.

Cavernous angiomas are more likely to cause symptoms such as focal signs, epilepsy and subarachnoid haemorrhage. They are seen grossly as a tangled mass of blood vessels in the cerebral hemisphere and less commonly in the cerebellum or spinal cord. Histologically, the important feature is that the vessels are not separated by normal brain.

Arteriovenous malformations are composed of a mixture of arteries and veins. They most commonly present in teenagers with neurological signs, epilepsy, subarachnoid or cerebral haemorrhage or headaches. The most common site is the supratentorial region, either in the meninges or in the cerebral substance. Pathologically, the tangle of arteries and veins is usually surrounded by an area of gliosis in which there is evidence of previous haemorrhages of different ages. When the lesions bleed they usually leave little neurological deficit, and subarachnoid haemorrhage due to an arteriovenous malformation carries a considerably better prognosis than that due to a ruptured berry aneurysm. CT scanning and angiography make the diagnosis, although a similar rapid circulation may also be seen in glioblastomas.

Excision is the treatment of choice and ligation of feeding vessels is less desirable. Embolization techniques may make the lesion smaller and permit surgery to be performed.

The Sturge–Weber syndrome consists of capillary angioma malformations of the brain surface with calcification of the underlying brain and haemangiomas in the skin of the ipsilateral side of the face.

Tumours of the Anterior Pituitary

Pituitary adenomas (*see Fig.* 20.24)

The majority of pituitary adenomas occur in adults and they may be either hormone secreting (about 75%) or non-hormone secreting (about 25%). Hormone secreting tumours usually present with symptoms referable to the production of a single hormone (for example, acromegaly or Cushing's disease), or rarely two

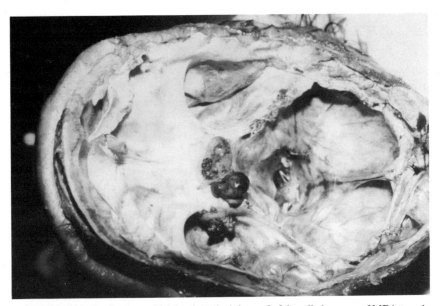

Fig. 20.24. Pituitary adenoma which has breached the roof of the sella in a case of MEA type 1. (Same patient as *Fig.* 8.9.)

hormones. Non-hormone secreting tumours are more likely to present as space occupying lesions or as panhypopituitarism. It is now realized that many adenomas which were originally thought to be hormonally inactive do in fact secrete prolactin and are responsible for some cases of infertility.

GROWTH HORMONE SECRETION: This is responsible for gigantism in prepubertal children and acromegaly in adults. In acromegaly there is characteristically enlargement of the hands, feet and jaws, together with metabolic abnormalities which lead to diabetes mellitus, osteoporosis and hypertension.

PROLACTIN SECRETION: Affected females often present in infertility clinics with amenorrhoea and galactorrhoea. In males, the condition can be clinically silent or it may cause infertility and decreased libido.

ACTH SECRETION: This is the cause of Cushing's disease (see p. 480).

OTHER HORMONES: Adenomas producing thyroid stimulating hormone, luteinizing hormone and follicle stimulating hormone are exceedingly rare.

PRESSURE EFFECTS: Non-secreting adenomas tend to produce symptoms at a late stage when they are large. Symptoms may be caused by compression of the optic chiasma or hypothalamus. Progressive destruction of the remainder of the pituitary eventually causes a panhypopituitarism.

Grossly, adenomas which are 10 mm in diameter or less are termed microadenomas; larger adenomas may be up to 10 cm in diameter. Pituitary adenomas are poorly encapsulated and although benign, they can erode surrounding structures, thus causing the characteristic enlargement of the sella turcica and erosion of the clinoid processes as seen on skull X-ray. On cut section, they are soft and show areas of haemorrhage and infarction; about 40% are cystic.

Histologically, the pattern of normal pituitary is lost and replaced by tumour cells growing in sheets or nests or in various patterns, including pseudoglandular and papillary. The cells are usually regular and very similar to normal anterior pituitary cells although in some lesions considerable cellular pleomorphism is seen.

There is some correlation between hormone secretion and cell type. Acidophilic adenomas tend to produce growth hormone and/or prolactin; basophil adenomas tend to produce ACTH; chromophobe adenomas which show no staining characteristics with haematoxylin and eosin tend to be non-hormone producing. More recently, pituitary adenomas have been characterized by immunohistochemistry in which the stains used are labelled with antibodies to individual hormones. Using this technique, a close correlation is found between hormone secretion and the histochemical type of adenoma. Electron microscopy is also helpful in demonstrating the different type of hormone containing granules within the tumour cells.

Most pituitary tumours are treated by surgery via the trans-sphenoidal route using the operating microscope. In cases of microadenoma, selective removal with preservation of normal pituitary function can be undertaken.

Most tumours are radiosensitive and some centres treat chromophobe adenomas solely by this method. Others use radiation if there has been incomplete removal or if the patient is unfit for surgery. Some centres use bromocriptine as the treatment of choice for prolactin-secreting adenomas but it probably does not cure the lesion and selective removal may be better.

Pituitary carcinomas

Carcinoma of the anterior pituitary is very rare. Invasion of local structures and anaplasia can both be seen in pituitary adenomas and therefore the only reliable criterion of malignancy for pituitary tumours is the presence of metastases.

Metastatic Tumours in the CNS

These are blood-borne either via the arterial supply or via the vertebral veins which are valveless and therefore allow retrograde flow.

The commonest source is bronchogenic carcinoma, followed by breast carcinoma and renal cell carcinoma. The deposits are usually discrete and occur in the cerebral hemispheres, frequently in the distribution of the middle cerebral artery or in the cerebellar hemispheres. Dural deposits may also occur.

Grossly, they are sharply circumscribed tumour masses with characteristic surrounding oedema. Central necrosis is common and surgical aspiration in these cases reveals pus-like material.

Deposits in the ventricular ependyma or choroid plexus are likely to give rise to CSF dissemination and carcinomatosis of the meninges. This may give rise to a low grade meningitis with cranial nerve palsies.

Angiography of a cerebral secondary deposit shows a circumferential halo of vessels with an avascular centre if there is necrosis. Removal of solitary secondaries often gives useful palliation. Steroids are useful to decrease cerebral oedema but chemotherapy and radiotherapy have little to offer.

Spinal Tumours

Spinal tumours may be classified according to their relationship with the dura and spinal cord.

Extradural tumours arise in the space between the dura and the vertebral column. Unlike the cranial cavity, the dura within the vertebral column is not firmly attached to bone and this results in a connective tissue filled extradural space. This may be the site of secondary tumours (either carcinoma or lymphoma) or, rarely, neurofibromas or meningiomas.

Intradural tumours may be either within the spinal cord (intramedullary) or outside the spinal cord (extramedullary).

The main intramedullary intradural tumours are ependymomas, astrocytomas and angiomas, all of which cause localized enlargement of the cord.

Extramedullary intradural tumours include meningiomas (the commonest) and schwannomas. Schwannomas arise in the posterior roots of the spinal nerves and typically spread through the adjacent intervertebral foramen to produce a dumb-bell shaped lesion.

Primary and secondary tumours of the vertebrae, especially when complicated by a pathological fracture, may also affect the spinal cord.

Clinically the symptoms of spinal tumours are related to the spinal cord (due either to direct pressure or to interference with the vascular supply) or to the spinal nerve roots. Spinal cord symptoms include spastic weakness below the lesion, followed by sensory loss and finally sphincter disturbances. Sphincter disturbances occur early in lesions of the conus medullaris. Involvement of anterior nerve roots causes a lower motor neurone type of weakness, whereas involvement of the posterior root causes pain in the relevant distribution.

Diagnosis is aided by myelography and CT scan.

Compression of the spinal cord may be relieved by laminectomy with or without removal of the tumour. Benign tumours may be completely removed and removal of the bulk of a metastatic deposit may be useful. Acute compression of the cord is a surgical emergency and complete sensory and motor loss of greater than half an hour's duration is often permanent.

Often little can be done for intramedullary tumours, except when they are cystic in which case release via an incision in the posterior median raphe may improve symptoms.

Tumours of Peripheral Nerves

Schwannomas

These are tumours of Schwann cells which occur on peripheral nerves throughout the body. The most important site is on the VIIIth cranial nerve; the pathology is discussed on p. 632.

Neurofibromas

Neurofibromas consist of a mixture of Schwann cells together with other cell types. They are found in the skin, related to deep nerves and at other sites.

Grossly, in the skin they appear as soft nodules. When related to deep nerves they may form large irregular plexiform masses within which the nerve appears to become entangled.

Histologically, the tumour consists of a mass of fibroblasts, Schwann cells and other cells together with nerve fibres which cross the lesion. They may occasionally undergo malignant change.

In some cases, neurofibromas are associated with von Recklinghausen's disease (neurofibromatosis). This is inherited as an autosomal dominant disorder with variable penetration. These patients develop areas of skin pigmentation (*café-au-lait* spots) and cutaneous neurofibromas which may be very large and undergo sarcomatous change. A widespread area of cutaneous involvement gives rise to elephantiasis nervosa. The patient may also have central nervous system malformations including stenosis of the aqueduct of Sylvius. They are also liable to develop neural tumours, including acoustic neuromas, meningiomas and gliomas.

References

Beyerl B., Black P. McL. (1984) Posttraumatic hydrocephalus. *Neurosurgery* **15**, 257–61.
Di Rocco C., Di Trapani G., Maira G., Bentivoglio M., Macchi G., Rossi G. F. (1977) Anatomoclinical correlations in normotensive hydrocephalus. Reports on three cases. *J. Neurol. Sci.* **33**, 437–52.

Fishman R. A. (1975) Brain edema. *N. Engl. J. Med.* **293**, 706–11.

Gentleman D., Jennett B. (1981) Hazards of inter-hospital transfer of comatose head-injured patients. *Lancet* **2**, 853–5.

Gordon D. S. (1975) Missile wounds of the head and spine. *Br. Med. J.* **1**, 614–16.

Kernohan J. W., Mabon R. F., Svien H. J., Adson A. W. (1949) Symposium on new and simplified concept of gliomas; simplified classification of gliomas. *Proc. Staff Meet. Mayo Clin.* **24**, 71–5.

Kistler J. P., Ropper A. H., Heros R. C. (1984) Therapy of ischemic cerebral vascular disease due to atherothrombosis (Part 1). *N. Engl. J. Med.* **311**, 27–34.

Kistler J. P., Ropper A. H., Heros, R. C. (1984) Therapy of ischemic cerebral vascular disease due to atherothrombosis (Part 2). *N. Engl. J. Med.* **311**, 100–5.

Loftus C. M., Quest D. O. (1983) Current status of carotid endarterectomy for atheromatous disease. *Neurosurgery* **13**, 718–23.

Mendelow A. D., Teasdale G. M. (1983) Pathophysiology of head injuries. *Br. J. Surg.* **70**, 641–50.

Miller J. D., Becker D. P. (1982) Secondary insults to the injured brain *J. R. Col. Surg. Edinb.* **27**, 292–8.

Modan B., Baidatz D., Mart H., Steinitz R., Levin S. G. (1974) Radiation-induced head and neck tumours. *Lancet* **1**, 277–9.

Oppenheimer D. R. (1968) Microscopic lesions in the brain following head injury. *J. Neurol. Neurosurg. Psychiat.* **31**, 299–306.

Seddon H. J. (1943) Three types of nerve injury *Brain* **66**, 237–88.

Strich S. J. (1956) Diffuse degeneration of the cerebral white matter in severe dementia following head injury. *J. Neurol. Neurosurg. Psychiat.* **19**, 163–85.

Strong A. J., Ingham H. R. (1983) Brain abscess. *Br. J. Hosp. Med.* **30**, 396–403.

Teasdale G., Jennett B. (1974) Assessment of coma and impaired consciousness. A practical scale. *Lancet* **2**, 81–4.

Williams B. (1981) Chronic herniation of the hindbrain. *Ann. R. Coll. Surg. Engl.* **63**, 9–17.

Chapter 21

Renal Transplantation

Claire M. Hill

Introduction

Transplantation is now an established method of treatment for end stage renal failure. The results are comparable to those of long-term dialysis but the quality of life is infinitely better.

The arrival of renal transplantation as a clinical reality was due to several factors. The pioneer work of Ullman (1902) and Carrel and Guthrie (1905) showed that the operation was technically feasible and that the kidney could recover from the trauma of harvesting and re-implantation. The basic immunology of transplantation was studied by Medawar using skin grafts in rabbits (Medawar 1944). Further information which led to tissue typing as a means of matching was gained from experiments on tumour transplantation between animals of different strains and species (Bittner 1935; Snell 1948). Early methods of immunosuppression such as total body irradiation and thoracic duct ligation proved too toxic. The introduction of combined therapy with corticosteroid and azathioprine proved an important milestone in permitting transplantation between non-related individuals (Murray *et al.* 1963). Rejection could be controlled by this means whilst the patient retained the ability to combat infections, which had been a major cause of death in early transplantation attempts. A more recent advance was the recognition of cyclosporin A (Cy A) as a potent immunosuppressive agent (Borel 1976). This drug is useful in all types of organ transplantation. However, it is nephrotoxic and the distinction between nephrotoxicity and rejection of a renal transplant may be difficult. It has also been suggested that Cy A can lead to progressive fibrosis of the renal interstitium (Myers *et al.* 1984). The drug has not been in use sufficiently long for this problem to be evaluated in the clinical situation.

Pre-transplant blood transfusion has been shown clinically and experimentally to have a definite beneficial effect on graft survival. The mechanism is not clear though it is probably a form of immunological enhancement. The transfusion has usually been from random donors who may or may not share antigens with the eventual organ donor. A deliberate policy of transfusing all patients awaiting kidney transplant has greatly improved the results from many centres (Morris 1984).

Selection of Recipients

Patients requiring a renal transplant are in end stage renal failure, most commonly as a result of glomerulonephritis. Other main causes are polycystic kidneys, pyelonephritis/reflux nephropathy, megacystis megaureter, hypertension and diabetes mellitus. In some parts of the world analgesic nephropathy is a major aetiological factor. Other less frequently observed diseases are renal dysplasia and metabolic conditions such as cystinosis. Some patients undergo pre-transplant bilateral nephrectomy. The main indications for this procedure are dialysis-resistant hypertension and large polycystic kidneys, if they are liable to interfere mechanically with the transplant operation or if they are the site of persistent infection. In some centres bilateral nephro-ureterectomy is performed if there are large refluxing ureters. When resources were even more limited than they are today the presence of atherosclerotic vascular disease, particularly of the coronary arteries, was an important contraindication. This no longer holds true as such patients may have coronary artery bypass before their kidney transplant. Important contraindications are malignant disease or a recent history of tuberculosis.

Whilst the presence of a potentially functioning urinary bladder was previously considered of vital importance, many patients have now been transplanted into an ileal bladder, usually constructed in advance.

Nomenclature

Most kidney transplants are 'allografts', that is the donor and recipient are not immunologically identical. In the rare circumstance where the donor is the recipient's identical twin the transplanted organ is an 'isograft'. Transplants from donors of other species are 'xenografts'. Kidney transplants are anastomosed into the iliac fossa (heterotopic site). In contrast, liver and heart transplants are usually placed in the site vacated after removal of the diseased organ at the time of transplantation (orthotopic site).

Matching

The commonest type of kidney transplant in the UK is from an unrelated cadaver donor, with a smaller number from living related donors. In some parts of the world live donors are the main source of kidneys. Each potential recipient is blood grouped and tissue typed. Matching for the major ABO (but not Rhesus) antigens was shown early on to be essential for graft survival (Starzl 1964). The role of tissue typing is less clear. The antigens concerned in man belong to a system of human leucocyte antigens (HLA) situated on the 6th chromosome. Initially the A and B antigens of the HLA system were thought to be important but more recently those related to the D locus (DR antigens) have been shown to play a major role in graft rejection. For tissue typing a sample of whole blood is required in order to provide leucocytes and serum for analysis. The most generally used system of tissue typing is the Teraski microlymphocytotoxicity method (Teraski and McClelland 1964). Potential recipients are tissue typed and tested for cytotoxic antibody to HLA antigens as they enter a transplant programme. In the UK the National Organ Matching Service stores these results on computer. This allows organ sharing between the participating centres in this country, and occasionally Europe where similar data banks exist.

Donors

Cadaver transplant donors are brain-dead individuals with normal kidneys. In practical terms they fall into two groups, traumatic and non-traumatic. The trauma cases have severe head injuries, often from road traffic accidents, without involvement of abdominal viscera. Non-trauma donors generally have suffered a major intracerebral catastrophe such as cerebral haemorrhage or have an untreatable primary brain tumour. Extracranial malignancy, infection or any generalized disease which might involve the kidneys are contraindications to organ donation. The criteria for establishing brain death are laid down in detail in a Working Party Report (Health Departments of Great Britain and Northern Ireland 1983).

As far as possible a history of donor disease is sought and potential donors are examined carefully for abnormalities other than the main cause of brain death. Undetected tumours, either primary or secondary, transplanted with a kidney have led to recipient death in a number of cases (Penn 1978; Forbes *et al.* 1981).

Harvesting and Perfusion of Donor Kidneys

This critical part of the procedure is usually undertaken by a specially trained surgical team. Donors who have died as a result of trauma will require a coroner's autopsy. It is therefore necessary for the harvesting surgeon to record his findings in the hospital chart. If there is evidence of injury to the kidneys then they are not used for transplantation. Kidneys which are scarred or have a complex blood supply are less suitable though in some cases aortic or venous patches can be used to make transplantation possible.

It is necessary to flush out the donor blood, particularly the leucocytes, and hold the kidney in a satisfactory state of electrolyte balance until it is re-anastomosed and has a blood supply. Several perfusion fluids have been tried, but those commonly used are Collins' and hypertonic citrate solutions introduced through an arterial cannula. Immediately after perfusion the kidney is placed in a sealed sterile polythene bag and placed inside a bag of ice for transportation. Machine perfusion is used extensively in the USA but is not in widespread clinical use in Europe. It may cause endothelial damage and changes which are histologically similar to hyperacute rejection (Hill *et al.* 1976).

Table 21.1 Definition of ischaemic times

	Begins	Ends
Anoxia	Respiratory arrest	Cardiac arrest
Initial warm ischaemia	Cardiac arrest	Kidney cooled in ice
Cold ischaemia	Kidney cooled	Kidney removed from ice
Operative ischaemia (warm)	Kidney removed from ice	Vascular clamps released
Total ischaemia	Cardiac arrest	Circulation re-established

The ischaemic times (*Table* 21.1) are carefully recorded in each case. They should be as short as possible, but the two periods of warm ischaemia are the most critical. The kidney is transplanted into the recipient's iliac fossa, most often on the contralateral side. The renal artery and vein are anastomosed to the iliac vessels and ureter to the bladder. (The surgical details are beyond the scope of this book).

Renal Transplant Biopsies

Due to its extraperitoneal location in the iliac fossa it should be relatively easy to obtain biopsy samples from a transplanted kidney percutaneously using a Tru-cut or other similar needle. In practical terms the kidney is often surrounded by fibrous tissue, particularly if there has been a capsulotomy or a haematoma, making the biopsy procedure more difficult in these cases.

The biopsy is carried out under local anaesthesia with the patient supine. Ideally the core of renal tissue is composed of cortex and medulla, permitting analysis of the cortico-medullary blood vessels which are a prime target for the rejection process.

A renal transplant biopsy should include samples for light and electron microscopy as well as immunohistology, and at least two cores should be taken. For optimum results the tissue is fixed immediately in freshly prepared solutions. The details of these vary according to local policy. This should be discussed in advance with the pathologist who will also arrange snap freezing of samples for immunohistology at the time of biopsy. The results of immunofluorescence are available within two hours and a rough assessment of the state of the kidney can be made from examination of a frozen section by light microscopy. It is unwise, however, to read too much into such a frozen section, particularly as to the nature and severity of a cellular infiltrate. It is better to wait for the definitive paraffin sections unless the pathology is very florid, such as in a necrotic kidney. The changes in a transplant may be rather focal so that biopsies should be from several areas. This can be achieved to some extent by altering the angle of the needle after the first biopsy core has been taken.

In the early years of clinical renal transplantation biopsies were taken electively at pre-specified times. This practice led to the rapid accumulation of knowledge regarding the histological appearances of a transplanted kidney with stable as well as unstable function. This elective biopsy policy has largely been abandoned except in centres evaluating new forms of treatment.

If there is reason to suspect the existence of pathology within the kidney when it is perfused with blood, after completion of the anastomoses, a 'closure-biopsy' is taken. This can give valuable information as to the existence of renal scarring and arteriolosclerosis in the donor kidney, but is of little prognostic value with regard to tubular necrosis or subsequent rejection, with the exception of hyperacute rejection. In practice, transplant biopsies are taken to establish whether or not rejection is present and this is most common during the first month. Biopsy is also useful in the differential diagnosis of late transplant dysfunction, even after several years.

Fine Needle Cytology

The technique of fine needle aspiration cytology was first applied to renal transplants by Häyry and von Willebrand in Finland and has since been investigated by several groups in other countries. Cells from the kidney are aspirated through a fine needle. A smear is prepared for cytopathological assessment and part of the sample is stained with a range of monoclonal antibodies to lymphocyte subsets. Because the procedure is less damaging to the kidney than a biopsy, it can be repeated regularly and daily samples taken if necessary (von Willebrand 1980;

Häyry and von Willebrand 1981). Some workers consider that this technique can now replace biopsy in the differential diagnosis of rejection. Others are more sceptical (Morris 1984). Since the results of the monoclonal antibody studies from several centres vary, it would seem prudent to investigate functional instability by biopsy in addition to aspiration cytology until the results of the technique have been evaluated more fully.

The Pathology of Renal Allograft Rejection

Rejection is still the major cause of graft loss. The rejection process has two main immunological components—cellular and antibody mediated. These commonly occur together but their relative importance depends on the timing of the episode which can be classified as follows:

1. *Hyperacute rejection*: This occurs within minutes of completion of the anastomoses.
2. *Acute rejection*:
   i. *Cellular*—May occur during the first days or weeks, but may happen at any subsequent time.
   ii. *Humoral or vascular*—May occur from the second week onwards. Occasionally seen in an accelerated form during the first week.
3. *Chronic rejection*: This occurs after the first few weeks.

Hyperacute rejection

This is caused by preformed circulating antibody to antigens present in the transplant. It can largely be prevented by matching for blood group and by direct cross matching of recipient serum and donor cells. It is seen most floridly in xenografts but is now rare in human allografts.

Hyperacute rejection is recognized before completion of the transplant operation. The kidney perfuses with recipient blood and then becomes cyanotic and flaccid. The reaction is irreversible. The pathological findings depend on the time of nephrectomy. Initially, the glomeruli are stuffed with polymorphs and fibrin. There is rapid progression to thrombosis within glomeruli and in intra- and extrarenal blood vessels. If the kidney is left *in situ* it undergoes extensive infarction.

Acute rejection

Many transplants have at least one rejection episode and the majority of these occur during the first few weeks whilst the patient is still in hospital. The classical clinical features of acute rejection are fever, graft swelling and tenderness, fall in urinary output and reduction in renal function. These signs may be modified by the immunosuppressive therapy. Investigations such as isotope renography and ultrasound scan of the kidney give useful clinical information prior to biopsy.

i. *Cellular rejection*

Histological examination reveals kidney in which the tubules are pushed apart by a combination of oedema and an infiltrate of mononuclear cells (*see Fig.* 21.1).

Polymorphs in a transplanted kidney (other than in hyperacute rejection) signify either infection or necrosis. The cellular infiltrate is present diffusely throughout the interstitium or is aggregated around glomeruli or blood vessels. It has a particular affinity for peritubular capillaries which in the untreated case become ruptured. The infiltrating cells have been shown to be of donor origin. They are generally recognized as lymphocytes in various stages of transformation to immunoblasts (*see* p. 431). More recently macrophages, particularly dendritic cells, have been recognized as an important constituent of the cellular infiltrate. Experimental studies suggest that the interaction between antigen presenting cells, which in man are dendritic cells and vascular endothelium, and helper T-cells is the basis of the whole rejection process (Mason 1983). The histological appearances are in keeping with a cell-mediated immune reaction which can be transferred experimentally by lymphocytes but not by serum. The reaction is reversible by increased corticosteroid therapy unless a vascular component is present.

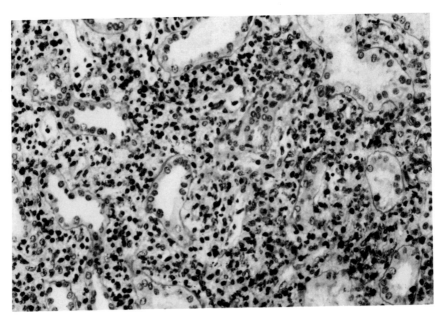

Fig. 21.1. Renal tubules separated by a dense mononuclear cell infiltrate in the interstitium. (PAS × 180)

ii. *Humoral or vascular rejection*

This process is thought to be mediated by antibody to donor antigens although, unlike hyperacute rejection, the antibody has developed after transplantation. Histologically, there is usually some evidence of cellular rejection but the main lesion is in the blood vessels, particularly interlobular and arcuate arteries. These show marked intimal oedema with frank necrosis in severe cases, associated with disruption of the elastic tissue. Infiltrating mononuclear cells may be seen in the wall of an affected vessel. One characteristic early change is in the endothelium which becomes swollen. The individual cells are very prominent and the lumen is narrowed. Arterioles are involved in this way and as the rejection episode continues they become necrotic (*see Fig.* 21.2). The necrosis also extends into adjacent glomeruli. At this stage the damage seems to be irreversible. As well as the intrarenal arterial branches, the main renal artery is rejected and the process stops abruptly at the anastomosis to the recipient iliac artery. The pathology in the artery wall is similar to that found within the kidney. The kidney becomes ischaemic and the changes on renography or histology resemble those caused by renal artery stenosis from any cause. Studies of transplant biopsy material have identified other bad prognostic features. In particular, interstitial haemorrhage and microinfarcts correlate with a poor outcome.

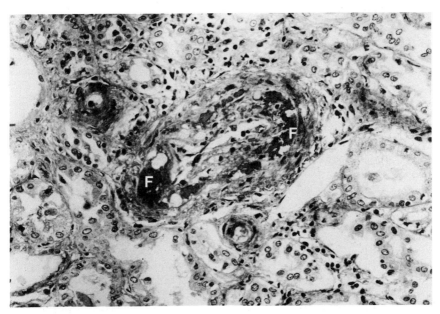

Fig. 21.2. In this acutely rejecting kidney there is accumulation of fibrin (F) in arteriolar walls. (MSB × 180)

Acute rejection causes a greatly enlarged oedematous kidney. When vascular changes are present the surface is mottled and 'flea-bitten' due to small foci of arteriolar or glomerular necrosis. On section the parenchyma is deeply congested and small infarcts may be visible on naked eye examination. The main renal vessels are sometimes thrombosed and histological examination should distinguish whether or not this is secondary to rejection or has occurred for mechanical or haemodynamic reasons.

Prompt anti-rejection treatment with additional corticosteroid either orally or as pulses of methylprednisolone arrests a rejection episode unless irreversible changes are present. The addition of plasma exchange to attempt to remove antibody may be useful. However, the healing process in blood vessels leads to further narrowing (*see Fig.* 21.3) with progressive ischaemic fibrosis and tubular atrophy in the parenchyma supplied by them.

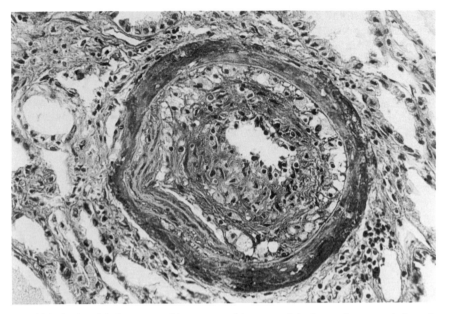

Fig. 21.3. An interlobular artery with a narrowed lumen, mainly due to the accumulation of pale foam cells in the wall. Acute rejection had been unsuccessfully treated and the section is from the nephrectomy specimen. (MSB × 180)

Chronic Rejection

The hallmark of so-called chronic rejection is severe fibrous thickening of small arteries and arterioles which develop an onion-skinned appearance. This lesion can be seen as early as a few weeks after transplantation as was described by Porter *et al.* (1963). The glomeruli become ischaemic with retracted tufts and wrinkled basement membranes. In addition other glomeruli contain increased mesangial matrix. The peripheral capillary loops have thick basement membranes with a wide subendothelial rarified zone, possibly due to fibrin deposition. Subendothelial deposits usually containing IgM are also seen. These glomeruli tend to be lobulated and in many respects similar to membranoproliferative glomerulo-nephritis on light microscopy. Using immunohistology and electron microscopy the distinction from recurrent disease is usually possible. In chronic rejection the tubules become atrophic and the extent of tubulo-interstitial scarring correlates with the severity of functional impairment. At this stage there may be little evidence of cellular rejection, though the interstitium often contains colllections of mature lymphocytes and fibroblasts in relation to the scarring.

On naked eye examination such a kidney is reduced in size and firm to cut. It is pale unless acute rejection has supervened, as sometimes happens if immuno-suppressive therapy is reduced prior to removal of the no-longer functioning transplant. The cortico-medullary blood vessels are easily seen due to their thickened walls and the cortex is reduced in width. The renal artery itself may be narrowed to a pin-point lumen. This is also seen in end-stage kidneys from patients maintained on dialysis, so that the original diagnosis is obscured by the pro-nounced proliferative vascular lesions.

The nature of the process known as chronic rejection is not clear. It is either the result of progressive healing of previous acute rejection, in which no additional immunological attack upon the kidney is occurring, or else it represents low grade continuing immunological damage of humoral type. If the latter is true, then additional immunosuppressive therapy should improve the situation, or at least arrest the functional deterioration. In many cases, however, anti-rejection therapy at this stage is not helpful and only increases the risk of morbidity due to side-effects.

Pathology of the Transplanted Ureter

Rejection in its various forms also involves the allografted ureter. In hyperacute rejection the ureter is cyanotic and necrotic along with the kidney. In the early post-transplant period, when cell-mediated rejection predominates, the ureter is oedematous and the wall is infiltrated by mononuclear cells (*see Fig*. 21.4). As a consequence, the wall is thickened and there is resistance to urinary drainage. This leads to renographic changes of obstruction and obscures the basic diagnosis of rejection. The ureteric arterial supply is involved in humoral rejection, acute or chronic. Progressive ischaemic fibrosis as a result of this may lead to stricture formation, requiring surgical intervention. Strictures may also follow trauma to the ureter or its blood supply at the time of harvesting and transplantation. A lymphocoele or a perirenal haematoma can press on the pelvis or the ureter causing obstruction. These are likely to be detected on ultrasound investigation.

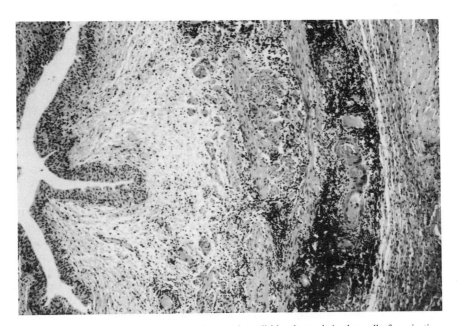

Fig. 21.4. Cellular infiltrate concentrated around small blood vessels in the wall of a rejecting ureter. (H and E × 75)

An interesting though rare cause of ureteric obstruction in renal transplant patients is BK virus infection. Typical inclusions of this polyoma virus have been found in the ulcerated urothelium of transplanted ureters at the site of stenosis. Similar inclusions were also present in the exfoliated cells in the urine from these patients (Coleman *et al.* 1978).

If surgical exploration is required for any of these complications it is useful to take an open biopsy of the kidney when it is exposed. This gives valuable information which can be used for future assessment of the transplant, particularly if the post-exploration function is not as good as expected.

The Differential Diagnosis of Rejection in a Transplanted Kidney

Although rejection is the most likely reason for impaired transplant function, it is of paramount importance to exclude other causes in order to avoid using unnecessarily high doses of immunosuppressive drugs.

In the early post-transplant period before stable function has been established the differential diagnosis must include factors related to the donor, perfusion, ischaemic times and technical problems at the vascular and ureteric anastomoses. Radiological investigations (including ultrasound scanning) have reduced the necessity for surgical exploration in a number of cases. The pathologist may be required to make a diagnosis on needle biopsy material—often a difficult task as the features tend to overlap. Transplant biopsy interpretation is a good example of a situation requiring the utmost co-operation and information sharing between clinician and pathologist.

Tubular necrosis

Acute tubular necrosis is very common in transplanted kidneys, particularly if the donor was hypotensive or if the ischaemia was prolonged. Acute tubular necrosis may result in post-transplant anuria or a fall off in urinary output after early function. In either situation the prognosis for the kidney is good in most cases. However, it is clearly very important to distinguish tubular necrosis from rejection as the former is managed conservatively and the latter requires therapeutic intervention.

Patients with tubular necrosis lack the typical clinical features of rejection such as pyrexia and hypertension, but even these are not always found in the immunosuppressed recipient. Biopsy of a transplanted kidney taken during the first week yields confirmatory evidence of tubular necrosis if tubulorrhexis (*see* p. 225) is present. However, tubular function may be considerably disordered in the absence of this feature, particularly on a small biopsy. The tubular epithelium may appear flattened with loss of nuclear detail. Interstitial oedema occurs in association with tubular necrosis but is much less marked than in early cellular rejection. Similarly, kidneys in which there is tubular necrosis have a sparse inflammatory infiltrate in the interstitium, whereas a cellular infiltrate is one of the hallmarks of acute cellular rejection. In later biopsies the tubular epithelium contains mitotic figures due to regeneration and it is more basophilic than normal due to its high RNA content.

It is important to remember that rejection can lead to tubular necrosis or the two processes can occur together. The histological distinction between them is often one of degree. Later review of such biopsies in the knowledge of the subsequent clinical course can give valuable information which is of use in evaluating similar histological findings from other patients.

Obstruction

The diagnosis of obstruction is occasionally made on renal biopsy when it has not been apparent clinically. Tubular dilatation is the most obvious feature but it has to be distinguished from apparent dilatation seen with the flattened epithelium of tubular necrosis. In an obstructed kidney the Bowman's spaces of the glomeruli are enlarged and prominent, without undue retraction of the glomerular tufts as would occur in ischaemic glomeruli. PAS positive material in obstructed Bowman's spaces is thought to be Tamm–Horsfall glycoprotein present at a more proximal level of the nephron than normal, because of back pressure. The features of obstruction may be seen without evidence of rejection but, as noted above, the two may co-exist since rejection of the ureter leads to obstructive changes in the kidney.

Pyelonephritis

The renal parenchyma may become the site of bacterial infection and unusual organisms such as Candida can cause tissue destruction in a kidney transplant without any significant symptomatology. Neutrophil polymorphs in the tubules and interstitium, in the absence of necrosis due to rejection or infarction, alert the pathologist to the presence of infection. In turn obstruction as a predisposing factor should be excluded and treated surgically if necessary.

When the recipient's own ureters have been the site of gross reflux it may be prudent to remove them and do pretransplant bilateral nephrectomy. This avoids the possibility of bladder urine from a new kidney refluxing into the old ureters which act as a reservoir for infection.

Glomerulonephritis

Glomerular lesions in a transplanted kidney may be part of the rejection process, as outlined. Less commonly they are due to glomerulonephritis (GN) either recurrent or *de novo*. Theoretically donor GN can be transplanted into a recipient, though this is usually excluded by the clinical evaluation of the donor.

Recurrent GN

Membranoproliferative GN of dense deposit type (Type II) is the pattern most likely to recur, though exact figures of the incidence of this complication are lacking, perhaps due to differences in biopsy policy. Patients with dense deposit disease are persistently hypocomplementaemic even after transplantation. It is thought that the abnormality in the complement system may predispose to this and other immune complex diseases.

The diagnosis of dense deposit disease is made by light microscopy and immunohistology. Ultrastructurally the glomeruli contain characteristic ribbon-like electron dense deposits in the basement membranes. When the disease recurs in a transplant the findings by all three types of microscopy are identical to those in the native kidneys. If additional features such as epithelial crescents were present, they also develop in the transplant. The clinical course of the recurrent disease is somewhat more protracted but renal failure occurs in months or years. The variant of membranoproliferative GN with subendothelial deposits recurs less frequently.

IgA nephropathy is becoming increasingly recognized as a major cause of renal failure. It has also been shown to recur in a transplant. This suggests that the abnormality is in the host rather than the kidney itself. Recurrent focal and segmental glomerulosclerosis may develop within a few days of transplantation in some cases. Crescentic GN associated with circulating antibody to glomerular basement membrane ('anti-GBM nephritis', or Goodpasture's disease if there is pulmonary haemorrhage as well) damages the new kidney if the patient is transplanted whilst antibody is still present in the serum. Radioimmunoassay is a sensitive method of antibody detection and can be used to diagnose patients with this form of renal failure even if they are too ill to have a renal biopsy. It is advisable to delay transplantation for some time after disappearance of anti-GBM antibody from the serum to avoid recrudescence in the donor kidney.

Live donor kidneys should not be used to treat patients with diseases likely to recur, unless other factors dictate extreme urgency of transplantation.

De novo GN

Interest has centred on the occurrence of membranous GN in a transplanted kidney. Transmission from the donor is unlikely. De novo disease of this type may be due to persistent hepatitis B virus infection. Another source of a chronic antigen load is malignancy, a potential hazard of immunosuppression. The diagnosis of membranous GN in a transplant should lead to a diligent search for a tumour, particularly of bronchus, gastrointestinal tract or the lymphoreticular system. In some cases membranous GN is a manifestation of rejection in which the antigen–antibody complexes include the incompatible HLA antigens. GN of any type may be complicated by renal vein thrombosis which in its chronic form is characterized by a sudden increase in urinary protein excretion.

Miscellaneous conditions which can recur

Patients with amyloidosis of the kidney tend to have a poor prognosis and succumb to a combination of infection, hypotension and heart failure. Their survival largely depends on the extent of extrarenal involvement. Those who receive a renal transplant are prone to develop amyloid within it. However, as with GN the course may be more protracted than was originally the case in that patient. Some recipients do not seem to develop recurrence of amyloid. It seems likely that the nature of the underlying cause, known or unknown, determines the outcome.

The renal lesions of diabetes mellitus recur and diabetic nephropathy has been shown both clinically and experimentally in transplants. Combined pancreatic and renal transplantation should in theory be preventive but this is not yet in widespread use. Diabetic patients in renal failure also tend to have advanced atheroma of their iliac arteries making the transplant operation technically more difficult and predisposing to renal damage from atheromatous emboli.

It seems logical that generalized metabolic abnormalities which lead to renal failure will also involve the transplant. However, in oxalosis satisfactory long-term graft function has been reported (Scheinman *et al.* 1984). Patients with cystinosis may also develop crystal deposits within the new kidney. This does not inevitably lead to renal failure and patients with cystinosis have been transplanted successfully. Living related donors should preferably be avoided as these may be carriers of the condition, making recurrence more likely.

Problems with Immunosuppression

Viral infection

Immunosuppressed transplant recipients are prone to develop opportunistic infection or to reactivation of a previously latent infectious agent. An example is disease due to cytomegalovirus (CMV) either acquired from the donor or reactivated. It is a common cause of fever in transplanted patients and some are very ill with marked leucopenia. Severe thrombocytopenia also occurs. The illness varies from a febrile episode to a life threatening or a fatal condition. It is frequently associated with reduced renal function so that it has to be differentiated from rejection. Rejection, however, may sometimes be stimulated by a viral infection either because the dosage of immunosuppressive drugs must be reduced (due to the leucopenia) or by some other unknown mechanism.

CMV inclusions in tubular epithelium or within glomerular cells are very rarely seen on biopsy. (They are more frequent in autopsy material—a reflection of sample size or severity of involvement.) The changes in the absence of co-existent rejection are rather non-specific. However, CMV glomerulitis has been described and small segments of glomerular necrosis in the absence of any vascular rejection are suggestive of this lesion (Richardson *et al.* 1981). When the tubular epithelium is heavily infected, CMV inclusions may be found on studying the urinary sediment cytologically. Current serological methods of diagnosis tend to give the evidence of infections retrospectively.

Histological changes due to immunosuppressive drugs

Reference has already been made to the problem of Cy A nephrotoxicity and to the lack of reliable histological parameters to distinguish between nephrotoxicity and rejection. Findings such as interstitial oedema and giant mitochondria in tubular epithelial cells are not specific though they occur more commonly in patients on Cy A than in those treated in the conventional manner with steroid and azathioprine (Mihatsch *et al.* 1983). Isometric vacuolation of proximal tubules seems to be the most consistent abnormality. There is also an arteriolar lesion which resembles hyaline arteriolosclerosis. The significance of this change is not certain—it bears some resemblance to the arteriolar lesion of rejection. Some workers consider that it is specific for Cy A toxicity but this is not generally agreed (Thiru 1984; Neild *et al.* 1985). It is hoped that additional evidence will come from the study of kidneys in patients treated with Cy A for another organ transplant, in which the kidney is not the site of the rejection process, and from animal models.

Anti-thymocyte globulin (ATG) is a potent immunosuppressive agent, which some consider unnecessarily toxic. However, since the advent of monoclonal antibody technology ATG is a purer preparation and side-effects are less likely. Local irradiation when given for rejection episodes tended to cause severe interstitial fibrosis in the kidney. This form of treatment is no longer in regular use in clinical renal transplantation.

General side-effects of immunosuppresion

Other than the desired effects of immunosuppressive agents on the transplant and on the immune system, they also have a wide range of unwanted side-effects on other body systems. Marrow toxicity, particularly to azathioprine, may require the dose to be reduced. Susceptibility to opportunistic infection has already been mentioned. Malignancy is more prevalent in immunosuppressed patients (Penn 1978). Initial reports showed that patients receiving Cy A were particularly likely to develop a malignant lymphoma. This does not, however, seem to have been borne out on longer follow-up of patients given lower doses of the drug than were first considered necessary (Stiller and Keown 1984). Cy A has other less troublesome side-effects such as gum hypertrophy and hirsutism.

Corticosteroid therapy leads to many complications which can be life-threatening. Gastrointestinal ulceration with perforation and haemorrhage may have atypical clinical features in these individuals with serious consequences. Unsuspected diabetes mellitus occasionally presents as severe metabolic upset and even coma in transplant recipients (Hill et al. 1974). Cushingoid facies and excessive weight gain are tolerable though not pleasant side-effects. The incidence of these problems can be dramatically diminished by cutting the steroid dosage to a level which does not impair graft survival and reduces the morbidity from complications of steroid therapy (McGeown et al. 1980).

Transplantation of Other Organs

The general principles outlined in this chapter can be applied to other organs. Those in current clinical use are cardiac, hepatic and bone marrow transplants. The programmes for pancreatic and heart–lung transplantation are at an earlier stage in their development.

The rejection of organs other than the kidney takes the same form though there is obviously a variation in its effect. Cardiac rejection may lead to sudden death due to arrhythmia, and the functional reserve of the heart is smaller than that of the kidney. In the liver, technical problems have been more prominent, although hepatic transplants are less aggressively rejected than either renal or cardiac transplants. Bone marrow transplants lead to graft versus host disease, whilst in the other cases it is the host which rejects the graft.

The problem of opportunistic infection is equally if not more important in these other transplants and such infections are frequently life-threatening. However, the advent of Cy A has improved survival rates considerably and reduced the incidence of opportunistic infection. Malignancy has not proved to be as much of a problem as was formerly feared when immunosuppressive drugs were used in higher dosage. Prolonged survival with a good quality of life can now be anticipated after transplantation.

References

Bittner J. J. (1935) A review of genetic studies on the transplantation of tumours. *J. Genet.* **31**, 471–87.

Borel J. F. (1976) Comparative study of *in vitro* and *in vivo* drug effects on cell-mediated cytotoxicity. *Immunology* **31**, 631–41.

Carrel A., Guthrie C. C. (1905) Functions of a transplanted kidney. *Science* **22**, 473.

Coleman D. V., Mackenzie E. F. D., Gardner S. D., Poulding J. M., Amer B., Russell W. J. I. (1978) Human polyomavirus (BK) infection and ureteric stenosis in renal allograft recipients. *J. Clin. Pathol.* **31**, 338–47.

Forbes G. B., Goggin M. J., Dische F. E. *et al.* (1981) Accidental transplantation of bronchial carcinoma from a cadaver donor to two recipients of renal allografts. *J. Clin. Pathol.* **34**, 109–15.

Häyry P., von Willebrand E. (1981) Monitoring of human renal allograft rejection with fine-needle aspiration cytology. *Scand. J. Immunol.* **13**, 87–97.

Health Departments of Great Britain and Northern Ireland (1983) *Cadaveric Organs for Transplantation, A Code of Practice Including the Diagnosis of Brain Death.* London, HMSO.

Hill C. M., Douglas J. F., Rajkumar K. V., McEvoy J., McGeown M. G. (1974) Glycosuria and hyperglycaemia after kidney transplantation. *Lancet* **2**, 490–2.

Hill G. S., Light J. A., Perloff L. J. (1976) Perfusion-related injury in renal transplantation. *Surgery* **79**, 440–7.

McGeown M. G., Douglas J. F., Brown W. A. *et al.* (1980) Advantages of low dose steroid from the day after renal transplantation. *Transplantation* **29**, 287–9.

Mason D. W. (1983) The mechanism of allograft rejection, progress and problems. *Transplant Proc.* **15**, 264–8.

Medawar P. B. (1944) The behaviour and fate of skin autografts and skin homografts in rabbits. *J. Anat.* **78**, 176–99.

Mihatsch M. J., Thiel G., Spichtin H. P. *et al.* (1983) Morphological findings in kidney transplants after treatment with Cyclosporine. *Transplant Proc.* **15**, 2821–35.

Morris P. J. (1984) Renal transplantation: current status. In: *Proceedings of the IX International Congress of Nephrology,* pp. 1627–43. New York, Springer-Verlag.

Murray J. E., Merrill J. P., Harrison J. H., Wilson R. E., Dammin G. J. (1963) Prolonged survival of human kidney homografts by immunosuppressive drug therapy. *N. Engl. J. Med.* **268**, 1315–23.

Myers B. D., Ross J., Newton L., Luetscher J., Perlroth M. (1984) Cyclosporine-associated chronic nephropathy. *N. Engl. J. Med.* **311**, 699–705.

Neild G. H., Reuben R., Hartley R. B., Cameron J. S. (1985) Glomerular thrombi in renal allografts associated with cyclosporin treatment. *J. Clin. Pathol.* **38**, 253–8.

Penn I. (1978) Malignancies associated with immunosuppressive or cytotoxic therapy. *Surgery* **83**, 492–502.

Porter K. A., Thomson W. B., Owen K. *et al.* (1963) Obliterative vascular changes in four human kidney homotransplants. *Br. Med. J.* **3**, 639–45.

Richardson W. P., Colvin R. B., Cheeseman S. H. *et al.* (1981) Glomerulopathy associated with cytomegalovirus viraemia in renal allografts. *N. Engl. J. Med.* **305**, 57–63.

Scheinman J. I., Najarian J. S., Mauer S. M. (1984) Successful strategies for renal transplantation in primary oxalosis. *Kidney Int.* **25**, 804–11.

Snell G. D. (1948) Methods for the study of histocompatibility genes. *J. Genet.* **49**, 87–103.

Starzl T. E. (1964) Patterns of permissible donor-recipient tissue transfer in relation to ABO blood groups. In: *Experience in Renal Transplantation,* 37–47. Philadelphia, W. B. Saunders.

Stiller C. R., Keown P. A. (1984) Cyclosporine therapy in perspective. In: Morris P. J., Tilney N. L. (eds.) *Progress in Transplantation,* pp. 11–45. Edinburgh, Churchill Livingstone.

Terasaki P. I., McClelland J. D. (1964) Microdroplet assay of human serum cytotoxins. *Nature* **204**, 998–1000.

Thiru S. (1984) Pathology of rejection—kidney. In: Calne R. Y. (ed.) *Transplantation Immunology, Clinical and Experimental,* 9–52. Oxford, Oxford University Press.

Ullman E. (1902) Experimentelle Nierentransplantation. Vorläufige Mittheilung. *Wien Klin. Wschr.* **15**, 281–2.

von Willebrand E. (1980) Fine needle aspiration cytology of human renal transplants. *Clin. Immunol. Immunopathol.* **17**, 309–22.

Chapter 22

Gynaecological Emergencies

J. M. Graham Harley

Introduction

Often in the absence of a gynaecologist the general surgeon may have to treat a known gynaecological condition, e.g. Bartholin's abscess, but more frequent are those occasions when he opens the abdomen believing the problem to be surgical and finds it is gynaecological. In this chapter the gynaecological problems most commonly encountered will be described and their management discussed so that the general surgeon will be provided with sufficient information to ensure the correct management of the patient.

Vulva and Vagina

Conditions involving these structures are usually so obvious that the patient is seldom seen by the general surgeon. However, there are conditions which may require the emergency services of the general surgeon.

Bartholin's abscess

This is the commonest vulval lesion which may require emergency surgery.

Clinical findings

The symptoms are vulval tenderness and introital dyspareunia. The pain may be so severe that the patient becomes distressed and requires urgent treatment. The gland is enlarged and fluctuant with the surrounding tissue reddened and oedematous. Diagnosis is usually obvious. However, a similar enlargement in a postmenopausal patient may have an underlying carcinoma and in these cases biopsy at the time of operation is important.

Pathogenesis

Bartholin's gland is situated deep in the posterior third of each labium majus with the opening of the duct, usually invisible, just external to the hymeal edge. Congenital narrowing, inspissated mucus or, more commonly, infection causes obstruction of the main ducts with the retention of secretion and dilatation of the gland, usually resulting in abscess formation. An important organism is *Neisseria gonorrhoea* (gonococcus) but this is perhaps not so common as *Escherichia coli* and mixed infections with aerobic and anaerobic organisms.

Management

Medical treatment with antibiotics and/or simple incision usually only provides temporary relief and recurrence is common because of the lack of permanent adequate drainage. To avoid this, marsupialization of the gland is preferred. The success of the marsupialization operation depends upon the correct operative technique so attention to the following details is essential.

To avoid possible subsequent dyspareunia, the incision should be sited correctly and at least 2 cm long; if made too small it will result in an increased risk of subsequent closure. The lining of the dilated gland or underlying cyst should be carefully identified and sutured with interrupted No. 0 chromic catgut to the skin edges. If this procedure is not carried out correctly then subsequent closure at the site of the incision will occur and there will be a recurrence of the abscess. At operation, swabs for bacteriology and a biopsy where indicated should be taken. Antibiotics may be considered if there is much inflammation of the surrounding tissues; however, this is rarely necessary.

Vulval haematoma

This is most often found in the female child who has slipped climbing over a fence or riding a bicycle. The haematoma of the vulva which may result can be of such a size that not only has the patient very severe pain but also she may be shocked and require resuscitation. If evacuation of the haematoma is necessary, this should be carried out as soon as possible and haemostasis achieved by the usual techniques.

Lacerations of the vaginal mucosa

These are uncommon but do occasionally occur and may require simple suturing with interrupted No. 1 catgut. Rarely, a laceration in the posterior fornix may have involved the peritoneal cavity and this possibility must be excluded by careful examination of the patient, including examination of the vagina by speculum.

Fibroids (Leiomyomas)

Fibroids are the most common tumours of the uterine corpus, occurring in about 15–20% of all women. They are usually asymptomatic and only discovered at a routine gynaecological check-up, or they are responsible for gynaecological symptoms which cause the patient's referral to a gynaecologist. Sometimes, however, they may cause acute abdominal symptoms, resulting in the patient's admission to a casualty or acute surgical unit. The two common conditions responsible are torsion of a 'pedunculated' fibroid or 'red' degeneration.

Little is known of the aetiology of fibroids although they may be at least partially under hormonal control. They tend to occur during reproductive life and regress after the menopause.

Clinical features

Symptoms of fibroids depend upon many factors, the most important of which are size, site and number, and whether or not the patient is pregnant. The symptoms are usually obviously gynaecological, but abdominal pain and clinical findings consistent with an acute abdomen may be produced by torsion or 'red' degeneration.

In the non-pregnant patient the common complication encountered by the general surgeon is 'torsion' of a 'pedunculated' intra-abdominal fibroid. In these patients the diagnosis prior to laparotomy may be impossible, for the findings of an abdominal or pelvic mass associated with the clinical picture of an acute abdomen may be due to other conditions such as a tubo-ovarian abscess, endometriosis, or one of the many other causes of ovarian enlargement. Very rarely, pain may be associated with sarcomatous changes in a fibroid.

During the second or third trimester, patients with uterine fibroids may present with abdominal pain which can be severe. The pain is due to 'red' degeneration and the diagnosis is usually easy if, on examination, an obvious painful, tender swelling is found in the uterine wall. In those cases where there is not an obvious fibroid palpable, the possibility of a placental abruption must always be considered and if possible excluded by sonography.

Sonography may also be helpful where a mass is discovered in close relation to the uterus and there is some doubt as to whether it is a fibroid or ovarian in origin. Mistakes, however, do occur and on at least two occasions the author has seen laparotomy performed to remove an ovarian cyst diagnosed by sonography and at operation a fibroid was found.

Morphology

Fibroids appear grossly as spherical masses which can be grouped as submucous, intramural or subserosal, according to site. Submucous fibroids may become pedunculated and grow into the endometrial cavity or even protrude through the cervical os. Subserosal fibroids may also become pedunculated and grow into the abdominal cavity. A subserosal fibroid may undergo torsion and become impacted. Occasionally it derives a new blood supply from peritoneum or omentum, discards its pedicle and becomes a parasitic fibroid.

Histologically, they are composed of spindle-shaped smooth muscle cells. The stroma may be hyalinized and calcification may be seen.

If the mass outgrows its blood supply it may become impacted. This is especially likely to occur during pregnancy, when the impacted fibroid appears as a red mass ('red' degeneration).

Malignant change in a fibroid is rare, occurring in only about 0·5% of cases.

Management

Torsion of a fibroid discovered at laparotomy in the non-pregnant patient should be removed by clamping the pedicle and transfixing it to obtain satisfactory haemostasis. (If the patient is pregnant, particularly in the early weeks, a similar procedure may be carried out.)

In the pregnant patient where the diagnosis of 'red' degeneration of a fibroid is made, laparotomy should not be carried out. Expectant management should be instituted with bed rest and sufficient sedation to control the pain until the acute episode subsides. Nearly always successful, this management can often be discontinued in a few days and the patient allowed home.

If a laparotomy has been carried out and a fibroid which has undergone 'red' degeneration is found, on no account should it be removed if it is intramural as haemostasis is very difficult and may not be possible. Only if there is a well defined pedicle present should removal, as previously described, be contemplated.

Pelvic Inflammatory Disease

Pelvic inflammatory disease (PID) is not only the most common gynaecological condition encountered by the general surgeon, but is also the most important because of its often serious consequences.

A great variety of clinical presentations can occur, depending upon whether the patient has a simple salpingitis or one complicated by septicaemic shock or a ruptured pelvic abscess.

Many diagnostic difficulties may be encountered due to the fact that the common presenting symptom is lower abdominal pain—a symptom often associated with peritoneal irritation—which results not only from infection but also from many other conditions such as perforation, haemorrhage, obstruction, torsion or ischaemic disease.

Clinical features

Early recognition and treatment are essential to minimize the dangerous consequences such as infertility, menorrhagia and chronic pelvic pain.

Symptoms often occur either with the onset or shortly after the menses but can occur at any time in the menstrual cycle. The pain is usually lower abdominal and varies in severity according to the extent of the disease; it is often bilateral although unilateral pain does not exclude the diagnosis. The patient may have headache, lassitude and nausea but vomiting is not common unless there is considerable peritonitis. A history of vaginal discharge is so common in these patients that it is of little diagnostic aid, but if present, may be of value in identifying the organism(s).

On examination the patient may look perfectly well, as is often the case in chronic PID and in some of the subacute cases. However, in the more acute forms of the disease the patient looks ill, toxic and may sometimes be shocked.

An invaluable clinical observation of great diagnostic value is that if the patient has peritonitis she will usually lie quietly and be apprehensive of any movement because it causes such increased pain, whereas the patient with intestinal or renal colic will be restless.

Pyrexia is usually present and its absence must alert the surgeon to the possibility of an ectopic pregnancy.

Palpation of the abdomen usually elicits tenderness on both sides of the lower abdomen, with varying degrees of guarding and rebound.

On pelvic examination any discharge should be noted for possible diagnostic features. The presence of any pus in the urethra, in Skene's or Bartholin's ducts, or coming from the cervix should be swabbed for laboratory investigation.

Bimanual examination will usually produce marked excitation tenderness on moving the cervix and uterus. Adnexal swellings are often absent or, if present, may be difficult to identify owing to the severity of the pain. Sometimes, a pelvic mass is present in the pouch of Douglas suggestive of an abscess.

Bacteriological investigations are usually not particularly valuable unless the purulent material demonstrates the gonococcus. The white cell count can be normal although a leucocytosis is often present, as is an elevated erythrocyte sedimentation rate.

The main differential diagnosis is appendicitis. Others include ectopic pregnancy, ruptured corpus luteum cyst, torsion of an adnexal mass, endometriosis, urinary tract infection and diverticulitis.

Pathogenesis

PID usually results from an ascending infection which is bacterial (aerobic and/or anaerobic), although viral, fungal and parasitic infection can occur. In some cases, *N. gonorrhoea* may be responsible for initiating the infection, but most cases are due to a mixture of organisms such as *E. coli* and bacteroides. Infection of the pelvic organs secondary to appendicitis, or other intra-abdominal inflammatory condition, is unusual. Rarely, certain diseases, such as tuberculosis, may gain access to the pelvic organs by blood spread.

PID may be acute, subacute or chronic and is often recurrent. It may involve the uterus, fallopian tubes, ovaries and adjacent pelvic tissue.

A previous history of pelvic surgery or delivery is sometimes encountered, but the ready availability of contraception, particularly the intrauterine contraceptive device, pregnancy termination and increasing promiscuity, have resulted in a much higher incidence associated with sexually transmitted diseases.

Morphology

Ascending infection at first attacks the lining of the genital tract, most commonly the lining of the fallopian tubes. At surgery the tube is seen to be hyperaemic, and if the infection has spread through the wall, there may be an exudate in the serosal surface and local peritonitis. The inflammatory reaction may cause agglutination of the fimbria at the end of the tube and the resultant obstruction leads to a pyosalpinx. Alternatively, pus may leak from the fimbrial end, leading to a pelvic abscess. In severe cases, infection may spread to the ovary, leading to a tubo-ovarian abscess. Occasionally, generalized peritonitis, ileus and bacteraemic shock may occur.

Histologically, the features are those of acute inflammation, with a polymorph infiltrate in the wall of the tube and pus in the lumen. In subacute and chronic cases the polymorphs are replaced by lymphocytes and histiocytes.

Management

In the majority of these patients the disease is of mild or moderate severity and they are treated by their own general practitioners with antibiotics, analgesics and bed rest. The management, if early, usually produces a satisfactory clinical response and surprisingly few cases of blocked or non-functioning fallopian tubes occur.

Hospitalization is essential for those who appear ill or where the diagnosis is in doubt. In hospital, parenteral therapy with penicillin or tetracycline together with metronidazole should be commenced and constant observation of the patient kept for signs of complications or deterioration.

Over 90% of the patients respond satisfactorily to therapy. However, exploratory laparotomy may be necessary if the patient's clinical condition is deteriorating. At operation, adnexal tubo-ovarian swellings should be left alone unless there is evidence of impending rupture of an abscess or isolated rupture has already occurred. In these patients only the affected structures should be removed.

In the patient where laparotomy has been performed and a diagnosis of PID has not been made prior to operation, peritoneal toilet with conservation of both tubes and ovaries is important unless such findings, as previously described, necessitating further surgery are present. It is most important that patients who have not yet had a family should have their ovaries conserved so that subsequent ovum retrieval may be carried out for *in vitro* fertilization. Patients with extensive PID who in the past would have had no chance of childbearing may, with correct treatment, now have some chance since removal of the ovaries is rarely necessary.

Extra-uterine (Ectopic) Pregnancy

The term 'ectopic' pregnancy usually indicates that the patient has an extra-uterine pregnancy implanted in the fallopian tube. This synonym is not unexpected because 90% of extra-uterine pregnancies do in fact occur in the fallopian tubes. It is important, however, to remember that extra-uterine pregnancies can occur in the ovary or anywhere in the abdominal cavity. The author has encountered them situated not only in the peritoneum of the abdominal wall, particularly that of the pouch of Douglas, but also in the broad ligament, bowel wall and omentum.

The incidence of tubal pregnancy is about 1 in 1150 pregnancies and is increasing because of the rising incidence of those factors most commonly associated with the condition. These are salpingitis, the intra-uterine contraceptive device, tubal surgery, including surgery for a previous ectopic (particularly if the tube is conserved) and increased numbers of tubal ligations with increased failures.

Patients with a history of infertility, perforated appendix or who have endometriosis are more prone to a tubal pregnancy, as are those in the lower socio-economic group and non-caucasians.

Clinical features

Ectopic pregnancies are notoriously difficult to diagnose because they may mimic many other conditions, and there are no specific symptoms or signs. It is essential always to remember the possibility of an ectopic pregnancy in any female patient who complains of abdominal pain, particularly if it is associated with some menstrual abnormality. This particularly applies to those patients who have a history of those conditions which predispose to an ectopic (*see* above).

Pain is the most common symptom and varies from an ache to a very severe sharp pain due to rupture and peritoneal irritation. Occasionally it may be colicky, if the tube is trying to expel the pregnancy. A period of amenorrhoea makes the diagnosis more likely but a menses which is not clearing up in its usual time, or which begins after the onset of the pain, may occur. The possibility of an early ectopic before a menstrual period is missed must never be forgotten. Shoulder pain is not a particularly valuable symptom because by the time it is present the signs of considerable intraperitoneal haemorrhage are obvious. Nausea and vomiting are less common than in any condition involving the bowel.

The general appearance of the patient may be quite normal or she may be showing the obvious signs of shock. Her pulse is usually increased and thready before there is any fall in blood pressure.

Examination of the abdomen may reveal nothing but there may be obvious localized tenderness, guarding and rebound tenderness in one or other iliac fossa or generalized in the lower or upper abdomen, or both. Surprisingly, the rigidity, if present, is less marked than if the patient has a perforated viscus.

On pelvic examination there may or may not be vaginal bleeding. On bimanual examination there is tenderness of varying severity which is often more severe on the side of the ectopic, particularly if rupture has not yet occurred. An adnexal mass may or may not be palpable, either because it is absent, too small, or the patient has too much pain to allow satisfactory examination. Excitation tenderness on moving the cervix is often described but is not diagnostic.

In the patient where all the findings are inconclusive but ectopic pregnancy cannot be excluded on the history, then laparoscopy may be helpful although the diagnosis in the patient with an early ectopic can be missed, even at laparoscopy. Laparoscopy should not be carried out in a shocked patient where intraperitoneal haemorrhage is considered to be present.

Morphology

There is little defence in the tubes against permeating trophoblast and so distension and rupture are common sequelae. The narrower the tube the earlier the rupture, and thus if implantation is at the isthmus end, rupture can occur even before the menses is missed, whereas at the ampullary or fimbrial end rupture may not occur until 10 to 12 weeks gestation. In some cases rupture does not occur and the products of conception are expelled from the tube at the fimbrial ostium—the so-called 'tubal abortion'. In others the pregnancy does not progress in the tube and the condition is referred to as a 'tubal mole'; many of these may go undetected and only those that give rise to symptoms are diagnosed.

At the time of laparotomy for a tubal pregnancy, blood is usually present in the pouch of Douglas, and the affected tube is distended, congested and possibly embedded in blood clot. Blood clot and placental villi may be seen within the tube or they may be seen prolapsing through a rupture in the tube.

Histologically, the tube is distended with blood clot. The diagnosis is confirmed by the finding of chorionic (placental) villi (*see Fig.* 22.1) or fetal parts. If tubal abortion or rupture occurred prior to surgery, the diagnosis may still be made by the finding of an implantation site of trophoblastic tissue in the tubal wall.

Where the implantation is outside the tube it is usually a primary abdominal pregnancy, although it may be secondary to a tubal rupture or abortion.

The corpus luteum of pregnancy continues as long as the pregnancy is alive and thus the usual hormonal changes occur together with their effects on the uterus where there is a decidual reaction in the endometrium. The Arias-Stella reaction is also commonly seen in the endometrium. This is a hypersecretory state in which the endometrial cells become enlarged and vacuolated. There is tufting of the epithelium within the endometrial glands. The presence of a decidual reaction and the Arias-Stella reaction without trophoblastic tissue in endometrial curetting suggests the possibility of an ectopic pregnancy, although this situation may also arise in an intra-uterine pregnancy in which the conceptus had been previously shed.

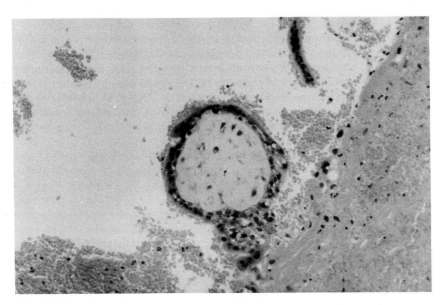

Fig. 22.1. Ectopic pregnancy. The presence of a chorionic villus in blood clot removed from the pelvis confirmed the diagnosis of ruptured ectopic pregnancy. (H and E × 70)

Management

If the diagnosis of ectopic pregnancy is made, laparotomy should be carried out immediately, as early control of the haemorrhage may be life-saving. Intravenous infusion with a plasma expander should be commenced if the patient is shocked, and whole blood given as soon as possible.

At laparotomy, if the tube is distorted or ruptured, removal of the tube by commencing clamping at the fimbrial end and working towards the uterus, should be carried out until the affected area of the tube has been passed; at this point the final clamp on the uterine side of the tube is applied. This procedure will allow, where possible, a portion of tube to be preserved should subsequent tubal surgery be required. Total salpingectomy should not be performed just to prevent a subsequent ectopic in the remaining portion of the tube.

In a tubal pregnancy, removal of the ovary on the affected side should be avoided. If the diagnosis is an ovarian pregnancy, which is very rare, then removal of the ovary is usually necessary.

Inspection of the other adnexa is mandatory and a careful record made of the condition of both tube and ovary. Any signs of infection should be treated with antibiotics.

Conservation of the tube in cases of tubal abortion or 'unruptured tubal pregnancy' may be possible in a few selected cases, but this decision can only be made by the individual operator at the time of surgery. Haemostasis is of paramount importance during this procedure.

Abdominal pregnancy

The incidence of abdominal pregnancy is rare in caucasians but is much more common in the African. It is usually primary but may be secondary to a ruptured ectopic or tubal abortion. A few continue until the fetus is viable but the diagnosis is usually missed unless the pregnancy is accompanied by certain unusual symptoms and signs such as a history of lower abdominal pain in early pregnancy or unexplained abdominal pain continuing throughout pregnancy. On abdominal examination, easily felt fetal parts and the so-called high-lying or 'flying fetus' may arouse suspicion.

Earlier diagnosis is now more likely as most patients have an ultrasound scan in the first trimester, but in areas where this is not available the symptoms and signs described should be noted, particularly if one is working in areas where extra-uterine pregnancy is common.

When diagnosed, irrespective of the period of gestation, laparotomy should be carried out and the fetus, cord and membranes removed. The placenta should *not* be removed unless haemostasis is going to be possible and this is unlikely.

Ovarian Conditions

The general surgeon will not have gone very far in his or her training or career before several conditions associated with the ovaries are encountered. It has been estimated that 25% of patients with ovarian malignancy present to a specialist other than a gynaecologist (Hudson 1973).

Ovarian conditions are traditionally classified into non-neoplastic and neoplastic. Before describing definite clinical entities, some generalizations are valuable and worth remembering, particularly as the diagnosis and treatment of any ovarian enlargement will usually involve making a distinction between malignant and benign.

The more marked the symptoms, the greater the chance that the ovarian swelling is benign, as malignant ovaries are often silent until palpable or evidence of secondaries are present. Simple non-neoplastic swellings such as a luteal or a follicular cyst, endometriosis or those resulting from infection, are usually symptomatic, producing pain and often disturbances in menstruation.

Although all ovarian enlargements are suspect, the following features, if present, make them more likely to be malignant:

1. The patient is postmenopausal.
2. Persisting over 60 days with a normal menstrual cycle.
3. More than 5 cm in diameter.
4. Reduced mobility.
5. Involvement of both ovaries.
6. Ascites present.

7. Nodules in the pouch of Douglas.
8. Irregular and solid mass.

Non-neoplastic ovarian conditions

Inflammatory adnexal swellings involving the ovaries
The subject of pelvic inflammatory disease has already been considered. It is important, however, to remember that acute oophoritis or primary ovarian abscess formation is very rare, the ovarian condition usually being part of a tubo-ovarian abscess. If an ovarian abscess is found as a distinct entity, tuberculosis should be considered.

A ruptured tubo-ovarian abscess usually causes an acute intra-abdominal condition requiring laparotomy and removal of the offending structure. On rare occasions, total hysterectomy and bilateral salpingo-oophorectomy may be necessary and life-saving.

In the chronic stages of tubo-ovarian infection the adnexal mass may arouse suspicion of a true neoplasm and laparotomy may be necessary to make the correct diagnosis. However, this chronic problem usually reaches the gynaecologist.

Luteal or follicular cysts
Luteal cysts occur when the central cavity of a corpus luteum is unusually large or they may result from a corpus luteum haematoma (due to excessive bleeding into a corpus luteum). A follicular cyst results from follicles which are partially matured and then become atretic.

The patient with an uncomplicated luteal or follicular cyst usually presents to the gynaecologist because of symptoms of menstrual irregularities or lower abdominal pain. Occasionally, as a result of sudden torsion or, more commonly, rupture of the cyst, the symptoms and signs are those of an acute abdomen with haemorrhage, and laparotomy is carried out by a general surgeon. At operation, a ruptured corpus luteum or follicular cyst should be carefully removed and haemostasis achieved at the site of removal by the insertion of deep interrupted plain catgut sutures. The ovary should not be removed unless satisfactory haemostasis is impossible.

If torsion of an ovary is found it should be unwound and ovarian cystectomy then carried out, although the presence of ischaemic changes requires ovariotomy (Taylor 1981).

Endometriosis
Endometriosis is defined as the presence of ectopic endometrial tissue outside the myometrium. It is commonly found in the ovaries, pouch of Douglas, broad ligament, etc. It may result from metaplasia of the peritoneum into endometrium or from retrograde menstruation of endometrium through the fallopian tubes and subsequent implantation.

The acute abdomen associated with endometriosis is not as common as the previous condition, mainly because endometriosis gives rise to many symptoms such as pelvic pain, menstrual abnormalities, dysmenorrhoea and dyspareunia, and these usually result in the patient's referral to a gynaecologist.

The rupture of an endometrioma into the peritoneal cavity, usually at the time of menstruation, causes severe peritoneal irritation and the patient presents with the clinical features of an acute abdomen. She may be admitted to a surgical unit where the differential diagnosis from a perforated viscus may be impossible and laparotomy is performed.

At the time of laparotomy endometriosis in the early stages appears as reddish-blue nodules. Some of these grow into cysts, up to 10 cm diameter, filled with altered blood (chocolate cyst). There are often gross adhesions between the areas of endometriosis and the surrounding tissues (*see Fig. 22.2*).

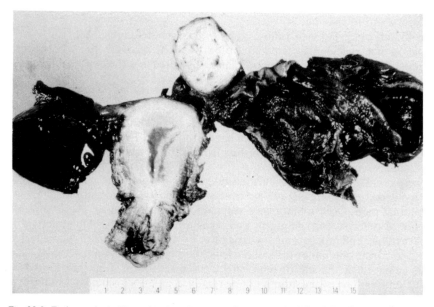

Fig. 22.2. Endometriosis. Note the chocolate cyst of ovary to the left of the photograph.

Histologically, the finding of endometrial glands with surrounding stroma confirms the diagnosis. Sometimes bleeding and subsequent fibrosis destroy any endometrial tissue, making histological diagnosis difficult.

At operation, if endometriosis is present, as many as possible of the endometriotic lesions on the ovary or ovaries are best removed but this should only be done if the operator is competent enough to do so with the conservation of as much healthy ovarian tissues as possible. If the uterus is retroverted uterine suspension should be carried out. Subsequent therapy with danazol for 6–9 months will probably be necessary together with gynaecological follow-up.

Neoplastic ovarian conditions

The classification of ovarian neoplasms proposed by the WHO has been widely accepted (Serov and Scully 1973). *Table* 22.1 is a modified version (Zaloudek and Kurman 1983). As these workers pointed out, ovarian neoplasms can be classified into three main categories: epithelial, stromal and germ cell. Of these, the epithelial neoplasms are by far the most important, accounting for 58% of all tumours and 90% of malignant ovarian tumours.

Table 22.1. Simplified histological classification of ovarian tumours*

I.	Epithelial tumours
	1. Serous tumours
	2. Mucinous tumours
	3. Endometrioid tumours
	4. Clear cell (mesonephroid) tumours
	5. Brenner (transitional cell) tumours
II.	Sex cord–stromal tumours
	1. Granulosa cell tumour
	2. Thecoma
	3. Fibroma
	4. Other tumours in fibroma/thecoma group
	5. Sertoli-Leydig cell tumours
III.	Germ cell tumours
	1. Dysgerminoma
	2. Endodermal sinus (yolk sac) tumour
	3. Choriocarcinoma
	4. Teratomas
IV.	Soft tissue tumours not specific to ovaries
V.	Lymphoma/leukaemia
VI.	Unclassified tumours
VII.	Metastatic tumours

* Adapted from Zaloudek and Kurman 1983.

Although some knowledge of the different types of tumour is essential, when the problem is encountered at operation by the general surgeon it is more important that he recognizes the features which would indicate malignancy (*see* p. 666) and observes the extent of the disease. *Table* 22.2 gives a description of the staging which is commonly accepted and should be of some help in making this possible (Zaloudek and Kurman 1983).

It is perhaps valuable at this stage to quote some statistics to highlight the dangers of ovarian neoplasm. By doing so the general surgeon will more readily appreciate his responsibilities in the correct management of the patient to give her a reasonable chance of survival.

Approximately 23% of all gynaecological cancers are ovarian and they account for 47% of deaths from genital tract cancer. Twelve out of every 1000 women in the United States and Europe over the age of 40 years will develop ovarian cancer but only two out of these will be cured (DiSaia 1983).

Table 22.2. Staging of ovarian cancer*

Stage I	Growth limited to the ovaries.
	Stage Ia: Growth limited to one ovary; no ascites. 1. No tumour on external surface and capsule intact. 2. Tumour present on external surface and/or ruptured.
	Stage Ib: Growth limited to both ovaries; no ascites. 1. No tumour on external surface and capsule intact. 2. Tumour present on external surface and/or ruptured.
	Stage Ic: Same as Ia or Ib but ascites or tumour cells in peritoneal washings.
Stage II	Growth involving one or both ovaries with pelvic extension.
	Stage IIa: Involves uterus and/or fallopian tubes.
	Stage IIb: Extension to other pelvic tissues.
	Stage IIc: Same as IIa or IIb but ascites or tumour cells in peritoneal washings.
Stage III	Growth involving one or both ovaries with intraperitoneal metastases outside the pelvis or positive retroperitoneal nodes, or both. Tumour limited to the true pelvis with histologically proven extension to small bowel or omentum.
Stage IV	Growth involving one or both ovaries with distant metastases. Pleural fluid containing malignant cells. Parenchymal liver metastases.

* From Zaloudek and Kurman 1983.

Epithelial tumours of the ovary

BENIGN: Several types are recognized. Serous tumours are often in the form of thin-walled unilocular cysts which contain straw-coloured fluid. The cell lining is a single layer of flattened or cuboidal cells. Serous tumours may also have a papillary or solid pattern. Mucinous tumours are often multiloculated and the cysts contain thick viscous material. The cell lining is a single layer of mucus secreting columnar cells (*see Fig.* 22.3). Rupture of a mucinous tumour may give rise to pseudomyxoma peritoneii. Brenner tumours typically show nests of epithelial cells set in a fibrous stroma. Benign endometrial or mesonephroid tumours are rare.

MALIGNANT: Each of the above benign epithelial tumours has a malignant counterpart, and all are grouped together as ovarian carcinomas. Serous and mucinous cystadenocarcinomas tend to have papillary and nodular excrescences on their surfaces and penetrating their capsules. Endometrioid carcinomas are masses which may be cystic or solid and are histologically similar to endometrial carcinomas. Mesonephroid adenocarcinomas are usually cystic and histologically are composed of clear cells in a tubular or papillary pattern. Malignant Brenner tumours are exceedingly rare.

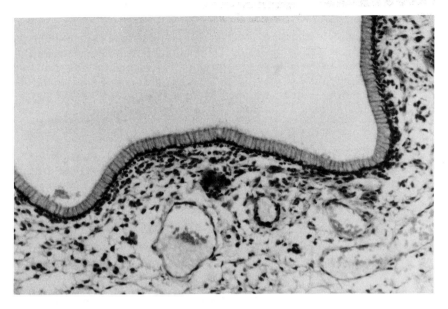

Fig. 22.3. Part of the wall of a mucinous cystadenoma. Note the mucus secreting epithelial lining. (H and E × 70)

BORDERLINE: This concept of 'borderline' tumours is now accepted by the International Federation of Gynaecology and Obstetrics (FIGO) and the World Health Organisation (WHO). They are described as 'neoplasms exhibiting an unusual degree of cellular proliferation, greater than that encountered in a benign form of the same type of tumour, but showing no destructive invasion of the stromal component' (Scully 1979). Features such as epithelial budding, multilayering of the epithelium, increased mitotic activity or nuclear atypia help to differentiate 'borderline' from 'benign', but the dividing line is not clearcut and is not universally agreed. The term 'borderline' usually refers only to serous or mucinous tumours.

Sex cord stromal tumours

Granulosa cell tumours occur mainly in premenopausal women. They are most commonly solid masses and about three-quarters of cases secrete oestrogens. The oestrogen secretion causes endometrial hyperplasia and, in a small proportion, endometrial carcinoma. Granulosa cell tumours are considered to be malignant although they are usually of low grade. Thecomas are also solid masses which secrete oestrogens. They are invariably benign. When a granulosa cell tumour or thecoma is suspected during a laparotomy, an endometrial curettage should be carried out to check for endometrial hyperplasia.

Androblastomas contain Sertoli cells or Leydig cells, or both, and they are often virilizing.

Germ cell tumours

These may be undifferentiated, in which case they are termed dysgerminomas and are similar to seminomas of the testes. Differentiation may take place into tissue not normally found in the embryo to form choriocarcinomas or yolk sac tumours. Alternatively, differentiation may be into tissue which is normally found in the embryo and this results in a teratoma. Many teratomas are benign and cystic (sometimes called a dermoid), although some may be malignant.

The presence of a neoplastic ovarian tumour at operation

The unexpected finding of a neoplastic tumour involving one ovary at the time of laparotomy by a general surgeon usually occurs in those patients where the indication for the laparotomy was an 'acute abdomen'. The common conditions responsible are:

1. torsion of a neoplastic ovarian cyst;
2. haemorrhage into a neoplastic ovarian cyst;
3. carcinoma of the ovary.

1. *Torsion of an ovarian cyst (see Fig. 22.4)*

At the time of operation the majority of twisted ovarian cysts are dark red in colour and there is obvious ischaemia which also involves the fallopian tube. In addition there is often a certain amount of bloodstained serous fluid in the peritoneal cavity.

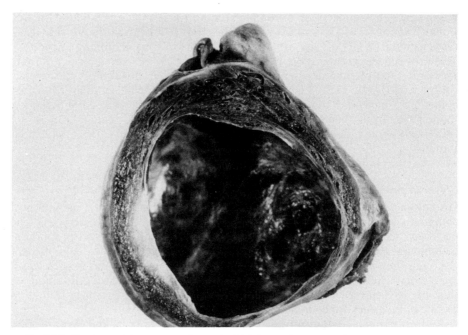

Fig. 22.4. Ovarian cyst (serous cystadenoma) which has undergone torsion.

Although the ovary may look very abnormal the tumour is usually benign.

Treatment is removal of ovary and tube. This may be relatively easy if the pedicle is narrow or difficult if it is very broad. Haemostasis is usually achieved by the careful positioning of the clamps, particularly if more than one is required for the pedicle. Ligature of the pedicle should be by transfixing and tying. All pedicles should be double tied.

If there are obvious signs of malignancy, or the patient is postmenopausal, then total hysterectomy should be carried out together with removal of the contralateral ovary and tube. The only exception would be in situations such as described below.

2. Haemorrhage into an ovarian cyst

In these patients, although the presenting symptoms and signs are similar to those with torsion, at operation the whole ovary may not be involved and removal of the cyst may be possible with conservation of some healthy ovarian tissue. The indications for hysterectomy and removal of the other ovary would be as previously described for torsion.

3. Carcinoma of the ovary

As emphasized earlier in this chapter, a knowledge of those features which are associated with malignancy and the staging of the condition allow for more adequate treatment. The age and reproductive status of the patient must also be considered.

The basic rule should be that if there is transcapsular extension to the broad ligament or the uterus then total hysterectomy and bilateral salpingo-oophorectomy should be carried out. As much as possible of the involved adjacent tissue should be removed, taking great care not to damage bowel. If the operator does not feel competent to remove the uterus, particularly in those cases where there is evidence of widespread metastases, then removal of as much of the ovarian mass as possible together with the other ovary should be carred out. Prophylactic removal of the omentum is still controversial; however, removal of as much omentum as possible, particularly if there are secondaries, is probably wise.

In a young woman whose reproductive capacity would be better preserved, if only one ovary with the capsule intact is involved, then removal of that ovary only should be considered.

Occasionally in a premenopausal woman only the ovarian tumour is removed because it was considered benign at the time of operation, although subsequent histopathological diagnosis is one of malignancy. The decision whether or not to reoperate in such a case is one which should only be made after consultation with the pathologist and gynaecologist.

The subsequent treatment of an ovarian carcinoma following the primary surgical procedure is best carried out by a gynaecological unit, preferably one that is experienced in oncology, as subsequent cytotoxic therapy will almost certainly be necessary. Radiotherapy may also be valuable in some cases. Unfortunately the prognosis for ovarian cancer remains poor and survival still depends largely on the clinical stage and the histopathology.

Conclusion

In a chapter such as this it would be impossible to cover every gynaecological emergency that might be encountered by the general surgeon. However, it is hoped that those which have been discussed will contribute towards satisfactory management of the patient.

References

DiSaia P. J. (1983) Ovarian cancer. (Forward). In : DiSaia P. J. (ed.) *Clinics in Obstetrics and Gynaecology*, Vol. 10, No. 2, pp. 153–4. Philadelphia, W. B. Saunders.

Hudson C. N. (1973) Surgical treatment of ovarian cancer. *Gynecol. Oncol.* **1**, 371–8.

Scully R. E. (1979) Tumors of the ovary and maldeveloped gonads. *Atlas of Tumor Pathology*, 2nd series, Fascicle 16. Washington D.C., Armed Forces Institute of Pathology.

Serov S. F., Scully R. E. (1973) Histological typing of ovarian tumours. *International Histological Classification of Tumours*, No. 9. Geneva, World Health Organisation.

Taylor R. W. (1981) Adverse menstrually-linked symptoms. In: Fisher A. M., Gordon H. (eds.) *Clinics in Obstetrics and Gynaecology*, Vol. 8, No. 1, pp. 111–20. Philadelphia, W. B. Saunders.

Zaloudek C., Kurman R. J. (1983) Recent advances in the pathology of ovarian cancer. In: DiSaia P. J. (ed.) *Clinics in Obstetrics and Gynaecology*, Vol. 10, No. 2, pp. 155–85. Philadelphia, W. B. Saunders.

Appendix

Surgery and Haemostasis

Elizabeth Mayne

Introduction

In recent years haemostasis has become more closely allied with modern surgery. Careful adjustment of the coagulability of the blood is necessary throughout cardiac by-pass procedures and is critical during the immediate postoperative period. Surgery is now acceptable in the haemostatically compromised patient. Today haemophilic patients undergo advanced orthopaedic operations; surgery for them is no longer confined to the emergency abdominal situation. Frequent correction of anticoagulant therapy is necessary to facilitate urgent surgery. The prevention of postoperative deep vein thrombosis is commonplace and many prophylactic regimes are advocated. Thus, the many advances in the field of blood coagulation have relevance for the surgeon. New knowledge has led to a better understanding of:

1. normal haemostasis;
2. haemostatic failure in acquired and inherited bleeding disorders;
3. the mode of action and limitations of current therapeutic and prophylactic anticoagulant therapy;
4. the place of thrombolytic therapy and role of fibrinolysis in the managment of thrombosis.

Background Physiology

Normally blood flows freely in the liquid state. Theoretically, at least, the maintenance of this steady state depends upon the equal but continuing opposing action of two enzyme systems. They are the coagulation or clot promoting system on the one hand and the fibrinolytic or clot dissolving system on the other. If the balance between the systems is upset pathologically, then increased coagulation or decreased fibrinolysis may result in intravascular thrombosis, whereas the converse, namely decreased coagulation or increased fibrinolysis may result in abnormal haemorrhage. Although this may be an oversimplification, it helps towards an understanding of the basic mechanisms of each system.

The coagulation system

There are three components which initiate physiological haemostasis in a phasic manner: blood vessels, blood platelets, and coagulation proteins (the clotting factors).

Immediately upon surgical or traumatic tissue injury (1) the vascular phase is initiated producing vasoconstriction, resulting in reduced blood flow. Simultaneously, (2) the particulate phase occurs; the blood platelets are activated. They adhere to the damaged capillary endothelium, sub-endothelial structures and to each other to form aggregates producing the temporary haemostatic plug. The third phase (3) is soluble and concerns the sequential activation of the protein factors. Prothrombin is activated to the proteolytic enzyme thrombin. It converts fibrinogen to the insoluble fibrin, which is laid down over and within the platelet plug, consolidating the sequence to produce permanent haemostasis.

Phase failure

Failure of (1) and (2) results in immediate persistent haemorrhage following injury, e.g. after dental extraction. This type of bleeding is characteristic of a low platelet count (less than $50 \times 10^9/l$) or severe platelet dysfunction, e.g. due to ingestion of aspirin or other antiplatelet drugs.

Failure of (3) results in delayed, persistent bleeding which may occur within the hour or up to several hours after the injury. In this situation (1) and (2) provide initial haemostasis but fibrin formation is delayed and weak. This type of bleeding is characteristic of the inherited 'haemophilia' states, liver disease and in the presence of oral anticoagulant therapy.

After completion of the three phases, the fibrinolytic mechanism exerts the major effect.

The fibrinolytic system

Physiological activation occurs during fibrin formation. The components of the system are also proteins but they are fewer in number compared with the coagulation system. Following stimulation an inactive precursor plasminogen is converted to another active proteolytic enzyme plasmin, which digests excess fibrin, clears it from the vascular bed and initiates the process of repair.

Excessive fibrinolytic activity may be associated with mental stress, severe shock and following strenuous exercise, but clinical bleeding is not usual in such situations. Many tissues in the body contain high levels of plasminogen activator, e.g. lung, uterus and prostate. Surgery of these organs can thus be associated with abnormal bleeding due to overactive fibrinolysis. Therapeutic activation of plasminogen can be achieved by i.v. infusion of streptokinase or urokinase. Recently tissue-type plasminogen activator has been isolated and characterized. It has aroused great interest as a potentially better thrombolytic agent and early studies indicate benefit in coronary artery thrombosis.

Clinical Haemostatic Problems

Defects associated with the coagulation system are more common than those arising from abnormal fibrinolysis. They are best considered in terms of the three phases of coagulation.

Vascular phase

There are only a few rare inherited disorders of collagen in this category, e.g. pseudoxanthoma elasticum and Ehler–Danlos syndrome, which, for the most part, can be disregarded.

Particulate phase

THROMBOCYTOPENIA: The most commonly encountered acquired abnormal bleeding is as the result of a low platelet count, usually $50 \times 10^9/l$ or less. In cases of suspected antiplatelet drug ingestion, e.g. aspirin, dipyridamole (Persantin) and the non-steroidal anti-inflammatory drugs, platelet aggregation studies should be performed. Correction of quantity or quality by platelet transfusion is readily available from most hospital blood banks. The only contraindication is in those patients with a known platelet antibody, e.g. multi-transfused patients or those suffering from autoimmune platelet disorders.

Soluble phase

Herein lies the largest and most common category of bleeding problems due to deficiency of one or more clotting proteins. The natural *in vivo* activation of coagulation is via tissue injury. The laboratory *in vitro* equivalent is contact with a plain glass surface. When freshly shed blood is placed in a glass tube, it solidifies and after 3–8 minutes the tube may be inverted without spilling. This represents the three phases of clotting and is known as the whole blood clotting time. It is a crude test, has fallen into disuse and has no place in the present day investigation of clotting defects. *In vivo* 'tissue juice', technically termed thromboplastin, can speed up the process of fibrin formation, e.g. amniotic fluid is the body's richest source of thromboplastin. If even a few millilitres are released into the maternal circulation, devastating acceleration of clotting occurs, with compensatory fibrinolysis and subsequent external bleeding. In miniature, different forms of thromboplastin are added to the patient's anticoagulated plasma in two test systems to yield the maximum information regarding defects.

Two clotting tests are commonly used as follows:

1. PT OR PROTHROMBIN TIME (utilizing brain thromboplastin): Normal time = 12 seconds $\pm$ 1 second. Prolongation of this result may indicate deficiency of: fibrinogen (factor I), prothrombin (factor II), or factors V, VII or factor X.

2. APTT OR ACTIVATED PARTIAL THROMBOPLASTIN TIME: Normal time = 35–50 seconds, depending on the individual laboratory. Prolongation indicates a deficiency of any clotting factor except factor VII. The test is specially sensitive to a deficiency of factors VIII, IX and X.

Equal prolongation of both tests suggests the presence of heparin or other circulating anticoagulant which can be verified by further specific tests. Individual factor assays are carried out for clarification of the problem.

Clotting Factor Disorders

Clotting factors are all proteins, except Factor III which is a lipid derived from platelets, and factor IV which is ionized calcium.

Six factors are synthesized in the liver: fibrinogen (factor I), prothrombin (factor II), and factors V, VII, IX and X. Four of these liver factors require vitamin K for their synthesis: prothrombin (factor II), and factors VII, IX and X.

The mode and sequence of these factors and how they are activated is shown in *Fig.* A1.1.

Disorders of clotting factors may arise in a variety of clinical situations, some of which are discussed below.

COAGULATION MECHANISM

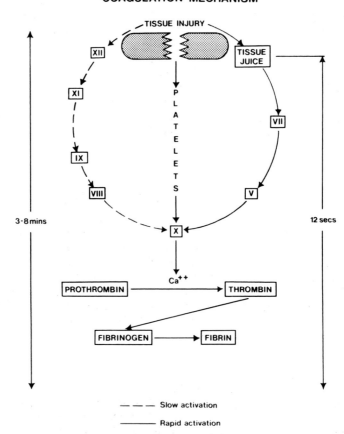

Fig. A1.1. Schematic diagram of normal haemostasis.

Liver disease

There is a variable defect of clotting factor synthesis dependent upon liver pathology, consequent upon the extent of damage to the hepatocyte. It is reflected by prolongation of the PT and, if severe, the APTT is also affected. If portal hypertension and splenomegaly are present, there may be additional thrombocytopenia due to hypersplenism. Diagnostic percutaneous biopsy should not be carried out without haemostatic cover if the PT is greater than 4 seconds longer than the control. Cover may be provided by fresh frozen plasma and platelets for either surgery or biopsy. Full coagulation studies should be carried out beforehand.

Vitamin K deficiency and correction of oral anticoagulant therapy

Malabsorption, obstruction to the common bile duct and oral anticoagulant therapy all prolong the prothrombin time due to vitamin K deficiency. The commonest oral anticoagulant in use is warfarin, derived from 4-hydroxycoumarin. Recommendations on reversal of its effect are influenced by the risks of introducing hepatitis from plasma concentrates and the dangers of over-correction with vitamin K, especially in patients with prosthetic or replacement heart valves. The use of fresh frozen plasma is advised with low dose vitamin K (2–5 mg). Doses in excess of 10 mg induce warfarin resistance as excess of the vitamin may remain within the circulation for up to three weeks. Plasma factor concentrates may be obtained in dire emergency. Vitamin K may be given to malabsorption patients but it has little benefit to offer patients with cirrhosis.

Massive blood transfusion

A unit of donor fresh blood contains active platelets and clotting proteins. Little or no platelet activity remains 72 hours after donation. After 21 days, 70% of all clotting activity is lost. Thus a bleeding patient may continue to haemorrhage despite receiving large quantities of blood due to lack of haemostatic content. It occurs after three-quarters to total blood volume replacement. It is advisable to use 'fresh' blood, not more than 48 hours old, after every 4–5 units of transfused old blood or packed cells. Platelets may be obtained separately as needed. Infusions of calcium are not necessary except in the case of liver disease, where citrate toxicity may be a problem. 10 ml 10% calcium gluconate should be given per litre of transfused blood. There is always enough ionised calcium in the body for haemostasis.

Disseminated intravascular coagulation (DIC)

Disseminated intravascular coagulation is a syndrome of multiple aetiologies, characterized by excessive bruising, with or without jaundice, external bleeding and—in its most severe form—incoagulable blood. Typical laboratory findings are reduced platelets, raised fibrin degradation products (FDP's) and depletion of all clotting factors to a variable degree. The common component of the underlying pathologies is the release of 'tissue juice' or thromboplastin into the circulation. Thus, intravascular clotting is initiated, fibrin is deposited within the capillaries, compensatory fibrinolysis attempts to reverse the balance and eventually overt haemorrhage occurs. The severity of the clinical problem depends upon the source, amount and potency of the thromboplastin released.

Severe DIC with extensive haemorrhage occurs in the following:

1. amniotic fluid embolism,
2. abruptio placenta,
3. multiple trauma such as crush injuries,
4. metastasizing carcinoma (adenomucinous tumours in particular),
5. progranulocytic leukaemia.

Moderate DIC with intravascular haemolysis occurs in the following:

1. prosthetic cardiac valves,
2. intracardiac defects, e.g. Fallot's tetralogy,
3. malignant hypertension and severe pre-eclampsia,
4. incompatible blood transfusion,
5. haemolytic uraemic syndrome,
6. snake bites.

Finally, DIC may have an infectious stimulus via the toxins of Gram-negative bacterial septicaemia, usually caused by coliforms or the meningococcus.

Treatment is that of dealing appropriately with the underlying disorder, accompanied by haemostatic support in the form of fresh frozen plasma and platelets. Initial treatment with heparin can be beneficial in cases of amniotic fluid embolism and during the early stages of repair in multiple trauma cases. A reduction in the standard dose of heparin is necessary in the presence of profound thrombocytopenia (less than $50 \times 10^9/l$). Normally, platelets contain a natural anti-heparin factor called platelet factor 4 (Hardisty and Ingram 1965).

Inherited bleeding disorders

These are genetic deficiencies of a single clotting factor. The most common are classical haemophilia and Christmas disease, the latter so called after Robert Christmas, the first patient diagnosed in 1952.

Haemophilia A (factor VIII deficiency) 1 : 25 000 population
Haemophilia B or
Christmas disease (factor IX deficiency) 1 : 100 000 population

Clinically, they are identical and have the same sex linked recessive mode of inheritance. The difference lies in the form of treatment.

Surgery is now commonplace in such patients. It varies from routine dental extraction to extensive orthopaedic joint replacement operations. All patients undergoing major surgery require to attain 100% circulating clotting factor beforehand. Replacement therapy is achieved by regular infusions of heat treated human factor VIII or factor IX concentrate.

Dose calculation

$$\text{Dose in no. of units required} = \frac{\% \text{ rise required} \times \text{weight in kg}}{k}$$

k = 1·5 for human VIII concentrate
k = 0·7 for IX material

Infusions are repeated at 8–12 hourly intervals, intravenously, until primary haemostasis and healing have commenced, usually for a minimum of 5–6 days. Thereafter they are continued daily for a full 14 days or longer, depending upon the type and extent of surgery. Antibiotic cover is also provided as any bleeding may serve as a ready culture medium for bacteria. The extraction of 2–3 teeth may be achieved by a simplified regime and the reader is referred to specialist manuals for further management details. Similarly, treatment of the other rare lifelong bleeding disorders is well documented (Bloom and Thomas 1981).

Therapeutic and Prophylactic Use of Heparin

As implied by the name, heparin was initially purified from liver. It is a naturally occurring sulphated glycosaminoglycan, produced by mast cells. Virtually all heparin in use in the United Kingdom is prepared from porcine intestinal mucosa.

Action

This results from the heparin binding to a naturally occurring inhibitor of clotting called antithrombin III. The binding neutralizes the activation of several clotting factors and interferes with thrombin formation, hence delaying the production of fibrin. The onset of action is rapid compared with oral drugs and is reversed by giving protamine sulphate.

Heparin does not cross the placenta and does not enter maternal milk. It is metabolized in the liver and a degraded form is excreted in the urine.

Mode of administration

Heparin must be administered parenterally, otherwise it would be inactivated by binding with gastric protein. It should not be given via an intramuscular route.

There are three modes of administration:

1. continuous i.v., thought to be the best method for established thrombi;
2. intermittent i.v.;
3. subcutaneously utilizing the adipose tissue of anterior abdominal wall.

Dose regimes

These are different depending on whether the patient has an established thrombus or whether the heparin is being given prophylactically, e.g. pre-surgery.

Established thrombosis

Give a loading dose of 5000 iu i.v. and continue with a further 35 000 units in a 24-hour period. Total = 40 000 units for average build 70 kg patient/24 hours.
Or—
10 000 units i.v. every 6 hours;
Or—
15 000 units i.v. every 8 hours.

Or—

15 000 units subcutaneously every 12 hours (this results in a wide variation of blood level of heparin).

MONITORING: Daily monitoring is advised at the same time each day. Many tests are available and at present the activated partial thromboplastin time is recommended (APTT). A broad guide is $1\frac{1}{2}$–$2\frac{1}{2}$ times the mean control reading. It should be emphasized that clinical assessment is more important than meticulous adherence to laboratory results. All samples of urine should be tested for blood, for early detection of overdosage.

ANTIDOTE FOR EXCESSIVE DOSAGE: 1 mg of protamine sulphate will neutralize 100 units heparin. A solution of 1% protamine sulphate is usually available in vials of 10 ml. Therefore 10 ml of 1% solution will neutralize 10 000 units of heparin. In cases of clinical haemorrhage it is customary to half neutralize a patient's 24-hour dose of heparin. Excess protamine sulphate is dangerous as it, in excess, may act as an anticoagulant.

Prophylactic use of heparin for prevention of deep vein thrombosis

There is a heparin co-factor circulating called anti-Xa. It has been found that very small doses of heparin enhance its activity to prevent generation of thrombin without impairing normal haemostasis at surgery:

     1 unit of Xa = 50 units thrombin

     1 µg of heparin can neutralize 32 units of Xa

thus   1 µg of heparin can prevent formation of 1600 units of thrombin.

DOSE: 5000 iu heparin subcutaneously $2\frac{1}{2}$ hours pre-operatively and no more until 8 hours post-surgery has elapsed, then 5000 iu subcutaneously 8-hourly until patient is up and well. The dose may be increased for patients over 70 kg body weight.

Excess Fibrinolysis

This condition seldom occurs spontaneously in isolation except in the rare cases of alpha$_2$ anti-plasmin deficiency. It may be associated with the DIC syndrome and occasionally it can complicate lung, uterine or prostatic surgery. Therapeutic fibrinolysis is an integral part of thrombolytic treatment utilizing streptokinase or urokinase. The diagnosis of excess fibrinolysis is established by:

1. reduced levels of fibrinogen, usually less than 0·70 g/l;
2. accelerated euglobulin lysis time, usually less than 100 minutes;
3. increased levels of fibrinogen degradation products (FDP's), usually greater than 160 µg/ml and up to 2560 µg/ml.

Treatment is by the administration of either oral or intravenous tranexamic acid, the antifibrinolytic drug cyclokapron (oral dose = 1·0 g q.d.s. duration 2–3 days to 1 week; intravenous dose = 15 mg/kg body weight hourly until bleeding stops or clotting tests are normalized).

Caution is needed in cases of haematuria or renal impairment and the advice of a haematologist should be sought. Likewise careful clinical and laboratory monitoring of thrombolytic therapy is essential to avoid haemorrhagic complications.

References

Bloom A. L., Thomas D. P. (1981) *Haemostasis and Thrombosis*, pp. 371–88. Edinburgh, Churchill Livingstone.

Hardisty R. M., Ingram G. I. C. (1965) *Bleeding Disorders (Investigation and Management)*, p. 138. Oxford, Blackwell Scientific Publications.

Index

Abdominal pregnancy, 666
Abscess
  cerebral, 607–8
  extradural, 608
  ovarian, 667
  paravertebral, 608
  spinal, 608
  subarachnoid, 608
  subdural, 608
  tubo-ovarian, ruptured, 667
Acalculous cholecystitis, 182–3
Achalasia, oesophageal, 31–3
  complications, 33
  secondary, 33
  treatment, 33
Achondroplasia (short limb dwarfism), 573
Acoustic neuroma, 632–3
Acquired immune deficiency syndrome (AIDS),
      424
  Kaposi's sarcoma, 10, 424
Acral lentiginous melanoma, 513
Actinic keratosis, 500
Actinomycosis
  breast, 294
  cervicofacial, 3
Activated partial thromboplastin time, 677
Adamantinoma, 564
Addison's disease (primary chronic adrenal
      insufficiency), 486
Adenomatoid tumour, paratesticular, 276
Adenomyomatosis, 186
Adrenals, 477–91
  acute insufficiency, 485
  adenoma
    Cushing syndrome due to, 481–2
    primary hyperaldosteronism due to, 483
    sex hormone overproduction, 485
  carcinoma
    Cushing's syndrome due to, 482
    primary hyperaldosteronism due to, 483
    sex hormone overproduction, 485
  chronic insufficiency
    primary (Addison's disease), 486
    secondary, 486
  congenital hyperplasia, 484–5
  cortex, 477, 478
    hypofunction, 485–6
    physiology, 477–8
  medulla, 477
    hyperplasia, 486
    physiology, 478
    tumours, 486–7
  myelolipoma, 491
  structure, 477
  traumatic necrosis post-surgery, 485

Adult hyaline membrane disease *see* Adult res-
      piratory distress syndrome
Adult respiratory distress syndrome (shock
      lung; pump lung; adult hyaline mem-
      brane disease; respirator lung; stiff
      lung syndrome), 397–400
  acute pancreatitis-induced, 202
  aetiology, 397–9
  associated conditions, 397 (table)
  clinical features, 399
  morphology, 399
  pathogenesis, 397, 398 (fig)
  prognosis, 399–400
Afferent loop obstruction, 62
Aflatoxins, 167
Air embolism, 358
Alcohol
  liver disease due to, 153–4; *see also* Cirrhosis
      of liver
  pancreatic juice in alcoholics/controls, 204
  pancreatitis due to, 197, 204
Allograft, 644
Alpha-1-antitrypsin, 156, 158
  deficiency, 390
Alpha-fetoprotein, 168, 170, 267
Alveolar duct, 378
Alveolar sac, 378
Alveolus, 378
Amazia, 293
Ameloblastoma, 10
Amoebic dysentery, 97
Amoebic hepatic abscess, 164
Amoebic pericarditis, 349
Amylase, 194
Amyloidosis, splenic, 441
Anal canal, 132–3
  malignant melanoma, 142
  squamous cell carcinoma, 140–1
  see also entries under Anorectal
Anal fissure, 135
Anal region
  basal cell carcinoma of margin, 140
  squamous carcinoma of margin, 139
Aneurysm(s), 362–9
  abdominal aortic, 363–5
  berry, 613–15
  dissecting, of aorta, 366–9
    complications, 368–9
    prognosis, 369
  false, 363
  femoral artery, 365
  mycotic, 615
  popliteal artery, 365
  splenic artery, 366
  subclavian artery, 365

Aneurysm(s) (*cont.*)
  thoracic aortic, 365
  traumatic, of cerebral vessels, 615
  true, 363
Aneurysmal bone cyst (multilocular haematinic
    bone cyst), 565–6
Angina pectoris, 332–3
  stable, 332
Angiodysplasia, 105–6
Angiofollicular hyperplasia, 434–5
Angioimmunoblastic lymphadenopathy, 434
Angiolipoma, 529
Angioma, cavernous, 637
Angiomyoma (vascular leiomyoma), 529
Angiosarcoma *see* Haemangiosarcoma
Ankylosing spondylitis, 582–3
Anorectal abnormalities, 133
Anorectal abscess, 135, 136 (fig)
Anorectal fistula, carcinoma of, 141
Anti-thymocyte globulin, 655–6
Antral G-cell hyperplasia, 63, 64
Aorta
  arch abnormalities, 328
  coarctation, 326–8
    postductal (adult), 326–7
    preductal (infantile), 327–8
Aortic regurgitation, 340
Aortic stenosis
  calcific, 326, 345
  congenital, 325–6
    subvalvular, 326
    supravalvular, 326
  rheumatic, 340
Aorto-coronary bypass graft pathology, 337–8
Apert's syndrome, 602
Aphthous ulcers (recurrent oral ulceration), 11
Appendicitis, 125–7
Appendix, 125
  mucocoele, 127
  tumours, 127–9
APUD cells, 108
Arachnoid mater, 600
Argentaffinoma *see* Carcinoma tumours
Arias-Stella reaction, 664–5
Arnold-Chiari malformation, 603, 604 (fig)
Arsenic, exposure to, 171
Arsenical keratosis, 501
Arterial embolism, 357–8
Arterial thrombosis, 356–7
Arteries, 351
Arterioles, 351
  arteriolosclerosis, 353
Arteriosclerosis, 353
Arteriovenous fistulas, 358–9
Arteriovenous malformations, cerebral, 638
Arthritis
  septic, 548–9
  tuberculous, 549–50
Asbestos, 402
  long tumour due to, 402

Asbestos (*cont.*)
  mesothelioma due to, 413–14
Aschoff bodies, 339–40
Ascites, 162
Aseptic (avascular) necrosis of bone, 592–3
Aspergilloma, 384, 385
Aspergillosis, 385
Aspergillus, 167
Astrocytoma, 626–7
  anaplastic, 628
  pilocytic, 627–8
  prognosis, 628
Atelectasis, 391
Atheroma, 352 (fig), 353–5
  morphology, 355
  pathogenesis, 354–5
Atrial septal defect, 321–3
  endocardial cushion, 323
  primum, 323
  secundum, 322, 323
  sinus venosus defect, 323
Axonotmesis, 622

Baker's cyst, 581
Balloon atrial septostomy (Rashkind), 330
Barrett's oesophagus, 38–9, 39–40
Barrett's ulcer, 37
Bartholin's abscess, 658–9
Basal cell papilloma (seborrhoeic keratosis),
    498–9
Basal ganglia, 598
Basilar artery, 599
  fusiform dilatation, 615
B-cells (lymphocytes), 421
  lymphomas, 431–2
  transformation, 431
Benign lymphoepithelial lesion, 16–18
Benzidine, 253
Berry aneurysm, 613–15
Beta-human chorionic gonadotrophin, 264
Beta-naphthylamine, 253
Bezoar, 78
Bile, supersaturation of, 177
Bile ducts
  atresia, 175–6
  benign tumours, 188
  carcinoma *see* Cholangiocarcinoma
  cysts/dilatations, 174–5
    type 1 (choledochal cyst), 175
    type 2, 175
    type 3 (choledochocoele), 175
    type 4 (Caroli's disease), 175, 181
  intrahepatic, congenital atresia, 147
  obstruction, 147
  papillomatous, 188
  strictures, 185–6
    post-inflammatory, 185
    stenosis of papilla, 186
    traumatic, 185–6

Bile gastritis, 63
Biliary atresia, 175–6
Biliary cirrhosis,
    primary, 147, 155, 158
        hepatocellular carcinoma associated, 167
    secondary, 155, 158, 181
Biliary colic, 178
Biliary-enteric fistula, 182
Biliary system, 173–91
Bilirubin, 145
Bizarre smooth muscle tumour (leiomyoblas-
    toma; epitheloid smooth muscle
    tumour), 76
B-K mole syndrome (familial atypical mole/ma-
    lignant melanoma syndrome), 509
Bladder
    adenocarcinoma, 257
    biopsy, 220
    carcinoma-in-situ, 256
    congenital abnormalities, 224
        diverticula, 241
        ectopia vesicae, 224
        persistent urachus, 224
    development, 219–20
    dysplasia, 257
    fistulas, 241
    metaplastic conditions, 234
    obstructive uropathy changes, 239
    proliferative conditions, 234
    squamous carcinoma, 257
    structure, 220
    transitional cell carcinoma, 253–6
        aetiology, 253
        clinical features, 254
        epidemiology, 253
        morphology, 254–5
        prognosis, 256
        recurrence, 256
        spread, 256
        staging, 255, 256 (fig)
    tuberculosis, 232
    vaginal-type epithelium, 234
Blalock-Taussig operation, 329
Blast lung see Adult respiratory distress
    syndrome
Blastoma, pulmonary, 410
Blood coagulation, 675–8
    phase failure, 676
Boerhaave's syndrome, 43
Bone, 543
    anatomy of long bones, 542, 543 (fig)
    aseptic (avascular) necrosis, 592–3
    blood supply, 544–5
    cells, 542–3
    inherited dysplasias, 573–6
        with dwarfism, 573–4
        without dwarfism, 574–5
    post-menopausal loss, 584
    tumours, 552–64
Bowenoid papulosis, 287

Bowen's disease, 287, 501
Bradykinin, 199
Brain, 597–9
    abscess, 607–8
    biopsy, 601–2
    blood supply, 599–600
    histology, 600–1
    see also entries under Cerebral
Branchial cyst, 35–6
Branchial fistula, 26
Branchial sinus, 26
Breast, 291–318
    abscess, 293
        retromammary, 293
    actinomycosis, 294
    biopsy, 292–3
    carcinoma see below Breast carcinoma
    congenital abnormalities, 293
    cystosarcoma phyllodes (phyllodes tumour),
        314–15
    fat necrosis, 295
    fibroadenoma, 299
        giant, 300
        juvenile, 300
    fibrocystic disease (fibroadenosis), 295–8
        aetiology, 296
        carcinoma in, 298
        clinical features, 296
        morphology, 296–8
    haematoma, 295
    male
        carcinoma, 316–17
        gynaecomastia, 316
    papillary lesions, 300–1
        intraduct papilloma, 301
        juvenile papillomatosis, 301
        papillary carcinoma, 301
    papillomatosis, 300
    sarcoma, 315–16
    tuberculosis, 293–4
Breast carcinoma
    classification, 306 (table), 307 (table)
    hormone receptors, 313–14
    in-situ, 302–4
        intraduct, 302–3
        lobular, 303–4
    invasive, 304–14
        adenoid cystic, 310
        aetiology, 305–6
        ductal, 308–9
        epidemiology, 304–5
        inflammatory, 311
        juvenile, 311
        lobular, 308
        medullary, with lymphoid stroma, 309
        mucoid, 310
        oestrogen window hypothesis, 305–6
        squamous, 310
        tubular, 310
        viral factors, 307

Breast carcinoma (*cont.*)
  male, 316–17
  minimal, 312
  papillary, 301
  prognosis, 312–13
Brock operation, 329
Brodie's abscess, 547
Bronchial arteries, 378
Bronchial biopsy, 379
Bronchial gland tumours, 411
Bronchial veins, 378
Bronchiectasis, 386–90
  aetiology, 387–8
  clinical features, 388
  congenital, 389
  follicular, 389
  morphology, 388–90
  pathogenesis, 387–8
  post-collapse, 389
  saccular, 389
Bronchioles, 377–8
Bronchitis, chronic, 390
Bronchogenic cysts, 380
Bronchopleural fistula, 413
Bronchopneumonia, 382
  tuberculous, 384
Bronchus, 377
Brown tumour, 585
Brucellosis, 551–2
Brunner's gland hyperplasia, 78–9
Brunn's nests, 234
Budd-Chiari syndrome, 161, 169
Buerger's disease (thromboangiitis obliterans),
  353, 361
Burkitt's lymphoma, 430, 432
Burns, 519–23
  aetiology, 519
  complications, 521–2
  morphology, 520–1
  pathogenesis, 519–20
  prognosis, 524

Cadmium, prostatic cancer related, 281
Calcifying epithelioma of Malherbe (pilomatri-
  coma), 518
Calcitonin, 584
Cancrum oris (noma), 3
Candida albicans
  oesophagitis, 44
  pulmonary infection, 385
  thrush, 3
Capillaries, 351
Carboxypeptidase, 194
Carcinogens, industrial, 253
Carcinoid syndrome, 345
Carcinoid tumours (argentaffinoma), 75
  appendiceal, 128
  gastric, 75

Carcinoid tumours (argentaffinoma) (*cont.*)
  lung, 410–11
  mucus secreting, 128–9
  small intestine, 109, 110 (fig)
Carcinosarcoma of lung, 410
Cardiac failure, left to right shunt, 324
Cardiogenic shock, 337
Cardiomyopathy, 345–6
  dilated, 346
  hypertrophic, 346
  restrictive/obliterative, 346
Caroli's disease, 174 (fig), 175, 189
Carotid body tumour, 26–8
Carpal tunnel syndrome, 622
Carr's concretions, 237
Cat-scratch disease, 423–4
C-cells, parafollicular, 450, 451
Cerebellum, 598
Cerebral biopsy, 601–2
Cerebral embolism, 610
Cerebral infarction, 610–11
Cerebral oedema, 618
Cerebral vascular disease, 608–15
Cerebrospinal fluid, 599
Cervical rib, 622
Chaga's disease, 34
Champagne-bottle leg, 474
Charcot-Bouchard microaneurysm, 610, 612
Charcot's joint, 551
Chemodectoma (paraganglioma), 27, 417
Chicken wire calcification, 559
Cholangiocarcinoma (carcinoma of bile ducts),
  188–91
  aetiology, 188–9
  epidemiology, 188–9
  clinical features, 189
  morphology, 189–90
  prognosis, 191
  spread, 191
Cholangiolocarcinoma, 190
Cholangitis
  ascending, 155, 158
    biliary obstruction-induced, 182
    liver abscess, 164
  primary sclerosing, 183–5
Cholecystitis
  acalculous, 182–3
  acute, 178–9
  chronic, 179–80
  emphysematous, 179
  gangrenous, 178
Cholecystohepatic duct, 173
Cholecystokinin, 174, 194
Choledochal cyst, 174 (fig), 175
Choledochal sphincter, 173
Choledochocoele, 174 (fig), 175
Choledochoenteric anastomosis, 173
Cholestasis, 146–7
  familial recurrent, 147
Cholesterolosis (strawberry gallbladder), 183

Chondroblastoma (epiphyseal chondroblastoma), 558–9
Chondrolysis, acute, 571
Chondroma, 557
Chondromyxoid fibroma, 539
Chondrosarcoma, 559–60
Chordee, 286
Chordoma, 563
Choriocarcinoma, 636
Choroid plexus tumour, 629
Christmas disease, 680–1
Chylomicrons, 354
Chylothorax, 413
Chymotrypsin, 194
Cigarette smoking
  carcinoma of bladder, 253
  carcinoma of pancreas, 209
Circle of Willis, 599, 600 (fig)
Cirrhosis of liver, 155–8
  aetiology, 155–6
  alcohol induced, 153–4
    morphology, 157, 158
  ascites, 162
  cryptogenic, 156
  hepatic failure due to, 158
  hepatocellular carcinoma, 167
  Indian childhood, 156
  morphology, 157–8
  pathogenesis, 156–7
  portal hypertension due to, 161
Clara cells, 377
Clonorchis sinensis, 178, 188
Clotting factor disorders, 678–81
  correction of oral anticoagulant therapy, 679
  disseminated intravascular coagulation, 679–80
  inherited bleeding disorders, 680
  liver disease, 678–9
  massive blood transfusion, 679
  vitamin K deficiency, 679
Clutton's joint, 551
Coccidioidomycosis, oral, 3
Coeliac artery compression, 358
Colitis
  indeterminate, 96
  infective, 97
  ischaemic, 103–4
  pseudomembranous, 97–8
  ulcerative, 89–90; *see also* Inflammatory bowel disease,
Collagen disease, pericarditis in, 349
Colloid cyst, 637
Colorectal cancer, 117–23
  adenoma-carcinoma sequence, 114–16
  aetiology/pathogenesis, 118
  complications, 122–3
  epidemiology, 117
  morphology, 119–20
  prognosis, 121–2
  spread, 120

Colovesical fistula, 102
Common bile duct, 173
  blood supply, 173
Condylomata accuminata, 139, 495
Congenital dislocation of hip, 568–9
Conn's syndrome (primary hyperaldosteronism), 482, 484 (fig)
Corolline thrombus, 373
Coronary artery(ies)
  anomalous origin, 328
  congenital aneurysm, 328
  fistula, 328
  intramural position, 332
  left, 333
    left dominance, 335–6
  right, 333–4
    right dominance, 334
  spasm, 332
Coronary thrombosis, 333
Courvoisier's sign, 209
Cranial nerves, 598–9
Craniopharyngioma, 636
Craniosynostosis, 602
Crigler-Najjar syndrome, 146
Crohn's disease, 91–2
  granulomas, 423
  mouth, 11
  see also Inflammatory bowel disease
Crouzon's syndrome, 602
Cryptococcosis, 386
Cushing's disease, 480–1
Curling's peptic ulcer, 55 (table), 56
Cushing's syndrome, 479–80
  adrenal adenoma-induced, 481–2
  adrenal carcinoma-induced, 482
Cutaneous horn, 501
Cylindroma, 411, 519
Cyst
  aneurysmal bone (multilocular haematinic bone cyst), 565–6
  colloid, 637
  dermoid, 12, 637
  solitary bone (simple/unicameral), 564–5
Cystic fibrosis, bronchiectasis in, 387
Cystic hygroma, 10
Cystinuria, 236, 238
Cystitis, 229
  follicular, 229
  ulcerative interstitial (Hunner's ulcer), 234
  see also Urinary tract infection
Cystitis cystica, 234
Cystitis glandularis, 234
Cytomegalovirus, in transplanted patients, 655
Cystosarcoma phyllodes (phyllodes tumour), 314

Da Nang lung *see* Adult respiratory distress syndrome

Dandy-Walker syndrome, 604
Dentigerous cyst, 10
Deoxyribonuclease, 194
De Quervain's thyroiditis (subacute thyroiditis),
    455
Dermatofibroma *see* Fibrous histiocytoma
Dermatofibrosarcoma protuberans, 531
Dermoid cyst, 12, 637
Descending perineal syndrome, 138–9
Desmoid
    abdominal (abdominal fibromatosis), 524–5
    extra-abdominal (extra-abdominal fibromato-
        sis), 525
Diabetes mellitus
    lower limb ischaemia, 353
    myocardial infarction, 332
    pancreatic carcinoma associated, 209
Diaphragmatic hernia, congenital, 380
Diastematomyelia, 605
Di-iodotyrosine, 451
Diphenylhydantoin (phenytoin), 435
Disappearing bone disease (massive osteolysis),
    562
Disseminated intravascular coagulation, 679–80
Diverticular disease of colon, 98–102
    aetiology, 99–100
    complications, 101–2
    epidemiology, 99
    morphology, 100
    pathogenesis, 99–100
Diverticulitis, acute, 101
Down's syndrome (trisomy-21), 54, 82, 221
Dressler's syndrome, 349
Dubin-Johnson syndrome, 146
Duchenne's muscular dystrophy, 321
Duct of Santorini, 192
Duct of Wirsung *see* Pancreatic duct
Duodenitis (pseudo-ulcer), 62
Duodenum
    Brunner's gland hyperplasia, 78–9
    congenital anomalies
        atresia, 54
        duplication, 54
        stenosis, 54
    diverticula, 78
    ulcer *see* Peptic ulcer
Dupuytren's contracture (palmar fibromatosis),
    524, 525 (fig)
Dura mater, 600
Dwarfism
    proportionate, 573
    short limb (achondroplasia), 573
Dysplasia, gastric, 68–9

Ebstein's anomaly, 325
Ecchondroma, 557
Ectopia vesicae, 224
Ectopic pregnancy *see* Extra-uterine pregnancy

Ehlers-Danlos syndrome, 321, 345, 359
Eisenmenger syndrome, 324
Elastase, 194, 199
Electrical osteogenesis, 543
Embolism, paradoxical, 324, 325
Emphysema, 390
    congenital lobar, 380
    surgical, 412
Empyema, 413
Encephalocoele, 602
Enchondroma, 557
Endodermal sinus tumour (yolk sac tumour),
    275, 636, 672
Endometriosis, 667–8
Endomyocardial fibrosis (Loeffler), 345
Entrapment syndromes, 358, 622–3
Eosinophilic granuloma, 567
Epididymis, 260–1
    abscess, 263
    cyst, 266
Epididymitis, 262–4
Ependymoma, 629
Epididymo-orchitis, 264
Epiphyseal chondroblastoma (chondroblas-
    toma), 558–9
Epispadias, 285
Epithelioid smooth muscle tumour (leiomyo-
    blastoma; bizarre smooth muscle
    tumour), 76
Epstein-Barr virus, 425, 428, 430
Epulis
    congenital, 12–13
    fibrous, 2
    giant cell, 12
Erdheim's cystic medial necrosis, 366
Erythroplakia, 5
Erythroplasia of Queyrat, 287
External carotid artery, fusiform dilatation, 615
Extradural abscess, 608
Extra-uterine (ectopic) pregnancy, 663–6
    clinical features, 663–4
    morphology, 664–5
    management, 665–6
Ewing's sarcoma, 561

False neuro-transmitters, 159–60
Familial atypical mole/malignant melanoma
        syndrome (B-K mole syndrome), 509
Fasciitis
    nodular (pseudosarcomatous), 523–4
    proliferative, 526
Fat embolism syndrome, 590–2
Fat necrosis, acute pancreatitis-induced, 203
Femoral artery, aneurysm of, 365
Femur
    shepherd's crook deformity, 566, 567 (fig)
    slipped upper epiphysis, 571
Fibrinolysis, 676

Fibrinolysis (*cont.*)
  excess, 682–3
Fibroid (leiomyoma), 659–61
Fibroma
  chondromyxoid, 559
  desmoplastic, 563
  non-ossifying (metaphyseal fibrous defect),
    566
Fibromatosis, 524–5
  abdominal (abdominal desmoid), 534–5
  extra-abdominal (extra-abdominal desmoid),
    525
  palmar (Dupuytren's contracture), 524, 525
    (fig)
  penile (Peyronie's disease), 524
  plantar, 524
Fibrosarcoma, 535
  bone, 563
  paratesticular, 276
Fibrous dysplasia, 566, 567 (fig)
Fibrous histiocytoma (dermatofibroma; scleros-
    ing haemangioma), 527–8
  malignant, 534–5
Fibroxanthoma, atypical, 531–2
Filariasis pericarditis, 349
Fistula-in-ano, 136–8
Floppy mitral valve syndrome (mitral valve pro-
    lapse) mid-systolic click syndrome),
    343–4
Floret giant cells, 529
Folliculitis, 494–5
Fournier's gangrene, 286–7
Frey's syndrome (gustatory sweating), 13
Friedreich's ataxia, 321
Functional renal failure (hepatorenal syn-
    drome), 158–9
Fusospirochetosis (acute necrotizing ulcerative
    gingivitis; Vincent's disease), 3

Galactosaemia, 156
Gallbladder, 173
  adenoma, 186
  adenomyoma, 186
  adenomyomatosis, 186
  benign tumours, 186
  blood supply, 173
  carcinoma, 186–8
    morphology, 187
    prognosis, 188
    spread, 187
    staging, 188
  congenital anomalies, 174
  empyema, 179
  mucocoele, 179, 180 (fig)
  papilloma, 186
  perforation, 179
  porcelain, 181
  Rokitansky-Aschoff sinuses, 180

Gallbladder (*cont.*)
  role in gallstones, 177
  strawberry (cholestrolosis), 183
Gallstones, 176–82
  cholesterol, 176–7, 177
  complications
    acute cholecystitis, 178–9
    ascending cholangitis, 182
    biliary cirrhosis, 181
    biliary colic, 178
    carcinoma of gallbladder, 186–7
    chronic cholecystitis, 179–80
    emphysematous cholecystitis, 179
    empyema of gallbladder, 179
    ileus, 182
    liver abscess, 182
    mucocoele of gallbladder, 179
    obstructive jaundice, 181
    pancreatitis, 197, 197–9, 202, 204
    perforation of gallbladder, 179
    porcelain gallbladder, 181
  mixed, 176–7, 177
  pigment (bilirubin), 177, 177–8
Gangliocytoma, 630
Ganglion (cutaneous), 498
Ganglioneuroblastoma, 490–1
  mediastinal, 417
Ganglioneuroma, 491
  mediastinal, 417
Gardner's syndrome, 117
Gastric atrophy, 67–8
  type A, 68
  type B, 68
Gastric carcinoma, 70–5
  adeno-squamous, 72
  aetiology, 70–1
  colloid, 71
  early, 73–5
    classification, 75
    prognosis, 75
  'epidemic' *vs* 'endemic', 71
  epidemiology, 70–1
  genetics, 71
  histological classification
    diffuse, 72
    intestinal, 72
  morphology, 71–2
  post-operative, 64–5
  pre-malignant conditions, 71
  prognosis, 72
  spread, 72–3
  stump, 64
  superficial spreading, 71
  squamous, 72
Gastric inhibitory peptide, 57
Gastrin, 215, 216
Gastrin cells, 212
Gastrinoma, 214–15
Gastritis, 66–8
  acute, 66–7

Gastritis (*cont*.)
  erosive, 66
  haemorrhagic, 66
  phlegmonous, 67
  chronic, 67–8
  atrophic, 67
  superficial, 67
  type A, 66, 68
  type B, 66, 68
Gastrocolic fistula, malignant, 71
Gastrointestinal haemorrhage, acute
    pancreatitis-induced, 203
Germ cell tumours
  intracranial, 636
  mediastinal, 417
  ovarian, 672
Germinoma, 636
Ghon complex, 384
Ghon focus, 384
Giant cell arteritis (temporal arteritis), 360
Giant cell tumour
  bone, 560–1
  tendon sheath, 531
Giant condylomata of Buschke and Loewen-
    stein, 495
Gilbert's syndrome, 146
Gingivitis, acute necrotizing ulcerative (Vin-
    cent's disease; fusospirochetosis), 3
Glioblastoma multiforme, 630, 631 (fig)
Glomus tumour, 77, 517, 562
Glossitis, median rhomboid, 11–12
Glottis, oedema, 3
Glucagonoma, 215
Glucocorticoids, 584
Glycogen tumour, 530
Goitre, 452
  non-toxic, 457–60
    aetiology, 457
    complications, 460
    malignant change, 460
    morphology, 459–60
    pathogenesis, 458
    sporadic, 459
  retrosternal, 460
  toxic nodular (thyrotoxicosis), 460, 462 (fig)
Gorlin's syndrome, 10
Granular cell myoblastoma, 13
Granuloma
  multifocal eosinophilic (Hand-Schüller-Chris-
    tian disease), 434
  pyogenic, 2, 517
  unifocal eosinophilic, 434
Grave's disease, 461
Gravitational (venous) ulcer, 374–5
Grawitz's tumour *see* Renal cell carcinoma
Gustatory sweating (Frey's syndrome), 13
Gynaecomastia, 316

Haemangioblastoma, 635

Haemangioendothelioma, 170, 562
Haemangiolymphangioma, 531
Haemangioma, 516–17
  bone, 562
  capillary, 516
  cavernous, 516–17
  hepatic, 170
  intestinal, 105
  juvenile, 516
  oral, 10
  sclerosing *see* Fibrous histiocytoma
  splenic, 443
Haemangiopericytoma, 532, 562
Haemangiosarcoma (angiosarcoma), 539, 563
  liver (Kupffer cell sarcoma), 170–1
  spleen, 444–5
Haematocoele, 266
Haematoma
  extradural, 618
  subdural
    acute, 618
    chronic, 618
Haemachromatosis, 155, 157, 158
  pancreatitis due to, 204
Haemophilia, 680–1
Haemorrhoids, 133–4
Haemosiderosis, 155
Haemostasis, 675–83
  problems, 676–7
    particulate phase, 677
    soluble phase, 677
    vascular phase, 677
Hairs, 494
Hamartoma, splenic, 443–4
Hand-Schüller-Christian disease (multifocal
    eosinophilic granuloma), 434, 567
Hashimoto's disease, 455–7
Hassall's corpuscles, 445, 446
  degeneration, 448
Head injuries, 615–21
  blunt: primary brain damage
    diffuse axonal injury, 617
    localized brain damage, 616
  blunt: prognosis, 621
  blunt: secondary brain damage, 617–21
    brain shifts, 620–1
    brain swelling, 618, 619 (fig)
    haematoma, 618
    epilepsy, 621
    hydrocephalus, 618, 621
    hypotension, 619
    hypoxia, 619
    infection, 618
    raised intracranial pressure, 620
    subarachnoid haemorrhage, 618
  penetrating, 621
Heart, 319–50
  congenital disease, 320–30
    acyanotic, with left to right shunt, 321–4
    acyanotic, without left to right shunt

Heart (*cont.*)
    left heart lesions, 325
    right heart lesions, 325–8
    causes, 321
    complications of left to right shunt, 324
    cyanotic, 328–30
    embryology, 321
    ischaemic disease, 331–7
        epidemiology, 331
        prognosis, 337
        risk factors, 331–2
    myxoma, 347–8
    rheumatic disease, 338–40
        aetiology, 338
        clinical features, 338–9
        epidemiology, 338
        morphology, 339–40
        prognosis, 340
    specific muscle disease, 345, 347
    tumours, 347
Heart valve prosthesis, 342–3
Heparin, 681–2
Hepatic encephalopathy, 159–60
Hepatic vein thrombosis, 161
Hepatitis
    alcoholic, 153, 154
    chronic active, 152–3, 158, 167
    chronic persistent, 152
    viral *see* Viral hepatitis
Hepatoblastoma, 170
Hepatocellular carcinoma, 166–70
    aetiology, 166–7
        cirrhosis of liver, 167
        hepatitis B, 166–7
        mycotoxins, 167
        oral contraceptives, 167
    epidemiology, 166
    clinical features, 167–8
    fibrolamellar variant, 170
    morphology, 168–9
    prevention, 169
    prognosis, 169
    spread, 169
Hepatolenticular degeneration (Wilson's disease), 156, 157, 158
Hepatoportal arteriovenous fistula, 161
Hepatorenal syndrome (functional renal failure), 158–9
Hereditary splenic hypoplasia, 437
Hereditary telangiectasia (Rendu-Weber-Osler disease), 10, 105
Herpangina, 3
Herpes simplex infection
    mouth, 2–3
    oesophagus, 44
Heterotopias, gastric, 69
Hiatus hernia, 39
    paraoesophageal (rolling hernia), 39
    sliding, presenting in infancy (partial thoracic stomach), 39–40

Hidradenoma papilliferum, 518
High density lipoproteins (HDL), 354–5
Hirschsprung's disease, 83–4
Histiocytoma, malignant fibrous, 534–5
Histiocytosis X, 434, 567
Histioplasmosis, 3, 386
Hodgkin's disease, 425–8
    prognosis, 428
    spread, 427
    stages, 427 (table)
    types, 425–7
Hodgkin's lymphoma of thymus, 448
Horn, cutaneous, 501
Howell-Jolly bodies, 437, 439, 441
Human T cell lymphotrophic virus type III (HTLV-III), 424
Hunner's ulcer (ulcerative interstitial cystitis), 234
Hunter's syndrome, 574
Hurler's syndrome, 573
Hürthle cell
    adenoma, 463, 464
    carcinoma, 467
Hutchinson's melanotic freckle (lentigo maligna), 510–11
Hydatid disease
    liver, 162–3
    spleen, 442
Hydatid of Morgagni torsion, 263
Hydrocalyx, 238
Hydrocephalus, 604–5
    normal pressure, 623–4
    post-head injury, 618, 621
Hydrocoele, 266
    infected, 263
Hydronephrosis, 238–9
    idiopathic, 239, 240 (fig)
Hydroureter, 238
Hyperaldosteronism
    primary (Conn's syndrome), 482–3
    secondary, 482
Hyperamylasaemia, 199
Hyperbilirubinaemia
    conjugated, 146–7
    unconjugated, 146
        congenital, 146
Hypercalcaemia, 235
Hypercalciuria, idiopathic, 235
Hypercholesterolaemia, 331
Hyperglycaemia, acute pancreatitis-induced, 203
Hyperlipidaemia, 331
Hypernephroma *see* Renal cell carcinoma
Hyperoxaluria, 235
Hyperparathyroidism (osteitis fibrosa cystica), 584–5
    intra-operative diagnosis, 474–5
    pancreatitis associated, 204
    primary, 472
    secondary, 475–6
    tertiary (persistent secondary), 476

Hypersplenism, 436–7
Hypertelorism, 602
Hyperthyroidism, 452, 584; *see also* Grave's disease
Hyperuricosuria, 235
Hypocalcaemia, acute pancreatitis-induced, 203
Hypoparathyroidism, 476
Hypospadias, 285–6
Hypothalamus, 598
Hypothyroidism, 452

Idiopathic mediastinal fibrosis, 418
IgA, in urine, 229
IgG, in urine, 229
Ileus, gallstone, 182
Immune deficiency states, bronchiectasis associated, 388
Immunoblast, 434
Immunosuppression problems, 655–6
Immunosuppressive drugs
   histological changes due to, 655–6
   side effects, 656
Impetigo, 484
Infectious mononucleosis, lymphadenopathy, 422–3
Infective endocarditis, 341–2
   left to right shunt, 324
Inflammatory bowel disease, 86–96
   aetiology/pathogenesis, 86–8
   complications, 93–5
   epidemiology, 86
   extra-intestinal manifestations, 95–6
   prognosis, 92–3
Infundibular pulmonary stenosis, 325
Insulinoma, 214
Internal carotid artery, 559, 560 (fig)
Interstitial cell tumour of testis (Leydig cell tumour), 274–5
Interstitial pneumonitis, 383
Intestinal bypass, liver disease following, 156
Intestinal failure, acute, 103
Intestinal ischaemia, 102–5
   chronic, 104
   focal ischaemia of small bowel, 105
Intestinal metaplasia, 68
Intracerebral haemorrhage, 612–13
Intracranial tumours
   metastatic, 640
   primary, 624–40
      aetiology, 624
      classification, 624, 625 (table)
      clinical features, 625–6
      epidemiology, 624
      location, 624–5
      malignancy, 626
      see also individual tumours
Intrarenal reflux, 227–8
Intussesception, 85–6

Islets of Langerhans, 194
Isograft, 644

Jaundice, 145–8
   acholuric, 145
   liver changes, 147
   obstructive, 181
   recurrent, of pregnancy, 147
   systemic effects, 147–8
Jod-Basedow effect, 460
Juvenile papillomatosis, 300

Kalliden, 199
Kallikrein, 199
Kaposi's sarcoma, 10, 424, 539–40
Kartagener's syndrome, 387
Kasai operation (porto-enterostomy), 176
Keloid, 528
Keratoacanthoma, 499–500
Keratosis
   actinic, 500
   arsenical, 501
   tar, 501
Kidney
   acute tubular necrosis, 159, 224–6
      aetiology, 224–5
      clinical features, 225
      morphology, 225–6
      pathogenesis, 225
      prognosis, 226
   biopsy, 220
   congenital abnormalities, 220–1
      bilateral agenesis (Potter's syndrome), 220
      calyceal cyst, 244
      contralateral fusion (horseshoe kidney), 221
      ectopic kidney, 221
      free supernumerary kidney, 221
      hypoplasia, 221
      ipsilateral fusion, 221
      unilateral agenesis, 220–1
   cystic dysplasia, 241–2
   cysts, 241–4
      calyceal, 244
      simple, 244
   development, 218
   function, 219
   functional failure (Hepatorenal syndrome), 158–9
   medullary cystia (nephronophthisis), 244
   medullary sponge, 244
   oncocytoma, 246
   polycystic disease
      adult, 243–4
      infantile, 242–3
   renal cell adenoma, 245
   renal cell carcinoma *see* Renal cell carcinoma

Kidney (*cont.*)
  structure, 218–19
  tuberculosis, 231
Killian's dehiscence, 44
Krukenberg tumour, 72
Kupffer cell sarcoma (haemangiosarcoma),
    170–1

Langerhans cells, 434
Laplace's law, 123, 363
Large intestine, 81–2
  cysts, 82
  duplication, 82
  endocrine tumours, 123
  lipoma, 124
  lymphoma, 123
  rotational abnormalities, 82
Lathyrism, 367
Leiomyoblastoma (epitheloid smooth muscle
    tumour; bizarre smooth muscle
    tumour), 76
Leiomyoma, 111–12, 123, 529
  gastric, 75–6
  hepatic, 170
  oesophageal, 45–6
  vascular (angiomyoma), 529
  uterine (fibroid), 659–61
Leiomyosarcoma, 536–7
  gastric, 75–6
  paratesticular, 276
Lentigo maligna melanoma, 510–11
Letterer-Siwe disease, 434, 567
Leukoplakia, 4–5
  penile, 287
Leydig cell tumour (interstitial cell tumour),
    274–5
Lichen planus, 3–4
Limb ischaemia, 352–3
  lower limb, 352–3
  upper limb, 353
Lines of Zahn, 357, 373
Linitis plastica, 71
Lipase, 194, 199
Lipid, 354–5
Lipodermatosclerosis, 374, 375
Lipoma, 528–9
  bone, 563
  hepatic, 170
  intermedullary, 529
  intramuscular, 529
  intraneural, 529
  pleomorphic, 529
  spindle-cell, 529
Lipoproteins, 354–5
Liposarcoma, 535–6, 563
Liver, 143–71
  abscess
    amoebic, 164

Liver (*cont.*)
    pyogenic, 164, 182
  adenoma, 165
  alcoholic disease, 153–4
  benign tumours, 170
  biopsy, 145
  cirrhosis *see* Cirrhosis of liver
  complications of advanced disease, 158–62
    encephalopathy, 159–60
    hepatic failure, 158
    renal, 158–9
  cyst
    hydatid, 162–3
    non-parasitic, 162
  development, 143
  fatty, 153, 154
  focal nodular hyperplasia, 165 (fig), 166
  function, 143–4
  haemangioendothelioma, 170
  haemangioma, 170
  haemangiosarcoma (Kupffer cell sarcoma),
      170–1
  hepatoblastoma, 170
  hepatocellular carcinoma *see* Hepatocellular
      carcinoma
  lipoma, 170
  partial nodular transformation, 166
  polycystic disease, 162
  secondary tumours, 171
  structure, 143–4
Liver fluke, 178, 188
Low density lipoproteins (LDL), 354–5
Lower limb ischaemia, 352–3
Ludwig's angina, 3
Lumbar disc degeneration/prolapse, 593–5
Lung
  abscess, 386
  accessory lobes, 381
  agenesis, 379
  atelectasis, 391
  benign tumours, 400–1
  biopsy, 379
  blood supply, 378
  bullous disease, 392
  congenital cystic adenomatoid malformation,
      380–1
  congenital/development abnormalities, 378
  cysts, 380
  development, 377
  hamartoma, 400
  hypoplasia, 380
  infections, 381–6
    fungal, 385–6
  lymph drainage, 378
  lymphoma, malignant, 412
  lymphomatoid granulomatosis, 412
  malignant tumours, 401–10
    adenocarcinoma, 406–7
    adenosquamous, 408
    aetiology, 401–2

Lung (*cont.*)
 blastoma, 410
 bronchial gland, 411
 bronchiolo-alveolar carcinoma (alveolar cell
  carcinoma), 407, 408 (fig)
 carcinoid, 410–11
 carcinosarcoma, 410
 clinical features, 403
 classification (WHO), 403 (table)
 large cell, 408
 morphology, 403–8
 mucoepidermoid, 411
 oat cell carcinoma, 406
 pathogenesis, 402
 prognosis, 409–10
 small cell carcinoma, 406
 spread, 408
 squamous carcinoma, 403–4, 405 (figs)
 staging, 409
 papillomatosis, 400
 pseudolymphoma, 412
 sequestration, 380
 structure, 377–8
Lymphadenitis
 non-specific, 422
 viral, 422–3
Lymphadenopathy
 angioimmunoblastic, 434
 dermatopathic, 435
 drug-induced, 435
 granulomatous, 423–4
 silicone, 435
Lymphangioma, 530–1
 spleen, 443
 tongue, 10
Lymph nodes, 420–1
 biopsy, 422
 granulomatous conditions, 422–4
 infective conditions, 422–4
Lymphoedema
 primary, 375
 secondary, 375
Lymphogranuloma venereum, 424
Lymphokines, 421
Lymphomatoid granulomatosis, 412
Lymphocytes, 421
Lymphoma
 B immunoblastic, 432
 Burkitt's, 430, 432
 follicle centre cell, 432
 gastric, 77
 histiocytic, 429
  true, 433
 increased incidence post-transplantations, 428
 large bowel, 123
 lymphocytic, 429, 431–2
 lymphoplasmacytic, 432
 lymphoplasmacytoid, 432
 mixed lymphocytic histiocytic, 430
 non-Burkitt's, 430

Lymphoma (*cont.*)
 primary malignant, 412, 634–5
 small bowel, 111
 splenic, 444
 T-cell, 433
 testicular, 274
 true histiocytic, 433
 undifferentiated, 430

Macroamylasaemia, 199
Macrophages, 421
Maffucci's syndrome, 557
Malakoplakia, 125, 233–4
Malignant fibrous histiocytoma, 534–5
Malignant melanoma
 anal canal, 142
 mouth, 9
 oesophagus, 50
 parotid metastases, 25
 skin, 509–15
Malignant mesothelioma of pericardium, 350
Mallory-Weiss syndrome, 43, 79
Mammary duct ectasia, 294–5
Marfan's syndrome, 321, 344, 345
 dissecting aneurysm of aorta, 366–7
Marjolin's ulcer, 374
Massive osteolysis (disappearing bone disease),
  562
Mastitis
 granulomatous, 294
 plasma cell, 295
Maxillary sinus, carcinoma, 10–11
Meckel's diverticulum, 82–3
Mediastinal fibrosis, idiopathic, 418
Mediastinitis, 418
Mediastinoscopy, 379
Mediastinum, 415–16
 developmental abnormalities, 416
 masses in 415 (table), 416–17
Medulla oblongata, 599
Medulloblastoma, 632
Megaduodenum, 66
Megalopenis, 284–5
Megaureter, primary obstructive (congenital),
  224, 240
Melanocyte disorders, 506–15
Melanoma
 acral lentiginous, 513
 desmoplastic, 513
 lentigo maligna (Hutchinson's melanotic
  freckle), 510–11
 malignant, 509–14
  prognosis, 514, 515 (table)
  spread, 514
  staging, 514 (table), 515 (fig)
 neurotrophic, 513
 nodular, 512 (fig), 513
 superficial spreading, 511, 512 (fig)
 unclassified, 513

Menétriér's disease, 77–8
Meninges, 600
Meningioma, 633–4
Meningitis
  bacterial, 605–7
  post-head injury, 618
Meningocoele, thoracic, 417–18
Merkel cell carcinoma, 519
Mesenchyme/Sertoli cell tumour, 274
Mesothelioma, malignant, 413–15
  peritoneal, 414
  pleural, 414
  staging, 415 (table)
Metabolic bone disease, 583–90
Metaphyseal fibrous defect (non-ossifying
    fibroma), 566
Metaplasia, intestinal, 68
Methotrexate, hepatic cirrhosis due to, 156, 157
Methyldopa, hepatic cirrhosis due to, 156
Michaelis-Gutmann bodies, 234
Micropenis, 283
Midbrain, 598
Mid-systolic click syndrome (floppy mitral valve
    syndrome; mitral valve prolapse),
    343–4
Mikulicz's syndrome, 16–18
Mitral valve
  congenital disease, 326
  miniaturization, 326
  prolapse (floppy mitral valve syndrome),
    343–4
  stenosis, 340
Mole, malignant changes, 510 (table); see also
    Melanoma
Molluscum contagiosum, 496
Mönckeberg's medial calcific sclerosis, 353
Mondor's disease, 295
Moniliasis (candidiasis), pulmonary, 385
Monocytes, 421
Mono-iodotyrosine, 451
Mucocoele, 15
Mucoepidermoid tumours, 411
Mucopolysaccaridoses, 573–4
Mucous glands, lack of in respiratory tract, 380
Multifocal eosinophilic granuloma
    (Hand-Schüller-Christian disease),
    454, 467
Multilocular haematinic bone cyst (aneurysmal
    bone cyst), 565–6
Multiple endocrine adenomatosis types 1 and 2,
    214, 475
Mural thrombosis, 337
Mustard operation, 330
Myasthenia gravis, 446–7
Mycetoma, 385
Mycotic aneurysm, 615
Mycotoxins, 167
Myelolipoma, 491
Myeloma, 562
Myoblastoma, granular cell, 13

Myocardial depressant factor (MDF), 202
Myocardial infarction, 333–6
  complications, 336–7
Myositis, proliferative, 526
Myxoma, cardiac, 347–8

Naevus
  white sponge, 3
  blue, 508
  compound, 507
  congenital, 509
  dysplastic, 509
  flammeus (salmon patch), 515
  halo, 508
  intradermal, 507, 508 (fig)
  junctional, 507
  spider, 516
  spindle cell (Spitz), 507–8
  strawberry, 516
Necrotizing sialometaplasia, 12
Nelson's syndrome, 481
Neonatal necrotizing enterocolitis, 84–5
Nephroblastoma see Wilms' tumour
Nephronophthisis (medullary cystic kidney), 244
Nerves, peripheral, 601
  injuries, 622–3
    neuronal response, 622
  tumours, 641
Neural tumour, mediastinal, 417
Neurilemmoma (schwannoma; neuroma), 632–3,
    641
  gastric, 77
  mediastinal, 417
Neuroblastoma, 489–90, 630
  mediastinal, 417
Neurofibroma, 633, 641
  gastric, 77
  mediastinal, 417
Neurofibrosarcoma, 417
Neuronal tumours, 630
Neuropraxia, 622
Neurotmesis, 622
Nipple
  absence, 293
  adenoma, 301
  Paget's disease, 311–12
  supernumerary, 293
Noma (cancrum oris), 3
Non-Cushing's stress ulcers, 55–6
Non-Hodgkin's lymphomas, 428–34
  classifications, 429–33
    Kiel, 430, 431–33
    Lukes-Collins, 430, 431
    Rappaport, 429–30
  prognosis, 433
  spread, 433
  stages, 427 (table), 433–4
  thymus, 448

Non-ossifying fibroma (metaphyseal fibrous defect), 566

Obstructive uropathy, 238–9
  prognosis, 239
Odontogenic epithelium, cysts/tumours, 10
Odontogenic keratocyst, 10
Oesophagitis
  candidal, 44
  herpes simplex virus, 44
  pre-malignant (Iran), 47
  reflux see Reflux oesophagitis
Oesophagus, 29–51
  achalasia see Achalasia
  anti-reflux mechanisms, 34–55
    failure, 35–6
  Barrett's, 38–9, 39–40
  benign tumours, 45–6
  carcinoma, 46–50
    aetiology, 46
    clinical features, 47
    epidemiology, 46
    morphology, 47–9
    pre-malignant conditions, 47
    prognosis, 49
    spread, 49
    staging, 50 (table)
  carcinosarcoma, 50
  Chaga's disease, 34
  congenital disorders
    atresia, 30–1
    cyst, 31
    duplication, 31
    stenosis, 31
    stricture, 31
    tracheo-oesophageal fistula, 30–1
    web, 31
  connective tissue disease, 34
  development, 30
  diffuse spasm, 33–4
  diverticula, 44–5
    epiphrenic, 45
    lateral pharyngeal, 44–5
    mid-oesophageal traction, 45
    pharyngeal, 44
  fibrous polyp, 45
  function, 29–30
  infections, 44
  leiomyoma, 45–6
  leiomyosarcoma, 50
  lower oesophageal sphincter, 30, 35
  malignant melanoma, 50
  oesophagitis see Reflux oesophagitis
  perforation, 43
  Schatzki's ring, 45
    squamous papilloma, 45
    varices, 40–3
      morphology, 40–1

Oesophagus (cont.)
  pathogenesis of bleeding, 41–2
  prognosis, 43
Oestrogen(s), 584
Oestrogen receptor (breast), 313–14
Ogilvie's syndrome, 125
Oligodendroglioma, 628–9
Ollier's disease, 557, 559
Oncocytoma of kidney, 246
Oophoritis, acute, 667
Opisthorchis viverrini, 188
Oral cavity, 1–13
  aphthous ulcers (recurrent oral ulceration), 11
  carcinoma-in-situ, 5
  connective tissue tumours, 10
  epithelial dysplasia, 5
  epulis
    congenital, 12–13
    fibrous, 2
    giant cell, 12
  fibro-epithelial polyp, 2
  fibrous hyperplasia, 1
  infections, 2–3
  pyogenic granuloma, 2
  spindle cell carcinoma, 9
  squamous carcinoma, 6–9
    aetiology, 6
    epidemiology, 6
    morphology, 6–9
    staging, 8
  squamous papilloma, 5
  traumatic ulcers, 1
  verrucous carcinoma, 9
  white lesions, 3–5
Oral contraceptives
  haemangiosarcoma (Kupffer cell sarcoma), 171
  hepatic adenoma, 165
  hepatocellular carcinoma, 167
  hepatic vein thrombosis, 161
Orchitis
  granulomatous, 264
  part of general infection, 264
  primary, 262–3
  syphilitic, 264
Osteitis fibrosa cystica see Hyperparathyroidism
Osteoarthrosis, 576–8
  aetiology, 576
  morphology, 577–8
  pathogenesis, 577
Osteoblast, 542–3
Osteoblastoma, 554
Osteocartilaginous exostosis (osteochondroma), 557–8
Osteochondritis, Parrot's syphilitic, 551
Osteochondroma (osteocartilaginous exostosis), 557–8
Osteoclast, 543
Osteogenesis imperfecta, 321, 345, 574–5
Osteoma, 553

Osteoma (*cont.*)
  osteoid, 553, 554 (fig)
Osteomalacia, 587
Osteomyelitis
  acute haematogenous, 545–7
  chronic, 547–8
  Garré's sclerosing, 547
  primary subacute, 547
  tuberculous, 549
Osteopetrosis, 574, 585–7
Osteosarcoma, 554–6
  Paget's disease associated, 557
  parosteal, 557
Ovary, 666–73
  androblastoma, 671
  carcinoma, 670 (table), 673
  epithelial tumours, 670–1
  follicular cyst, 667
  germ cell tumour, 672
  granulosa cell tumour, 671
  haemorrhage into cyst, 673
  inflammatory adnexae, 667
  luteal cyst, 667
  neoplasms, 669–73
    classification, 669 (table)
  sex cord stromal tumours, 671
  teratoma, 672
  thecoma, 671
  torsion of cyst, 672–3
Overwhelming post-splenectomy infection
  (post-splenectomy sepsis), 438, 439,
  440

Paget's disease of bone, 588–90
  osteosarcoma associated, 557, 590
Paget's disease of nipple, 311–12
Paget's disease of perianal skin, 139
Pancarditis, 339
Pancoast syndrome, 403
Pancreas, 192–217
  abscess, 203
  acinar cell carcinoma, 211
  annular, 66, 195
  autodigestion, 199
  biopsy
    intraoperative, 195
    preoperative, 194–5
  blood supply, 194
  carcinoma, 209–11
    acinar cell, 211
    aetiology, 209
    clinical features, 209
    epidemiology, 209
    morphology, 209–11
    prognosis, 211
    spread, 211
  congenital abnormalities, 195–6
  cysts, 206–8

Pancreas (*cont.*)
  congenital, 206
    neoplastic, 207
    non-epithelial (pseudocysts), 207–8
    retention, 207
  development, 192, 193 (fig)
  ectopic, 196
  endocrine tumours, 212–16
    clinical features, 212
    ectopic hormone production, 216
    gastrinoma, 214–15
    glucagonoma, 215
    insulinoma, 214
    morphology, 212–13
    non-functional, 212
    polypeptidoma, 215–16
    somatostatinoma, 215
    vipoma, 216
  exocrine tumours, 208–12
    carcinoma *see above* carcinoma
    dermoid cysts, 212
    fibrosarcoma, 212
    intraduct papilloma, 208
    leiomyosarcoma, 212
    lymphoma, 212
    mucinous cystic, 208–9
    neurogenic, 212
    pancreaticoblastoma, 212
    secondary carcinoma, 212
    serous cystadenoma, 208
    solid/cystic (papillary cystic neoplasms), 211
  functions, 194
  papillary cystic neoplasm, 211
  pseudocysts (non-epithelial cysts), 207–8
  structure, 192–4
  trauma, 197
Pancreas divisum, 195
Pancreatic duct (duct of Wirsung), 192
  rupture, 197
  variations, 192
Pancreatic juice, in alcoholics/controls, 204
Pancreaticoblastoma, 212
Pancreatic polypeptidoma, 215–16
Pancreatitis, 196–206
  acute, 196, 197–204
    aetiology, 197
    alcohol-induced, 197, 202
    children, 197
    clinical features, 199
    complications, 202–3
    fat necrosis, 200, 202 (fig)
    haemorrhage into pancreas, 202
    hereditary, 196, 209
    morphology, 200–2
    pathogenesis, 197–9
    prognosis, 203–4
    prognostic factors, 200
  chronic, 196, 204–6
    aetiology, 204
    Afro-Asian, 204

Pancreatitis (*cont.*)
    calcific, 205–6
    clinical features, 205
    complications, 206
    idiopathic, 204
    morphology, 205–6
    painless, 206
    pathogenesis, 204–5
  chronic relapsing, 196
  hereditary, 204
  classification, 196–7
  relapsing acute, 196
Papillary muscle rupture, 337
Paradoxical embolism, 324, 325
Paraganglioma (chemodectoma), 27
  mediastinal, 417
Paratesticular tumours, 276
Parathyroid, 471–7
  adenoma, 472–3
  blood supply, 471
  carcinoma, 474
  cyst, 476–7
  development, 471
  function, 471
  hyperplasia, 474
  mediastinal, 416
  structure, 471
  waterclear (*Wasserhelle*) cells, 474
  see also Hyperparathyroidism; Hypopara-
    thyroidism; Pseudohypoparathyroidism
Parathyroid hormone (parathormone), 471,
  583–4
Paravertebral abscess, 608
Parotitis, acute, 15
Parrot's syphilitic osteochondritis, 551
Partial thoracic stomach (sliding hiatus hernia
  presenting in infancy), 39–40
Paterson-Kelly syndrome (Plummer-Vinson syndrome), 6, 40
Pel-Ebstein fever, 425
Pelvic inflammatory disease, 661–3
Pendred's syndrome, 453
Penis, 284
  carcinoma, 287–8
  congenital/developmental abnormalities,
    284–5
Peptic ulcer, 55–65
  acute, 55–6
    causes, 55–6
    Curling's, 55 (table), 56
    Cushing's, 55, 56
  chronic, 56–62
    aetiology/pathogenesis, 57–9
      duodenal ulcer, 57–8
      gastric ulcer, 58–9
    complications, 60–2
      haemorrhage, 60–1
      malignancy, 61–2
      perforation, 61
      pyloric stenosis, 65

Peptic ulcer (*cont.*)
  epidemiology, 56–7
  morphology, 59–60
  post-operative pathology, 62–6
    afferent loop obstruction, 62–3
    bile gastritis, 63
    carcinoma, 64–5
    lesser curve necrosis, 62
    recurrent ulcer, 63–4
    pre-pyloric, 62
Pericarditis, 348–9
  acute non-specific, 348
  constrictive, 349
  infective, 348–9
Pericardium
  acquired defects/cysts, 348
  congenital defects/cysts, 348
  pseudocysts, 348
  tumours, 349–50
Periostitis, syphilitic, 551
Perisplenitis, 442
Peritonitis, spontaneous bacterial, 162
Persistent ischiadic artery, 358
Persistent ductus arteriosus, 324
Perthes' disease, 570–1
Peutz-Jeghers polyps, 70, 108
Peyronie's disease (penile fibromatosis), 286, 524
Phaeochromocyte, extra-adrenal, 417
Phaeochromocytoma, 487–8, 489 (fig)
Pharyngeal diverticulum (pouch), 44
  lateral, 44
Phimosis, 238, 285
Phlegmasia alba dolens, 374
Phlegmasia caerulea dolens, 374
Phenytoin (diphenylhydantoin), 435
Phospholipase, 194
Phospholipase A, 199, 202
Phylloides tumour (cystosarcoma phylloides),
  314–15
Phytobezoar, 78
Pia mater, 600
Pick's disease (chronic constrictive pericarditis),
  349
Pilomatricoma (calcifying epithelioma of Mal-
  herbe), 518
Pineal tumours, 629
Pituitary gland, 599
  adenoma, 638–40
  carcinoma, 640
Placental alkaline phosphatase, 268
Plagiocephaly, 602
Platelet derived growth factor, 354
Pleural, biopsy, 379
Pleuropericardial cyst (springwater cyst), 416
Plummer's disease (multiple toxic adenomata),
  460
Plummer-Vinson syndrome (Paterson-Kelly syn-
  drome), 6, 40
Plunging ranula, 15
Pneumatosis cystoides intestinalis, 124–5

Pneumonia
  atypical, 383
  bacterial, 381–2
  lobar, 382–3
  lymphoid interstitial, 412
  Pneumocystis carinii, 424
  staphylococcal, 412
Pneumothorax, 412
  tension, 412
Polyarteritis nodosa, 360
Polymazia, 293
Polyp
  colonic, 112–16
    hamartomatous, 112–13
    inflammatory, 113
    metaplastic, 113
    neoplastic, 113–16
  gastric *see under* Stomach
  lymphoid, rectal, 123
  Peutz-Jeghers, 70, 108
Polyposis coli
  familial, 116
  juvenile, 112–13
Pons, 599
Popliteal artery
  aneurysm, 365
  cystic degeneration, 362
  entrapment, 358
  idiopathic thrombosis/dissection, 362
Portal hypertension, 160–2
  causes, 160 (table)
  complications, 161
  extrahepatic, 160–1
  idiopathic, 161
  increased portal blood flow induced, 161
  intrahepatic, 161
  sectorial, 206
  spleen, 436 (fig)
  suprahepatic, 161
Portal tracts, pipe stem fibrosis, 161
Porto-enterostomy (Kasai operation), 176
Port wine stain, 516
Post-mastectomy lymphangiosarcoma (Stewart-
    Treves syndrome), 315 (fig), 316
Postphlebitic syndrome, 373–4
Post-splenectomy sepsis (overwhelming post-
    splenectomy infection), 438, 439, 440
Potter's syndrome (bilateral renal agenesis), 220
Pott's disease (tuberculous spondylitis), 550
Pregnancy tumours, 2
Priapism, 286
Proctitis, idiopathic, 96
Progesterone receptor (breast), 313
Progressive generalized lymphadenopathy, 424
Prostate
  benign nodular hyperplasia, 279–81
    aetiology, 279
    clinical features, 279–80
    epidemiology, 279
    morphology, 280–1

Prostate (*cont.*)
    pathogenesis, 279
    prognosis, 281
  biopsy, 277–8
  cancer, 281–4
    aetiology, 281
    clinical features, 282
    epidemiology, 281
    morphology, 282–3
    prognosis, 283, 284
    spread, 283
    staging, 283, 284 (table)
    terminology, 281
    treatment, 284
  structure, 276–7
Prostatitis
  acute bacterial, 278
  chronic bacterial, 278–9
  chronic non-bacterial, 279
  granulomatous, 279
Prothrombin time, 677
Psammoma, 467
Pseudo-hermaphrodite, 485
Pseudohypoparathyroidism, 476
Pseudolymphoma
  gastric, 76
  pulmonary, 412
Pseudo-obstruction, 125
Pseudotumour, 222
Pseudo-ulcer (duodenitis), 62
Pseudoxanthoma elasticum, 677
Pulmonary arteriovenous fistula, 381
Pulmonary artery, 378
  aplasia, 381
  stenosis, 325, 381
Pulmonary embolism, 392–6
  acute massive, 393
  acute minor, 393–4
  chronic, 394
  classification, 393–4
  groups I–V, 394
  morphology, 394–6
  pathophysiology, 393
  prognosis, 396
  pulmonary hypertension due to, 396
  submassive, 394
Pulmonary valve stenosis, 325
Pulmonary vascular resistence increase, 324
Pump lung *see* Adult respiratory distress syn-
    drome
Pyelonephritis
  acute, 229–30
  chronic, 230–1
  xanthogranulomatous, 231
  see also Urinary tract infection
Pyloric stenosis, 65–6
  adult hypertrophic, 65–6
  annular pancreas induced, 66
  infantile hypertrophic, 65
  peptic ulcer induced, 65

Pyloric stenosis (*cont.*)
  pre-pyloric web, 66
  tumour induced, 65
Pyogenic granuloma, 2, 517
Pyonephrosis, 229, 239
Pyopneumothorax, 413
Pyrrolizidine alkaloids, 161

Randall's plaques, 237
Raynaud's syndrome, 353, 361–2
  primary (Raynaud's disease), 361
  secondary (Raynaud's phenomenon), 361–2
Recklinghausen's disease, 641
  acoustic neuroma, 633
Rectal prolapse, 138
Recurrent oral ulceration (aphthous ulcers), 11
Reed-Sternberg cells, 425, 426 (fig)
Reflux
  intrarenal, 227–8
  nephropathy, 231 (fig)
  vesico-ureteric, 227
Reflux nephropathy, 231 (fig)
Reflux oesophagitis, 34–9
  clinical features, 36
  complications
    Barrett's oesophagus, 38–9
    Barrett's ulcer, 37
    peptic ulceration, 37
    stricture, 37
  morphology, 36–7
  pathogenesis, 34–5
    anti-reflux mechanisms, 34–5
    oesophageal factors, 36
Renal artery stenosis, 245
Renal cell carcinoma, (Grawitz's tumour; hyper-
    nephroma), 247–50
  aetiology, 247
  clinical features, 247
  epidemiology, 247
  morphology, 248–9
  prognosis, 250
  regression, 250
  spread, 249–50
  staging, 250, 250 (table)
Renal dysfunction, acute pancreatitis induced,
    203
Renal failure
  acute, 224
  pericarditis, 349
Renal papilla, refluxing/non-refluxing, 228
Renal pelvis, tumours 257
Renal transplantation, 643–57
  biopsy, 646
  BK virus infection, 652
  donors, 645
  fine needle cytology, 646–7
  harvesting of donor kidney, 645
  immunosuppression problems, 655–6
  immunosuppressive drug effects, 655–6

Renal transplantation (*cont.*)
  ischaemic times, 645 (table),
  matching, 644
  nomenclature, 644
  perfusion of donor kidney, 645
  recurrent conditions, 654–5
  rejection, 647–55
    acute, 647–9
      cellular, 647–8
      humoral, 648–9
    chronic, 650–1
    differential diagnosis, 652–4
      obstruction, 653
      glomerulonephritis, 653–4
      pyelonephritis, 653
      tubular necrosis, 652–3
    hyperacute, 647
    ureter, 651–2
  selection of recipients, 643
Rendu-Weber-Osler disease (hereditary telan-
    giectasia), 10, 105
Respirator lung *see* Adult respiratory distress
    syndrome
Respiratory complications of surgery, 390–2
  lung changes after surgery, 391–2
    adult respiratory distress syndrome, 392
    atelectasis, 391
    bronchopneumonia, 392
    exacerbation of pre-existing disease, 391
    pneumothorax, 392
    pulmonary embolus, 392
  predisposing factors, 390–1
    age, 391
    cigarette smoking, 390
    heart disease, 391
    inadequate analgesia, 391
    obesity, 391
    pre-existing pulmonary disease, 390
    reflex inhibition of diaphragm, 391
    type of incision, 391
  prevention, 392
Retromammary abscess, 293
Retroperitoneal fibrosis, 240, 526–7
Rhabdomyoma, 529–30
Rhabdomyosarcoma, 537–9
  paratesticular, 276
Rheumatic fever, 338
Rheumatoid arthritis, 578–82
  aetiology, 579
  clinical features, 579, 581–2
  heart valves, 345
  morphology, 580–1
  pathogenesis, 579
  pericarditis, 349
  treatment, 582
Ribonuclease, 194
Rickets, 587–8
Riedel's thyroiditis, 457
Right middle lobe syndrome, 389
Rokitansky-Aschoff sinuses, 180

Rolling hernia (paraoesophageal hiatus hernia), 39
Rotor syndrome, 146

Sabre tibia, 551
Salivary glands, 13–25
  biopsy, 15
  calculi, 16
  inflammatory disease, 15–16
  tumours, 18–25
    acinic cell, 23
    adenocarcinoma, 245
    adenoid cystic carcinoma, 23–4
    adenolymphoma, 21–2
    fibrosarcoma, 25
    haemangioma, 25
    lipoma, 25
    lymphangioma, 25
    lymphoma, 25
    metastatic, 25
    monomorphic adenoma, 21–2
    mucoepidermoid, 23
    non-epithelial, 25
    oxyphilic adenoma, 22
    pleomorphic adenoma (mixed salivary tumour), 19–20
      carcinoma in, 25
    squamous carcinoma, 24
    undifferentiated carcinoma, 24
Salmon patch (naevus flammeus), 515
Sarcoidosis, 423
Sarcoma
  Ewing's, 561
  irradiation, 557
  Kaposi's, 10, 424, 539–40
  paratesticular, 276
  soft tissue, 533–4
  synovial, 540
Scalded skin syndrome, 495
Scaphocephaly, 602
Schatzki's ring, 45
Schiller-Duval bodies, 275
Schistosomiasis, 233
  bladder carcinoma, 233, 253
  intrahepatic portal hypertension, 161
Schwannoma see Neurilemmoma
Sciatica, 594
  bony, 595
Sclerosing haemangioma see Fibrous histiocytoma
Scrotum, 284
  carcinoma, 288–9
Scleroderma see Systemic sclerosis
Seborrhoeic keratosis (basal cell papilloma), 498–9
Secretin, 194
Seminoma, 268–71
  extrascrotal, 271

Seminoma (cont.)
  morphology, 268, 269 (fig)
  prognosis, 270
  spermatocytic, 270
  spread, 268
  staging, 270
  teratoma combined, 274
Sepsis, post-obstructive jaundice surgery, 148
Sertoli-cell/mesenchyme tumour, 274
Sex hormones
  cholestasis due to, 147
  overproduction, 484–5
    adrenal adenoma-induced, 485
    adrenal carcinoma-induced, 485
Shock, acute pancreatitis-induced, 202
Shock lung see Adult respiratory distress syndrome
Sialadenitis
  acute, 15
  chronic recurrent, 16
Sialectasis, 16
Sicca syndrome, 16–18, 25
Silicone lymphadenopathy, 435
Sinus venosus defect, 323
Sjögren's syndrome, 16–18, 25
Skin
  appendage tumours, 517–19
    benign, 517–19
    malignant, 519
  basal cell carcinoma, 503–6
  benign tumours of epidermis, 498–500
  cysts
    dermoid, 498
    epidermal inclusion, 497
    pilar, 497
    sebaceous, 496
  infections
    bacterial, 494–5
    viral, 495–6
  melanocyte disorders, 506–15
  pre-malignant conditions of epidermis, 500–1
  squamous cell carcinoma, 501–3
  structure, 493–4
  tag, 498
  vascular lesions, 515–17
Slipped upper femoral epiphysis, 571–2
Small intestine, 81
  atresia, 82
  cysts, 82
  duplication, 82
  rotational abnormalities, 82
  stenosis, 82
  tumours, 107–11
    benign, 107–8
    carcinoma, 108
    endocrine, 109–11
Smegma, 287
Smooth muscle tumours (leiomyomatous tumours), 111–12, 123
Soft tissues, 524–41

Soft tissues (*cont.*)
  benign tumours, 527–31
  sarcoma, 533–4
  tumour-like conditions, 524–7
  tumours of intermediate malignant potential, 531–2
Solitary bone cyst (simple/unicameral bone cyst), 564–5
Solitary plasmacytoma, 562
Solitary rectal ulcer syndrome, 106
Somatostatinoma, 215
Spermatocoele, 266
Sperm granuloma, 264
Spider naevus, 516
Spina bifida
  cystica, 603
  dorsalis, 602–3
  occulta, 603
Spinal cord, 599
Spinal tumours, 640–1
Spleen, 435–45
  abscess, 442
  accessory tissue (spleniculi), 437
  amyloidosis, 441
  atrophy, 440–1
  congenital anomalies, 437
  cyst
    dermoid, 443
    epidermoid, 443
    parasitic, 442
    simple (congenital, serous), 443
  enlargement, *see* Splenomegaly
  functions, 436
  haemangioma, 443
  haemangiosarcoma (angiosarcoma), 444–5
  hamartoma, 443–4
  herditary hypoplasia, 437
  infarction, 441
  lymphangioma, 443
  lymphoma, 444
  pseudocyst, 442
  torsion, 442
  trauma, 437–9
  tumours
    benign, 443–4
    malignant, 444–5
      secondary (metastatic), 445
Splenectomy
  effects, 439–40
  mortality, 440
  partial, 438
  prophylaxis against infection, 438
  sepsis after, 438, 439, 440
Splenic artery
  aneurysm, 366
  false aneurysm, 203
Splenic vein thrombosis, 206
Splenomegaly, 436–7
  portal blood flow increase, 161
Splenorrhaphy, 438

Splenosis, 441
Splenunculi, 437
Springwater cyst (pleuropericardial cyst), 416
Steatorrhoea, 206
Stewart-Treves syndrome (post-mastectomy lymphangiosarcoma), 315 (fig), 316, 539
Stiff lung *see* Adult respiratory distress syndrome
Stomach, 52–79
  acute dilatation, 77
  anatomy, 52–3
  biopsy, 54
  cancer *see* Gastric carcinoma
  carcinoid tumours, 75
  congenital anomalies, 54
  diverticula, 78
  endocrine tumours, 75
  erosion, 53, 54
  epithelioid smooth muscle tumour (leiomyoblastoma; bizarre smooth muscle tumour), 76
  glomus tumours, 77
  leiomyoma, 75–6
  leiomyosarcoma, 75–6
  lesser curve necrosis, 62
  lymphoma, 77
  neurilemmoma (Schwannoma), 77
  neurofibroma, 77
  outlet obstruction *see* Pyloric stenosis,
  polyps, 69–70
    carcinomatous, 69
    eosinophilic granulomatous, 70
    epithelial, 69
    hamartomas, 70
    heterotopias, 69
    hyperplastic (regenerative), 69
    inflammatory fibroid, 70
    juvenile, 70
    neoplastic (adenomatous), 69
    Peutz-Jeghers, 70
  pre-pyloric web, 66
  pseudolymphoma, 76
  secretion, 53–4
  ulcer *see* Peptic ulcer
  volvulus, 78
Stone protein, 204
Stroke, 610–13
Sturge-Weber syndrome, 516, 638
Subarachnoid abscess, 608
Subarachnoid haemorrhage, 613
  post-head injury, 618
Subclavian artery
  aneurysm, 365
  compression, 358
Subcutaneous nodules, 581
Subdural abscess, 608
Sucquet-Hoyer canals, 494
Superior mesenteric artery occlusion, 103
Subphrenic abscess, 413

Sweat glands, 494
Synovial sarcoma, 540
Syphilis
　bone, 550–1
　joint, 550–1
　mouth, 3
Systemic lupus erythematosus, heart valves, 345
Systemic sclerosis (scleroderma), oesophageal,
　34

Takayasu's arteries, 361
Tardy ulnar paralysis, 622
Tar keratosis, 501
T-cells (-lymphocytes), 421, 446
　lymphoma, 433
　transformation, 431
Telangiectasis, capillary, 657
Temporal arteritis (giant cell arteritis), 360
Tendon sheath giant cell tumours, 531
Teratoma
　cerebral, 636
　mediastinal, 417, 448
　thymus, 447–8
　testicular, 271–4
　　appearance, 271–3
　　differentiated, 271–3
　　malignant intermediate, 272 (fig), 273
　　malignant trophoblastic, 273
　　malignant undifferentiated, 273
　　prognosis, 273–4
　　seminoma combined, 274
　　spread, 273
　　staging, 273
　　terminology, 271
Testis
　development, 260
　maldescended, 261–2
　　complications, 262
　structure, 260
　torsion, 264–5
　tumours, 267
　　carcinoma-in-situ, 276
　　classification, 267
　　clinical features, 267
　　interstitial cell tumour (Leydig cell tumour),
　　　274–5
　　lymphoma, 274
　　markers, 267–8
　　origins, 267
　　paratesticular, 276
　　seminoma see Seminoma
　　Sertoli cell/mesenchyme, 274
　　teratoma see Teratoma, testicular
　　yolk sac tumour (endodermal sinus
　　　tumour), 275
Tetralogy of Fallot, 328–9
Thalamus, 598
Thoracic duct obstruction, 413

Thoracic outlet syndrome, 622
Thromboangiitis obliterans (Buerger's disease),
　353, 361
Thrombocytopenia, 677
Thrombophlebitis
　migrans, 375
　superficial, 375
Thrush, 3
Thymoma, 447–8
Thymopoietin, 446
Thymus, 445–8
　aplasia, 446
　carcinoma, 447
　cysts, 448
　development, 445
　functions, 446
　Hodgkin's lymphoma, 448
　hyperplasia, 446
　hypoplasia, 446
　malignant tumours invading, 448
　non-Hodgkin's lymphoma, 448
　teratoma, 448
　tumours, 447–8
Thyroglossal cyst, 454
Thyroglossal duct, 454
　carcinoma, 454
Thyroglossal sinus, 454
Thyroglossal tract abnormalities, 454
Thyroid, 450–71
　absence, 453
　adenoma, 462–5
　　atypical, 464
　　autonomously functioning, 464–5
　　complications, 464–5
　　follicular, 463–4
　　haemorrhage into, 465
　　Hürthle cell, 463, 464
　　morphology, 463–4
　　papillary, 464
　biopsy, 451
　carcinoma, 464–70
　　anaplastic, 468–9
　　follicular, 467–8
　　Hürthle cell, 467
　　medullary, 469–70
　　papillary, 465–7
　　squamous, 469
　cyst, 465
　descent, 450, 453 (fig)
　development, 450
　dyshormonogenesis, 453
　ectopia, 452–3
　function, 450–1
　hypoplasia, 453
　lateral aberrant, 454
　malignant lymphoma, 470–1
　mediastinal, 416
　multiple toxic adenomas (Plummer's
　　disease), 460
　presentation of disease, 452

Thyroid (*cont.*)
   retrosternal, 416
   structure, 450
   tumour classification, 462 (table)
Thyroiditis, 452
   infective, 454
   Riedel's, 457
   subacute (de Quervain's), 455
Thyroid-stimulating hormone (TSH; thyrotro-
      phin), 451
Thyrotoxicosis (toxic nodular goitre), 460, 462
      (fig)
Thyrotrophin (thyroid-stimulating hormone;
      TSH), 451
Thyroxine (T4), 450–1
Tongue
   geographic, 12
   lymphangioma, 10
Total anomalous pulmonary venous connection,
      330
Toxic megacolon, 92, 97
Toxoplasmosis
   lymphadenopathy, 424
   pericarditis, 349
Trachea, 377
   carina
      bifurcation, 377
      widening, 377
Tracheo-oesophageal fistula, 30–1
Transient ischaemic attacks, 608–9
Transplantation, 656; *see also* Renal transplan-
      tation
Transposition of great arteries, 329–30
   corrected, 330
Traumatic aneurysms of cerebral vessels, 615
Traumatic wet lung *see* Adult respiratory dis-
      tress syndrome
Trichobezoar, 78
Tricuspid valve stenosis, 340
Tri-iodothyronine (T3), 450–1
Trisomy-21 (Down's syndrome), 54, 82, 321
Trotter's syndrome, 11
Trypsin, 194, 199
Trypsinogen, 194
Tryptophan, abnormal metabolism, 253
Tuberculosis
   bone, 549–50
   breast, 293–4
   endobronchial, 384
   endotracheal, 384
   epididymis, 263
   gastrointestinal, 98
   genitourinary, 231–2
   joint, 549–50
   lymph nodes, 423
   miliary, 384
   oral, 3
   ovarian, 667
   paravertebral abscess, 608
   pericarditis, 349

Tuberculosis (*cont.*)
   pulmonary, 383–4
      primary infection, 384
      secondary infection, 384
   spondylitis (Pott's disease), 550, 608
   ureteric, 232
Turban tumour, 519
Turcot's syndrome, 117
Turner's syndrome, 321
Tyrosinosis, congenital, 156

Ulcerative colitis, 89–90; *see also* Inflammatory
      bowel disease
Ulcerative interstitial cystitis (Hunner's ulcer),
      234
Upper limb ischaemia, 353
Urachus, persistent, 224
Ureter, 219
   congenital abnormalities, 222–4
      diverticula, 224
      duplication with ectopic ureter, 223
      duplication with ectopic ureterocoele, 223
      megaureter, 224
      postcaval ureter, 223
      simple complete duplication, 222–3
      simple partial duplication, 222
      valves, 223
   development, 221–2
   rejection, 651–2
   tuberculosis, 232
   tumours, 258
Ureterocoele, ectopic, 222 (fig), 223
Urethra
   carcinoma, 288
   congenital stenosis of external meatus, 285
   congenital stricture, 285
   diverticulum, 285
   duplication,m 285
   papillomatosis, 288
   posterior valves, 285
   tumours, 258
Urinary stones, 234–8
   calcium, 235, 238
   complications of renal stones, 238
   cystine, 236, 238
   epidemiology, 234–5
   infective, 236
   morphology, 237–8
   pathogenesis
      matrix theory, 236–7
      supersaturation theory, 236
   prognosis, 238
   radio-opacity, 238
   recurrence, 238
   screening procedures for metabolic defect,
      238
   staghorn, 236, 238
   uric acid, 235–6, 238

Urinary tract infection, 226–31
  aetiology, 226
  clinical features, 229
  morphology, 229–31
    acute pyelonephritis, 229–30
    chronic pyelonephritis, 230–1
    cystitis, 229
  pathogenesis, 227–9
    anatomical, 227
    bacterial factors, 229
    immunological features, 229
    intrarenal reflux, 227–8
    mechanical washout, 228
    vesico-ureteric reflux, 227

Vaginal mucosa laceration, 659
Varicocoele, 266–7
Varicose veins
  primary, 369–70
  secondary, 70
Vasculitis, 359–60
  hypersensitivity, 360
VATER syndrome, 30
Veins, 351–2
Veno-occlusive disease, 161
Venous thrombo-embolism, 370–4
  clinical features, 372–3
  complications, 373–4
  morphology, 373
  pathogenesis, 372
  risk factors, 370–1
Venous (gravitational) ulcer, 374–5
Ventricular aneurysm, 337
Ventricular septal defect, 323–4
Ventricular wall rupture, 336
Venules, 351
Verner-Morrison syndrome (WDHA syndrome),
  216
Verruca, Libman and Sach's, 345
Verruca plana, 495
Verruca vulgaris, 495
Very low density lipoproteins (VLDL), 354
Vertebral artery, 599, 600 (fig)
Vesico-cutaneous fistula, 241
Vesico-enteric fistula, 241
Vesico-umbilical fistula, 224
Vesico-ureteric reflux, 227
Vesico-uterine fistula, 241
Vesico-vaginal fistula, 241
Vincent's disease (acute necrotizing ulcerative
    gingivitis; fusospirochetosis), 3
Vinylchloride monomer, 170–1
Vipoma, 216

Viral hepatitis, 148–51
  hepatitis A, 148
  hepatitis B, 148–9, 155
    hepatocellular carcinoma, 166–7
    vaccine, 151
  clinical features, 150
  delta agent, 149
  fulminant, 150
  morphology, 150
  non-A non-B, 150, 155
  outcome, 150–1
  precautions, 151
Virchow's triad, 372
Vitamin D, 584
Vitamin K, 679
Volvulus
  caecal, 124
  gastric, 78
  sigmoid, 124
Vulval haematoma, 659

Waldenström's lymphoma, 429
Wang test, 475
Warfarin, 679
Waterhouse-Friderichsen syndrome, 440, 485,
  605
WDHA syndrome (Verner-Morrison syndrome),
  216
Whipple's disease, 345
Whipple's triad, 214
Wilkie's syndrome, 66
Wilms' tumour (nephroblastoma), 250–2
  prognosis, 252
  spread, 251–2
  staging, 252 (table)
Wilson's disease see Hepatolenticular degener-
  ation
Wolff-Parkinson-White syndrome, 325
Wolff's law, 542

Xenograft, 644

Yersinia infection, 424
Yersinia enteritis, 96
Yolk sac tumour (endodermal sinus tumour),
  275, 636, 672

Zollinger-Ellison syndrome, 63, 75, 215